Difficult Decisions in Thoracic Surgery

Mark K. Ferguson, Ed.

Difficult Decisions in Thoracic Surgery

An Evidence-Based Approach

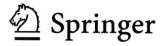 Springer

Mark K. Ferguson, MD
Professor, Department of Surgery
The University of Chicago
Head, Thoracic Surgery Service
The University of Chicago Hospitals
Chicago, IL, USA

British Library Cataloguing in Publication Data
Difficult decisions in thoracic surgery
   1. Chest — Surgery — Decision making   2. Chest — surgery
   I. Ferguson, Mark K.
   617.5′4
ISBN-13: 9781846283840
ISBN-10: 1846283841

Library of Congress Control Number: 2006926462

ISBN-10: 1-84628-384-1   e-ISBN 1-84628-470-0   Printed on acid-free paper
ISBN-13: 978-1-84628-384-0

9 8 7 6 5 4 3 2 1

springer.com

To Phyllis, a decision that has withstood the test of time.

Preface

Why do thoracic surgeons need training in decision making? Many of us who have weathered harrowing residencies in surgery feel that, after such experiences, decision making is a natural extension of our selves. While this is no doubt true, *correct* decision making is something that many of us have yet to master. The impetus to develop a text on evidence-based decision making in thoracic surgery was stimulated by a conference for cardiothoracic surgical trainees developed in 2004 and sponsored by the American College of Chest Physicians. During that conference it became clear that we as thoracic surgeons are operating from a very limited fund of true evidence-based information. What was also clear was the fact that many of the decisions we make in our everyday practices are not only uninformed by evidence-based medicine, but often are contradictory to existing guidelines or evidence-based recommendations.

The objectives of this book are to explain the process of decision making, both on the part of the physician and on the part of the patient, and to discuss specific clinical problems in thoracic surgery and provide recommendations regarding their management using evidence-based methodology. Producing a text that will purportedly guide experienced, practicing surgeons in the decision-making process that they are accustomed to observe on a daily basis is a daunting task. To accomplish this it was necessary to assemble a veritable army of authors who are widely considered to be experts in their fields. They were given the unusual (to many of them) task of critically evaluating evidence on a well-defined topic and provide two opinions regarding appropriate management of their topic: one based solely on the existing evidence, and another based on their prevailing practice, clinical experience, and teaching. Most authors found this to be an excellent learning experience. It is hoped that the readers of this book will be similarly enlightened by its contents.

How should a practicing surgeon use this text? As is mentioned in the book, wholesale adoption of the stated recommendations will serve neither physician nor patient well. The reader is asked to critically examine the material presented, assess it in the light of his or her own practice, and integrate the recommendations that are appropriate. The reader must have the understanding that surgery is a complex, individualized, and rapidly evolving specialty. Recommendations made today for one patient may not be appropriate for that same patient in the same situation several years hence. Similarly, one recommendation will not serve all patients well. The surgeon must use judgment and experience to adequately utilize the guidelines and recommendations presented herein.

To produce a text with timely recommendations about clinical situations in a world of rapidly evolving technology and information requires that the editor, authors, and publisher work in concert to provide a work that is relevant and up-to-date. To this end I am grateful to the authors for producing their chapters in an extraordinarily timely fashion. My special thanks go to Melissa Morton, Senior Editor at Springer, for her rapid processing and approval of the request to develop this book, and to Eva Senior, Senior Editorial Assistant at Springer, for her tireless work in keeping us all on schedule. My thanks go to Kevin Roggin, MD, for sharing the T.S. Eliot lines and the addendum to them. Finally, the residents with whom I have had the opportunity and privilege to work during the past two decades continually reinforce the conviction that quality information is the key to improved patient care and outcomes.

Mark K. Ferguson, MD

Contents

Contributors

Naveed Z. Alam, MD, FRCS
Department of Surgical Oncology
Peter MacCallum Cancer Centre
Melbourne, VIC, Australia

Marco Alifano, MD
Unité de Chirurgie Thoracique
Centre Hospitalier Universitaire
Paris, France

Nasser K. Altorki, MD
Department of Cardiothoracic Surgery
Weill-Medical College of Cornell University
New York, NY, USA

Nobutoshi Ando, MD
Department of Surgery
Tokyo Dental College Ichikawa General
   Hospital
Ichikawashi, Japan

Anirban Basu, MS, PhD
Section of General Internal Medicine
Department of Medicine
The University of Chicago
Chicago, IL, USA

Richard J. Battafarano, MD, PhD
Department of Surgery
Division of Cardiothoracic Surgery
Washington University School of Medicine
St. Louis, MO, USA

Faiz Y. Bhora, MD
Division of Cardiothoracic Surgery
Department of Surgery
Philadelphia Veterans Affairs Medical Center
Hospital of the University of Pennsylvania
Philadelphia, PA, USA

Daniel J. Boffa, MD
Department of Thoracic and Cardiovascular
   Surgery
Cleveland Clinic Foundation
Cleveland, OH, USA

Jeffrey A. Bogart, MD
Department of Radiation Oncology
SUNY Upstate Medical University
Syracuse, NY, USA

Vera Bril, BSc, MD, FRCPC
Division of Neurology
Toronto General Hospital
University Health Network
University of Toronto
Toronto, Ontario, Canada

Glenda G. Callender, MD
Department of Surgery
The University of Chicago
Chicago, IL, USA

Alan G. Casson, MB ChB, MSc, FRCSC
Division of Thoracic Surgery
Department of Surgery
Dalhousie University
QEII Health Sciences Centre
Halifax, NS, Canada

Lindsey A. Clemson, MD
Department of General and General Thoracic
   Surgery
The University of Texas Medical Branch
Galveston, TX, USA

Jean-Marie Collard, MD, PhD, MHonAFC
Unit of Upper Gastro-Intestinal Surgery
Louvain Medical School
St-Luc Academic Hospital
Brussels, Belgium

Thomas A. D'Amato, MD, PhD
Heart, Lung and Esophageal Surgery Institute
University of Pittsburgh Medical Center
Presbyterian – Shadyside
Pittsburgh, PA, USA

Thomas A. D'Amico, MD
Division of Thoracic Surgery
Duke University Medical Center
Durham, NC, USA

Antonio D'Andrilli, MD
Department of Thoracic Surgery
University La Sapienza
Sant Andrea Hospital
Rome, Italy

Subrato J. Deb, MD
Department of Cardiothoracic Surgery
National Naval Medical Center
Bethesda, MD, USA

Malcolm M. DeCamp Jr., MD
Division of Cardiothoracic Surgery
Beth Israel Deaconess Medical Center
Harvard Medical School
Boston, MA, USA

Claude Deschamps, MD
Division of General Thoracic Surgery
Mayo Clinic College of Medicine
Rochester, MN, USA

Frank C. Detterbeck, MD
Division of Thoracic Surgery
Department of Surgery
Yale University School of Medicine
New Haven, CT, USA

Robert J. Downey, MD
Thoracic Service
Department of Surgery
Memorial Sloan-Kettering Cancer Center
New York, NY, USA

Jo Ann Broeckel Elrod, PhD
Department of Surgery
University of Washington
Seattle, WA, USA

Nathaniel R. Evans, MD
Division of General and Gastrointestinal
  Surgery
Massachusetts General Hospital
Harvard Medical School
Boston, MA, USA

Farhood Farjah, MD
Department of Surgery
University of Washington
Seattle, WA, USA

Mark K. Ferguson, MD
Department of Surgery
The University of Chicago
Chicago, IL, USA

Hiran C. Fernando, MBBS, FRCS
Minimally Invasive Thoracic Surgery
Department of Cardiothoracic Surgery
Boston Medical Center
Boston University
Boston, MA, USA

Christine Fisher, MD
Department of Surgery
The University of Texas Medical Branch
Galveston, TX, USA

Raja M. Flores, MD
Department of General Surgery
Memorial Sloan-Kettering Cancer Center
New York, NY, USA

David R. Flum, MD, MPH
Department of Surgery
University of Washington
Seattle, WA, USA

Seth D. Force, MD
Lung Transplantation
Division of Cardiothoracic Surgery
Emory University School of Medicine
Atlanta, GA, USA

Carlos A. Galvani, MD
Department of Surgery
Lapososcopic and Robotic Surgery
University of Illinois at Chicago
Chicago, IL, USA

Philip P. Goodney, MD
Department of General Surgery
Dartmouth-Hitchcock Medical Center
One Medical Center Drive
Lebanon, NH, USA

Andrew J. Graham, MD, MHSc, FRCSC
Department of Surgery
Division of Thoracic Surgery
University of Calgary
Calgary, AB, Canada

Sarah E. Greer, MD
Department of General Surgery
Dartmouth-Hitchcock Medical Center
Lebanon, NH, USA

Sean C. Grondin, MD, MPH, FRCSC
Department of Surgery
Division of Thoracic Surgery
University of Calgary
Calgary, AB, Canada

Christian A. Gutschow, MD
Department of Surgery
University of Cologne
Cologne, Germany

Jeffrey A. Hagen, MD
Division of Thoracic/Foregut Surgery
Keck School of Medicine
University of Southern California
Los Angeles, CA, USA

Zane T. Hammoud, MD
Department of Cardiothoracic Surgery
Indiana University
Indianapolis, IN, USA

David H. Harpole, Jr., MD
Division of Thoracic Surgery
Duke University Medical Center
Cardiothoracic Surgery
Durham Veterans Affairs Medical Center
Durham, NC, USA

Jay T. Heidecker, MD
Division of Pulmonary, Critical Care, Allergy,
   and Sleep Medicine
Medical University of South Carolina
Charleston, SC, USA

Fernando A. Herbella, MD
Gastrointestinal Surgery
Department of Surgery
University of California San Francisco
San Francisco, CA, USA

Luis J. Herrera, MD
Cardiothoracic Surgery
Department of Thoracic and Cardiovascular
   Surgery
University of Texas
MD Anderson Cancer Center
Houston, TX, USA

Santiago Horgan, MD
Minimally Invasive Surgery Center
University of Illinois
Chicago, IL, USA

Charles B. Huddleston, MD
Washington University School of Medicine
Children's Hospital
St. Louis, MO, USA

Jan B.F. Hulscher, MD
Department of Surgery
Academic Medical Center at the University of
   Amsterdam
Amsterdam, the Netherlands

Mark D. Iannettoni, MD, MBA
Department of Cardiothoracic Surgery
University of Iowa Hospitals and Clinics
Iowa City, IA, USA

David M. Jablons, MD
Department of Thoracic Surgery
Division of Cardiothoracic Surgery
University of California
San Francisco, CA, USA

Michael T. Jaklitsch, MD
Division of Thoracic Surgery
Brigham and Women's Hospital
Harvard Medical School
Boston, MA, USA

Loay Kabbani, MD
Division of Cardiothoracic Surgery
University of Wisconsin
Madison, WI, USA

Jedediah A. Kaufman, MD
Department of Surgery
University of Washington Medical Center
Seattle, WA, USA

Shaf Keshavjee, MD, MSc, FRCSC
Division of Thoracic Surgery
Toronto General Hospital
University of Toronto
Toronto, Ontario, Canada

Kenneth A. Kesler, MD
Department of Cardiothoracic Surgery
Indiana University
Indianapolis, IN, USA

Ara Ketchedjian, MD
Department of Cardiothoracic Surgery
Boston Medical Center
Boston University
Boston, MA, USA

Anthony W. Kim, MD
Department of Cardiovascular-Thoracic Surgery
Rush University Medical Center
Chicago, IL, USA

Leslie J. Kohman, MD
Department of Surgery
SUNY Upstate Medical University
Syracuse, NY, USA

Robert J. Korst, MD
Division of Thoracic Surgery
Department of Cardiothoracic Surgery
Weill Medical College of Cornell University
New York, NY, USA

Jasleen Kukreja, MD, MPH
Division of Cardiothoracic Surgery
University of California
San Francisco, CA, USA

Rodney J. Landreneau, MD
Heart and Lung Esophageal Surgery Institute
University of Pittsburgh Medical Center
Pittsburgh, PA, USA

Christine L. Lau, MD
Section of Thoracic Surgery
University of Michigan Medical Center
Ann Arbor, MI, USA

France Légaré, MD, MSc, PhD, CCMF, FCMF
Centre Hospitalier Universitaire de Québec
Hôpital St-François d'Assise
Québec, QC, Canada

Amy G. Lehman, MD, MBA
Department of Surgery
The University of Chicago
Chicago IL, USA

Richard W. Light, MD
Division of Allergy, Pulmonary, and Critical
    Care Medicine
Vanderbilt University Medical Center
Nashville, TN, USA

Alex G. Little, MD
Wright State University Boonshoft School of
    Medicine
Department of Surgery
Dayton, OH, USA

Maria Luisa Lugaresi, MD, PhD
Department of Surgery, Intensive Care, and
    Organ Transplantation
Division of Esophageal and Pulmonary Surgery
University of Bologna
Bologna, Italy

Douglas J. Mathisen, MD
General Thoracic Surgery Division
Massachusetts General Hospital
Boston, MA, USA

Sandro Mattioli, MD
Department of Surgery, Intensive Care, and
    Organ Transplantation
Division of Esophageal and Pulmonary Surgery
University of Bologna
Bologna, Italy

Bryan F. Meyers, MD, MPH
Division of Cardiothoracic Surgery
Washington University School of Medicine
St. Louis, MO, USA

Shari L. Meyerson, MD
Division of Thoracic Surgery
Duke University Medical Center
Durham, NC, USA

Keith S. Naunheim, MD
Division of Cardiothoracic Surgery
Department of Surgery
Saint Louis University School of Medicine
St. Louis MO, USA

Annette M. O'Connor, RN, MScN, PhD
School of Nursing and Clinical Epidemiology
    Program
University of Ottawa and Ottawa Health
    Research Institute
Ottawa, ON, Canada

Brant K. Oelschlager, MD
Department of Surgery
The Swallowing Center
Center for Videoendoscopic Surgery
University of Washington Medical Center
Seattle, WA, USA

Raymond P. Onders, MD
Minimally Invasive Surgery
University Hospitals of Cleveland
Case Western Reserve University
Cleveland, OH, USA

Kalpaj R. Parekh, MD
Department of Cardiothoracic Surgery
University of Iowa Hospitals and Clinics
Iowa City, IA, USA

Ashish Patel, MD
Department of Surgery
Beth Israel Deaconess Medical Center
Harvard Medical School
Boston, MA, USA

Marco G. Patti, MD
Department of Surgery
University of California San Francisco
San Francisco, CA, USA

Douglas E. Paull, MD
Wright State University School of Medicine
Veterans Administration Medical Center
Surgical Service
Dayton, OH, USA

Christian G. Peyre, MD
Department of Surgery
Division of Thoracic/Foregut Surgery
Keck School of Medicine
University of Southern California
Los Angeles, CA, USA

Giuseppe Portale, MD
Department of General Surgery and Organ
   Transplantation
University of Padova School of Medicine
Padova, Italy

Joe B. Putnam, Jr., MD
Department of Thoracic Surgery
Vanderbilt University Medical Center
Nashville, TN, USA

David W. Rattner, MD
Division of General and Gastrointestinal Surgery
Massachusetts General Hospital
Harvard Medical School
Boston, MA, USA

Erino A. Rendina, MD
Department of Thoracic Surgery
University La Sapienza
Sant Andrea Hospital
Rome, Italy

Thomas W. Rice, MD
Section of General Thoracic Surgery
Department of Thoracic and Cardiovascular
   Surgery
The Cleveland Clinic Foundation
Cleveland, OH, USA

Hyde M. Russell, MD
Department of Surgery
The University of Chicago
Chicago, IL, USA

Steven A. Sahn, MD, FCCP, FACP, FCCM
Division of Pulmonary, Critical Care, Allergy,
   and Sleep Medicine
Medical University of South Carolina
Charleston, SC, USA

Jarmo A. Salo, MD, PhD
Division of General Thoracic and Esophageal
   Surgery
Department of Cardiothoracic Surgery
Helsinki University Central Hospital
Helsinki, Finland

Richard J. Sanders, MD
Vascular Surgery
University of Colorado
Health Sciences Center
Denver, CO, USA

Joseph B. Shrager, MD
Division of General Thoracic Surgery
University of Pennsylvania Health System
Philadelphia Veterans Affairs Medical Center
Philadelphia, PA, USA

Terrell A. Singleton, MD
Department of General Surgery
The University of Texas Medical Branch
Galveston, TX, USA

Joshua R. Sonett, MD
Lung Transplant Program
Department of Surgery
Columbia University
New York Presbyterian Hospital
New York, NY, USA

Lisa Spiguel, MD
Department of Surgery
The University of Chicago
Chicago, IL, USA

Dawn Stacey, RN, MScN, PhD
School of Nursing
University of Ottawa
Ottawa, ON, Canada

Stacey Su, MD
General Surgery
Brigham and Women's Hospital
Harvard Medical School
Boston, MA, USA

David J. Sugarbaker, MD
Division of Thoracic Surgery
Brigham and Women's Hospital
Harvard Medical School
Dana Farber Cancer Institute
Boston, MA, USA

John E. Sutton, MD
Trauma Services
Department of General Surgery
Dartmouth-Hitchcock Medical Center
Lebanon, NH, USA

Lee L. Swanstrom, MD
Oregon Health Sciences University
Division of Minimally Invasive Surgery
Legacy Health System
Portland, OR, USA

Michelle D. Taylor, MD
Esophageal Surgery
Division of Minimally Invasive Surgery
Legacy Health System
Portland, OR, USA

Karl Fabian L. Uy, MD
Division of Thoracic Surgery
University of Massachusetts
Boston, MA, USA

J. Jan B. van Lanschot, MD, PhD
Department of Surgery
Academic Medical Center at the University of
  Amsterdam
Amsterdam, the Netherlands

Nirmal K. Veeramachaneni, MD
Department of Surgery
Division of Cardiothoracic Surgery
Washington University School of Medicine
St. Louis, MO, USA

Federico Venuta, MD
Department of Thoracic Surgery
University La Sapienza
Sant Andrea Hospital
Rome, Italy

Thomas K. Waddell, MD, MSc, PhD, FRCS
Division of Thoracic Surgery
Toronto General Hospital
University of Toronto
Toronto, ON, Canada

Garrett L. Walsh, MD, FRCS
Department of Thoracic and Cardiovascular
  Surgery
University of Texas
MD Anderson Cancer Center
Houston, TX, USA

William H. Warren, MD
Thoracic Surgical Associates
Chicago, IL, USA

Tracey L. Weigel, MD
Section of Thoracic Surgery
Division of Cardiothoracic Surgery
University of Wisconsin
Madison, WI, USA

Todd S. Weiser, MD
General Thoracic Surgery Division
Massachusetts General Hospital
Boston, MA, USA

David C. White, MD
Division of Thoracic Surgery
Duke University Medical Center
Durham, NC, USA

Lara J. Williams, MD
Division of Thoracic Surgery
Department of Surgery
Dalhousie University
Halifax, NS, Canada

Cameron D. Wright, MD
Department of Thoracic Surgery
Massachusetts General Hospital
Boston, MA, USA

Giovanni Zaninotto, MD
Department of General Surgery and Organ
  Transplantation
University of Padova School of Medicine
Padova, Italy

Joseph B. Zwischenberger, MD
Department of Cardiothoracic and Ceneral
  Thoracic Surgery
The University of Texas Medical Branch
Galveston, TX, USA

Part 1
Background

1
Introduction

Mark K. Ferguson

Dorothy Smith, an elderly and somewhat portly woman, presented to her local emergency room with chest pain and shortness of breath. An extensive evaluation revealed no evidence for coronary artery disease, congestive heart failure, or pneumonia. A chest radiograph demonstrated a large air–fluid level posterior to her heart shadow, a finding that all thoracic surgeons recognize as being consistent with a large paraesophageal hiatal hernia. The patient had not had similar symptoms previously. Her discomfort was relieved after a large eructation, and she was discharged from the emergency room a few hours later. When seen several weeks later in an outpatient setting by an experienced surgeon, who reviewed her history and the data from her emergency room visit, she was told that surgery is sometimes necessary to repair such hernias. Her surgeon indicated that the objectives of such an intervention would include relief of symptoms such as chest pain, shortness of breath, and postprandial fullness, and prevention of catastrophic complications of giant paraesophageal hernia, including incarceration, strangulation, and perforation. Ms. Smith, having recovered completely from her episode of a few weeks earlier, declined intervention, despite her surgeon's strenuous encouragement.

She presented to her local emergency room several months later with symptoms of an incarcerated hernia and underwent emergency surgery to correct the problem. The surgeon found a somewhat ischemic stomach and had to decide whether to resect the stomach or just repair the hernia. If resection was to be performed, an additional decision was whether to reconstruct immediately or at the time of a subsequent operation. If resection was not performed, the surgeon needed to consider a variety of options as part of any planned hernia repair: whether to perform a gastric lengthening procedure; whether a fundoplication should be constructed; and whether to reinforce the hiatal closure with nonautologous materials. Each of these intraoperative decisions could importantly affect the need for a subsequent reoperation, the patient's immediate survival, and her long-term quality of life. Given the dire circumstances that the surgeon was presented with during the emergency operation, perhaps it would have been optimal if the emergent nature of the operation could have been avoided entirely. In retrospect, which was correct in this hypothetical situation, the recommendation of the surgeon or the decision of the patient?

Decisions are the stuff of everyday life for all physicians; for surgeons, life-altering decisions often must be made on the spot, frequently without what many might consider to be necessary data. The ability to make such decisions confidently is the hallmark of the surgeon. However, decisions made under such circumstances are often not correct or even well reasoned. All surgeons (and many of their spouses) are familiar with the saying "…often wrong, but never in doubt." As early as the 14th century, physicians were cautioned never to admit uncertainty. Arnauld of Villanova wrote that, even when in doubt, physicians should look and act authoritative and confident.[1] In fact, useful data do exist that impact on many of the individual decisions regarding elective and emergent management of giant paraesophageal hernia outlined above. Despite the existence of these data, surgeons tend to make decisions based on their own personal experience, anecdotal tales of good or bad outcomes, and unquestioned adherence to dictums from their mentors or other respected leaders in the field, often to the exclusion of objective data. It is believed that only 15% of medical decisions are scientifically based,[2] and it is possible that an even lower percentage of thoracic surgical decisions are so founded. With all of our modern technological, data processing, and communication skills, why do we still find ourselves in this situation?

1.1. Early Surgical Decision Making

Physicians' diagnostic capabilities, not to mention their therapeutic armamentarium, were quite limited until the middle to late 19th century. Drainage of empyema, cutting for stone, amputation for open fractures of the extremities, and mastectomy for cancer were relatively common procedures, but few such conditions were diagnostic dilemmas. Surgery, when it was performed, was generally indicated for clearly identified problems that could not be otherwise remedied. Some surgeons were all too mindful of the warnings of Hippocrates: "…physicians, when they treat men who have no serious illness,…may commit great mistakes without producing any formidable mischief…under these circumstances, when they commit mistakes, they do not expose themselves to ordinary men; but when they fall in with a great, a strong, and a dangerous disease, then their mistakes and want of skill are made apparent to all. Their punishment is not far off, but is swift in overtaking both the one and the other."[3] Others took a less considered approach to their craft, leading Hunter to liken a surgeon to "an armed savage who attempts to get that by force which a civilized man would get by stratagem."[4]

Based on small numbers of procedures, lack of a true understanding of pathophysiology, frequently mistaken diagnoses, and the absence of technology to communicate information quickly, surgical therapy until the middle of the 19th century was largely empirical. For example, by this time fewer than 90 diaphragmatic hernias had been reported in the literature, most of them having been diagnosed postmortem as a result of gastric or bowel strangulation and perforation.[5] Decisions were based on dogma promulgated by word of mouth. This has been termed the "ancient era" of evidence-based medicine.[6]

An exception to the empirical nature of surgery was the approach espoused by Hunter in the mid-18th century, who suggested to Jenner, his favorite pupil, "I think your solution is just, but why think? Why not try the experiment?"[4] Hunter challenged the established practices of bleeding, purging, and mercury administration, believing them to be useless and often harmful. Theses views were so heretical that, 50 years later, editors added footnotes to his collected works insisting that these were still valuable treatments. Hunter and others were the progenitors of the "renaissance era" of evidence-based medicine, in which personal journals, textbooks, and some medical journal publications were becoming prominent.[6]

The discovery of X rays in 1895 and the subsequent rapid development of radiology in the following years made the diagnosis and surgical therapy of a large paraesophageal hernia, such as that described at the beginning of this chapter, commonplace. By 1908, the X ray was accepted as a reliable means for diagnosing diaphragmatic hernia, and by the late 1920s surgery had been performed for this condition on almost 400 patients in one large medical center.[7,8] Thus, the ability to diagnose a condition was becoming a prerequisite to instituting proper therapy.

This enormous leap in physicians' abilities to render appropriate ministrations to their patients was based on substantial new and valuable objective data. In contrast, however, the memorable anecdotal case presented by a master (or at least an influential) surgeon continued to dominate the surgical landscape. Prior to World War II, it was common for surgeons throughout the world with high career aspirations to travel Europe for a year or two, visiting renowned surgical centers to gain insight into surgical techniques, indications, and outcomes. In the early 20th century, Murphy attracted a similar group of surgeons to his busy clinic at Mercy Hospital in Chicago. His publication of case reports and other observations evolved into the Surgical Clinics of North America. Seeing individual cases and drawing conclusions based upon such limited exposure no doubt reinforced the concept of empiricism in decision making in these visitors. True, compared to the strict empiricism of the 19th century there were more data available upon which to base surgical decisions in the early 20th century, but information regarding objective short-term and long-term outcomes still was not readily available in the surgical literature or at surgical meetings.

Reinforcing the imperative of empiricism in decision making, surgeons often disregarded valuable techniques that might have greatly improved their efforts. It took many years for anesthetic methods to be accepted. The slow adoption of endotracheal intubation combined with positive pressure ventilation prevented safe thoracotomy for decades after their introduction into animal research. Wholesale denial of germ theory by U.S. physicians for decades resulted in continued unacceptable infection rates for years after preventive measures were identified. These are just a few examples of how ignorance and its bedfellow, recalcitrance, delayed progress in thoracic surgery in the late 19th and early 20th centuries.

1.2. Evidence-based Surgical Decisions

There were important exceptions in the late 19th and early 20th centuries to the empirical nature of surgical decision making. Among the first were the demonstration of antiseptic methods in surgery and the optimal therapy for pleural empyema. Similar evidence-based approaches to managing global health problems were developing in nonsurgical fields. Reed's important work in the prevention of yellow fever led to the virtual elimination of this historically endemic problem in Central America, an accomplishment that permitted construction of the Panama Canal. The connection between the pancreas and diabetes that had been identified decades earlier was formalized by the discovery and subsequent clinical application of insulin in 1922, leading to the

awarding of a Nobel prize to Banting and Macleod in 1923. Fleming's rediscovery of the antibacterial properties of penicillin in 1928 led to its development as an antibiotic for humans in 1939, and it received widespread use during World War II. The emergency use of penicillin, as well as new techniques for fluid resuscitation, were said to account for the unexpectedly high rate of survival among burn victims of the Coconut Grove nightclub fire in Boston in 1942. Similar stories can be told for the development of evidence in the management of polio and tuberculosis in the mid-20th century. As a result, the first half of the 20th century has been referred to as the "transitional era" of evidence-based medicine, in which information was shared easily through textbooks and peer-reviewed journals.[6]

Among the first important examples of the used of evidence-based medicine is the work of Semmelweiss, who in 1861 demonstrated that careful attention to antiseptic principles could reduce mortality associated with puerperal fever from over 18% to just over 1%. The effective use of such principles in surgery was investigated during that same decade by Lister, who noted a decrease in mortality on his trauma ward from 45% to 15% with the use of carbolic acid as an antiseptic agent during operations. However, both the germ theory of infection and the ability of an antiseptic such as carbolic acid to decrease the risk of infection were not generally accepted, particularly in the United States, for another decade. In 1877, Lister performed an elective wiring of a patellar fracture using aseptic techniques, essentially converting a closed fracture to an open one in the process. Under practice patterns of the day, such an operation would almost certainly lead to infection and possible death, but the success of Lister's approach secured his place in history. It is interesting to note that a single case such as this, rather than prior reports of his extensive experience with the use of antiseptic agents, helped Lister turn the tide towards universal use of antiseptic techniques in surgery thereafter.

The second example developed over 40 years after the landmark demonstration of antiseptic techniques and also involved surgical infectious problems. Hippocrates described open drainage for empyema in 229 B.C.E., indicating that "when empyema are opened by the cautery or by the knife, and the pus flows pale and white, the patient survives, but if it is mixed with blood and muddy and foul smelling, he will die."[3] There was little change in the management of this problem until the introduction of thoracentesis by Trusseau in 1843. The mortality rate for empyema remained at 50% to 75% well into the 20th century.[9] The confluence of two important events, the flu pandemic of 1918 and the Great War, stimulated the formation of the U.S. Army Empyema Commission in 1918. Led by Graham and Bell, this commission's recommendations for management included three basic principles: drainage, with avoidance of open pneumothorax; obliteration of the empyema cavity; and nutritional maintenance for the patient. Employing these simples principles led to a decrease in mortality rates associated with empyema to 10% to 15%.

1.3. The Age of Information

These surgical efforts in the late 19th and early 20th centuries ushered in the beginning of an era of scientific investigation of surgical problems. This was a period of true surgical research characterized by both laboratory and clinical efforts. It paralleled similar efforts in nonsurgical medical disciplines. Such research led to the publication of hundreds of thousands of papers on surgical management. This growth of medical information is not a new phenomenon, however. The increase in published manuscripts, and the increase in medical journals, has been exponential over a period of more than two centuries, with a compound annual growth rate of almost 4% per year (Figure 1.1).[10] In addition, the quality and utility of currently published information is substantially better than that of publications in centuries past.

Currently, there are more than 2000 publishers producing works in the general field of science, technology, and medicine. The field comprises more than 1800 journals containing 1.4 million peer-reviewed articles annually. The annual growth rate of health science articles during the past two decades is about 3%, continuing the trend of the past two centuries and adding to the difficulty of identifying useful information (Figure 1.2).[10] When confronting this large amount of published information, separating the wheat from the chaff is a daunting task. The work of assessing such information has been assumed to some extent by experts in the field who perform structured reviews of information on important issues and meta-analyses of high quality, controlled, randomized trials. These techniques have the potential to summarize results from multiple studies and, in some instances, crystallize findings into a simple, coherent statement.

An early proponent of such processes was Cochrane, who in the 1970s and 1980s suggested that increasingly limited medical resources should be equitably distributed and consist of interventions that have been shown in properly designed evaluations to be effective. He stressed the importance of using evidence from randomized, controlled trials, which were likely to provide much more reliable information than other sources of evidence.[11] These efforts ushered in an era of high-quality medical and surgical research. Cochrane was posthumously honored with the development of the Cochrane Collabora-

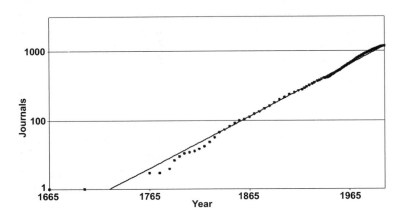

FIGURE 1.1. The total number of active refereed journals published annually. (Data from Mabe.[10])

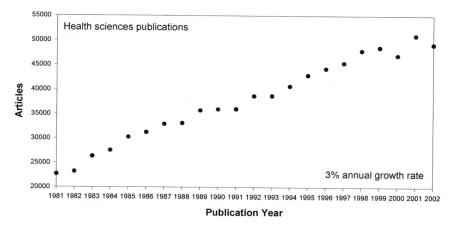

FIGURE 1.2. Growth in the number of published health science articles published annually. (Data from Mabe.[10])

tion in 1993, encompassing multiple centers in North America and Europe, which "produces and disseminates systematic reviews of health-care interventions, and promotes the search for evidence in the form of clinical trials and other studies of the effects of interventions."[12]

Methods originally espoused by Cochrane and others have been codified into techniques for rating the quality of evidence in a publication and for grading the strength of a recommendation based on the preponderance of available evidence. This methodology is described in detail in Chapter 2. The clinical problems addressed in this book have been assessed using one of two commonly employed rating systems, one from the Scottish Intercollegiate Guidelines Network (Table 1.1) and the other from the Oxford Centre for Evidence-Based Medicine (Table 1.2).[13,14] Each has its own advantages and disadvantages, and each has been shown to function well in a variety of settings, providing consistent results that are reproducible. The latter system is explained in detail in Chapter 2.

Techniques such as those described above for synthesizing large amounts of quality information were introduced for the development guidelines for clinical activity in thoracic surgery, most commonly for the management of lung cancer, beginning in the mid-1990s. An example of these is a set of guidelines based on current standards of care sponsored by the Society of Surgical Oncology for managing lung cancer. It was written by experts in the field without a formal process of evidence collection.[15] A better technique for arriving at guidelines is the consensus

statement, usually derived during a consensus conference in which guidelines based on published medical evidence are revised until members of the conference agree by a substantial majority in the final statement. The problem with this technique is that the strength of recommendations, at times, is sometimes diluted until there is little content to them. The American College of Chest Physicians recently has issued over 20 guideline summaries in a recent supplement to their journal that appear to have avoided this drawback.[16] Similar sets of guidelines have recently been published for appropriate selection of patients for lung cancer surgery,[17] for multimodality management of lung cancer,[18] and for appropriate follow-up of lung cancer patients having received potentially curative therapy,[19] to name but a few. In addition to lung cancer management, guidelines have been developed for other areas of interest to the thoracic surgeon.

Despite the enormous efforts expended by professional societies in providing evidence-based algorithms for appropriate management of patients, adherence to these published guidelines, based on practice pattern reports, is disappointing. Focusing again on surgical management of lung cancer, there is strong evidence that standard procedures incorporated into surgical guidelines for lung cancer are widely ignored. For example, fewer than 50% of patients undergoing mediastinoscopy for nodal staging have lymph node biopsies performed. In patients undergoing major resection for lung cancer, fewer than 60% have mediastinal lymph nodes biopsied or dissected.[20] There are also important regional variations in the use of standard staging techniques and in the use of surgery for stage I lung cancer patients, patterns of activity that are also related to race and socioeconomic status.[21–23] Failure to adhere to accepted standards of care for surgical lung cancer patients results in higher postoperative mortality rates; whether long-term survival is adversely affected has yet to be determined.[24,25]

TABLE 1.1. Scottish Intercollegiate Guidelines Network evidence levels and grades of recommendations.

Level	Description
1++	High-quality meta-analyses, systematic reviews of RCTs, or RCTs with a very low risk of bias
1+	Well-conducted meta-analyses, systematic reviews of RCTs, or RCTs with a low risk of bias.
1−	Meta-analyses, systematic reviews or RCTs, or RCTs with a high risk of bias
2++	High-quality systematic reviews of case-control or cohort studies
	or
	High-quality case-control of cohort studies with a very low risk of confounding, bias, or chance and a high probability that the relationship is causal
2+	Well-conducted case-control or cohort studies with a low risk of confounding, bias, or chance and a moderate probability that the relationship is causal
2−	Case-control or cohort studies with a high risk of confounding, bias, or chance and a significant risk that the relationship is not causal
3	Non-analytic studies, e.g. case reports, case series
4	Expert opinion

GradeH	Description
A	At least one meta-analysis, systematic review, or RCT rated as 1++ and directly applicable to the target population
	or
	A systematic review of RCTs or a body of evidence consisting principally of studies rated as 1+ directly applicable to the target population and demonstrating overall consistency of results
B	A body of evidence including studies rated as 2++ directly applicable to the target population and demonstrating overall consistency of results
	or
	Extrapolated evidence from studies rated as 1++ or 1+
C	A body of evidence including studies rated as 2+ directly applicable to the target population and demonstrating overall consistency of results
	or
	Extrapolated evidence from studies rated as 2++
D	Evidence level 3 or 4
	or
	Extrapolated evidence from studies rated as 2+

Abbreviation: RCT, randomized, controlled trial.
Source: Harbour and Miller.[13]

TABLE 1.2. Oxford Centre for Evidence-Based Medicine levels of evidence and grades of recommendations for therapeutic interventions.

Level	Description
1a	SR (with homogeneity) of RCTs
1b	Individual RCT (with narrow confidence interval)
1c	All or none
2a	SR (with homogeneity) of cohort studies
2b	Individual cohort study (including low quality RCT; e.g., < 80% follow-up)
2c	"Outcomes" research; ecological studies
3a	SR (with homogeneity) of case-control studies
3b	Individual case-control studies
4	Case series (and poor quality cohort and case-control studies)
5	Expert opinion without explicit critical appraisal, or based on physiology, bench research, or "first principles"

Grade	Description
A	Consistent level 1 studies
B	Consistent level 2 or 3 studies or extrapolations from level 1 studies
C	Level 4 studies or extrapolations from level 2 or 3 studies
D	Level 5 evidence or troublingly inconsistent or inconclusive studies at any level

Abbreviations: RCT, randomized, controlled trials; SR, systematic review.
Source: Oxford Centre for Evidence-Based Medicine.[14]

The importance of adherence to accepted standards of care, particular those espoused by major professional societies, such as the American College of Surgeons, The Society of Surgical Oncology, the American Society of Clinical Oncology, the American Cancer Society, the National Comprehensive Cancer Network, is becoming clear as the United States Centers for Medicare and Medicaid Services develops processes for rewarding adherence to standards of clinical care.[26] This underscores the need for surgeons to become familiar with evidence-based practices and to adopt them as part of their daily routines. What is not known is whether surgeons should be rewarded for their efforts in following recommended standards of care, or for the outcomes of such care. Do we measure the process, the immediate success, or the long-term outcomes? If outcomes are to be the determining factor, what outcomes are important? Is operative mortality an adequate surrogate for quality of care and good results? Whose perspective is most important in determining success, that of the patient, or that of the medical establishment?

1.4. The Age of Data

We have now entered into an era in which the number of data available for studying problems and outcomes in surgery is truly overwhelming. Large clinical trials involving thousands of subjects render databases measured in megabytes. As an example, for the National Emphysema Treatment Trial (NETT), which entered over 1200 patients, initial data collection prior to randomization consisted of over 50 pages of data for each patient.[27] Patients were subsequently followed for up to 5 years after randomization, creating an enormous research database. The size of the NETT database is dwarfed by other databases in which surgical information is stored, including the National Medicare Database, the Surveillance Epidemiology and End Results (SEER; 170,000 new patients annually), Nationwide Inpatient Sample (NIS; 7 million hospital stays annually), and the Society of Thoracic Surgeons (STS) database (1.5 million patients).

Medical databases are of two basic types: those that contain information that is primarily clinical in nature, especially those that are developed specifically for a particular research project such as the NETT, and administrative databases that are maintained for other than clinical purposes but that can be used in some instances to assess clinical information and outcomes, an example of which is the National Medicare Database. Information is organized in databases in a hierarchical structure. An individual unit of data is a field; a patient's name, address, and age are each individual fields. Fields are grouped into records, such that all of one patient's fields constitute a record. Data in a record have a one-to-one relationship with each other. Records are complied in relations, or files. Relations can be as simple as a spreadsheet, or flat file, in which there is a one-to-one relationship between each field. More complex relations contain many-to-one, or one-to-many, relationships among fields, relationships that must be accessed through queries rather than through simple inspection. Examples are multiple diagnoses for a single patient or multiple patients with a single diagnosis.

In addition to collection of data such as those above that are routinely generated in the process of standard patient care, new technological advances are providing an exponential increase in the amount of data generated by standard studies. An example is the new 64-slice computed tomography (CT) scanner, which has quadrupled the amount of information collected in each of the x–y–z-axes as well as providing temporal information during a routine CT scan. The vast amount of additional information provided by this technology has created a revolutionary, rather than evolutionary, change in diagnostic radiology. Using this technology, virtual angiograms can be performed, three-dimensional reconstruction of isolated anatomical entities is possible, and radiologists are discovering more abnormalities than clinicians know what to do with.

A case in point is the use of CT as a screening test for lung cancer. Rapid low-dose CT scans were introduced in the late 1990s and were quickly adopted as a means for screening high-risk patients for lung cancer. The results of this screening have been mixed. Several reports suggest that the number of radiographic abnormalities identified is high compared to the number of clinically important findings. For example, in the early experience at the Mayo Clinic, over 1500 patients were enrolled in an annual CT screening trial, and in the 4 years of the trial, over 3100 indeterminate nodules were identified, only 45 of which were found to be malignant.[28] Many additional radiographic abnormalities other than lung nodules were also identified.

1.5. What Lies in the Future?

What do we now do with the plethora of information that is being collected on patients? How do we make sense of these gigabytes of data? It may be that we now have more information than we can use or that we even want. Regardless, the trend is clearly in the direction of collecting more, rather than less, data, and it behooves us to make some sense of the situation. In the case of additional radiographic findings resulting from improved technology, new algorithms have already been refined for evaluating nodules and for managing their follow-up over time, and have yielded impressive results in the ability of these approaches to identify which patients should be observed and which patients should undergo biopsy or surgery.[29] What, though, of the reams of numerical and other data that pour in daily and populate large databases? When confronting this dilemma, it useful to remember that we are dealing with an evolutionary problem, the extent of which has been recognized for decades. Eliot aptly described this predicament in *The Rock* (1934), lamenting:[30]

Where is the wisdom we have lost in knowledge?
Where is the knowledge we have lost in information?

To those lines one might add:

Where is the information we have lost in data?

One might ask, in the presence of all this information, are we collecting the correct data? Evidence-based guidelines regarding indications for surgery, surgical techniques, and postoperative management are often lacking. We successfully track surgical outcomes of a limited sort, and often only in retrospect: complications, operative mortality, and survival. We do not successfully track patient's satisfaction with their experience, the quality of life they are left with as a result of surgery, and whether they would make the same decision regarding surgery if they had to do things over again. Perhaps these are important questions upon which physicians should focus. In addition to migrating towards patient-focused rather than institutionally focused data, are we prepared to take the greater leap of addressing more important issues requiring data from a societal perspective, including cost effectiveness and appropriate resource distribution (human and otherwise) and utilization? This would likely result in redeployment of resources towards health prevention and maintenance rather than intervention. Such efforts are already underway, sponsored not by medical societies and other professional organizations, but by those paying the increasingly unaffordable costs of medical care.

Insurance companies have long been involved, through their actuarial functions, in identifying populations who are at high risk for medical problems, and it is likely that they will extend this actuarial methodology into evaluating the success of surgical care on an institutional and individual surgeon basis as more relevant data become available. The Leapfrog Group, representing a consortium of large commercial enterprises that covers insurance costs for millions of workers, was founded to differentiate levels of quality of outcomes for common or very expensive diseases, thereby potentially limiting costs of care by directing patients to better outcome centers. These efforts have three potential drawbacks from the perspective of the surgeon. First, decisions made in this way are primarily fiscally based, and are not patient focused. Second, policies put in place by payers will undoubtedly lead to regionalization of health care, effectively resulting in de facto restraint of trade affecting those surgeons with low individual case volumes or comparatively poor outcomes for a procedure, or who work in low volume centers. Finally, decisions about point of care will be taken from the hands of the patients and their physicians. The next phase of this process will be requirements on the part of payers regarding practice patterns, in which penalties are incurred if proscribed patterns are not followed, and rewards are provided for following such patterns, even if they lead to worse outcomes in an individual patient.

Physicians can retain control of the care of their patients in a variety of ways. First, they must make decisions based on evidence and in accordance with accepted guidelines and recommendations. This text serves to provide an outline for only a fraction of the decisions that are made in a thoracic surgical practice. For many of the topics in this book there are preciously few data that can be used to formulate a rational basis for a recommendation. Practicing physicians must therefore become actively involved in the process of developing useful evidence upon which decisions can be made. There are a variety of means for doing this, including participation in randomized clinical trials, entry of their patient data (appropriately anonymized) into large databases for study, and participation in consensus conferences aimed at providing useful management guidelines for problems in which they have a special interest. Critical evaluation of new technology and procedures, rather than merely adopting what is new to appear to the public and referring physicians that one's practice is cutting edge, may help reduce the wholesale adoption of what is new into patterns of practice before its value is proven.

1.6. Conclusion

Decisions are the life blood of surgeons. How we make decisions affects the immediate and long-term outcomes of care of individual patients. Such decisions will also, in the near future, affect our reimbursement, our referral patterns, and possibly our privileges to perform certain operations. Most of the decisions that we currently make in our surgical practices are insufficiently grounded in adequate evidence. In addition, we tend to ignore published evidence and guidelines, preferring to base our decisions on prior training, anecdotal experience, and intuition as to what is best for an individual patient.

Improving the process of decision making is vital to our patients' welfare, to the health of our specialty, and to our own careers. To do this we must thoughtfully embrace the culture of evidence-based medicine. This requires critical appraisal of reported evidence, interpretation of the evidence with regards to the surgeon's target population, and integration of appropriate information and guidelines into daily practice. Constant review of practice patterns, updating management algorithms, and critical assessment of results is necessary to maintain optimal quality care. Documentation of these processes must become second nature. Unless individual surgeons adopt leadership roles in this process and thoracic surgeons as a group buy into this concept, we will find ourselves marginalized by outside forces that will distance us from our patients and discount our expertise in making vital decisions.

References

1. Kelly J. *The Great Mortality. An Intimate History of the Black Death, the Most Devastating Plague of All Time.* New York: Harper Collins; 2006.
2. Eddy DM. Decisions without information. The intellectual crisis in medicine. *HMO Pract* 1991; 5:58–60.
3. Hippocrates. *The Genuine Works of Hippocrates.* Adams CD, trans-ed. New York: Dover; 1868.
4. Moore W. *The Knife Man: The Extraordinary Life and Times of John Hunter, Father of Modern Surgery.* New York: Broadway Books; 2005.
5. Bowditch HI. A treatise on diaphragmatic hernia. *Buffalo Med J Monthly Rev* 1853,9:65–94.
6. Claridge JA, Fabian TC. History and development of evidence-based medicine. *World J Surg* 2005;29: 547–553.
7. Hedblom C. Diaphragmatic hernia. A study of three hundred and seventy-eight cases in which operation was performed. *JAMA* 1925;85:947–953.
8. Harrington SW. Diaphragmatic hernia. *Arch Surg* 1928;16:386–415.
9. Miller JI Jr. The history of surgery of empyema, thoracoplasty, Eloesser flap, and muscle flap transposition. *Chest Surg Clin N Am* 2000;10:45–53.
10. Mabe MA. The growth and number of journals. *Serials* 2003;16:191–197.
11. Cochrane AL. *Effectiveness and Efficiency. Random Reflections on Health Services.* London: Nuffield Provincial Hospitals Trust; 1972.
12. Cochrane Collaboration website. Available from http://www.cochrane.org/. Accessed 18 Marh 2006.
13. Harbour R, Miller J. Scottish Intercollegiate Guidelines Network Grading Review Group. A new system for grading recommendations in evidence based guidelines. *Br Med J* 2001;323:334–336.
14. Oxford Centre for Evidence-Based Medicine. Available from http://cebm.net/levels_of_evidence. asp. Accessed 26 March 2006.
15. Ginsberg R, Roth J, Ferguson MK. Lung cancer surgical practice guidelines. Society of Surgical Oncology practice guidelines: lung cancer. *Oncology* 1997;11:889–892, 895.
16. McCrory DC, Colice GL, Lewis SZ, Alberts WM, Parker S. Overview of methodology for lung cancer evidence review and guideline development. *Chest* 2003;123(suppl 1):3S–6S.
17. British Thoracic Society; Society of Cardiothoracic Surgeons of Great Britain and Ireland Working Party. BTS guidelines: guidelines on the selection of patients with lung cancer for surgery. *Thorax* 2001;56:89–108.
18. Ettinger D, Johnson B. Update: NCCN small cell and non-small cell lung cancer Clinical Practice Guidelines. *J Natl Compr Cancer Network* 2005; (suppl 1):S17–S21.
19. Saunders M, Sculier JP, Ball D, et al. Consensus: the follow-up of the treated patient. *Lung Cancer* 2003;42(suppl 1):S17–S19.
20. Little AG, Rusch VW, Bonner JA, et al. Patterns of surgical care of lung cancer patients. *Ann Thorac Surg* 2005;80:2051–2056.

21. Greenwald HP, Polissar NL, Borgatta EF, McCorkle R, Goodman G. Social factors, treatment, and survival in early-stage non-small cell lung cancer. *Am J Public Health* 1998;88:1681–1684.

22. Bach PB, Cramer LD, Warren JL, Begg CB. Racial differences in the treatment of early-stage lung cancer. *N Engl J Med* 1999;341:1198–1205.

23. Lathan CS, Neville BA, Earle CC. The effect of race on invasive staging and surgery in non-small-cell lung cancer. *J Clin Oncol* 2006;24:413–418.

24. Birkmeyer NJ, Goodney PP, Stukel TA, Hillner BE, Birkmeyer JD. Do cancer centers designated by the National Cancer Institute have better surgical outcomes? *Cancer* 2005;103:435–441.

25. Goodney PP, Lucas FL, Stukel TA, Birkmeyer JD. Surgeon specialty and operative mortality with lung resection. *Ann Surg* 2005;241:179–184.

26. Polk HC Jr. Renewal of surgical quality and safety initiatives: a multispecialty challenge. *Mayo Clin Proc* 2006;81:345–352.

27. Naunheim KS, Wood DE, Krasna MJ, et al., and the National Emphysema Treatment Trial Research Group. Predictors of operative mortality and cardiopulmonary morbidity in the National Emphysema Treatment Trial. *J Thorac Cardiovasc Surg* 2006;131:43–53.

28. Crestanello JA, Allen MS, Jett JR, et al. Thoracic surgical operations in patients enrolled in a computed tomographic screening trial. *J Thorac Cardiovasc Surg* 2004;128:254–259.

29. Henschke CI. Computed tomography screening for lung cancer: principles and results. *Clin Cancer Res* 2005;11:4984s–4987s.

30. Eliot TS. The Complete Poems and Plays 1909–1950. Orlando, FL. Narcourt Brace & Company, 1950.

2
Evidence-Based Medicine: Levels of Evidence and Grades of Recommendation

Andrew J. Graham and Sean C. Grondin

Evidenced-based medicine (EMB) is a philosophical approach to clinical problems introduced in the 1980s by a group of clinicians with an interest in clinical epidemiology at McMaster University in Canada. The concepts associated with this approach have been widely disseminated and described by many as a paradigm shift. Others, however, have debated the usefulness of this approach.

In this chapter, we will provide a definition and rationale for an evidence-based approach to clinical practice. The central role of systems that grade clinical recommendations and levels of evidence will be outlined. Readers interested in a more in-depth review are advised to consult the *Users' Guide to the Medical Literature: A Manual for Evidence-Based Clinical Practice*.[1]

2.1. What Is Evidence-Based Medicine

Evidence-based medicine is a philosophical approach to clinical problems that has arisen from the physician's need to offer proven therapies to patients. In 1996, Sackett and colleagues more formally defined EBM as "the conscientious, explicit, and judicious use of current best evidence in making decisions about the care of individual patients."[2] The goal of this approach is to be aware of the evidence supporting a particular approach to a clinical problem, its soundness, and the strength of its inferences. More recently, the term *evidence-based clinical practice* (EBCP) has been used instead of EBM to indicate that this approach is useful in a variety of disciplines. In this chapter the terms are used interchangeably.

Two fundamental principles of EBM have been proposed.[1] The first is that evidence alone is never enough to guide clinical decision making. Clinical expertise is required to place the evidence in context and advise individual patients while considering their unique values and preferences. The second principle is that a hierarchy of evidence exists that is determined by the soundness of the evidence and the strength of the inferences that can be drawn from it.

It has been recognized that clinicians can embrace the philosophy of EBM either as practitioners of EBM or as evidence users.

A practitioner would adhere to the following five steps:

1. Form clinical questions so that they can be answered.
2. Search for the best external evidence for its validity and importance.
3. Clinically appraise that evidence for its validity and importance.
4. Apply it to clinical practice.
5. Self-evaluate performance as a practitioner of evidence-based medicine.

The evidence user searches for pre-appraised or preprocessed evidence in order to use bottom-line summaries to assist patients in making decisions about clinical care.

2.2. Why Use an Evidence-Based Approach?

Proponents of EBCP report that the advantages to the physician who use an EBCP approach are that the practitioner acquires the ability to obtain current information, is able to perform a direct review of the evidence, and utilizes a interactive form of continuing medical education.[3]

2.2.1. Obtain Current Evidence

The traditional method of acquiring information has been the review of textbooks and ongoing review of medical journals. Traditional texts have been shown to go out of date quickly. In one study, for example, the delay in the recommendation of thrombolytic therapy for myocardial infarction was up to 10 years from when the published literature suggested it was advisable.[4] Due to the huge number and variety of journals, however, it is challenging even for the most diligent practitioner to stay current. With the development of modern technology that allows easy and rapid access to Medline and other full-text rapid internet access sites, an increasing number of busy practitioners have been able to obtain current evidence.

2.2.2. Direct Review of Evidence

Developing and maintaining critical assessment skills is essential in order to have an EBCP. The ability to perform a direct review of the evidence by the individual practitioner is felt to be a superior method for appraising the literature compared to traditional review articles by experts.[5] In many instances, reviews by experts have been revealed to be of low scientific quality and felt to be influenced unfavorably by potentially unsystematic hierarchal authority. Given the time required to critically appraise the literature, however, preprocessed sources of EBM have been necessary for most surgeons to incorporate EBM into their practice.

2.2.3. Interactive Learning

Many consider an evidence-based approach to clinical practice an interactive form of learning designed to improve physician performance. Studies designed to examine the effectiveness of continuing medical education have found that traditional didactic approaches are inferior to interactive forms of learning at changing physician performance.[6] Once the learner has acquired the necessary skills for EBCP, interactions with students and fellow learners reinforces the active process of learning and becomes the starting point for self-appraisal.[7]

Ironically, the evidence that EBM works is from observational studies that have suggested that recommendations arising from an evidence-based approach are more consistent with the actual evidence than traditional approaches.[4] The second piece of evidence suggested to demonstrate the effectiveness of EBM is gathered from studies that show that those patients who get the treatment supported by high-quality evidence have better outcomes than those who do not.[8,9]

2.3. What Is the Role of Grades of Recommendation and Levels of Evidence?

An evidence-based approach to clinical practice is said to have two fundamental principles. First, evidence alone is never enough to make a clinical decision, and, second, a hierarchy of evidence exists to guide decision making.

The proponents of an evidence-based approach define evidence very broadly as any empirical observation about the apparent relation between events. Thus, evidence can come from unsystematic clinical observations of individual clinicians to systematic reviews of multiple randomized clinical trials. The different forms of evidence may each provide recommendations that result in good outcomes for patients but it is clear that some forms of evidence are more reliable than others in giving guidance to surgeons and their patients. It is for this reason that a hierarchy of the strength of evidence has been proposed to further guide decision making. The assumption is that the stronger the evidence the more likely the proposed treatment or diagnostic test will lead to the predicted result.

TABLE 2.1. Hierarchy of strength of evidence for treatment decisions.

N of 1 randomized, controlled trial

Systematic reviews of randomized trials

Single randomized trial

Systematic review of observational studies addressing patient-important outcomes

Physiological studies (studies of blood pressure, cardiac output, exercise capacity, bone density, and so forth)

Unsystematic observations

The hierarchy of strength of evidence for treatment decisions (as opposed to diagnostic tests) is shown in Table 2.1.

The hierarchy represents a combination of reasoning and the study of different methodologies used to study treatments. The highest level of evidence will not be familiar to most thoracic surgeons. *N* of 1 trials were developed to address the finding that no single treatment is always effective for every patient. *N* of 1 trials involve a patient and his/her physician, usually treating a stable chronic illness, being blinded to randomized periods of taking a placebo or an active medication in random sequence and then deciding if the drug was or was not effective. Clearly, *N* of 1 trials have no relevance for patients having surgical procedures!

Given that *N* of 1 randomized, controlled trials are not feasible for thoracic surgical procedures, the fundamental underpinning of the hierarchy is the superiority of well-done, randomized, controlled trials (RCT) as compared to observational studies, physiological studies, and unsystematic observations. The majority of surgical and thoracic surgical research consists of observational or physiological studies or unsystematic observations. The superiority of randomized trials as compared to observational studies is still debated by some methodologists and some thoracic surgeons, as seen in debates regarding the National Emphysema Treatment Trial (NETT) for Lung Volume Reduction Surgery.[10–13]

The supporters of evidence-based clinical practice would define the observations of an experienced clinician as unsystematic observations. They acknowledge that profound clinical insights can come from experienced colleagues but that these are limited by small sample size

and "deficiencies in human process of making inferences."[1] Physiological studies are defined as studies in which the measured outcome is a physiological parameter such as blood pressure, forced expiratory volume in 1s (FEV_1), and exercise capacity, rather than patient important end points such as quality of life, frequency of hospitalizations, morbidity, and mortality.

Why do evidence-based advocates place such emphasis on RCT for selecting treatment for patients? First, observational studies are not an experimental design, so each patient is deliberately chosen, not randomly selected, thus leading to an unavoidable risk of selection bias. The selected patients may, therefore, have systematic differences in outcome that are due not to the given treatment but rather the selection process.[12]

Second, is the observation that the results of RCT have not been predicted by prior observational or physiological studies. We would like to outline examples in which RCT provided surprising results in relation to both the general medical literature and to studies of adjuvant treatments of lung cancer.

The classic example often given to demonstrate the potentially misleading conclusions drawn from studies with physiological end points is the study of the anti-arrhythmic drugs flecainide and encainide, in which nonrandomized studies were shown to decrease the physiological end point of frequency of ventricular arrhythmias in patients after myocardial infarction. The RCT subsequently carried out using a patient-important end point of cardiac deaths and arrests found a relative risk (RR) of 2.64 [95% confidence interval (CI), 1.60–4.36]; a substantially increased risk among patients on the active drug versus those on placebo.[14]

An example drawn from thoracic surgery demonstrates the limitations of lower forms of evidence and highlights the important contributions thoracic surgeons have made toward proving the importance and power of RCT and validating the evidence hierarchy. The studies of adjuvant intrapleural bacillus Calmette–Guerin (BCG) for stage I non-small cell lung cancer (NSCLC) demonstrate the limitations nicely. The initial studies suggesting that an infectious immune stimulant would improve survival in the treatment of lung cancer came from observational studies that suggested that postoperative empyema improves survival in lung cancer.[15] An elegant pathophysiological mechanism of immune stimulant was proposed. This was followed by supportive animal physiological studies and a small randomized trial in which a subgroup analysis suggested that immune stimulation via BCG would confer a survival advantage as adjuvant therapy for lung cancer.[16] Unfortunately, this was not shown to be the case when the theory was tested in a well-conducted RCT by the Lung Cancer Study Group.[17]

The evidence-based approach to surgery implies that physiological rationale or observational studies usually predict the results of RCT. However, this may not always be the case. Thus, the hierarchy of evidence has ranked RCT above other forms of study. The evidence-based approach hierarchy is, however, not proposed as an absolute. For example, in the case where observational studies show an overwhelming advantage for treatment, such as insulin for the treatment of ketoacidosis, RCT are not required. The majority of treatments, however, do not demonstrate an overwhelming advantage for a particular form of treatment and major treatment decisions of common problems therefore require evidence from RCT in order to provide the best advice to patients.

2.4. Grading Systems of Recommendations and Levels of Evidence

The hierarchy of evidence has been formulized by a wide variety of groups into different classifications of levels of evidence and grades of recommendation. The proliferation of such classifications, each being slightly different from each other, has led to the formation of an international working group whose mandate is to reach agreement on a standardized classification.[18]

Given that a single classification has not been universally accepted, we have suggested the use of the Oxford Centre for Evidence-based Medicine Grades of Recommendations and Levels of Evidence (Table 2.2). The strengths of this classification are that it was developed by leaders in

the field of EBM, it allows assignment of studies for not only therapy but for diagnostic tests as well, and it has been used in studies exploring methodology in thoracic surgery.[19,20] The limitations are that it is detailed and may appear complex to those not familiar with the field.

A number of aspects of the Oxford Centre for Evidence-based Medicine Grades of Recommendations and Levels of Evidence are worthy of highlighting. The bottom line for an evidence-based user is the grades of recommendation A through D. In the clinical setting, the levels of evidence of applicable studies are determined and then examined to assign the grade of recommendation. An A level recommendation is the strongest possible.

For those surgeons who have an interest in a deeper understanding, the initial step is to determine the methodological nature of the clinical question. Thoracic surgeons will likely be interested in questions regarding the choice of therapy or diagnostic test. For example, a surgeon may wish to advise a patient regarding the role of adjuvant chemotherapy following lung cancer resection. The surgeon would then examine existing studies and use the first column of the table to assign the appropriate level of evidence.

The surgeon will note that level 1a is assigned to systematic reviews with homogeneity of RCT. It is critical to understanding the table that surgeons appreciate that systematic reviews are not the same as traditional narrative reviews. Systematic reviews of published and unpublished data are carried out in an explicit fashion. The criteria for locating articles, assigning methodological criteria, and combing data are explicitly stated and are repeatable by another investigator. Following the location of evidence regarding adjuvant chemotherapy for lung cancer, a level of evidence could be assigned to each paper and then a grade of recommendation determined. Given a secure understanding of the soundness of the proposed treatment, the thoracic surgeon can use his/her clinical expertise to determine if the proposed treatment is appropriate for an individual patient after due consideration of factors such as local expertise, patient values, and patient preferences.

Depending on the nature of the clinical question, the surgeon may find high levels of evidence

TABLE 2.2. Oxford Centre for Evidence-based Medicine Levels of Evidence (May 2001).

Level	Therapy/prevention, etiology/harm	Prognosis	Diagnosis	Differential diagnosis/symptom prevalence study	Economic and decision analyses
1a	SR (with *homogeneity**) of RCTs	SR (with *homogeneity**) of inception cohort studies; *CDR†* validated in different populations	SR (with *homogeneity**) of level 1 diagnostic studies; CDR† with 1b studies from different clinical centres	SR (with *homogeneity**) of prospective cohort studies	SR (with *homogeneity**) of level 1 economic studies
1b	Individual RCT (with narrow *Confidence Interval‡*)	Individual inception cohort study with ≥80% follow-up; *CDR†* validated in a single population	Validating** cohort study with good††† reference standards; or CDR† tested within one clinical center	Prospective cohort study with good follow-up****	Analysis based on clinically sensible costs or alternatives; systematic review(s) of the evidence; and including multiway sensitivity analyses
1c	*All or none§*	All or none case-series	Absolute SpPins and SnNouts††	All or none case-series	Absolute better-value or worse-value analyses††††
2a	SR (with *homogeneity**) of cohort studies	SR (with *homogeneity**) of either retrospective cohort studies or untreated control groups in RCTs	SR (with *homogeneity**) of level >2 diagnostic studies	SR (with *homogeneity**) of 2b and better studies	SR (with *homogeneity**) of level >2 economic studies
2b	Individual cohort study (including low quality RCT; e.g., <80% follow-up)	Retrospective cohort study or follow-up of untreated control patients in an RCT; derivation of *CDR†* or validated on split-sample§§§ only	Exploratory** cohort study with good††† reference standards; CDR† after derivation, or validated only on split-sample§§§ or databases	Retrospective cohort study, or poor follow-up	Analysis based on clinically sensible costs or alternatives; limited review(s) of the evidence, or single studies; and including multiway sensitivity analyses
2c	"Outcomes" research; ecological studies	"Outcomes" research		Ecological studies	Audit or outcomes research
3a	SR (with *homogeneity**) of case-control studies		SR (with *homogeneity**) of 3b and better studies	SR (with *homogeneity**) of 3b and better studies	SR (with *homogeneity**) of 3b and better studies
3b	Individual case-control study		Nonconsecutive study; or without consistently applied reference standards	Nonconsecutive cohort study, or very limited population	Analysis based on limited alternatives or costs, poor quality estimates of data, but including sensitivity analyses incorporating clinically sensible variations.
4	Case-series (and *poor quality cohort and case-control studies§§*)	Case-series (and *poor quality prognostic cohort studies****)	Case-control study, poor or nonindependent reference standard	Case-series or superseded reference standards	Analysis with no sensitivity analysis
5	Expert opinion without explicit critical appraisal, or based on physiology, bench research, or "first principles"	Expert opinion without explicit critical appraisal, or based on physiology, bench research, or "first principles"	Expert opinion without explicit critical appraisal, or based on physiology, bench research, or "first principles"	Expert opinion without explicit critical appraisal, or based on physiology, bench research, or "first principles"	Expert opinion without explicit critical appraisal, or based on economic theory or "first principles"

Produced by Bob Phillips, Chris Ball, Dave Sackett, Doug Badenoch, Sharon Straus, Brian Haynes, Martin Dawes since November 1998.

Users can add a minus sign "−" to denote the level of that fails to provide a conclusive answer because of:

- EITHER a single result with a wide confidence interval (such that, for example, an ARR in an RCT is not statistically significant but whose confidence intervals fail to exclude clinically important benefit or harm)
- OR a systematic review with troublesome (and statistically significant) heterogeneity.
- Such evidence is inconclusive, and therefore can only generate grade D recommendations.

*By homogeneity we mean a systematic review that is free of worrisome variations (heterogeneity) in the directions and degrees of results between individual studies. Not all systematic reviews with statistically significant heterogeneity need be worrisome, and not all worrisome heterogeneity need be statistically significant. As noted above, studies displaying worrisome heterogeneity should be tagged with a "−" at the end of their designated level.

†Clinical Decision Rule. (These are algorithms or scoring systems which lead to a prognostic estimation or a diagnostic category.)

‡See note #2 for advice on how to understand, rate and use trials or other studies with wide confidence intervals.

Met when *all* patients died before the Rx became available, but some now survive on it; or when some patients died before the Rx became available, but *none* now die on it.

§§By poor quality *cohort* study we mean one that failed to clearly define comparison groups and/or failed to measure exposures and outcomes in the same (preferably blinded), objective way in both exposed and non-exposed individuals and/or failed to identify or appropriately control known confounders and/or failed to carry out a sufficiently long and complete follow-up of patients. By poor quality *case-control* study we mean one that failed to clearly define comparison groups and/or failed to measure exposures and outcomes in the same (preferably blinded), objective way in both cases and controls and/or failed to identify or appropriately control known confounders.

§§§Split-sample validation is achieved by collecting all the information in a single tranche, then artificially dividing this into "derivation" and "validation" samples.

††An "Absolute SpPin" is a diagnostic finding whose Specificity is so high that a Positive result rules-*in* the diagnosis. An "Absolute SnNout" is a diagnostic finding whose Sensitivity is so high that a Negative result rules-*out* the diagnosis.

‡‡Good, better, bad, and worse refer to the comparisons between treatments in terms of their clinical risks and benefits.

†††*Good* reference standards are independent of the test, and applied blindly or objectively to applied to all patients. *Poor* reference standards are haphazardly applied, but still independent of the test. Use of a nonindependent reference standard (where the "test" is included in the "reference," or where the "testing" affects the "reference") implies a level 4 study.

††††Better-value treatments are clearly as good but cheaper, or better at the same or reduced cost. Worse-value treatments are as good and more expensive, or worse and the equally or more expensive.

***Validating studies test the quality of a specific diagnostic test, based on prior evidence. An exploratory study collects information and trawls the data (e.g., using a regression analysis) to find which factors are "significant."

***By poor quality prognostic cohort study we mean one in which sampling was biased in favor of patients who already had the target outcome, or the measurement of outcomes was accomplished in <80% of study patients, or outcomes were determined in an unblinded, nonobjective way, or there was no correction for confounding factors.

****Good follow-up in a differential diagnosis study is >80%, with adequate time for alternative diagnoses to emerge (e.g., 1–6 months acute, 1–5 years chronic).

Grades of recommendation

A	consistent level 1 studies
B	consistent level 2 or 3 studies **or** extrapolations from level 1 studies
C	level 4 studies **or** extrapolations from level 2 or 3 studies
D	level 5 evidence **or** troublingly inconsistent or inconclusive studies of any level

"Extrapolations" are where data is used in a situation which has potentially clinically important differences than the original study situation.

Source: The Centre for Evidence-Based Medicine. Levels of evidence and grades of recommendation. Oxford: The Centre. Available from http://www.cebm.net/levels_of_evidence.asp. Accessed 25 August 2005.

and grades of recommendation. Many thoracic surgical procedures only have level 4 or 5 evidence.[20] This does not invalidate the process, but rather allows the surgeon to be aware of limitations of the data and potentially to identify critical areas where further higher level studies could be performed.

2.5. Limitations of EBCP and Preprocessed Evidence

Most medical and surgical specialties have embraced the principles of EBM. However, discussions persist among doctors as to whether or not EBM represents a time-consuming "cookbook" approach to patient care that ignores patient values. Although EBCP has a number of limitations, we feel these limitations are outweighed by the advantages of an evidence-based approach.

One of the biggest concerns among busy practicing surgeons is the large amount of time required to develop and maintain an EBCP. Increasingly, surgeons must juggle a significant operative workload, clinical visits, hospital patient care, on-call responsibilities, research, and administrative duties. Adding the time and cost to acquire a variety of new skills, such as critically appraising the literature and grading current evidence, is overwhelming if not impossible. A potential solution is to become a knowledgeable user of EBM using preprocessed evidence such as the evidence-based summaries in this book. This text combines the selected authors' individual clinical expertise with an evidence-based summary of the literature to provide the reader with information on the management of complex thoracic surgery problems.

Another limitation to EBCP is that it places less weight on hierarchical authority and nonsystematic clinical observations; a concept which is counterintuitive to traditional surgical training and practice. This observation, combined with the fact that many surgeons do not embrace the best evidence because of their personalities (self-confidence, the need for rapid clinical decisions, and decisive actions during surgery), may lead to a diminished willingness to incorporate EBM principles into their practice.[21]

Although the limitations that have been discussed are significant, we believe they can be overcome. Improving the number and quality of available research trials and teaching the principles of EBM in undergraduate and graduate medical training will be important for establishing the widespread use of EBM.

References

1. Guyatt G, Drummond R. *User's Guide to the Medical Literature. A Manual for Evidence-Based Clinical Practice.* Chicago: AMA Press, 2002.
2. Sackett DL, Rosenberg WM, Gray JA, Haynes RB, Richardson WS. Evidence based medicine: what it is and what it isn't. *BMJ* 1996;312:71–72.
3. Sackett D, Richardson S, Rosenberg W, Haynes R. *Evidence-based Medicine; How to Practice and Teach EBM.* 1st ed. Edinburgh: Churchill Livingston; 1998.
4. Antman EM, Lau J, Kupelnick B, Mosteller F, Chalmers TC. A comparison of results of meta-analyses of randomized control trials and recommendations of clinical experts. Treatments for myocardial infarction. *JAMA* 1992;268:240–248.
5. Oxman AD, Guyatt GH. The science of reviewing research. *Ann N Y Acad Sci* 1993;703:125–133; discussion 133–134.
6. Davis D, O'Brien MA, Freemantle N, Wolf FM, Mazmanian P, Taylor-Vaisey A. Impact of formal continuing medical education: do conferences, workshops, rounds, and other traditional continuing education activities change physician behavior or health care outcomes? *JAMA* 1999;282:867–874.
7. Fingerhut A, Borie F, Dziri C. How to teach evidence-based surgery. *World J Surg* 2005;29:592–595.
8. Krumholz H, Radford M, Wang Y, Chen J, Heiat A, Marciniak T. National use and effectiveness of β-blockers for the treatment of elderly patients after acute myocardial infarction. *JAMA* 1998;280:623–630.
9. Krumholz HM, Radford MJ, Ellerbeck EF, et al. Aspirin for secondary prevention after acute myocardial infarction in the elderly: prescribed use and outcomes. *Ann Intern Med* 1996;124:292–298.
10. Benson K, Hartz AJ. A comparison of observational studies and randomized, controlled trials. *N Engl J Med* 2000;342:1878–1886.
11. Concato J, Shah N, Horwitz RI. Randomized, controlled trials, observational studies, and the hierarchy of research designs. *N Engl J Med* 2000;342:1887–1892.

12. Pocock SJ, Elbourne DR. Randomized trials or observational tribulations? *N Engl J Med* 2000;342:1907–1909.

13. Ciccone AM, Meyers BF, Guthrie TJ, et al. Long-term outcome of bilateral lung volume reduction in 250 consecutive patients with emphysema. *J Thorac Cardiovasc Surg* 2003;125:513–525.

14. Echt DS, Liebson PR, Mitchell LB, et al. Mortality and morbidity in patients receiving encainide, flecainide, or placebo. The Cardiac Arrhythmia Suppression Trial. *N Engl J Med* 1991;324:781–788.

15. Ruckdeschel JC, Codish SD, Stranahan A, McKneally MF. Postoperative empyema improves survival in lung cancer. Documentation and analysis of a natural experiment. *N Engl J Med* 1972;287:1013–1017.

16. McKneally MF, Maver C, Kausel HW. Regional immunotherapy of lung cancer with intrapleural B.C.G. *Lancet* 1976;1:377–379.

17. Mountain CF, Gail MH. Surgical adjuvant intrapleural BCG treatment for stage I non-small cell lung cancer. Preliminary report of the National Cancer Institute Lung Cancer Study Group. *J Thorac Cardiovasc Surg* 1981;82:649–657.

18. Schunemann HJ, Best D, Vist G, Oxman AD. Letters, numbers, symbols and words: how to communicate grades of evidence and recommendations. *CMAJ* 2003;169:677–680.

19. Graham AJ, Gelfand G, McFadden SD, Grondin SC. Levels of evidence and grades of recommendations in general thoracic surgery. *Can J Surg* 2004;47:461–465.

20. Lee JS, Urschel DM, Urschel JD. Is general thoracic surgical practice evidence based? *Ann Thorac Surg* 2000;70:429–431.

21. Slim K. Limits of evidence-based surgery. *World J Surg* 2005;29:606–609.

3
Decision Analytic Techniques

Anirban Basu and Amy G. Lehman

Accumulation of new and more reliable information has been monumental over the last decades, mediated via unprecedented growth in biomedical and associated social sciences research.[1] This research has certainly played a key role in the tremendous improvement of health throughout the world. It has also complicated decision making, both at the individual and at the policy level, by presenting clinicians with an increasing number of medical technologies and strategies for the management of a given medical situation. A fundamental concern in clinical decision making is how to synthesize information about the effect of a medical intervention on patients with specific characteristics. Furthermore, an additional critical step involves integrating population level evidence about outcomes with patient-level values for these outcomes in order to produce individualized care. Thus, individualized decisions for patients demand a systematic approach to sort through the evidence and to incorporate patients' and their family members' values and preferences into the decision-making processes, so as to combine the much-acclaimed evidence-based medicine[2] with the pragmatism of shared decision making.[3]

In this context, the decision analytic model (DAM) has proven to be a successful tool that can provide a systematic approach for decision makers.[4-6] These models enable the clinicians to apply a systematic, quantitative approach called decision analysis and thereby assess the relative value of one or more options or strategies to approach a particular medical problem. Furthermore, the approach allows them to pool evidence from a variety of settings, including randomized

clinical trials, as well as incorporate patients' preferences to inform the final decision. There are several published reviews and books that are entirely devoted to this topic. Interested readers are pointed to these references.[4-8] This chapter is intended to provide a succinct description of the fundamental theory and methods of decision analysis to clinicians, and to illustrate a stylized example of building a DAM based on a clinical choice problem in thoracic surgery.

3.1. Theoretical Foundations

The goal of a DAM is simple – it compares two or more treatment decisions or strategies for dealing with the same problem, and applies a set of rules to identify the preferred decision that would produce the maximum benefit or the minimum loss. Expected utility theory is the most commonly used rule to calculate the final outcome in terms of benefits (or loss). Under this theory, the final outcome resulting from a treatment decision is given by

$$B = \sum_{l=1}^{L} p_l \cdot b_l \qquad (3.1)$$

where payoff values (b_l) are associated with each level ($l = 1, 2, \ldots, L$) of success (or failure). The expected outcome is then calculated by summing over all levels, the product of the probability of a specific level of success (p_l) with its corresponding payoffs. Expected utility theory suggests that the preferred treatment decision is the one with the maximum expected benefit (or minimum expected loss).

Although almost all DAM perform under the auspices of this simple theoretical intuition, any DAM that attempts to model a practical clinical situation can become complicated very quickly. Each level of success at the end depends on a sequence of chance outcomes and various intermediate decisions that, in turn, may depend on further chances and decisions. Therefore, understanding, defining, and structuring the decision process is essential for clinical decision analysis. In this pursuit, a fundamental decision tool is a decision tree that helps the clinician to systematically display the temporal and logical structure of the decision problem and to thus carry out the analysis. In order to facilitate explanation of each part of this process in more detail, we begin with a stylized example of clinical decision making in thoracic surgery.

3.2. A Motivating Example

Let us begin with a common problem in thoracic surgery – the solitary pulmonary nodule – that can illustrate the basic principles of decision analysis. Suppose we have a patient referred to a thoracic surgery clinic. She is a 65-year-old woman who presents with an incidentally found solitary pulmonary nodule discovered on chest X ray taken in an emergency room after a minor motor vehicle collision. She has a 35 pack-year smoking history, but quit smoking 6 years ago. She has well-controlled hypertension, no heart disease, and no diabetes. She has no previous chest X ray with which to compare to this new abnormal one. The patient underwent a computed tomography (CT) scan scheduled by her primary care doctor, and this scan shows an 8-mm peripheral nodule with no enlarged lymph nodes. Let us further specify that due to the size of her lesion, positron emission tomography (PET) scan is nondiagnostic, and that due to her particular anatomy, she is not a candidate for a video-assisted thorascopic resection (VATS) biopsy. How shall we advise this patient? We are now faced with a choice in recommendations: watchful waiting, or perform open diagnostic thoracotomy. There are several considerations that inform our decision that have been discussed in detail elsewhere[9]; namely, we must consider

the pretest probability of cancer, the risk of surgical complications, and whether the appearance of the nodule on CT suggest benign or malignant disease. Finally, what are the patient's preferences given the possibility of adverse outcomes of open surgery? A DAM can help in the systematic integration of all this information in order for the surgeon to make an individualized and informed decision. A simple, stylized decision tree to address this clinical decision is illustrated in Figure 3.1. We now discuss in detail each part that goes into making up this decision tree and how one would arrive at the final result.

3.3. Elements of the Decision Analytic Approach

3.3.1. Identify and Bound the Decision Problem

The first step in decision analysis is to understand the decision problem at hand and the particular issues associated with making that decision. To do this, one must define the set of alternative actions under consideration and the primary outcome measure based on which decision will be made, determine the perspective and the time frame of the analysis, and consider several factors, such as the clinical characteristics of the patient, which may influence the primary outcome measure. These considerations can be broadly classified into the following:

1. *Define the set of alternative actions.* Decision analysis always presumes that there is more than one action for the same decision problem. If this were not the case, there would be no decision to make. Note that one of these alternative actions may, and often does, include the option to do nothing. In our stylized example, the alternatives are watchful waiting versus thoracotomy.

2. *Perspective.* The most common perspective taken in clinical decision making is that of the patient, whose welfare is the fundamental outcome for the decision at stake. This is also the perspective we take in our example. Chapter 4 (this book) explores the implications of the patient perspective in greater detail. Nevertheless, it is easy to foresee that a clinical decision based on a patient's perspective will be integrally

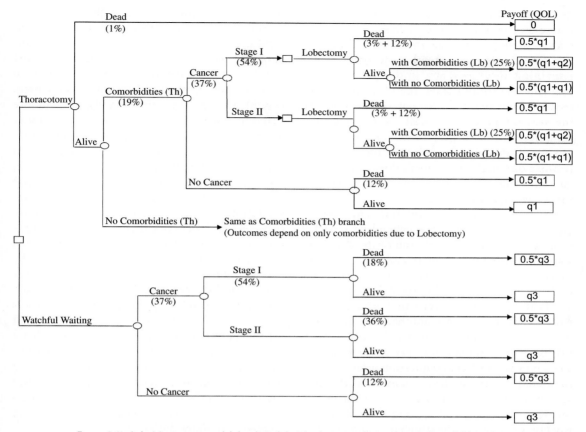

FIGURE 3.1. A decision tree to model the clinical decision between thoracotomy and watchful waiting.

tied with the preferences of that individual patient. Comprehending an individual patient's preferences and incorporating them in the decision process is essential for optimal decision making. However, in certain acute conditions, where the patient's preferences are unknown, alternative preferences of family members or sometimes those of clinicians may be used as proxies. More broadly, depending on the types of questions asked, perspectives of different stakeholders – for example, the hospital, the health insurance company, and even society at large – may become relevant in the analyses.[10] For example, from the hospital's perspective, reducing inpatient mortality may be more important than a patient's potentially diminished quality of life due to side effects of treatments. Outcomes such as costs and cost effectiveness may be more relevant to health insurance companies than to individual patients.

3. *Clinical conditions and demographics of patient(s).* Several risk factors affect patient outcomes and therefore are important to consider when choosing between alternative therapies. A patient's clinical condition constitutes the fundamental source of information for appropriate medical care. For example, surgeons require clinical information on the stage, and often grade, of a cancer before performing a surgical resection. Often, information on comorbidities, such as genetic susceptibilities to malignancy, becomes critical for prescribing appropriate treatment. Demographics also play a key role in determining outcomes. For example, pretest probability of cancer would depend on a patient's gender, smoking history, age, and possibly many other factors.

4. *Time frame of analysis.* The time frame of analysis should reflect the time over which the consequences of the clinician's choices have the potential to influence the patient's survival and

quality of life. In some acute conditions, the time frame may be the time until the patient is sent home from inpatient care. In chronic conditions, the time frame may extend up to the patient's remaining life expectancy. In the clinical choice problem that we illustrate, the ideal time frame should be the lifetime of the patient because both the disease process as well as the potential complications of surgery influence the patient's quality of life over her entire lifetime. However, because our analysis is a mere illustration of the concepts and not a substantive analysis, we will use a time frame of 1 year.

5. *Primary outcome of interest.* The optimal clinical decision may vary depending on what type of benefits the patients and/or the clinicians want to maximize. Identifying the primary outcome on which the final decision is made is perhaps the most crucial issue in decision analysis. Is the primary concern the survival of the patient over the next few months, or is the overall quality of life for the patient over his/her remaining life expectancy the most relevant measure to dwell on? Answering this question often involves incorporating the patient's preference and perspective, as well as determining the overall goal of medical treatment. It also uniquely determines what type of analysis the clinician is interested in. The types of analyses can be broadly classified into four categories based on the types of outcomes being evaluated: (1) clinical outcomes; (2) patient's values about the clinical outcomes; (3) costs, and (4) both costs and outcomes.[11]

Outcomes Analysis: In such analysis, neither costs nor patient preferences are used to choose the optimal decision. Instead, the focus is entirely on one of the clinical outcomes (e.g., survival or length of hospital stay) that are used as the primary outcome of interest. The optimal treatment is selected based on the most beneficial clinical outcome (e.g., lowest mortality or shortest length of hospital stay).

Utility Analysis: In these analyses, costs are not incorporated in the decision-making process; however, a patient's preferences are included, in conjunction with the relevant clinical outcomes. Most clinical decisions have an effect not only on life and death, but also on the quality of life of patients, mediated through a variety of health states. In utility analyses, the value of any par-

ticular health state to the patient, popularly known as *utility* or *quality of life* (QOL) *weight*, is measured using either a time-tradeoff or standard gamble method.[10,12,13] The utility for any health state is constructed to lie between 0 (representing death) and 1 (representing perfect health). In time-tradeoff methods, patients are asked to trade-off a longer time in a particular health state for a shorter time in perfect health. In standard gamble methods, patients are asked to choose between living with a particular health state and a gamble between perfect health and death. The utility for the health state under consideration is obtained at the point of indifference between the choices in either method. These utilities, multiplied with the duration of time that the person is in that health state under a specific decision choice, form the *quality-adjusted life-years* (QALYs) corresponding to that decision. The decision producing the maximum QALYs is chosen to be the optimal one. The advantage of utility analyses over outcomes analyses is that a variety of outcomes that influence the patient's overall quality of life can be summarized using one generic measure such as the QALYs, and therefore the effects of a decision on multiple outcomes can be simultaneously determined and compared to other decisions.

We use QALYs as the primary outcome of interest in our analysis.

Cost Analysis: In these analyses, only the costs of alternative treatments form the primary outcome of interest and the least costly treatment is recognized as the optimal choice.[14] Such analyses are carried out when the clinical outcomes of the alternative treatments are not a contentious issue – a situation that is becoming increasingly less common in clinical practice.

Cost-effectiveness Analysis: Cost-effectiveness analysis (CEA) compare both the resources used (costs) and the health benefits achieved (e.g., QALYs or simply life years) among alternative treatments, making these trade-offs explicit to both the clinician and to the patient so that together they can make the optimal decision for the patient.[15,16] The practice of cost-effectiveness analysis when comparing two interventions, for example, a new treatment versus standard care, can be summarized as follows: the first step is to calculate the mean costs incurred and the mean benefits produced by each intervention; next, an incremental cost-effectiveness ratio (ICER) is formed by dividing the difference in the mean costs over the difference in the mean benefits between the new and standard interventions. The ICER represents the additional costs required by the new intervention in producing one extra unit of benefit over that produced by the standard intervention. The ICER is then compared with the threshold value that represents the maximum a decision maker is willing to pay for an additional unit of benefit.[17] If the ICER is lower than this threshold value then the new intervention is deemed to be cost effective.

Because, in most cases, a substantial portion of the costs of health care is often borne by health insurance and not the patient, several interesting normative issues arise when an attempt is made to compare both costs and benefits simultaneously. A widely debated question revolves around whose perspective is most appropriate to consider when the burden of costs is distributed amongst patients, healthcare providers, and third-party payers. Furthermore, obtaining a threshold value that represents the maximum willingness-to-pay for an additional unit of benefit is difficult to ascertain at the individual patient level. However, in order to preserve some notion of fairness, one can uniformly apply a societal threshold to all patients. Such discussions are beyond the scope of this chapter but interested readers are encouraged to explore this important literature.[5,6]

6. *Other considerations.* Several other considerations may influence treatment choices. They include information on how much weight patients place on outcomes that will arise in the future compared to those at present time (this is popularly summarized by the concept of the *discount rate*),[10,11] whether consideration of the effects of patients outcomes on the family members are important,[18] and how patient demographic characteristics, health insurance status, and out-of-pocket payments influence the primary outcome of interest.[19,20]

3.3.2. Structure the Decision Problem over Time

Although choosing between alternative actions is the primary goal of a decision analysis, often the decision problem will involve a temporal sequence of choices that inevitably influence the final choice of action. Moreover, these choices may themselves depend on certain chance outcomes that may or may not be controlled by previous decisions. Therefore, the second step in decision analysis is to identify the components of the decision problem. To do this, one defines a structure for the temporal and logical sequence of choices, chances, and outcomes, as well as their interactions, which would lead to the final outcome of interest as defined in the previous step. A decision tree helps to structure this temporal decision problem in a systematic format. An excellent primer for building decision trees is given by Detsky and colleagues.[21]

Figure 3.1 illustrates the decision tree for our simple example on the choice between proceeding to open thoracotomy and watchful waiting. Each point in the decision tree that leads to multiple outcomes or decisions is called a node. There are two types of nodes: (1) a decision node is indicated by a square box, and (2) a chance node is indicated by a circle. A decision node represents the alternative choices that are available to the clinician. A chance node represents the alternative outcomes and patient's responses that are possible. Each chance node is associated with a probability with which a specific outcome is realized, thereby accounting for the inherent uncertainties in such processes. The rightmost column of the decision tree illustrates the final payoffs or outcomes associated with each possible branch of the decision tree. Each branch can be visualized as a level of success given the initial choice of treatment, and is defined by the sequence of events starting with the initial treatment choice and leading up to the final outcome.

In our example, we assume that the clinician makes a decision aiming to maximize the patient's QALYs over the next 1-year period after considering the potential risks and benefits of each choice. If the patient undergoes open thoracotomy, the benefits will include definitive diagnosis (cancer or no cancer), as well as pathological staging and a potential curative resection (lobectomy) with or without adjuvant therapy if the nodule is indeed malignant. The risks include possible morbidity and mortality from both thoracotomy and lobectomy (if needed). These outcomes generally depend on a number of issues, including the experience of the surgeon and the patient's other medical comorbidities, as well as the risk of development of other chronic problems such as a post-thoracotomy chronic pain syndrome that would affect the patient's quality of life.

If the patient undergoes watchful waiting, she avoids the comorbidities associated with thoracotomy. However, the patient is then subjected to a higher mortality risk if the nodule is indeed malignant; she may also suffer from the anxiety of not knowing whether she has cancer, and therefore a reduced quality of life. Please note that the time frame of 1 year does not permit the increased risk of mortality associated with a cancer diagnosis and the choice of watchful waiting to become fully realized in the real world. We have arbitrarily chosen this time frame to simplify our tree, and facilitate the model. Therefore, the reader should be cautioned to not use this model for actual clinical decision making, as it is not clinically accurate.

The non-cancer yearly mortality risk applies irrespective of the choice. The associate payoffs include the quality of life weights of the patient. Death from thoracotomy happens at the beginning of the period and so is assigned a QOL value of 0. Death from lobectomy or natural death is assumed to occur at the middle of the year; so half year of life is weighted by the patient's QOL during that time. Under the thoracotomy arm, if the patient stays alive for the year, her QOL depends on the presence or absence of comorbidities. Under watchful waiting, death from cancer or natural death is also assumed to occur at the middle of the year. If the patient stays alive, then her quality of life is determined by her level of anxiety about cancer.

Note again, that the model in Figure 3.1 is illustrative and uses a very simplified and stylized version of an actual decision-making process. Several additional factors, such as the sensitivity and specificity of detecting cancer through thoracotomy, differences between clinical staging, and the true pathological stage and recurrence of cancer post-lobectomy, to name a few, must be considered for developing a comprehensive model that can appropriately represent this clinical situation.

3.3.3. Characterize the Information to Fill in the Structure

Once the clinician has identified the sequence of choices to be made and the sequence of chance nodes and their associated outcomes determined by these choices, the next step is to obtain information on these chances and outcomes. Choices at each step of the decision process can be made based on this information. This is the critical part of the decision model because the quality of information that goes into these chance nodes entirely determines the credibility of the decision model and the decision it generates.

Bayes' formula provides the key theoretical insight for determining what types of information are required.[22,23] The classic example for application of the Bayes' formula lies in the interpretation of results from a diagnostic test. For example, given that a diagnostic test correctly detects a clinical problem 90% of the time (specificity – a measure of *prior belief*) and correctly detects the absence of a clinical problem 85% of the time (sensitivity – also a measure of *prior belief*), what is the probability that the patient has the problem (*posterior belief* about *success in diagnosis*) given a positive or negative test result (*evidence*)? This question is readily answered using the Bayes' formula. We now provide a more intuitive discussion on the Bayes' formula.

A clinician is often interested in knowing about the probability of success (at any chance node) associated with a treatment decision for a patient, based on the current evidence on success rates with that decision. However, the clinician can only observe, from published research and his or her own experience, the likelihood of evidence given some underlying prior belief about success rates. Bayes' formula, as shown below, helps the clinician to go from the latter quantity to the former one.

$$\begin{aligned} &\Pr(Success|Evidence) \\ &= \frac{\Pr(Evidence|Success) \times \Pr(Success)}{\Pr(Evidence)} \end{aligned} \quad (3.2)$$

where $\Pr(x|y)$ represents probability of x conditional on or given y. Here, $\mathrm{P}_r(Evidence|Success)$ indicates the likelihood (or probability) of observing the data that clinicians observe in practice or in clinical trials given a specific hypothesis about the prior belief on success rates. Often, there will be uncertainty regarding the true success rates and there may be more than one prior belief. However, once new evidence (e.g., observed data in clinical trials) is revealed, the likelihood of that evidence under a variety of prior beliefs becomes known. Consequently, one can feel more confident to restrict the beliefs on success rates to those ranges that correspond to the highest likelihood for the evidence. These new updated beliefs then form the evidence-based posterior beliefs based on which that particular chance node in the model can be informed.

Note that although this exposition of Bayes' formula suggests a prospective process of updating beliefs and information about specific parameters in the model, it also can be readily applied to generate a current estimate of success rates that seem most likely given all the evidence that has accumulated to date. Thus, the role of evidence is important because more evidence would tend to strengthen the posterior beliefs and dispel a larger part of uncertainty associated with prior beliefs. Incorporating all relevant evidence into the model is accomplished by a detailed search on the published and possibly unpublished research literature that point to evidence for the specific parameters in the model. Posterior estimates of parameters are generally weighted by the quality of evidence as defined by sample size, study design, and use of robust analytical methods.

Information gathering for decision analysis almost always uses one or more of the following: literature review, meta-analysis, primary data collection, and consultation with experts.[5,6]

The relevant information for our model and their sources are outlined in Table 3.1. Because we are using a stylized example, we will use point estimates for our model parameters that reasonably lie within the widely disparate ranges that are reported in the literature concerning morbidity and mortality from thoracic procedures. In a more formal treatment of this problem, one has to pay considerable attention to pooled and meta-analyzed available evidence so as to obtain estimates that more closely reflect true values and also properly account for uncertainties from multiple sources. We discuss these sorts of issues further in section 3.5.

Attention should also be paid to the timeliness of information. For example, estimates given in Table 3.1 do not account for the fact that published literature shows a consistent trend over time toward lower morbidity and mortality from thoracic procedures, probably resulting from a combination of improved technique, improved anesthesia, and improved performance by dedicated thoracic surgeons, as well as the vast improvements in adjuvant chemotherapy therapy now available to patients.

TABLE 3.1. Information on parameters for the choice between thoracotomy and watchful waiting.

Description	Value	References
Pr(death due to thoracotomy)	1%	24
Pr(cancer|patient characteristics)	37%	25
Pr(stage I|cancer, patient characteristics)	54%	26
Pr(death|lobectomy, stage I cancer)[a]	3% + 12%	27
Pr(co-morbidities|lobectomy, no death)	25%	28
Pr(death|lobectomy, stage II cancer)[a]	5% + 12%	27
Pr(comorbidities|thoracotomy, no death)	19%	29
Pr(death|watchful waiting, stage I cancer)	18%	30, 31
Pr(death|watchful waiting, stage II cancer)	36%	30, 31
Pr(death|watchful waiting, no cancer, patient characteristics)	12%	32, 33, 34
QOL(alive with no comorbidity & no cancer)	1	Standard
QOL(comorbidities due to lobectomy) = $q2$	= $0.9*q1$	Assumed
QOL(comorbidities due to thoracotomy) = $q1$	0.90	Assumed
QOL(alive with the anxiety of knowing that cancer might be present) = $q3$	0.80	Internal data
QOL(death)	0	Standard

[a]We model this probability as inclusive of the probability of natural death given no cancer, i.e., Pr(death\|lobectomy, stage I cancer) = Pr(death due to lobectomy) + Pr(death\|watchful waiting, no cancer, patient characteristics).

3.3.4. Apply Decision Analysis

The final step is to synthesize the information gathered and the choices made in the process of decision making. This will allow us to obtain estimates of the primary outcome of interest that can be directly compared, in order to choose among alternative actions. This is accomplished by working backwards, that is, from right to left, on our decision tree for which we have filled in probability values for nodes. At decision nodes, we *roll back* (alternatively, the term *fold back* is also used[5]) along the best choices – in effect, the choices that maximize gain or minimize harm. At chance nodes, we average out along all branches, yielding an expected value, such as QALYs, expected number of days of hospital stay, or expected risk of postoperative survival, etc.

Consider the expected QALYs of lobectomy for the patient after she survives thoracotomy with comorbidities and is detected with stage I cancer and undergoes lobectomy. Let the $q1$ and $q2$ be utility weights for comorbidities due to thoracotomy and lobectomy, respectively. As mentioned previously, we also assume that death occurs on average at the middle of the year. The levels of outcomes possible are (1) death from lobectomy (payoff = $0.5 * q1$); (2) survive with comorbidities from lobectomy (payoff = $0.5 * q1 + 0.5 * q2$); and (3) survive without comorbidities from lobectomy (payoff = $q1$). The overall expected payoff is then calculated using the formula in Equation 3.1, by multiplying the corresponding probability of each level of outcome (Table 3.1) with it corresponding payoffs. This process is repeated for each possible level of outcome under thoracotomy and under watchful waiting.

Based on the parameter estimates in Table 3.1, thoracotomy produces an expected QALY of 0.899 while watchful waiting produces an expected QALY of 0.731. This is our baseline result, which reveals that thorocotomy may be the optimal decision for this patient.

3.3.5. Sensitivity Analysis

Clinical decision making using a DAM is usually followed by an assessment of the strength of the final decision that can be accomplished by quantitatively assessing the sensitivity of the final decision to the structural assumptions of the models and feasible alternative information sets. This is done by substituting a range of values for those parameters that are believed to be the most variable in practice. If the conclusions of the model are robust over a range of values for each node, then one can feel very comfortable with the decision that the model suggests. If the decision changes as values are varied, then one must be pay closer attention to those parameters and try to get a better sense of the parameters for the case at hand. This exercise will produce a threshold value where two decisions stand at equipoise. In this latter case, the strength of the data used to generate the parameter estimates becomes exceedingly important.

In our case, we vary the QOL of the patient anxiety and that of the comorbidities of thoracotomy to see how our baseline result change. Figure 3.2 shows the phase diagram for this sensitivity analysis. In the diagram, the y-axis represents different levels of QOL for anxiety, while the x-axis represents different levels of QOL for thoracotomy-related comorbidities. The area in the graph identifies the regions where, conditional of the respective QOL weights, either thoracotomy or watchful waiting is more beneficial. As evident from Figure 3.2, a patient with high levels of anxiety [i.e., low QOL(Anxiety)] would benefit from thoracotomy. A patient with low anxiety [i.e., high QOL(Anxiety)] but low QOL(complications of thoracotomy) would benefit from watchful waiting. Such phase diagrams can help clinicians identify where their patient lie in this graph so that they can make an informed decision about treatment choices.

Phase diagrams, as in Figure 3.2, can be produced based on several other parameters in the model. However, multiple phase diagrams can easily make the decision as complicated as it was to begin with, and hence lose the utility of DAMs. Such scenarios, where there are considerable uncertainties and heterogeneity in several parameters in the model, can be addressed using probabilistic analysis, which we discuss in section 3.5.

FIGURE 3.2. Sensitivity analysis of the baseline QALY result with respect to QOL weights for patient's anxiety and of thoracotomy-related comorbidities. The shaded and the blank areas in the graph identify the values of QOL weights for which thoracotomy or watchful waiting produces the maximum expected QALY, respectively.

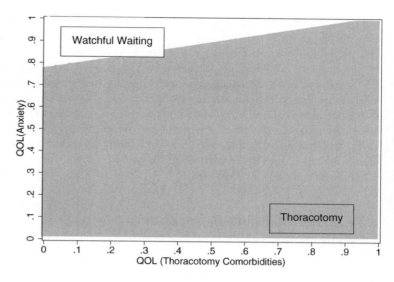

3.4. Clinical Decision Analysis in Thoracic Surgery

Heretofore, DAMs have been used to address a number of issues and/or problems in thoracic surgery. Many of these issues and controversies will be more thoroughly explored in the context of this book. Some examples of models that have been published in the past include those that evaluate different surgical techniques,[35] whether or not to proceed to more invasive and/or aggressive treatments given a common problem in thoracic surgery,[36,37] and appropriate management of certain types of metastases,[38] to name a few. The perspectives that have been used include: the patient's perspective (as we have, and is most common in clinical DAMs); the treating hospital's perspective; and the government's perspective, via Medicare and Medicaid programs. Many DAMs use clinical conditions of patients that have been somewhat simplified, although this may change as older, sicker patients undergo thoracic procedures, and new data are generated about their outcomes. Time frames tend to be dominated by traditional markers of success or failure in surgery; that is, 30-day morbidity and mortality or 1- to 5-year survival. There are centers,[39] however, that have published long-term data. Such information will become increasing relevant and important as outcomes of interest expand to include measures like QALYs and cost-effectiveness ratios that usually require long time frames for appropriate conclusions to be drawn. These longer term time horizons are more commonly found when a DAM incorporates data from sources like the Surveillance, Epidemiology, and End Results database or the Veterans Administration Hospitals extensive database, where patients are followed for many years. Several different primary outcomes of interest have been measured, including mortality, particular morbidities for certain operations, and length of hospital stay, as well as QOL, cost effectiveness, and patient satisfaction.

The chief problem with many of the published DAMs revolves around the fact that almost all point estimates are generated from a few retrospective studies or blinded, prospective, randomized trials, mostly comprised of a handful of patients. The robustness of these estimates can be greatly improved by meta-analyzing the data across studies and properly accounting for the uncertainties arising out of different sources. For example, one DAM compares three choices concerning optimal management for patients undergoing esophagectomy for carcinoma of the esophagus[40] and bases all probabilities on a single, randomized, prospective trial that compared the use of pyloroplasty with non-use.[41] However, in the 72 patients enrolled, there was no statistically significant difference demonstrated between

populations. In addition, there was little exploration of the potential negative side effects of both
procedure non-use and use from the patient's perspective; that is, which might decrease quality of
life more: delayed gastric emptying or dumping
syndrome? Though the model is very insightful,
it is also quite hypothetical – just as our example
is in this chapter. Therefore, to overcome these
sorts of limitations, one can employ more
advanced techniques that have been developed by
practitioners of decision analysis.

3.5. Advanced Issues in Decision Analytic Techniques

The discussions below are an attempt to provide a
general understanding of the advanced issues in
modeling and analysis. It does not, in any way, serve
to provide a comprehensive review of these topics.
More importantly, we recommend that clinicians
interested in taking advantage of these advanced
techniques consult with professionals who are well
versed with the nuances of these methods.

3.5.1. Markov Models

Although decision trees provide intuitive repre-
sentation of the disease process and the consequences of choice over a short time period, they
can get extremely complicated when extended
over long periods of time. To address this situation, one can use a Markov process that is a modeling technique based on matrix algebra. The

fundamental idea behind these models is that,
instead of considering health state transitions
over a short period of time, as in decision trees,
a Markov process is concerned with transitions
during a series of short time intervals or cycles.

For example, consider the watchful waiting
arm of the decision tree in Figure 3.1. One can
revise the model to include a bi-annual follow-up
for detecting whether the lesion is growing or
not. The probability that the clinician would find
an advanced lesion in the next follow-up will be
based on the natural progression of cancer over
time. In order to model the progression of cancer,
the cancer can be delineated into mutually exclusive health states based on its stage and grade. An
example of such a model, borrowed from our col-
league David Meltzer's work in prostate cancer,
is shown in Figure 3.3, also known as a bubble
diagram. Each health state, defined by a combination of stage and grade, is represented by a
bubble. The figure represents progression of
cancer by stage and grade leading up to cancer-
related death. The patient begins in one of these
bubbles and in every cycle, with some transition
probabilities, either stays in that bubble or moves
to another bubble representing an advanced
health state. The sum of all transition probabilities in a cycle must add up to one because, by
definition, a patient has to be in one of the
mutually exclusive health states. The transition
probabilities can vary with time (or number of
cycles) and also with patient characteristics such
as age of diagnosis. The transition probabilities
determine the progression of the disease over

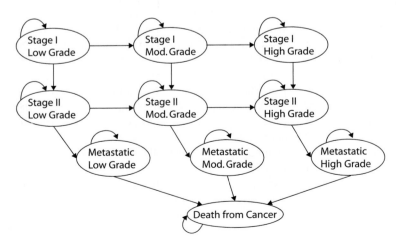

FIGURE 3.3. Structure of a Markov model for cancer progression

time, and therefore are critical in evaluating the costs and outcomes of any intervention at a particular point in time. We refer interested readers to some of the applications of Markovian processes in decision models available in the literature.[42-46]

3.5.2. Probabilistic Analysis

Uncertainty remains an integral part of any analysis. Although a part of this uncertainty is reflected in the probability estimates used in decision models (e.g., such as those in Table 3.1), they do not reflect the overall uncertainty for an outcome. For example, if we say that Mrs. X has a 40% chance of having cancer, we make a statement about a population comprised of millions of Mrs. X clones in which 40% of them will have cancer and 60% will not. When the clinician is faced with one Mrs. X from that population, her true cancer status is not known with certainty. But by incorporating the point estimate of 40%, the clinician can characterize the uncertainty that she might fall in the part of the population who has cancer. This type of model, as the one we illustrate above, is called a deterministic model as one uses predetermined point estimates for probabilities to reflect the uncertainty.

However, we seldom know how many patients in that population truly have cancer; instead, we rely on a random sample from the population to determine how many patients in that sample have cancer. If we find 40% of patients in the sample have cancer, it gives us a reasonable estimate for the population, but not the exact estimate. That is, 35% of patients in the population may truly have cancer, while in the random sample we have chosen, 40% show up with cancer. The bigger the sample size, the closer will be the sample estimate to the population estimate. Hence, there remains a degree of uncertainty about the true value of the population parameter because we almost always infer based on a fraction of that population.

The traditional way to deal with uncertainty is to a perform sensitivity analysis by varying the parameter of interest across a range of values and observing the changes in outcomes associated with it, as we have shown in our stylized example. However, there are several limitations to this method. One-way or two-way sensitivity analysis may severely undermine the effect of uncertainty in a multiparameter model. Multiple-way sensitivity analysis can easily become extremely complicated as to disallow straightforward interpretation. Even in the absence of complicated analysis, traditional sensitivity analysis can identify the optimal decision if only the true values of the parameters are known, as, for example, in the case of patient preferences that can be directly measured. This poses problems for the clinicians who may often find it hard to use sensitivity analysis results in clinical decision making due to lack of guidance and uncertainty about the true value of many clinical parameters.

Probabilistic analyses help to characterize these uncertainties in the model parameters and to arrive at the final decision by simultaneously averaging out the uncertainties in multiple parameters. In these models, instead of specific point estimates of different parameters in the model, one specifies distributions for these input parameters where these distributions might center on the point estimates. Using Monte Carlo techniques, a patient is then propagated through the model several times (iterations), each time with random values of a parameter drawn from its respective distribution. The costs and outcomes are then averaged over all iterations and compared across treatment options.

A good example of a probabilistic analysis can be found Andrew Brigg's work on gastroesophageal reflux disease.[47]

3.5.3. Bayesian Meta-analysis

Bayesian meta-analysis is a sophisticated hierarchical modeling approach that utilizes the concept of Bayes' theorem discussed earlier. It summarizes and integrates the findings of research studies in a particular area. One can obtain the posterior distribution of Pr(Success| Evidence), that is the current distribution of belief about success rates given all the past evidence, and directly use it as an input in a probabilistic analysis. Such an approach provides a combined analysis of studies that indicate the overall strength of evidence for a success while properly accounting for multiple sources of uncertainty.

For example, suppose there are four studies with varying sample sizes indicating that a woman with a smoking history similar to that in our example has a pretest probability of cancer of 60%, 45%, 30%, and 75%, respectively. Perhaps we also know, from even bigger studies, that women are 1.5 times more likely than men to have a lung cancer unrelated to their smoking, while a person with a significant smoking history is 9 times more likely to have cancer than a never-smoker. A Bayesian meta-analysis can combine this prior information on the effects of gender and smoking history with the data from the four samples to produce the posterior distribution of the pretest probability of cancer for this female patient given all relevant evidence.

With the advent of the Society of Thoracic Surgeons General Thoracic Surgery Database, these methods will be most relevant for the field of thoracic surgery in order to synthesize information arising out of a large number of prospectively collected data.

Several books on Bayesian estimation and meta-analysis have been written and several examples of Bayesian meta-analysis can be found in the literature. Interested readers are encouraged to explore Peter Congdon's book on this topic.[48] Of interest to the readers of this book may be the work by Tweedie and colleagues, who perform a Bayesian meta-analysis of the published literature to determine the association between incidence of lung cancer in female never smokers and exposure to environmental tobacco smoke.[49] Bayesian meta-analysis can be most conveniently implemented using freely available software called the WinBUGS (http://www.mrc-bsu.cam.ac.uk/bugs).

3.5.4. Value of Information Analyses

As we discussed earlier, probabilistic models often can provide a more efficient way to address uncertainty in decision models. It provides the clinician with a sense of the strength of evidence for an optimal decision after accounting for multiple sources of uncertainty. It also provides the basis for conducting value of information analysis on specific parameters. In these analyses, uncertainties in parameter estimates that trans-late into uncertainties surrounding the outcome of interest can be used to establish the value of acquiring additional information by conducting further research. Information is valuable because it reduces the expected costs of uncertainty surrounding a clinical decision. The expected costs of uncertainty are determined by the probability that a treatment decision based on existing information will be wrong and by the consequences (or costs) if the wrong decision is made. The expected costs of uncertainty can also be interpreted as the expected value of perfect information (EVPI), because perfect information (an infinite sample) can eliminate the possibility of making a wrong decision. It is also the maximum a decision maker should be willing to pay for additional evidence to inform this decision in the future. Such analyses can identify research priorities by focusing on those parameters where more precise estimates would be most valuable.[50–52]

Additionally, an analogous type of calculation may be done on heterogeneous parameters such as quality of life weights and patient's preferences and attitudes towards treatment. Knowing this information can help clinicians make individualized decisions by incorporating patients' values and preferences into the process of making treatment decisions. Concretely, clinicians might pursue this approach using a variety of decision aids that are designed to facilitate transmission of information on patients' values and preferences to physicians. These decision aids are often expensive in terms of program development and implementation as well as in time costs for patients and physicians.[53] Therefore, in order to decide how to best allocate limited resources towards decision aids and similar approaches to implementing individualized care, it is important to have information on the potential social value of such endeavors and which dimensions of patient preference are most valuable to elicit. This is accomplished by the Expected Value of Individualized Care (EVIC) analysis.[54] EVIC represents the expected costs of ignorance of patient-level heterogeneity. It is the potential value of research, as compared to optimal population level decision making, to elicit information on heterogeneous parameters so that individualized information about each patient can be conveyed to the physician.

3.6. Conclusions

Decision analytic modeling is a systematic approach to integrating information about a variety of different aspects of clinical decision making. It helps the clinician to make an objective decision by incorporating both the population-level evidence on outcomes and also the individual-level preferences in the decision-making process. It is worthwhile to issue a reminder at this point that the sole purpose of DAM is to provide information in a systematic way so as to facilitate decision making based on best and comprehensive evidence. Decision analytic modeling, although viewed by some clinician and researchers as *prescriptive*, only prescribes the consideration of a decision to be optimal and *should not* be viewed as the final prescription for the patient. Decision analytic modeling in no way serves to make a decision for the clinician, who must utilize his/her own expertise to interpret the evidence placed in front him/her and determine the relevance of this evidence in the context of an individual patient's case.

The tension inherent in any DAM lies between the desire to create a model that is conceptually rich – to more accurately reflect the complexity of real-world decision making – that is also somewhat data poor, versus creating a more simple model which utilizes few, highly reliable estimates. However, if real-world decision making does demand a richer model, we believe that it is more appropriate to develop such a model, even if subjective decisions and estimates inform some parts of this model. We say this because often in real-world clinical practice, such subjective decisions and estimates do play a part in clinical decision making. Decision analytic modeling helps to translate these subjective estimates into a formal statement about uncertainty and help clinicians understand the implications of these uncertainties in the decision process. It also helps clinicians to identify priorities in research areas and patient preferences that are most critical for patient outcomes.

Most DAMs in thoracic surgery have focused on information from clinical data. Such information is certainly crucial and forms the backbone of a DAM. However, any attempt to translate efficacy information available from clinical trials and other studies into effectiveness for a given patient requires a careful examination of patient preferences and behavior. Therefore, creating models that accurately reflect the choices at hand requires a fusion of several types of information. This information can be crudely divided into two categories – information that is derived from biological science, and that derived from social science. As we learn more about the genetic behavior and cell biology of tumors, as well as genetic information about individual patients, clinical decision making will most certainly be impacted. But this sort of information must be contextualized within the study of actual human behaviors – information that is captured by fields as diverse as behavioral and classical economics to statistics to political science to epidemiology. Consequently, it is imperative that surgeons and practitioners in these other fields collaborate if DAMs are to function as nuanced, effective tools to improve the clinical outcomes, and indeed the lives, of patients.

Acknowledgments. We are grateful to Caleb G. Alexander, William Dale, and Mark Ferguson at the University of Chicago for helpful comments and suggestions.

References

1. Meltzer D. Can medical cost-effectiveness analysis identify the value of research? In: Murphy KM, Topel RH, eds. *Measuring the Gains from Medical Research: An Economic Approach.* Chicago: The University of Chicago Press; 2003:206–247.
2. Sackett DL, Rosenberg WM, Gray JA. Evidence based medicine: what it is, what it isn't. *BMJ* 1996;312:71–72.
3. Coutler A. Partnerships with patients: the pros and cons of shared clinical decision-making. *J Health Serv Res* 1997;2:112–121.
4. Pauker SG, Kassirer JP. Decision analysis. *N Engl J Med* 1987;316:250–257.
5. Weinstein MC, Fineberg HV. *Clinical Decision Making.* Philadelphia: Saunders; 1980.
6. Petitti DB. *Meta-analysis, Decision Analysis and Cost-Effectiveness Analysis.* New York: Oxford University Press; 1994.
7. Detsky AS, Naglie G, Krahn MD, et al. Primer on medical decision analysis: getting started. *Med Decis Making* 1997;17:123–125.

8. Eddy D. *Clinical Decision Making: From Theory to Practice.* Boston: Jones & Bartlett; 1996.

9. Ost D, Fein A. Management strategies for the solitary pulmonary nodule. *Curr Opin Pulm Med* 2004;10:272–278.

10. Gold MR, Siegel JE, Russell LB, Weinstein MC. *Cost-effectiveness in Health and Medicine.* New York: Oxford University Press; 1996.

11. Drummond M, Stoddard G, Torrence G. *Methods of Economic Evaluation of Health Care Programmes.* Oxford: Oxford University Press; 1987:6–26.

12. Torrence GW. Utility approach to measuring health-related quality of life. *J Chron Dis* 1987;40:593–600.

13. Torrence GW. Measurement of health state utilities for economic appraisal: a review. *J Health Econ* 1986;5:1–30.

14. Lowson KV, Drummond MF, Bishop JM. Costing new services: long-term domiciliary oxygen therapy. *Lancet* 1981; ii:1146–1149.

15. Weinstein MC, Stason WB. Foundation of cost-effectiveness analysis for health and medical practices. *N Eng J Med* 1977;296:716–721.

16. Garber A, Phelps C. Economic foundations of cost-effectiveness analysis. *J Health Econ* 1997;16:1–32.

17. Weinstein M, Zeckhauser R. Critical ratios and efficient allocation. *J Pubic Econ* 1973;2:147–158.

18. Basu A, Meltzer D. Implications of spillover effects within the family for medical cost-effectiveness analysis. *J Health Econ* 2005;24:751–773.

19. Alexander GC, Casalino LP, Meltzer DO. Patient-physician communication about out-of-pocket costs. *JAMA* 2003;290:953–958.

20. Alexander GC, Casalino LP, Meltzer DO. Physician strategies to reduce patients' out-of -pocket prescription costs. *Arch Intern Med* 2005;165:633–636.

21. Detsky AS, Naglie G, Krahn MD, et al. Primer on medical decision analysis: building a tree. *Med Decis Making* 1997;17:126–135.

22. Bayes T. An essay towards solving a problem in the doctrine of chances. *Philos Trans R Soc* 1763;330–418. Taken from: *Biometrika* 1958;45:293–315.

23. Pratt JW. Bayesian interpretation of standard inference statements (with discussions). *J R Stat Soc B* 1965;27:169–203.

24. Dominioni L, Imperatore A, Rovera F, et al. Stage I non-small cell lung carcinoma, analysis of survival and implications for screening. *Cancer* 2000;89:2334–2344.

25. Swensen SJ, Silverstein MD, Ilstrup DM, et al. The probability of malignancy in solitary pulmonary nodules. Application to small radiologically indeterminate nodules. *Arch Intern Med* 1997;157:849–855.

26. Wisnivesky JP, Yankelevitz D, Henschke CI. Stage of lung cancer in relation to its size. *Chest* 2005;127:1136–1139.

27. Ginsberg RJ, Hill LD, Eagan RT, et al. Modern thirty-day operative mortality for surgical resections in lung cancer. *J Thorac Cardiovasc Surg* 1983;86:654–658.

28. Stéphan F, Boucheseiche S, Hollande J, et al. Pulmonary complications following lung resection: a comprehensive analysis of incidence and possible risk factors. *Chest* 2000;118:1263–1270.

29. Barrera R, Shi W, Amar D, et al. Smoking and timing of cessation: impact on pulmonary complications after thorocatomy. *Chest* 2005;127:1977–1983.

30. Chadha AS, Ganti AK, Sohi JS, et al. Survival in untreated early stage non-small cell lung cancer. *Anticancer Res* 2005;25:3517–3520.

31. McGarry RC, Song G, des Rosiers P, et al. Observation-only management of early stage, medically inoperable lung cancer: poor outcome. *Chest* 2002;121:1155–1158.

32. U.S. Department of Health and Human Services. *The Health Consequences of Smoking: A Report of the Surgeon General.* Washington, DC: U.S. Department of Health and Human Services, Centers for Disease Control and Prevention, National Center for Chronic Disease Prevention and Health Promotion, Office on Smoking and Health; 2004.

33. Arias E. *United States Life Tables, 2002. National Vital Statistics Reports.* Hyattsville, MD: National Center for Health Statistics; 2004:53.

34. English DR, Holman CDJ, Milne E, et al. *The Quantification of Drug Caused Morbidity and Mortality in Australia.* Canberra: Commonwealth Department of Human Services and Health; 1995.

35. Ferguson MK, Lehman AG. Sleeve lobectomy or pneumonectomy: optimal management strategy using decision analysis techniques. *Ann Thorac Surg* 2003;76:1782–1788.

36. Morimoto T, Tsuguya F, Koyama H, et al. Optimal strategy for the first episode of primary spontaneous pneumothorax in young men. *J Gen Intern Med* 2002;17:193–202.

37. Falcoz PE, Binquet C, Clement F, et al. Management of the second episode of spontaneous pneumothorax: a decision analysis. *Ann Thorac Surg* 2003;76:1843–1848.

38. Porter G, Cantor S, Walsh G, et al. Cost-effectiveness of pulmonary resection and systemic

chemotherapy in the management of metastatic soft tissue sarcoma: a combined analysis from the University of Texas M.D. Anderson and Memorial Sloan-Kettering Cancer Centers. *J Thorac Cardiovasc Surg* 2004;127:1366–1372.

39. Martini N, Rusch V, Bains, MS et al. Factors influencing ten-year survival in resected stages I to III a non-small cell lung cancer. *J Thorac Cardiovasc Surg* 1999;117:32–36.

40. Olak J, Detsky A. Surgical decision analysis: esophagectomy/esophagogastrectomy with or without drainage? *Ann Thorac Surg* 1992;53:493–497.

41. Cheung HC, Siu KF, Wong J. Is pyloroplasty necessary in esophageal replacement by stomach? A prospective, randomized controlled trial. *Surgery* 1987;102:19–24.

42. Goldie SJ, Kuntz KM, Weinstein MC, et al. Cost-effectiveness of screening for anal squamous intraepithelial lesions and anal cancer in human immunodeficiency virus-negative homosexual and bisexual men. *Am J Med* 2000;108:634–641.

43. Goldie SJ, Weinstein MC, Kuntz KM, et al. The costs, clinical benefits, and cost-effectiveness of screening for cervical cancer in HIV-infected women. *Ann Intern Med* 1999;130:97–107.

44. Goldie SJ, Kuhn L, Denny L, et al. Policy analysis of cervical cancer screening strategies in low-resource settings: clinical benefits and cost-effectiveness. *JAMA* 2001;285:3107–3115.

45. Zeliadt SB, Etzioni RD, Penson DF, et al. Lifetime implications and cost-effectiveness of using finasteride to prevent prostate cancer. *Am J Med* 2005;118:850–857.

46. Manser R, Dalton A, Carter R, et al. Cost-effectiveness analysis of screening for lung cancer with low dose spiral CT (computed tomography) in the Australian setting. *Lung Cancer* 2005;48:171–185.

47. Briggs AH, Goeree R, Blackhouse G, et al. Probabilistic analysis of cost-effectiveness models: choosing between treatment strategies for gastroesophageal reflux disease. *Med Decis Making* 2002;22:290–308.

48. Congdon P. *Bayesian Statistical Modeling.* New York: Wiley; 2001.

49. Tweedie RL, Scott DJ, Biggerstaff BJ, et al. Bayesian meta-analysis, with application to studies of ETS and lung cancer. *Lung Cancer* 1996;14(suppl 1):S171–S194.

50. Meltzer D. Addressing uncertainty in medical cost-effectiveness analysis: implications of expected utility maximization for methods to perform sensitivity analysis and the use of cost-effectiveness analysis to set priorities for medical research. *J Health Econ* 2001;20:109–129.

51. Claxton K. The irrelevance of inference: a decision making approach to the stochastic evaluation of health care technologies. *J Health Econ* 1999;18:341–364.

52. Claxon K, Neumann PJ, Araki S, et al. Bayesian value of information analysis: An application to a policy model of Alzheimer's disease. *Int J Tech Assoc Health Care* 2001;17:38–55.

53. Kennedy AD, Sculpher MJ, Coulter A, et al. Effects of decision aids for menorrhagia on treatment choices, health outcomes, and costs: a randomized controlled trial. *JAMA* 2002;288:2701–2708.

54. Basu A. Value of information on preference heterogeneity and individualized care. In: *Three Essays in Cost-Effectiveness Analysis* [master's thesis]. Chicago: University of Chicago; 2004.

4
Nonclinical Components of Surgical Decision Making

Jo Ann Broeckel Elrod, Farhood Farjah, and David R. Flum

Examining surgical trends before the National Emphysema Treatment Trial (NETT) demonstrates the importance of nonclinical determinants of care. The number of lung volume reduction surgery (LVRS) claims increased dramatically after 1994 despite the fact that there was considerable uncertainty in the available evidence base.[1] Favorable media reports and testimonials from patient advocacy groups may have influenced both patient and surgeon attitudes about LVRS.[2] Some surgeons felt that investigations prior to the NETT demonstrated clear and dramatic improvements in quality of life, sufficient to justify Medicare reimbursement for the procedure.[3] Accordingly, they believed the NETT was a form of coercion because patients who refused to enroll in the study would not have financial coverage of their LVRS or receive the operation from a NETT surgeon. Furthermore, even if patients enrolled, the study deprived half of them a procedure with "established" benefits. Surgeons less comfortable with this level of scientific uncertainty may have decided against performing the procedure. Nonsurgeon observers proposed that surgeons were motivated by financial gains, as the procedure was relatively inexpensive and reimbursement was generous.[2] In addition to potential patient and surgeon influence, third-party coverage had an effect on decision making as evidenced by the dramatic decrease in the number of operations upon suspension of Medicare reimbursement in December 1995.[4] Because many third-party payers base their coverage plans on Centers for Medicare and Medicaid Services (CMS) guidelines, this policy likely affected many non-Medicare patients and provid-

ers as well. Whether surgeons stopped performing the operation because of lack of reimbursement or as an acknowledgement of scientific uncertainty is unclear. It is clear, however, that the sharp decline in the number of procedures was temporally related to CMS intervention. Subsequent CMS policy partly limited surgical decision making because reimbursement was limited to eligible patients and surgeons.

Professional organizations can also play a role in decision making by effectively regulating surgeon-directed clinical practice in the setting of clinical uncertainty. For example, through educational and advisory statements, the American Society of Colorectal Surgeons strongly influenced its membership to avoid performing laparoscopic procedures for colorectal cancer despite the use of these interventions by many surgeons for benign disease. There was no similar "prohibition" by thoracic surgical professional organizations in 1994, and these circumstances may have "permitted" surgeon-level, non-evidence–based decision making to flourish with LVRS. The case of LVRS reveals that many nonclinical factors involving patients, surgeons, and the practice environment can influence surgical decision making.

4.1. Methodology for Evaluating Nonclinical Factors of Decision Making

Previous investigations of nonclinical factors influencing clinical decision making have used qualitative or semiquantitative research methodologies – such as surveys, case vignettes, and decision-analytic modeling – all of which have important methodological limitations.[5] Clinicians often find qualitative research (i.e., focus groups and key informant interviews) difficult to interpret because the question of generalizability is more problematic and because this approach does not test hypotheses. Rather, qualitative research helps develop hypotheses that may then be evaluated using semiquantitative evaluations such as surveys. Surveys are difficult to interpret because of their limited generalizability to those who respond, the degree to which the question being asked is understood by the respondent, and, in the case of physician surveys, the extent of socially normative responses. Socially normative responses occur when members of a group provide "acceptable" answers to questions when the "real" answer would generate negative social judgments. These socially normative answers can also occur in the setting of anonymous surveys but are more common when the individuals are identified. In quantitative evaluations of these issues, such as in a prospective cohort that includes data on beliefs and attitudes of the surgeon and patient, the number of variables of interest and potential for confounding may be overwhelming. Methods less familiar to surgeons, such as the factorial experimental design, may partly overcome these obstacles. Factorial design allows comparisons of differential groupings of categorical variables. For example, five dichotomized variables have 32 (2^5) unique groupings that one can analyze using hierarchical logistic regression. In essence, factorial design can estimate the individual and combined effects of many variables, allowing some control of confounding, and may facilitate studies trying to quantify the influence of clinical and nonclinical variables. The complexity of the calculations rises with the number of variables and combinations of variables, and thus even this study design has practical limits in terms of the number of variables it can analyze. Of greatest importance to the surgeon interested in assessing this complicated line of research is the need to collaborate with behavioralists and biostatisticians with relevant knowledge and experience in alternative research methods.

4.2. Surgeon Factors Related to Clinical Decision Making

As demonstrated in the LVRS example, the clinical decision-making process appears to be influenced by surgeons factors. These factors include the surgeon's tolerance of uncertainty, how willing they are to take risks in clinical care, the demographic characteristics of the surgeon, and their level and type of training.

4.2.1. Impact of Risk-Taking Attitude on Clinical Decision Making

Because clinical decisions are made under conditions of uncertainty, reactions to uncertainty and attitudes toward risk taking may have important implications on clinical decision making. There is a limit in our understanding of the degree to which this issue influences surgical care.[6] Several investigators have developed instruments to assess risk taking among physicians. Nightingale and colleagues[7-9] have developed a two-question test that has been frequently used to assess the degree to which physicians view themselves as risk seeking or risk averse. In Nightingale's study, respondents' willingness to gamble for their patients in both the face of gain and in the face of loss is measured. Those who refuse to gamble in the face of loss are considered risk averse. The first question:

(1) Choose between two new therapies for a healthy person:
  (A) 100% chance of living 5 years more than the average person
  0% percent chance of living 0 years more than the average person
  Or
  (B) 50% chance of living 10 years more than the average person
  50% chance of living 0 years more than the average person

If the physician selects A, there is a moderate gain and no chance of failure. If they select option B, there is a chance for significant gain, but also a risk of complete failure. The second question is stated in a similar manner, but evaluates the willingness to accept loss for the patient:

(2) Choose between two new therapies for a sick person:
  (A) 100 % chance of living 5 years less than the average person
  0% chance of living 10 years less than the average person
  Or
  (B) 50% chance living just as long as the average person
  50% chance of living 10 years less than the average person

Answer A minimizes loss while answer B subjects the patient to a smaller risk of great loss and a possible risk of no loss. The same question is posed in two different ways to determine a person's willingness to gamble in the face of gain (the first case) and in the face of loss (the second case). One set of studies[7-9] performed by Nightingale examined physicians' risk preferences and the relationship of such preferences to laboratory test usage, critical care decision making, and emergency room admissions. Although no significant association was found between the item "dealing with a gamble in the face of gain" and resource utilization, in all three of Nightingale's studies, a significant correlation was found between resource utilization and risk preference in the face of loss. The more often physicians chose the second gamble, the more likely they were to utilize additional medical resources to rule out uncertain conditions than those who chose the certain outcome. Therefore, when faced with possible loss, the physician preferred to minimize loss and fail in half of these attempts than accept a certain loss. Other authors[10] have found that the "fear of failure" paradigm in risk taking is less consistent but varies based on the mode of testing[10] or across different cultures.[11] They also found that physicians who chose to gamble in the face of loss were also more likely to order more testing procedures.

4.2.2. Surgeon Age

Although little data exist on the extent to which surgical decision making is related to risk taking behavior and comfort with ambiguous situations, a recent study by Nakata and colleagues[12] explored the relationship between risk attitudes and demographic characteristics of surgeons and anesthesiologists. The authors distributed a survey on clinical decision making and expected life years to 122 physicians in Japan. Participants were asked to read a brief scenario designed to produce certainty equivalents for two gambles, one framed as though the respondent were a patient (of the participant's same age) and the other framed as though the respondent were a physician. Both scenarios ask the respondent to state their willingness (yes or no) to undergo a treatment with a success rate of 80% (i.e., the probability of failure is 20%) with the assumption that they will live for 20 years if the treatment is successful but will die immediately if the treatment fails. The scenario also states that they will be guaranteed to survive 18 years if they do not choose the treatment. The questions were repeated with 2-year differences in expected longevity. Based on the certainty equivalents from the responses, participants were defined as risk averse, risk neutral, and risk seeking. Results from the 93 physicians who completed the questionnaire (38 anesthesiologists and 55 surgeons) showed no significant differences in the number and percentage of risk seekers between groups. Comparisons by gender and specialty did not reveal any significant differences in risk preference, nor was risk attitude affected by how the question was framed (as a physician or patient). However, results did indicate that the physician's age was a statistically significant predictor of risk attitude. Specifically, the older the physician, the more risk averse they were. The authors interpreted this to mean that based on experience and judgment, older physicians may shy away from risk and younger physicians may be more willing to gamble.

4.2.3. Surgeon Gender

Clinical decisions may also be affected by surgeon demographics, such as physician gender, and, given the paucity of female thoracic surgeons (2.2% of all thoracic surgeons reportedly are female[13]), this may be a significant issue for this field. Several studies have documented the varying communication styles of male and female physicians.[14] Specifically, female clinicians are more likely to actively facilitate patient participation in medical discussions by engaging in more positive talk, more partnership building, question asking, and information giving.[12-16] Female physicians also tend to be less dominant verbally during clinic visits than male physicians,[14] and, although patients of female physicians talk proportionately more during a medical visit than do patients of male physicians, female doctors engage in discussion more with patients than male doctors.[16] While female doctors spend more time with their patients,[17] this difference may be better attributed to gender distribution and health status of their patients. Women physicians tend to see more female patients and female patients tend to have longer medical visits than males.[18] Furthermore, because female physicians engage in more discussion of emotional and psychosocial issues than male clinicians,[16] it has been hypothesized that female doctors are more responsive to the nonclinical components of decision making that derive from the patients.[14]

Clinical decision making with regard to cancer screening is also affected by physician gender. Specifically, women patients of female physicians have higher rates of screening by Pap smear and mammography than patients of male physicians.[19] It is unclear how these gender differences impact decision making in thoracic surgery but they may be relevant in the comparative use of screening and staging techniques for thoracic malignancies and other entities.

4.2.4. Impact of Training on Clinical Decision Making

Surgeon specialization has been studied in the context of mortality, and specialty training has been shown to predict postoperative outcomes among high-risk operations.[20] For example, Dimick and colleagues[21] found that specialty board certification in thoracic surgery was independently associated with lower operative mortality rates after esophageal resection in the national Medicare population (from 1998 through 1999). Goodney and colleagues[22] showed that board-certified thoracic surgeons have lower rates of operative mortality with lung resection compared to general surgeons, although they noted that surgeon and hospital characteristics, in particular volume, also influenced a patient's operative risk of mortality. Some of this effect

may be mediated by the volume of procedures performed by differently trained surgeons, but process of care variables are often different in specialty trained surgeons and it is very likely that other components of decision making are influenced by training factors.

Surgeon specialization, however, has not been rigorously studied as it relates to clinical decision making. Training and specialization undoubtedly impact decision making by physicians. Specialty-trained thoracic surgeons may be more recently trained than non-specialty–trained surgeons and therefore may include more recently developed evidence-based protocols in their decision making. Conversely, after a lifetime of experience, older surgeons (more likely to be non-fellowship–trained) are undoubtedly influencing decision making through a separate group of experience-based care guidelines. It remains to be seen if subspecialty-trained clinicians are more risk seeking in their treatment options given their additional training. The maxim "a surgeon with lots of experience got that way by having lots of bad experiences" underlies the way that collective professional experience influences decision making. While most try not to unduly influence their behavior by their last unsuccessful outcome, the lessons learned from unfortunate decisions must influence surgeon decision making. The potential effects of this influence may include the way we discuss risk with patients, or may consist of modulation of risk taking if we have had a recent bad outcome related to prior risk taking. The interesting issue related to past experience is how little we understand about how it affects clinical decision making. If one goal of quality improvement (QI) activities is to limit variation then we must better understand and regulate the influence of non-evidence–driven factors, such as past experiences, if we are to achieve that goal.

4.3. System Factors

Clinicians do not make decisions in a vacuum. Systems including colleagues, employers, payers, healthcare systems, and QI staff all review our decision making and thereby influence it. These system factors may be as limited as a group of colleagues with whom we share decision making.

These "coverage" partners may influence our decision making in that they share the consequences of decision making through "on-call coverage." Sometimes decisions about who returns to the operating room to rule out problems (rather than taking a wait-and-see approach) or what types of diagnostic testing we obtain to evaluate for potential problems are influenced by the day of the week, cross-coverage patterns, and expectations for on-call responsibilities.

Organized health systems may also influence decision making because significant variability in process and outcome of care also has important implications for payers and hospitals. For example, in some health maintenance organizations (HMOs) there are rigid guidelines for the treatment of patients that may limit individual surgeon decision making. This can be as innocuous as the limits some HMOs have put on formularies of drugs to influence the use of drugs for our patients. In other systems the types of devices surgeons can use are limited, thereby limiting surgeon autonomy in decision making. Hospitals have also been expanding the use of guidelines, treatment pathways, and care plans. These are all interventions aimed at limiting decision making variability. The extent to which these approaches are used and effective in limiting hospital stay, the use of resources, and variability in care demonstrate the impact of nonclinical components of care in systems that do not have such interventions.

4.3.1. Characteristics of the Environment and Clinical Decision Making

For over a decade, surgeons in the Veterans Administration hospitals have participated in a systematic data-gathering and feedback system of outcomes after major surgery. The National Surgical Quality Improvement Project (NSQIP) works to decrease variation in clinical outcomes by demonstrating to surgeons when their center is an "outlier" in performance. This system allows hospitals to target QI activities that may influence components of care and may also influence surgeon decision making. A potential unintended consequence of any ranking system is that it may also impact a surgeons' willingness to operate on patients who have particularly high risk of

adverse outcome, especially if the risk adjustment strategy is not considered adequate. This influence on surgical decision making needs further investigation to determine its importance.

Other system factors that cannot be excluded relate to the value of surgeon performance to a system. For example, in systems such as the Canadian National Healthcare System and in Scandinavia, where surgeons are given a fixed salary and procedure volume is not tied to reimbursement, there is a considerably lower use of operative procedures and considerably less population-level variability in the use of procedures. Clearly, this is a health system influence on surgeon decision making and it clearly challenges the notion that surgical decision making is driven exclusively by clinical factors.

4.4. Social Factors

4.4.1. Patient Interest

In a more paternalistic era, decision making was driven exclusively by the physician, but patient autonomy has become a central feature of modern medical ethics. Informed patients will bring to the decision-making process a perspective that sometimes completely affirms the surgeon's primacy in decision making but other times may challenge this primacy. Empowered patients may bring to the decision-making process their interest in quality of life and functional outcomes that may be less important in physician-directed decision making. Alternatively, helping patients develop a realistic risk assessment of an intervention can be challenging, especially in the setting of unfamiliar diagnoses, medical terms, and prognostic information. Acknowledging that the patient may be a major determinant of care decisions is an important step to understanding the variability we see in clinical care. However, it also raises the challenge of adequately informing our patients about the components of decision making without overwhelming them. The challenge is extended by the use of web-based resources that may both inform and misinform patients and the unique experiences patients, their loved ones, and friends may have had with similar conditions.

One interesting evolution in our understanding of nonclinical factors that influence decision making comes from research in shared decision making in cancer patients. Decision aids have been developed to improve communication between the cancer patients and the physicians and to allow patients to express their preference for treatment by providing information on the outcomes relative to their health status. The interactive nature of these tools allows patient values and interests to be incorporated into decision making. For example, decisions about adjuvant therapy that include a discussion of the risks of chemotherapy (e.g., hair loss) may not be relevant to certain patients (e.g., patients who have no hair) while for others it may be an outcome that they are not willing to tolerate even if it has implications for survival. While some may disagree with the decisions that patients make, acknowledging their autonomy and empowerment may help in the delivery of care that is appropriate to each patient and meet each patient's needs. These decision aids have been quite successful. In fact, Whelen and colleagues,[23] in a randomized trial of 20 surgeons and 201 breast cancer patients, demonstrated that patients whose physician used this tool had greater knowledge of breast cancer, treatment, and treatment outcomes, had lower decisional conflict, and expressed higher satisfaction with their decision following a consultation with their physician. Because these tools are increasingly available,[24] decision aids will likely become useful for a greater number of patients, physicians, and treatment options.

4.4.2. Public Disclosure of Report Cards and Clinical Decision Making

The impact of disclosure of outcome data [such as the reporting of hospital and surgeon risk-adjusted mortality rates for coronary artery bypass graft (CABG) on decision making has been controversial. Although outcome data were rarely published prior to the mid-1980s,[25] the first release of hospital risk-adjusted mortality rates in December 1990[26] and the first formal public release published in December 1992[27] ushered in a new era of public reporting. These performance reports, sometimes called "physician scorecards," have become more prevalent in recent years.[28,29] Advocates of this form of reporting believe they

provide information about quality of care that consumers, employers, and health plans can use to improve their decision making and to stimulate quality improvement among providers.[30]

These reports have raised concern regarding their effect on patient care and surgeon decision making. Most of the problems surgeons have with public reporting are that the risk adjustment schemes intended to "level the playing field" are considered inadequate to tease out how their patients differ from others. If there is not complete confidence in the risk adjustment strategy, then publication of procedural mortality rates may cause physicians to withhold offering a procedure to high-risk patients. To address this issue, Narins and colleagues[29] assessed the attitudes and experiences of cardiologists by administering an anonymous questionnaire to all physicians who were included in the Percutaneous Coronary Interventions (PCI) in New York State 1998–2000 report.[31] The physicians were sent nine statements/questions regarding the New York report and were asked to rate their level of agreement with each statement/question. Of the 120 physicians (65% response rate) who responded, the vast majority indicated that the PCI in New York State report influences their clinical decision-making process. Eighty-three percent agreed or strongly agreed that "patients who might benefit from angioplasty may not receive the procedure as a result of public reporting of physician specific mortality rates." As well, 79% agreed or strongly agreed that the presence of the scorecard influences whether they decide to treat a critically ill patient with a high expected mortality rate. Further analyses showed that physicians performing coronary angioplasty procedures at a major university teaching hospital were significantly more likely than other physicians to agree that "the publication of mortality statistics factors into their decision on whether to intervene in critically ill patients with high expected mortality rates." The authors concluded that while the scorecards were developed to improve healthcare outcomes, they may instead adversely affect the healthcare decisions for individual patients, particularly those with a high expected mortality rate. In fact, migration of high-risk patients outside of the reporting sphere of influence has been found to occur. Omoigui and coworkers[32] reviewed 9442 isolated coronary artery bypass operations performed at the Cleveland Clinic between 1989 and 1993 to compare mortality rates for patients from New York who underwent CABG at the Cleveland Clinic with those treated in New York. Results indicated that patients from New York had a higher expected mortality and experienced higher morbidity and mortality than other patients operated on at this clinic. However, although physicians may be paying attention to the scorecards, evidence suggests that patients are not. In a survey of nearly 500 patients who had undergone CABG surgery during the previous year, only 20% reported awareness of their state's CABG performance reports, and only 12% knew of this guide prior to undergoing surgery. Furthermore, less than 1% of these patients knew the correct rating for their surgeon or hospital.[30]

4.4.3. Medical–Legal Issues and Clinical Decision Making

Another important social factor that may influence behavior is the medicolegal climate in which surgeons practice. Fear of lawsuits appears to influence behavior in many specialties such as obstetrics and neurosurgery. In many states where insurance rates have soared, these practitioners have often stopped practicing. This has led to surgeon-specialists shortage in many regions. Short of stopping the practice of surgery, it is also likely that surgeons may be influenced by the medicolegal risk associated with certain operations in certain populations. Although the extent of this influence is unclear, in thoracic surgery it would be surprising if this did not influence care to some extent. The effect of medicolegal challenges on decision making in thoracic surgery has not been well explored but may be important given that a significant percentage of cardiothoracic surgeons will face such a challenge in their career.

4.5. Summary

Surgeons may like to believe that evidence drives clinical decision making, but a host of nonclinical factors likely influence the care we direct.

This is a possible explanation for the widespread variability in the use and types of clinical care across different regions and between countries. While the research methodology used to understand these effects is limited, further investigation into these factors may help explain and control variability in clinical care and outcomes. Broad areas of nonclinical influences include surgeon-specific features (attitudes about risk taking, demographics, and training), system-specific factors (incentives, guidelines, and scrutiny of outcomes), and social factors (patient perspectives of nonclinical components of care, public reporting of performance, and medicolegal issues). Surgeons need to better assess and limit these nonclinical components of decision making as we aim to provide rationale, consistent, and appropriate care to our patients.

References

1. Cooper JD, Trulock EP, Triantafillou AN, et al. Bilateral pneumectomy (volume reduction) for chronic obstructive pulmonary disease. *J Thorac Cardiovasc Surg* 1995;109:106–116; discussion, 116–109.
2. Ramsey SD, Sullivan SD. Evidence, economics, and emphysema: Medicare's long journey with lung volume reduction surgery. *Health Aff (Millwood)* 2005;24:55–66.
3. Cooper JD. Paying the piper: the NETT strikes a sour note. National Emphysema Treatment Trial. *Ann Thorac Surg* 2001;72:330–333.
4. Huizenga HF, Ramsey SD, Albert RK. Estimated growth of lung volume reduction surgery among Medicare enrollees: 1994 to 1996. *Chest* 1998;114:1583–1587.
5. Clark JA, Potter DA, McKinlay JB. Bringing social structure back into clinical decision making. *Soc Sci Med* 1991;32:853–866.
6. Tubbs EP, Broeckel Elrod JA, Flum DR. Risk taking and tolerance of uncertainty: implications for surgeons. *J Surg Res* 2006;131:1–6.
7. Nightingale SD. Risk preference and laboratory use. *Med Decis Making* 1987;7:168–172.
8. Nightingale SD. Risk preference and admitting rates of emergency room physicians. *Med Care* 1988;26:84–87.
9. Nightingale SD. Risk preference and decision making in critical care situations. *Chest* 1988;93:684–687.
10. Holtgrave DR, Lawler F, Spann SJ. Physicians' risk attitudes, laboratory usage, and referral decisions:

the case of an academic family practice center. *Med Decis Making* 1991;11:125–130.

11. Zaat JOM. General practitioners' uncertainty, risk preference, and use of laboratory tests. *Med Care* 1992;30:846–854.

12. Nakata Y, Okuno-Fujiwara M, Goto T, Morita S. Risk attitudes of anesthesiologists and surgeons in clinical decision making with expected years of life. *J Clin Anesth* 2000;12:146–150.

13. Hartz RS. "The XX files": demographics of women cardiothoracic surgeons. *Ann Thorac Surg* 2001; 71(suppl 2):S8–S13.

14. Roter DL, Hall JA. Why physician gender matters in shaping the physician-patient relationship. *J Womens Health* 1998;7:1093–1097.

15. Roter D, Lipkin M Jr, Korsgaard A. Sex differences in patients' and physicians' communication during primary care medical visits. *Med Care* 1991;29: 1083–1093.

16. van den Brink-Muinen A, Bensing JM, Kerssens JJ. Gender and communication style in general practice. Differences between women's health care and regular health care. *Med Care* 1998;36:100–106.

17. Lurie N, Margolis KL, McGovern PG, Mink PJ, Slater JS. Why do patients of female physicians have higher rates of breast and cervical cancer screening? *J Gen Intern Med* 1997;12:34–43.

18. Bertakis KD, Helms LJ, Callahan EJ, Azari R, Robbins JA. The influence of gender on physician practice style. *Med Care* 1995;33:407–416.

19. Franks P, Clancy CM. Physician gender bias in clinical decisionmaking: screening for cancer in primary care. *Med Care* 1993;31:213–218.

20. Cowan JA Jr, Dimick JB, Thompson BG, Stanley JC, Upchurch GR Jr. Surgeon volume as an indicator of outcomes after carotid endarterectomy: an effect independent of specialty practice and hospital volume. *J Am Coll Surg* 2002;195:814–821.

21. Dimick JB, Goodney PP, Orringer MB, Birkmeyer JD. Specialty training and mortality after esopha-

geal cancer resection. *Ann Thorac Surg* 2005;80:282–286.

22. Goodney PP, Lucas FL, Stukel TA, Birkmeyer JD. Surgeon specialty and operative mortality with lung resection. *Ann Surg* 2005;241:179–184.

23. Whelan T, Levine M, Willan A, et al. Effect of a decision aid on knowledge and treatment decision making for breast cancer surgery: a randomized trial. *JAMA* 2004;292:435–441.

24. Whelan TJ, Loprinzi C. Physician/patient decision aids for adjuvant therapy. *J Clin Oncol* 2005;23: 1627–1630.

25. Topol EJ, Califf RM. Scorecard cardiovascular medicine. Its impact and future directions. *Ann Intern Med* 1994;120:65–70.

26. Hannan EL, Kilburn H Jr, O'Donnell JF, Lukacik G, Shields EP. Adult open heart surgery in New York State. An analysis of risk factors and hospital mortality rates. *JAMA* 1990;264:2768–2774.

27. Health NYSDo. *Coronary Artery Bypass Surgery in New York State: 1989–1991.* Albany, NY: New York Department of Health; 1992.

28. Epstein A. Performance reports on quality – prototypes, problems, and prospects. *N Engl J Med* 1995;333:57–61.

29. Narins CR, Dozier AM, Ling FS, Zareba W. The influence of public reporting of outcome data on medical decision making by physicians. *Arch Intern Med* 2005;165:83–87.

30. Schneider EC, Epstein AM. Use of public performance reports: a survey of patients undergoing cardiac surgery. *JAMA* 1998;279:1638–1642.

31. Health NYSDo. *Percutaneous Coronary Interventions (PCI) in New York State 1998–2000.* Albany, NY: New York Department of Health; 2003.

32. Omoigui NA, Miller DP, Brown KJ, et al. Outmigration for coronary bypass surgery in an era of public dissemination of clinical outcomes. *Circulation* 1996;93:27–33.

5
How Patients Make Decisions with Their Surgeons: The Role of Counseling and Patient Decision Aids

Annette M. O'Connor, France Légaré, and Dawn Stacey

Recent studies of patient decision making about surgical options that involve making trade-offs between benefits and harms underscore major gaps in decision quality.[1] Following standard counseling, patients' score D on knowledge tests and F on their understanding of the probabilities of benefits and harms. Moreover, there is a mismatch between the benefits and harms that patients' value most and the option that is chosen. Patients participate in decision making less than they prefer; some have high levels of decisional discomfort which is an independent predictor of downstream dissatisfaction, regret, and the tendency to blame their doctor for bad outcomes.[2,3] The underlying mechanisms explaining the poor decision quality with standard counseling is (1) patients' difficulties recalling facts and understanding probabilities and (2) surgeons' difficulties judging the values that patients' place on benefits versus harms. There is a clear need to improve the way patients are prepared to participate in decision making and the way surgeons counsel patients about options.

The goal of evidence-based medicine is to integrate clinical expertise with patient's values using the best available evidence.[4] Some decisions are straightforward because there is strong scientific evidence that the benefits are large and the risks are minimal. Others are more difficult because (1) there is insufficient scientific evidence on the benefits, risks, and side effects; and/or (2) patients differ on how they value the benefits, risks, and scientific uncertainties. These decisions are said to be preference sensitive or values sensitive.[5,6] For example, patients with similar demographic and clinical characteristics who become informed about treatment options might differ on their preferred treatment for diseases such as breast cancer (mastectomy vs. breast conserving therapy), angina (coronary artery bypass vs. medical therapy), thoracoabdominal aneurysm (corrective surgery vs. watchful waiting), benign uterine bleeding (hysterectomy vs. endometrial ablation vs. medical treatment), and herniated disk (discectomy vs. medical treatment).

In the past, when patients faced these difficult decisions, surgeons acted as agents in the best interest of their patients by deciding whether benefits outweighed the harms.[7] Today, surgeons are still considered experts in problem solving: diagnosing, identifying treatment options, and explaining the probabilities of benefits and harms.[8,9] However, patients are increasingly recognized as the best experts for judging the personal value of benefits versus harms.[7,10,11] The principles of passive informed consent are evolving into active informed choice or shared decision making. Shared decision making is defined as a decision-making process jointly shared by patients and their healthcare providers.[12] It aims at helping patients play an active role in decisions concerning their health,[13] to reach the ultimate goal of patient-centered care.[14] Shared decision making rests on the best evidence of the risks and benefits of all the available options.[15] Thus, communication techniques that enable the patient to adequately weigh the risks and benefits associated with the treatment choices are skills essential to shared decision making.[16] Shared decision making takes into account the establishment of a context in which the values and preferences of the patient are sought and his/her opinions valued.

Shared decision making does not completely exclude a consideration of the values and preferences of the physician or other health practitioners involved in the decision.[12,15] It occurs through a partnership in which the responsibilities and rights of each of the parties are explicit and the benefits for each party are made clear. Therefore, with growing patient interest to participate in decision making about options, evidence-based decision aids have been developed to supplement (not replace) surgeons' counseling. These tools prepare patients to discuss options which the clinician has judged as clinically appropriate by helping them to (1) understand the probable benefits, risks, side effects, and scientific uncertainties of options; (2) consider and clarify the value they place on the benefits, risks, and scientific uncertainties; and (3) participate in decision making with their surgeons in ways they prefer. The goal of shared decision making is to reach agreement on the option that best matches the informed patients' values for benefits, risks, and scientific uncertainties.

This chapter discusses practical and effective methods to help patients become involved in decision making. First, we present evidence on how patients currently make decisions. Second, we describe patient decision aids including their underlying conceptual framework, structural elements, and evidence of efficacy. Next, we outline current international standards for developing and evaluating patient decision aids. Finally, we propose strategies for using patient decision aids in clinical practice.

5.1. Current Status of Patient Decision Making

To our knowledge, the decisional needs and decision making behavior of patients facing specific difficult thoracic surgery decisions have not been studied. For other surgical decisions, the best evidence comes from the Cochrane systematic review of randomized trials of patient decision aids[1] when patients were randomized to receive usual counseling. The obvious limitation of the data is that trial participants may not be similar

to nontrial participants. Nevertheless, until data from more representative cohorts are published,[17] data from trials provide some insight into patients' decision-making behavior when facing diverse surgical decisions.

5.1.1. Primary Data Source

The Cochrane systematic review of 34 trials of patient decision aids found 9 trials of patients who were facing major elective surgical treatment options: 2 coronary artery disease, 2 benign prostate hypertrophy, 2 breast cancer, 1 menorrhagia, 1 prostate cancer, and 1 herniated disc or spinal stenosis.[1] We report the behavior of patients following usual counseling from their surgeons with no additional patient decision aids. These data are supplemented with evidence from several nonrandomized, controlled trial studies.

5.1.2. Did Patients Want to Participate in Decisions?

Yes, the majority of patients want to participate in decision making. However, there is a minority of patients who report that surgeons made the decision; rates range from 33% of men for decisions about prostate cancer surgery[18] to 41% for those focused on cardiac revascularization.[19] Although not specifically related to surgery, an international survey confirmed that the majority of patients in United States, Canada, United Kingdom, South Africa, Japan, and Germany want to actively participate in major decisions affecting their health.[20] The percentage preferring a more passive role (e.g., deferring to the physician to make the decision on their behalf) ranged from 10% in South Africa to 3% in Germany. However, at the time of diagnosis and without decision support resources, patients may be less likely to participate in decision making to the level they prefer.

5.1.3. What Was the Quality of the Decisions?

In the groups of patients receiving standard counseling, the quality of their decisions was inadequate using the definition of the 2005 International Patient Decision Aid Standards Collaboration (http://www.ipdas.ohri.ca). Decision quality was defined as (1) informed (knows key facts about options and has realistic perceptions of the probabilities of positive and negative outcomes) and (2) based on patients' values (chooses an option that matches the benefits and risks that the patient values most).[12,21-25]

In the three trials of patient decision aids that evaluated how informed the patients were, those who received usual counseling about surgical options only scored 54% to 62% on knowledge tests.[19,26,27] Although the accuracy of patient perceptions of the chances of benefits and harms were not measured specifically in trials of patient decision aids for surgical decisions, other trials indicated an accuracy ranging from 27% to 66%. None of the surgical decision-making trials measured the agreement between values and choice. However, in three trials focused on hormone replacement therapy, agreement between values and choice was poor in the control counseling arms of the trials.[28-30]

5.1.4. What Was the Quality of the Process of Decision Making?

The quality of the decision-making process is determined using measures of decisional conflict and satisfaction with this process. Two trials of decision aids that measured decisional conflict in patients receiving usual counseling about surgical options indicated that the degree of decisional conflict ranged from 28% to 33%.[19,31] Furthermore, for every one unit increase in decisional conflict, patients were 3 times more likely to fail a knowledge test, 23 times more likely to delay their decision, 59 times more likely to change their mind about the chosen option, 5 times more likely to regret their decision, and 19% more likely to blame their doctors for poor outcomes.[2,3]

Overall, patients were satisfied with the usual counseling they received when considering surgical treatment options; satisfaction scores ranged from 67.2% to 80.0% across trials.[1] These high levels of satisfaction could be due to patients' satisfaction being strongly influenced by the relationship with the practitioner and/or patients may not be aware of the decision support they did not receive.

It is clear that there are serious problems with the current approach to counseling about options.

The majority of patients have unrealistic expectations of benefits and harms and about one third have high levels of decisional discomfort leading to higher regret and tendency to blame others. Complications and poor outcomes are a reality of surgery and patients' expectations need to be realigned with the evidence. This does not mean that patients should not hope for the best, but they do need to be prepared for the worst. From a legal perspective, the biggest predictor of lawsuits is not bad outcomes but a combination of bad outcomes with poor communication. More effective methods are needed to improve surgeon–patient communication and deliberation about treatment options.

5.2. Conceptual Framework and Key Elements Underlying Patient Decision Aids

When there is no clearly indicated "best" therapeutic option, shared decision making is perceived as the optimal process of decision making between practitioners and patients. Shared decision making is the process of interacting with patients who wish to be involved in arriving at an informed, values-based choice among two or more medically reasonable alternatives (which may include watchful waiting). Shared decision-making programs, also known as patient decision aids (PtDAs), are standardized, evidence-based tools intended to facilitate that process. They are designed to *supplement* rather than replace patient–practitioner interaction. Patient decision aids help prepare patients to discuss the options by providing information, values clarification, and structured guidance in the steps of collaborative decision making. The goal of these interventions is to improve the quality of the decision-making process by addressing the suboptimal intermediary modifiable determinants of decision making. This decisional process does not aim at the adoption of a decision determined a priori by the expert. It seeks to ensure that the decision made together with the patient is informed by the best evidence and consistent with the patient's values.

Patient decision aid development has been guided by several different decision theories, risk communication, and transactional frameworks from economics, psychology, and sociology.[1] They have been delivered using diverse print, video, or audio media, but there is a current shift toward internet-based delivery systems. Patient decision aids are self-administered or practitioner administered; they are used in one-to-one or group situations. Most are designed to prepare patients for personalized counseling; however, the timing of their integration into the process of care depends on practitioners' usual counseling practices and feasibility constraints.

5.2.1 Structural Elements of Patient Decision Aids

Regardless of the framework, medium, or implementation strategy, there are three key elements common to their design:

1. *Information and risk communication.* For a given clinical condition, decision aids include high-quality, up-to-date information about the condition or disease stimulating the need for a decision, the available healthcare options, the likely outcomes for each option (e.g., benefits, harms, side effects, and inconveniences), the probabilities associated with these outcomes, and the level of scientific uncertainty. The information is clearly presented as a choice situation, in a balanced manner so as not to persuade the viewer toward any particular option and in sufficient detail to permit choosing among the options.

2. *Values clarification.* Several methods are used to help patients sort out their values (i.e., the personal desirability/undesirability of different features of the available options). First, patients are better able to judge the value of options when they are familiar and easy to imagine. Therefore, PtDAs describe what it is like to experience the physical, emotional, and social consequences of the procedures involved and the potential benefits and harms. Second, balanced examples of how others' values influenced their choices help patients learn how their values matter in decisions. Third, some PtDAs directly engage patients in explicitly revealing their values using rating techniques such as balance scales or trade-off techniques. For example, in balance scales, patients use the familiar 1-to-5 star rating system

to deliberate about the degree of personal importance associated with each of the possible benefits and harms. Visual ratings like this also help family members and the practitioner understand at a glance which benefits and harms are most/least salient to the patient in this particular decision situation.

3. *Structured guidance or coaching in deliberation and communication.* Patient decision aids are designed to improve patients' confidence and skills by guiding them in the steps involved in decision making. This involves helping them become informed, weighing their specific options, and showing them how to communicate values and personal issues to families and practitioners. Personal coaching by nurses or other professionals can also be used to prepare patients to deliberate and communicate with their surgeon.[32] Once patients understand what is at stake in a close-call situation and appreciate the importance of clarifying their personal values, they can meaningfully decide and communicate whether they wish to be actively involved in the healthcare decision.

5.2.2. Evidence of Effectiveness of Patient Decision Aids

The International Cochrane Collaboration Review Group on Decision Aids updated its ongoing systematic review of randomized, controlled trials of treatment and screening PtDAs; there are 34 published trials and another 30+ trials are ongoing.[1] We briefly describe the main results from this 80-page technical document, focusing on decision quality and uptake of the options.

5.2.2.1. Decision Quality

The systematic review indicated that, when PtDAs are used as adjuncts to counseling, they have consistently demonstrated superior effects relative to usual practices on the following indicators of decision quality:

- Increased knowledge scores, by 19 points out of 100 [95% confidence interval (CI), 13–24], which moves patients' tests scores from a barely passing D to a B+.

- Improvements in the proportion of patients with realistic perceptions of the chances of benefits and harms, by 40% (95% CI, 10%-90%), moving patients' scores from a failing grade F to a barely passing D.
- Lowered scores for decisional conflict (psychological uncertainty related to feeling uninformed) by 9 points out of 100 (95% CI, 6–12).
- Reduced proportions of patients who are passive in decision making by 32% (95% CI, 10%–50%).
- Reduced proportions of people who remain undecided after counseling by 57% (95% CI, 30%–70%).
- Improved agreement between a patient's values and the option that is actually chosen. Three of three trials,[6] all focusing on menopause hormone decisions, found that decision aids were better than educational interventions in improving the match between values and choices. A cohort study by Barry and colleagues also showed that men who were especially bothered by their urinary symptoms are seven times more likely to choose surgery for benign prostate disease than those who are not. Men who were especially bothered by the prospect of sexual dysfunction as a complication of surgery are one fifth as likely to choose it compared to as those who are not.[33]

These improvements in decision quality were accomplished without deleterious effects on patient satisfaction or anxiety.[1] Moreover, the amount of time spent by the physician and nurse counseling patients during the initial consultation or second visit 1 week later did not differ between patients who received usual care compared to those who used the PtDA in a more recent study.[34]

5.2.2.2. Rates of Uptake of Different Options

Of the 34 trials in the systematic review, 7 measured rates of different procedures involving major elective surgery (see Table 5.1).[19,26,27,31,32,35,36] Six of these 7 trials demonstrated 21% to 44% reductions in the use of the more invasive surgical option in favor of more conservative surgical or medical options without adverse effects on health outcomes. For example, the rates of mastectomy declined in favor of breast-conserving surgery and the rates of hysterectomy for menorrhagia declined in favor of surgical ablation or medical therapy. The underlying mechanism of this effect is likely in moderating expectations and communicating values. When patients face a major health issue, their first inclination is to "cut it out" or "get rid of" the offending organ. When they begin to appreciate that there are alternatives and that there are potential harms associated with the aggressive procedures, some decide on the simpler procedure. The remainder stay with their original view, but their expecta-

TABLE 5.1. Effect of PtDAs on specific decisions about major elective surgeries.

Decision (source)	PtDA group		Comparison group		Weight (%)	Relative risk (RR; 95% CI)
	N	% choosing option	N	% choosing option		
PtDA versus usual care						
Coronary revascularization[19]	86	52.3%	95	66.3%	37.3	0.79 (0.62–1.01)[a]
Coronary revascularization[27]	61	41.0%	48	58.3%	16.4	0.70 (0.48–1.03)
Hysterectomy[32]	253	32.4%	244	41.4%	41.8	0.78 (0.62–0.99)[a]
Prostatectomy[26]	103	7.7%	116	13.8%	3.9	0.56 (0.25–1.26)
Prostatectomy[31]	54	11.1%	48	2.1%	0.6	5.33 (0.67–42.73)
Pooled RR, 0.77 (0.66–0.90)[a]						
Detailed PtDA with probabilities of outcomes versus simple PtDA						
Breast cancer surgery[35]	30	23.3%	30	40.0%	15.2	0.58 (0.27–1.28)
Back surgery[36]	171	25.7%	173	32.9%	84.8	0.78 (0.56–1.09)
Pooled RR, 0.75 (0.55–1.01)						

[a]$p < 0.05$.

tions are more realistic. They place more value on the peace of mind from removing the organ than the potential complications and side effects. In the case of the hysterectomy study,[32] a video decision aid alone did not have an effect on rates of procedures as much as the combination of the video with nurses' coaching to encourage patients to clarify and communicate to their surgeon (1) the value they placed on keeping their uterus and (2) the role they wished to take in decision making. Therefore, in this arm of the study, surgeon follow-up counseling about options was enhanced with better communication of what informed women valued most and their preferred role in decision making.

Do PtDAs always dampen patients' enthusiasm for surgery? In Table 5.1, the one trial which showed a nonsignificant trend toward increasing the rates of prostate surgery also had the lowest rate of surgery in the control group (2%). This was a U.K. study that had low referral rates by general practitioners due to a shortage of urologists. This observation suggests that PtDAs may promote uptake in surgery when rates are arguably too low. Therefore, PtDAs may address both underuse as well as overuse of options, thereby reflecting the true underlying distribution of informed patients' preferences.[6,37]

5.3. Current Standards for Patient Decision Aids

In 2005, the International Patient Decision Aid Standards (IPDAS) Collaboration undertook a two-stage modified Delphi approach to reach consensus on the important criteria for judging the quality of patient decision aids (http://www.ipdas.ohri.ca). This initiative was driven by the rapid explosion in the development of patient decision aids since 1999, many of which are easily available on the Internet. As well, there was recognition of the difficultly judging the quality of these types of decision support resources when there is no agreed-upon standards to guide their development and evaluation.

The following summarizes the approved IPDAS Standards based on voting by 122 participants from 14 countries. These voters represented four key stakeholder groups: patients/consumers, policy makers, health professionals, and patient decision aid developers/researchers. The broad categories of criteria endorsed were:

I. Patient Decision Aid Specific Criteria
   1.1. Essential decision support elements criteria

The patient decision aid contains the following:
- **Facts** on the health condition, options, benefits, harms, and side effects.
- **Risk communication** to help patients develop realistic expectations of the chances of benefits, harms, and side effects. For example, using event rates with comparable denominators, time periods, and scales; describing uncertainty around estimates; using multiple methods (words, numbers, diagrams); placing probabilities in context; and using mixed positive and negative frames.
- **Values clarification** to help patients clarify and communicate the features of options that matter most to them.
- **Structured guidance** to help patients deliberate and discuss options with others.
- **Balanced display** of information to facilitate comparing positive and negative features across options.

1.2 Effectiveness criteria

There is evidence that patient decision aids lead to:
- A quality decision that is informed and based on patients' values (primary outcome).
- Improved process of decision making as indicated by outcomes such as lower decisional conflict and higher satisfaction (secondary outcomes).

II. Generic Criteria
- **Systematic development process** is used to assess needs of users, field test the decision aid with potential users, and obtain expert review.
- **Up-to-date evidence** using references to scientific studies and with a policy for ongoing update to incorporate new evidence.
- **Disclosure of interests** requires identification of funding sources and conflicts of interest.

- **Plain language** principles are used to ensure patient decision aids can be understood by intended users and includes ways to help patients, other than only reading, understand the information (e.g., in person discussion, audio, video).

These criteria can assist practitioners and patients to judge the quality of patient decision aids.

5.4. Examples of How Patient Decision Aids Are Used

An example of a very simple decision aid is included in Appendix 5.A. It guides patients to prepare for discussing decisions with their practitioners by assessing their individual decision making needs and comparing their options. The steps include (1) verifying the decision: options, rationale, timing, and stage in decision making; (2) clarifying the patient's preferred role in decision making; (3) reviewing the options being considered, including relevant pros and cons for each option. Patients are invited to add additional pros and cons before clarifying their values by rating the importance they attach to each outcome using a 1-to-5 star rating system. The final question asks patients for their overall leaning for or against the option. (4) Assessing current decision making needs and uncertainty using the Decisional Conflict Scale. (5) Planning the next steps.

Patients can be encouraged to share their completed Ottawa Personal Decision Guide with their practitioner as a way to communicate knowledge and values associated with a health-related decision at a glance. Alternatively, the guide can be completed together with the practitioner to structure the process of decision making. A similar guide is being used as part of the process of care in nurse call centers and patient information services located in the United States, Australia, Britain, and Canada. However, referrals to these types of services are intended to compliment and streamline the decision-making process rather than replace discussion with the patient's physician. Most patients have made it clear that individual consultation with their practitioner about options is extremely important.[10,20]

This Decisional Conflict Scale, used within this decision guide (see Appendix 5.A), was developed to determine whether a patient is experiencing uncertainty about the best course of action to identify the modifiable factors contributing to decisional conflict (e.g., feeling uninformed, unclear about values, unsupported in decision making).[23] Decisional conflict is a state of uncertainty about the course of action to take and is frequently characterized by difficulty in making a decision, vacillation between choices, procrastination, being preoccupied with the decision, and having signs and symptoms of distress or tension.

5.5. How Do Clinicians Integrate Decision Aids into Their Practice?

Practitioners are essential for clarifying the decision, identifying patients in decisional conflict or requiring decision support, referring patients to the appropriate resources including decision aids as part of the process of care, and following up on patients' responses in the decision aids to facilitate progress in decision making. Patients prefer face-to-face contact with a practitioner to individualize the information and guide them in decision making.[11] Patient decision aids are designed to enhance this interaction rather than replace it.

To use decision aids in practice, the following steps can be followed by your team:

1. *Clarify the decision* including specific options the patient needs to consider.

   a. *Refer patients to the decision aid.* Endorsement of patient information from one's personal practitioner is highly valued by patients.[11] Direct patients to the website (http://www.ohri.ca/decisionaid) to access a decision aid or provide them with copies. If no decision aids exist for specific health decisions, the Ottawa Personal Decision Guide can be combined with quality patient education resources.

2. *Explain how the decision aid is used in your practice.* Ask the patient to complete the decision aid in preparation for a follow-up discussion.

3. *Refer to the decision aid at follow-up discussion.* It is important that the practitioner acknowledge patients' responses to their decision aid. It can serve as a communication tool to focus the patient–practitioner dialogue. At a glance, you can quickly learn how your patients see the decision. You can

a. assess decisional conflict (uncertainty)
b. clarify their understanding of the benefits and harms
c. acknowledge their values as revealed by the patient's rating of importance on the balance scale
d. answer their questions
e. facilitate decision making according to the patient's preference for decision participation and leaning toward options.

This information helps you judge how quickly you can move from facilitating decision making to implementing the chosen option.

4. *Screen for residual decisional conflict.* Based on what is currently known on the downstream effects of patients presenting with decisional conflict, practitioners would benefit from rescreening for any residual decisional conflict and its sources before arriving at a final decision. After using patient decision aids, most patients have unresolved needs for advice and continued uncertainty, that only gets resolved following counseling with their surgeons.

These steps can be completed by the individual practitioner or shared among team members. When shared within a clinical team, it is better to determine who on the team will be responsible for each part of the process. In the absence of staff to help with this process, referral to nurse call centers or patient information services may be an option to prepare patients for a dialogue. Decision aids can also be used by patients when discussing their options and preferences with important others such as a spouse, family member, or friend.

Surgeons at Dartmouth Hitchcock Medical Center in Lebanon, New Hampshire, have created electronic versions of the Ottawa Personal Decision Guide that patients use after viewing a video decision aid. Using patient data-entry programs and touch-screen tablets, a 1-page summary is created for the surgeon indicating, not only patients' self-reported history and functional status but also their understanding of options, values, and preferred participation role. In this way, surgeons' can appreciate at a glance what the patient knows as a basis for shared deliberation about options.

5.6. Conclusions

Based on systematic review evidence, patients facing difficult decisions, as well as their practitioners, need help beyond standard counseling.[1,38] Decision aids improve the quality of patient decision making, facilitate the integration of patient values into evidence-based medical practice, and enhance the practitioner–patient interaction. The challenge is developing best practices for implementing decision aids as part of the process of care that will lead to better evidence-based decision making that matches patients' values.

References

1. O'Connor AM, Stacey D, Entwistle V, et al. *Decision Aids for People Facing Health Treatment or Screening Decisions* [Cochrane Review]. Oxford: Update Software; 2003.
2. Gattellari M, Ward JE. Men's reactions to disclosed and undisclosed opportunistic PSA screening for prostate cancer. *Med J Aust* 2005;182: 386–389.
3. Sun Q. *Predicting Downstream Effects of High Decisional Conflict: Meta-analysis of the Decisional Conflict Scale* [master's thesis]. Ottawa: University of Ottawa; 2004.
4. Sackett DL, Straus SE, Richardson WS, et al. *Evidence-Based Medicine. How to Practice and Teach EBM.* Edinburgh: Churchill Livingstone; 2000.
5. O'Connor AM, Légaré F, Stacey D. Risk communication in practice: the contribution of decision aids. *BMJ* 2003;327:736–740.
6. Wennberg JE. Unwarranted variations in healthcare delivery: implications for academic medical centres. *BMJ* 2002;325:961–964.
7. Gafni A, Charles C, Whelan T. The physician-patient encounter: the physician as a perfect agent

for the patient versus the informed treatment decision-making model. *Soc Sci Med* 1998;47:347–354.

8. Deber RB. Physicians in health care management: 7. The patient-physician partnership: changing roles and the desire for information. *CMAJ* 1994;151:171–176.

9. Deber RB. Physicians in health care management: 8. The patient-physician partnership: decision making, problem solving and the desire to participate [review]. *CMAJ* 1994;151:423–427.

10. Martin S. 'Shared responsibility' becoming the new medical buzz phrase. *CMAJ* 2002;167:295.

11. O'Connor AM, Drake ER, Wells GA, et al. A survey of the decision-making needs of Canadians faced with complex health decisions. *Health Expect* 2003;6:97–109.

12. Briss P, Rimer B, Reilley B, et al. Promoting informed decisions about cancer screening in communities and healthcare systems. *Am J Prev Med* 2004;26:67–80.

13. Wetzels R, Geest TA, Wensing M, et al. GPs' views on involvement of older patients: an European qualitative study. *Patient Educ Counsel* 2004;53:183–188.

14. Howie JG, Heaney D, Maxwell M. Quality, core values and the general practitioner consultation: Issues of definition, measurement, and delivery. *Family Pract* 2004;21:458–468.

15. Towle A, Godolphin W. Framework for teaching and learning informed shared decision making. *BMJ* 1999;319:766–771.

16. Edwards A, Elwyn G. How should effectiveness of risk communication to aid patients' decisions be judged? A review of the literature. *Med Decis Making* 1999;19:428–434.

17. Moore C, Collins E, Clay K, et al. Can decision support be successfully integrated into clinical care? *Med Decis Making* 2005;24:E48.

18. Davison BJ, Degner L. Empowerment of men newly diagnosed with prostate cancer. *Cancer Nurs* 1997;20:187–196.

19. Morgan MW, Deber RB, Llewellyn-Thomas H, et al. Randomized, controlled trial of an interactive videodisc decision aid for patients with ischemic heart disease. *J Gen Intern Med* 2000;15:685–699.

20. Magee M. Relationship-based Health Care in the United States, United Kingdom, Canada, Germany, South Africa, and Japan. A Comparative Study of Patient and Physician Perceptions Worldwide. World Medical Association Annual meeting: Patient Safety in Care and Research; Helsinki, Finland, Sept II, 2003.

21. Kennedy AD. On what basis should the effectiveness of decision aids be judged? *Health Expect* 2003;6:255–268.

22. IPDAS. *International Patient Decision Aid Standards Collaboration*. Ottawa: IPDAS; 2005.

23. O'Connor AM. Validation of a decisional conflict scale. *Med Decis Making* 1995;15:25–30.

24. Ratliff A, Angell M, Dow R, et al. What is a good decision? *Effect Clin Pract* 1999;2:185–197.

25. Sepucha KR, Fowler FJ, Mulley AG. Policy support for patient-centered care: the need for measurable improvements in decision quality. *Health Affairs* 2004.

26. Barry MJ, Cherkin DC, Chang Y, et al. A randomized trial of a multi-media shared decision-making program for men facing a treatment decision for benign prostatic hyperplasia. *Dis Manage Clin Outcomes* 1997;1:5–14.

27. Bernstein SJ, Skarupski KA, Grayson CE, et al. A randomized controlled trial of information-giving to patients referred for coronary angiography: effects on outcomes of care. *Health Expect* 1998;1:50–61.

28. Dodin S, Légaré F, Daudelin G, et al. Prise de décision en matière d hormonothérapie de remplacement: Essai clinique randomisé. *Can Family Physician* 2001;47:1586–1593.

29. O'Connor AM, Wells G, Tugwell P, et al. The effects of an 'explicit' values clarification exercise in a woman's decision aid regarding postmenopausal hormone therapy. *Health Expect* 1999;2:21–32.

30. Rothert ML, Holmes-Rovner M, Rovner D, et al. An educational intervention as decision support for menopausal women. *Res Nurs Health* 1997;20:387.

31. Murray E, Davis H, Tai SS, et al. Randomized controlled trial of an interactive multimedia decision aid on benign prostatic hypertrophy in primary care. *BMJ* 2001;323:493–496.

32. Kennedy A, Sculpher MJ, Coulter A, et al. Effects of decision aids for menorrhagia on treatment choices, health outcomes, and costs. A randomized controlled trial. *JAMA* 2002;288:2701–2708.

33. Barry MJ. Watchful waiting vs. immediate transurethral resection for symptomatic prostatism: the importance of patients' preferences. *JAMA* 1988;259:3010–3017.

34. Whelan T, Sawka C, Levine M, et al. Helping patients make informed choices: a randomized trial of a decision aid for adjuvant chemotherapy in lymph node negative breast cancer. *J Natl Cancer Inst* 2003;95:581–587.

35. Street RLJ, Voigt B, Geyer CJ, et al. Increasing patient involvement in choosing treatment for early breast cancer. *Cancer* 1995;76:2285.

36. Deyo RA, Cherkin DC, Weinstein J, et al. Involving patients in clinical decisions: Impact of an interactive video program on use of back surgery. *Med Care* 2000;38:959–969.

37. Wennberg JE, Peters PG Jr. Unwarranted variations in the quality of health care: can the law help medicine provide a remedy/remedies? *Sepc Law Dig Health Care Law* 2004;305:9–25.

38. Guimond P, Bunn H, O'Connor AM, et al. Validation of a tool to assess health practitioners' decision support and communication skills. *Patient Educ Counsel* 2003;50:235–245.

Appendix 5.A. Ottawa Personal Decision Guide Adapted for Early Stage Breast Cancer Surgery Decision

Case Situation: *Mrs. Jones is a 60-year-old woman newly diagnosed with stage I breast cancer. Her surgeon has offered her the option of mastectomy or lumpectomy plus radiation therapy. Mrs. Jones' responses to the decision aid are indicated below.*

1. **What decision do you face?**   <u>*Mastectomy versus Lumpectomy plus Radiation*</u>
   Both options have the same chance of survival
   1.1 What is your reason for making the decision?   <u>*Stage 1 Breast Cancer*</u>
   1.2 When does the decision have to be made?   <u>*within a few weeks*</u>
   1.3 How far along are you with this decision? [*Check ✓ the box that applies to you*]
      ❑ not started thinking about the options   ❑ close to choosing one option
      ☑ is considering the options   ❑ already made a choice
2. **What role do you prefer to take in decision making?** [*Check ✓ the box that applies to you*].
   ❑ decide on my own after listening to the opinions of others
   ☑ share the decision with: <u>*my surgeon*</u>
   ❑ someone else to decide for her, namely: _____
3. **Details about how you see the options right now**
   3.1 What I know: List the options and their pros and cons. Underline the pros & cons that are most likely to happen.
   3.2 What's Important to Me: Show how important each pro and con is to you using one (*) star for a little important to five (*****) stars for very important

Reasons to Choose Mastectomy	Personal Importance	Reasons to Choose Lumpectomy plus Radiation	Personal Importance
After 10 years, 92 out of 100 women will be <u>free of cancer</u> in the breast area. Treatment may take less time because several weeks of radiation are not needed Other reasons, please specify:_____	(★ ★ ★ ★ ★) (★)★ ★ ★ ★ ★ ★ ★ ★	After 10 years, 90 out of 100 women will be <u>free of cancer</u> in the breast area. Most of the breast is saved unless the surgeon is not satisfied that all the tumor was removed the first time There is <u>no need for a prosthesis or reconstructive surgery</u> Other reasons, please specify:_____	(★ ★ ★ ★ ★) (★ ★ ★ ★ ★) (★ ★ ★ ★)★ ★ ★ ★ ★ ★

Show which option you think is best for you:

❑ I am leaning toward   ❑ I am unsure   ☑ I am leaning toward
   Mastectomy   **Lumpectomy plus Radiation**

4. What are your current decision making needs? *[Circle your answers to these questions]* Decisional Conflict Scale © A. O'Connor 1993, Revised 2004.

What I Know	Do you know which options you have? Do you know both the good **and** bad points of each option?	(Yes) No (Yes) No
What's important	Are you clear about which good and bad points matter most to you?	(Yes) No
How others help	Do you have enough support and advice to make a choice? Are you choosing without pressure from others?	Yes (No) (Yes) No
How sure I feel	Do you feel sure about what to choose?	Yes (No)

Note: If you have many 'no' answers, talk to your doctor.

5. What steps do you need to take to meet your needs?

   Talk to my surgeon & other women who have been in this position

Part 2
Lung

Part 2
Lung

6
Radiographic Staging of Lung Cancer: Computed Tomography and Positron Emission Tomography

Frank C. Detterbeck

The issue of how to preoperatively stage patients with known or suspected lung cancer is complex, and remains confusing despite a large number of publications on the subject. Part of the confusion arises from the multiplicity of available tests, but more importantly from the fact that the question to be addressed varies in different patient groups. There are different subgroups of patients, particularly with respect to mediastinal staging. The patients considered in one study may not be the same as those in another study, and often arguments are made for a particular approach in some patients using data that is not applicable because it pertains to a different subgroup. Another major obscuring factor is the frequent difference in perspective of authors and practicing clinicians. In general, papers addressing the value of a procedure have retrospectively included all patients who underwent the procedure, and not defined the characteristics of the patients. The clinician, on the other hand, is faced with a patient in whom he can define clinical and radiographic characteristics, but then has trouble using the published literature to find data that specifically applies to this type of patient.

In this chapter, the approach taken is that from the perspective of the clinician, by considering the patient characteristics first, and then using what can be gleaned from the literature to guide us on how to further evaluate the patient. The focus of the chapter is on the role of positron emission tomography (PET) imaging. More specifically, the question is posed whether situations can be defined in which the initial clinical staging is sufficiently reliable (further confirmation by

PET or invasive tests are not needed), or, conversely, when staging by clinical evaluation and imaging studies are clearly not sufficiently reliable.

Clinical staging, as officially defined, includes any and all staging information available before the initiation of treatment (pathological staging is available only after a *resection*). More specifically, clinical staging includes the clinical evaluation (history and physical exam), imaging tests [e.g., computed tomography (CT) and PET], as well as any biopsies (e.g., mediastinoscopy, needle aspiration of nodes, etc.). Thus, clinical staging can be based on physical signs and symptoms, on radiographic studies, or on invasive procedures.

This chapter assumes that patients have had a clinical evaluation and focuses on the reliability of imaging tests, particularly the role of PET imaging. This in turn defines the need for invasive clinical staging tests (e.g., mediastinoscopy, needle aspiration of nodes, etc.), but a full discussion of the advantages and disadvantages of different invasive clinical staging tests is beyond the scope of this chapter.

In this chapter it is assumed that patients with a known or suspected lung cancer have had a chest CT scan. Although the chest CT can itself be viewed as a staging tool, it is done in order to better characterize an abnormality on a chest radiograph (CXR). The chest CT provides a great deal of diagnostic information, and in general, the combination of the patient's risk factors, presentation, and the CT appearance usually allow a presumptive clinical diagnosis to be made with a high degree of accuracy. This chapter will focus on the patients in whom a diagnosis of lung cancer is strongly suspected, and will not pertain to those thought more likely to have another disease process (e.g., sarcoidosis, pneumonia, etc.).

6.1. General Considerations

Positron emission tomography scanning has clearly been shown to be a useful tool in evaluating patients with a wide variety of malignancies. This is to a large extent because PET can distinguish tissues based on differences in cellular metabolism, rather than primarily anatomical size as is true for CT and, to a large extent, also conventional magnetic resonance imaging (MRI). The cost of PET scanning has decreased substantially, although it is still a more expensive test than CT. Furthermore, the availability of PET has become quite commonplace in the United States, although in many instances it involves a mobile PET scanner.

In many communities, it has become quite routine to obtain a PET scan in any patient suspected of having a lung cancer. This is often done by the family practitioner simply because it is thought to be indicated in patients with lung cancer, but without a clear definition of the questions to be addressed by the test, or an understanding of how the results are to be interpreted. This practice is deplored. Although PET is clearly a dramatically useful test in many cases, and although the test itself is safe, it does come at a cost of healthcare dollars, and, most importantly, is associated with a risk of misinterpretation or misapplication that has great potential for harm in some patients.

Defining appropriate indications for PET scanning in patients with suspected lung cancer is often confusing because PET has four different uses. Although any one is sufficient to justify a PET, it is best to have a clear understanding of what question is to be addressed primarily by the scan. The first use of PET is to aid in making a presumptive diagnosis of the primary lesion. This is of little use in patients in whom the probability of lung cancer is very high based on the radiographic appearance and the clinical assessment (risk factors, presentation), because the PET

will likely not rule out lung cancer, and a positive PET result will not obviate the need for tissue for a histological or cytological diagnosis. PET for diagnosis is primarily useful in patients with a nodule that has an intermediate risk of lung cancer, provided it is greater than 1 cm in diameter.[1] The role of PET for diagnosis will not be discussed further in this chapter because of the low utility in patients with a strong suspicion of cancer and because patients with a low or intermediate suspicion of cancer are not the focus of this chapter.

The second use of PET is for the detection of distant metastases in asymptomatic patients or those with more subtle symptoms.[2] The third potential use of PET imaging is for confirmation of the presence or absence of mediastinal involvement.[2] These two uses of PET are central to the subject of this chapter and will be discussed in detail. The fourth use of PET is to guide therapeutic interventions.[3] This includes prognostication, radiotherapy treatment planning, and assessment of response to chemotherapy. Such indications for PET are beyond the scope of this chapter.

A caveat of PET imaging is in the interpretation of the results. There is a widespread tendency to view PET as black and white (positive or negative) with nothing in between. The reality is that PET scans often show areas of indeterminate uptake. There is little doubt that the interpretation of these areas of PET uptake is significantly influenced by the clinical information and judgment, although there is no literature that quantifies it. The PET radiologist that is interpreting the scan with only limited (sometimes incorrect) clinical information passed on by clerical staff is at a disadvantage. This is particularly true for mobile PET scans, where there is little opportunity for the cancer clinician to discuss the PET findings with the radiologist in order to combine the clinical with the radiographic judgment to arrive at a correct interpretation. Furthermore, the quality of the PET images is also variable. There is clear data that shows that interpretation of PET without a CT scan is inferior, and furthermore that a dedicated PET/CT results in improved accuracy. Therefore, as PET scans are more widely available, the expertise of those reading the scans, the ability to correlate this with CT findings and clinical judgment, and the quality of the scans themselves have become much more variable. The applicability of the published data may not apply to many settings because this data almost invariably involves dedicated PET experts interpreting scans in an optimal setting.

6.2. Clinical Stage IV

The first step in evaluating a patient who is strongly suspected to have a non-small cell lung cancer (NSCLC) is always to talk with the patient. This is an important part of making a clinical diagnosis of lung cancer (based on risk factors for lung cancer and local symptoms such as cough or hemoptysis). A crucial factor in staging the patient is to assess whether there are any signs or symptoms of distant metastases. This includes both constitutional symptoms (fatigue, anorexia, weight loss) as well as organ-specific symptoms, particularly with regards to bone and brain metastases (pain, headache, etc.). It is clear that the physician must listen carefully and pay attention to even subtle symptoms.[4]

Some patients will have quite obvious signs of distant metastases (severe localized bone pain, focal neurological findings, palpable metastases). In this case, a PET scan is rarely justified. In general, the presence of distant metastases can be confirmed by a directed test that is much less expensive and can usually be done that same day. Examples are a brain MRI or CT in the patient with focal neurological findings, a plain film of a site of significant bone pain, or a needle aspiration of palpable supraclavicular nodes or subcutaneous metastasis. Similarly, if the patient has a significant pleural effusion, thoracentesis and cytology is the next appropriate step because palliative chemotherapy is the treatment for patients with a malignant pleural effusion regardless of whether other metastases are demonstrated as well. If the directed test shows typical findings (osteolytic bone lesions, brain metastases) in a patient with marked typical symptoms, the diagnosis of stage IV disease can be made with confidence without more extensive testing.[5]

Patients with more subtle symptoms of possible distant metastases should clearly undergo confirmatory imaging.[5] Although the sensitivity of a carefully done clinical evaluation for distant metastases is high, additional confirmation is needed because of a false-positive rate of approximately 70%.[5] Positron emission tomography is ideal because it is more likely to find distant metastases than other imaging studies.[6,7] (A brain MRI or CT should also be done because of PET limitations in detecting brain metastases.) Several studies have shown that in a direct comparison, PET scanning is more sensitive and specific than bone scanning.[8,9] Hence, PET imaging should be preferred, and there is no justification for obtaining a bone scan if a PET has already been done.

A small but significant subgroup of patients presents without signs and symptoms of distant metastases, but with a solitary suspicious lesion noted on the chest CT scan. This is usually either an enlarged adrenal gland or a second pulmonary lesion in another lobe. It must be borne in mind that benign lesions are frequent (adrenal adenomas occur in 3%–4%, hepatic cysts or adenomas in 2% of normal patients,[5] and pulmonary nodules in 16% of patients with lung cancer, of which the vast majority are benign.[10,11]) Furthermore, patients with a satellite focus of cancer in the same lobe have an good prognosis, and should undergo evaluation and treatment without further investigation of the satellite nodule.[12] Thus, in many cases further testing is not necessary if the lesion is typical of a normal benign finding. In those patients in whom a significant suspicion of a metastasis exists, a PET scan is generally very useful in sorting out how to approach these patients. Besides demonstration of the presence or absence of uptake in the suspicious lesion, PET is useful because most patients with a metastasis will have additional lesions noted on PET (including in mediastinal nodes). Alternatively, if the suspicion is high enough, a biopsy of the lesion may be warranted instead of PET imaging, which cannot deliver a histological specimen.

Patients who have a solitary site of distant metastasis by PET scan should undergo biopsy confirmation of metastatic disease.[13,14] This is because a substantial number (10%–50%) of these presumed solitary metastases are in fact benign lesions.[15–17] Finally, it must be remembered that occasionally patients with a solitary distant metastasis and no nodal involvement should be considered for a curative approach with resection of the primary and the metastasis.[12]

6.3. Clinical Stage III

The patients addressed in this section have enlarged mediastinal nodes on a chest CT scan, but are asymptomatic with regards to either constitutional or organ-specific symptoms (i.e., the definition of clinical stage III). The questions to be addressed are how reliable the negative clinical evaluation is with regards to distant metastases, and how reliable the CT appearance of mediastinal node involvement is. It should be noted that the CT criteria for a suspiciously enlarged mediastinal node is a node that is greater than 1 cm in the short axis dimension on a transverse CT image.

There is consistent data from multiple sources indicating that asymptomatic clinical stage III patients should undergo further testing to identify possible distant metastases.[2] The false-negative rate of the clinical evaluation in these patients is about 15% to 30%.[5] Several studies have confirmed that PET will detect distant metastases in 25% to 30% of stage cIII patients.[7,18,19] It has already been mentioned that PET is more sensitive than bone scan to detect bone metastases; furthermore only a minority of the distant metastases found involve the bone.[18] Hence, a very strong argument can be made for obtaining a PET scan to look for distant metastases in stage III patients (without a pleural effusion).

The role of either PET or invasive biopsy of mediastinal nodes is more confusing. This is in part because there are different groups of patients with potential mediastinal involvement and the reported data has not always described which groups were included in the analysis. The following paragraphs attempt to arrive at recommendations for each group because of the applicability to clinical care, realizing though that the data is often imperfect. It is assumed in the next paragraphs in this section that patients do undergo a PET scan (and brain MRI/CT) for the detection of distant metastases; furthermore it is assumed that no distant metastases were found.

Patients with known or suspected lung cancer without symptoms of distant metastases can be divided into four general groups on the basis of the chest CT characteristics (Figure 6.1). Group A has very extensive mediastinal infiltration, to the point where discrete lymph nodes can no longer be discerned or measured, or where mediastinal structures (i.e., vessels, trachea, etc.) are encircled (infiltrative stage cIIIa,b). Group B involves patients with discrete enlarged mediastinal lymph nodes by CT scan (nodal stage cIIIa or cIIIb). Groups C and D do not have radiographic mediastinal node involvement (by CT), and will therefore be discussed in the sections on clinical stage I and II.

In patients with stage cIII NSCLC with extensive mediastinal infiltration (Group A, infiltrative stage cIIIa,b), clinical experience suggests that this appearance on CT is quite reliable for malignant involvement.[20] However, there is no data substantiating this because biopsies to confirm malignancy have not been felt to be necessary. In these situations, PET scanning invariably demonstrates significant uptake. Because the CT appearance alone is accepted as reliable without further biopsy, there is no reason to pursue a biopsy to confirm PET uptake in the mediastinum either. (A biopsy may be necessary simply to confirm the diagnosis and define the cell type, but that is a different issue than obtaining a biopsy because the mediastinal staging is in question.)

Patients with enlargement of discrete mediastinal nodes represent another group (group B, nodal stage cIIIa or cIIIb). In these patients it is well documented that reliance on the CT appearance alone is notoriously inaccurate because approximately 40% of patients do not have mediastinal involvement.[21] Again, such patients should undergo PET imaging to detect distant metastases. However, the value of PET to define the status of the mediastinal nodes is debatable because the data suggests that either a positive or a negative PET result in the mediastinum should be confirmed by a tissue biopsy.[2]

It is generally agreed that positive PET uptake in the mediastinum should be confirmed by biopsy[20] because of a false-positive rate of 13% to 23%.[21-24] Most clinicians would be uncomfortable relying on a negative PET scan in the face of

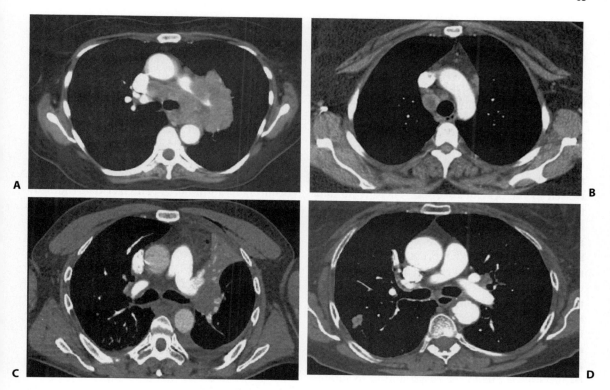

Figure 6.1. Different categories of patients with regards to mediastinal staging by CT. (A) Group A, infiltrative stage cIIIa,b. Patients with mediastinal infiltration of tumor, making individual lymph nodes impossible to distinguish. (B) Group B, nodal stage cIIIa or cIIIb. Patients with enlargement of discrete mediastinal nodes. (C) Group C, stage cII or central stage cI. Patients with a central tumor or evidence of N1 nodal enlargement, but with a normal mediastinal CT. (D) Group D, peripheral stage I. Patients with a peripheral clinical stage I tumor and a normal mediastinal CT.

clearly enlarged mediastinal nodes, although data that pertains to this is limited. One study suggested the false-negative rate of PET in patients with enlarged mediastinal nodes was 8%,[22] but a meta-analysis suggests that the probability of N2,3 involvement after a negative PET scan is approximately 30%, given a pretest probability of 60% (for enlarged nodes by CT).[24] Thus, in patients with enlarged mediastinal nodes tissue confirmation should generally be obtained, regardless of the PET results. This can be accomplished either by a traditional mediastinoscopy or by needle aspiration [using esophageal ultrasound, endobronchial ultrasound, or simple landmark-guided transbronchial aspiration (TBNA)].[20] Each of these procedures has reasonably good sensitivity (with the lowest being for blind TBNA), but the false-negative rate of the needle aspiration techniques is 20% to 30%.[20]

6.4. Clinical Stage II

The role of PET imaging for distant staging in patients with a clinical stage II NSCLC is unclear. Only one study has specifically reported on such patients (involving only 18 cII patients), and found that PET detected distant metastases in 18% of patients.[18] Thus, PET can be justified in these patients. Another approach is to argue that the data relating to CT scans in patients with cII NSCLC indicates that approximately 20% have mediastinal node involvement despite normal-sized nodes on CT.[21] This approach argues that mediastinoscopy should be done first; if it is positive then a PET would be indicated to look for distant metastases, whereas if it is negative, then the PET could be omitted. However, it must be acknowledged that there is very little data to define an evidence-based approach.

Similarly, the role of PET in staging of the mediastinum in patients with cII NSCLC is unclear. There is ample evidence of a 20% to 25% chance of N2,3 nodal involvement despite normal-sized mediastinal nodes in these patients.[21] This is true both for patients with enlarged N1 nodes as well as in patients with central tumors. These patients are classified as Group C in Figure 6.1 (stage cII or central stage cI). In this group, PET uptake in a mediastinal node should be confirmed, based on the 20% false-positive rate discussed in the previous section. There is no data that directly defines the false-negative rate of PET in the mediastinum in these patients, although a false-negative rate of greater than 5% for PET can be estimated when the pretest probability of malignant involvement is 20% to 25%.[24]

In the absence of direct data for PET, one rational approach is to pursue invasive biopsy of the mediastinum in cII patients, given what is known from studies involving only CT imaging. In this example, the procedure of choice would be mediastinoscopy rather that a needle aspiration technique. This is due to the easier ability to sample multiple mediastinal nodes in the most prominent nodal areas, and due to the higher false-negative rate (20%–30%) for needle aspiration techniques, especially in normal-sized nodes.[23] Another rational approach is to perform PET imaging in cII patients and omit mediastinoscopy if the PET is negative in the mediastinum (and for distant metastases). The advantage of the approach involving mediastinoscopy is that it is based on data that is directly derived from this group of patients, and also yields a tissue biopsy for diagnosis should there be mediastinal involvement.

6.5. Clinical Stage I

There is little role for PET in asymptomatic patients with a peripheral clinical stage I tumor. If the clinical evaluation is negative, traditional staging tests (bone scan, brain CT, upper abdominal CT) detect distant metastases in less than 5% of patients.[5] Positron emission tomography imaging also detects distant metastases in less than 5% of patients, as demonstrated by multiple studies (although some included a proportion of cII patients or did not document a negative clinical evaluation).[7,16,18,25,26] In fact, the chance of a false-positive PET finding is higher than the chance of identifying an actual metastasis, which underscores a danger of obtaining a PET scan in these patients.[16] Thus, there is little justification for PET to detect distant metastases in patients with clinical stage I tumors.

Similarly, the data does not strongly support the value of PET scanning to evaluate the mediastinum in patients with peripheral cI tumors (Group D in Figure 6.1).[2] The fact that thoracotomy and node dissection discloses less than 10% with positive mediastinal nodes argues against the use of PET for mediastinal staging in these patients.[21] Less than 5% of 84 stage cI patients who underwent PET were found to have N2,3 node involvement in one study.[26] Moreover, 60% of the positive PET results in the mediastinum turned out to be false positives,[26] underscoring the drawbacks of pursuing such imaging if the incidence of disease is low.

6.6. Summary

Table 6.1 is a general guideline regarding the need for PET imaging in patients with lung cancer. This algorithm assumes the patient has had a careful history and physical exam by a physician experienced in dealing with lung cancer patients, and assumes the patient has had a chest CT scan. This schema represents a rational approach based on the available evidence. It is recognized that no approach is 100% accurate. There must be a balance between the risk of subjecting a patient to futile resection (by missing unsuspected metastases) versus denying the patient a curative approach (because of presumed metastases that are not truly present). Furthermore, the process of staging requires judgment about the incremental benefit versus the risks of further testing (morbidity and potential detriment by misleading results).

The text of this chapter provides a numerical assessment of the reliability of particular assessments (false-positive and false-negative rates), so that the clinician can weigh the pros and cons of adding another layer of testing in a particular patient. This weighing of pros and cons is the

TABLE 6.1. Overview of recommended staging tests in patients with NSCLC.

Clinical scenario	Next step	Justification
cIV		
Strong clinical symptoms	Directed radiographic study or biopsy	Expediency
Subtle clinical symptoms	PET, brain MRI/CT	70% FP rate of clinical evaluation
Specific radiographic issue (e.g., pulmonary nodule, adrenal)	PET, brain MRI/CT (vs. biopsy)	Settle specific issue, rule in/out additional mets
cIII (asymptomatic)		
Mediastinal infiltration	PET, brain MRI/CT	30% chance of distant metastases
Discrete nodal enlargement	PET, brain MRI/CT	25%–30% chance of distant metastases
EUS-NA, TBNA (vs. Med) if no distant mets		20% FP, ~20% FN rate of PET in mediastinum
cII (asymptomatic, normal mediastinum on CT)		
Central tumor or cN1 on CT	Mediastinoscopy	20% FN rate of CT in mediastinum, 30% FN rate of TBNA, EUS-NA; unclear value of PET for distant mets or mediastinal assessment
	PET, brain MRI/CT if Med +	20%–30% chance of distant metastases
	Resection if Med −	<5% chance of distant metastases
cI (asymptomatic, normal mediastinum on CT)		
cI (peripheral lesion)	Resection	<5% chance of distant mets, <10% chance of N2,3 mets

Abbreviations: CT, computed tomography; EUS-NA, esophageal ultrasound and needle aspiration; FN, false negative; FP, false positive; Med, mediastinoscopy; mets, metastases; MRI, magnetic resonance imaging; NSCLC, non-small cell lung cancer; PET, positron emission tomography; TBNA, transbronchial needle aspiration.

process of clinical judgment and represents the art of medicine. Table 6.1 does not allow all these nuances to be represented, and inherently involves judgments about what degree of accuracy is acceptable. In general terms, a less than 5% chance of changing the stage is considered acceptable in avoiding another imaging test, and a less than 10% chance acceptable for avoiding an invasive test.

In patients with very obvious signs of metastatic disease, there is little role for PET imaging, and a directed radiographic study or biopsy is usually more expedient and sufficient. Patients with subtle signs of possible distant metastases need to be investigated more carefully, and PET represents an ideal test in this situation (as well as a brain MRI; level of evidence 1+; recommendation grade B). Furthermore, PET imaging is frequently useful in patients in whom a possible metastasis has been detected by the chest CT. In any of these scenarios, if PET imaging shows multiple areas of uptake that are typical for metastases, this is sufficient; however, a solitary site of possible metastasis by PET or an atypical radiographic appearance or clinical presentation requires a biopsy of the site in question (level of evidence 2+; recommendation grade D).

In patients with obvious metastatic disease, there is little role for PET imaging; patients with subtle signs of possible distant metastases need to be investigated more carefully, and PET represents and ideal test in this situation (level of evidence 1+; recommendation grade B).

A solitary site of possible metastasis by PET requires a biopsy of the site in question (level of evidence 2+; recommendation grade D).

Asymptomatic patient with radiographic stage cIII tumors (by CT) should undergo a PET and brain MRI/CT because there is a 25% to 30% chance of finding distant metastases (level of evidence 2+; recommendation grade C). Patients with discrete nodal enlargement on CT should undergo tissue confirmation of these nodes regardless of the PET findings (level of evidence 2++; recommendation grade B).

Patients with stage cIII tumors (by CT) should undergo a PET (level of evidence 2+; recommendation grade C).

Patients with discrete nodal enlargement on CT should undergo tissue confirmation of these nodes regardless of the PET findings (level of evidence 2++; recommendation grade B).

Two different approaches to patients with central tumors or stage II lung cancer can be justified, in part because the data for this stage is limited. One strategy involves an initial mediastinoscopy, and a PET scan is obtained only if it is positive (level of evidence 3; recommendation grade D). This is based on a high incidence of positive N2,3 involvement in normal-sized nodes, which may well not show up on PET (the data regarding the false-negative rate of PET in this situation is unclear). An alternative would be to do a PET scan first, and perform mediastinoscopy only if it is positive in the mediastinum (level of evidence 3; recommendation grade D).

Neither a PET scan nor mediastinoscopy is recommended for patients with peripheral stage I tumors (level of evidence 2+; recommendation grade C).

Patients with central tumors or stage II lung cancer can undergo (1) an initial mediastinoscopy with a PET scan obtained only if it is positive; or (2) a PET scan first with mediastinoscopy only if the PET is positive in the mediastinum (level of evidence 3; recommendation grade D).

Neither a PET scan nor mediastinoscopy is recommended for patients with peripheral stage I tumors (level of evidence 2+; recommendation grade C).

These recommendations are as evidence-based as possible. However, little data exists for some clinical scenarios. Perhaps future studies will address this so that PET imaging as well as invasive testing can be used in a rational, logical manner, avoiding overuse and misinterpretation of results.

Acknowlegments. This work was performed at the Yale University.

References

1. Detterbeck F, Falen S, Rivera M, Halle J, Socinski M. Seeking a home for a PET, part 1: defining the appropriate place for Positron Emission Tomography imaging in the diagnosis of pulmonary nodules or masses. *Chest* 2004;125:2294–2299.
2. Detterbeck F, Falen S, Rivera M, Halle J, Socinski M. Seeking a home for a PET, part 2: defining the appropriate place for Positron Emission Tomography imaging in the staging of patients with suspected lung cancer. *Chest* 2004;125:2300–2308.
3. Detterbeck FC, Vansteenkiste JF, Morris DE, Dooms CA, Khandani AH, Socinski MA. Seeking a home for a PET, part 3: emerging applications of positron emission tomography imaging in the management of patients with lung cancer. *Chest* 2004;126:1656–1666.
4. Guyatt GH, Cook DJ, Griffith LE, et al. Surgeons' assessment of symptoms suggesting extrathoracic metastases in patients with lung cancer. *Ann Thorac Surg* 1999;68:309–315.
5. Detterbeck FC, Jones DR, Molina PL. Extrathoracic staging. In: Detterbeck FC, Rivera MP, Socinski MA, Rosenman JG, eds. *Diagnosis and Treatment of Lung Cancer: An Evidence-Based Guide for the Practicing Clinician.* Philadelphia: Saunders; 2001:94–110.
6. Marom EM, McAdams HP, Erasmus JJ, et al. Staging non-small cell lung cancer with whole-body PET. *Radiology* 1999;212:803–809.
7. Weder W, Schmid RA, Bruchhaus H, Hillinger S, von Schulthess GK, Steinert HC. Detection of extrathoracic metastases by positron emission tomography in lung cancer. *Ann Thorac Surg* 1998;66:886–893.
8. Bury T, Barreto A, Daenen F, Barthelemy N, Ghaye B, Rigo P. Fluorine-18 deoxyglucose positron emission tomography for the detection of bone metastases in patients with non-small cell lung cancer. *Eur J Nucl Med* 1998;25:1244–1247.
9. Cheran SK, Herndon JE 2nd, Patz EF Jr. Comparison of whole-body FDG-PET to bone scan for detection of bone metastases in patients with a new diagnosis of lung cancer. *Lung Cancer* 2004;44:317–325.
10. Keogan MT, Tung KT, Kaplan DK, Goldstraw PJ, Hansell DM. The significance of pulmonary nodules detected on CT staging for lung cancer. *Clin Radiol* 1993;48:94–96.
11. Kunitoh H, Eguchi K, Yamada K, et al. Intrapulmonary sublesions detected before surgery in patients with lung cancer. *Cancer* 1992;70:1876–1879.
12. Detterbeck FC, Jones DR, Kernstine KH, Naunheim KS. Special treatment issues. *Chest* 2003;123:244S–258S.
13. Rivera MP, Detterbeck F, Mehta AC. Diagnosis of lung cancer: the guidelines. *Chest* 2003;123:129S–136S.

14. Silvestri GA, Tanoue LT, Margolis ML, Barker J, Detterbeck F. The noninvasive staging of non-small cell lung cancer. *Chest* 2003;123:147S–156S.
15. Patchell RA, Tibbs PA, Walsh JW, et al. A randomized trial of surgery in the treatment of single metastases to the brain. *N Engl J Med* 1990;322:494–500.
16. Reed C, Harpole D, Posther K, et al. Results of the American College of Surgeons Oncology Group Z0050 Trial: the utility of positron emission tomography in staging potentially operable non-small cell lung cancer. *J Thorac Cardiovasc Surg* 2003;126:1943–1951.
17. Lardinois D, Weder W, Roudas M, et al. Etiology of solitary extrapulmonary positron emission tomography and computed tomography findings in patients with lung cancer. *J Clin Oncol* 2005;23:6846–6453.
18. MacManus MP, Hicks RJ, Matthews JP, et al. High rate of detection of unsuspected distant metastases by PET in apparent stage III non-small-cell lung cancer: Implications for radical radiation therapy. *Int J Radiat Oncol Biol Phys* 2001;50:287–293.
19. Eschmann SM, Friedel G, Paulsen F, et al. FDG PET for staging of advanced non-small cell lung cancer prior to neoadjuvant radio-chemotherapy. *Eur J Nucl Med Mol Imaging* 2002;29:804–808.
20. Detterbeck FC, DeCamp MM Jr, Kohman LJ, Silvestri GA. Invasive staging: the guidelines. *Chest* 2003;123:167S–175S.
21. Detterbeck FC, Jones DR, Parker LA Jr. Intrathoracic staging. In: Detterbeck FC, Rivera MP, Socinski MA, Rosenman JG, eds. *Diagnosis and Treatment of Lung Cancer: An Evidence-Based Guide for the Practicing Clinician.* Philadelphia: Saunders; 2001:73–93.
22. Dietlein M, Weber K, Gandjour A, et al. Cost-effectiveness of FDG-PET for the management of potentially operable non-small cell lung cancer; priority for a PET-based strategy after nodal-negative CT results. *Eur J Nucl Med* 2000;27:1598–1609.
23. Toloza EM, Harpole L, Detterbeck F, McCrory D. Invasive staging of non-small cell lung cancer: a review of the current evidence. *Chest* 2003;123:157S–166S.
24. Gould MK, Kuschner WG, Rydzak CE, et al. Test performance of positron emission tomography and computed tomography for mediastinal staging in patients with non-small-cell lung cancer: a meta-analysis. *Ann Intern Med* 2003;139:879–892.
25. Viney RC, Boyer MJ, King MT, et al. Randomized controlled trial of the role of positron emission tomography in the management of stage I and II non-small-cell lung cancer. *J Clin Oncol* 2004;22:2357–2362.
26. Farrell MA, McAdams HP, Herndon JE, Patz EFJ. Non-small cell lung cancer: FDG PET for nodal staging in patients with stage I disease. *Radiology* 2000;215:886–890.

7
Routine Mediastinoscopy for Clinical Stage I Lung Cancer

Karl Fabian L. Uy and Thomas K. Waddell

Cervical mediastinoscopy is a widely used procedure in the invasive staging of non-small cell lung cancer (NSCLC). It is a safe invasive diagnostic procedure that has been shown to have a morbidity rate of 1.7%, a mortality rate of 0.07%, and an emergency thoracotomy rate of 0.12%.[1-5] Most commonly, it is done after noninvasive staging modalities have demonstrated no advanced disease, and is the final step in the determination of the benefit of surgical resection. Mediastinoscopy policies differ among countries, institutions, and surgeons, but generally it is done either selectively or routinely. There is a strong consensus for performing this in patients with enlarged mediastinal lymph nodes, but there is less than widespread acceptance for performing it in the setting of normal-sized nodes. Certainly, the prevalence of N2 or N3 disease is lower when both hilar and mediastinal lymph nodes are not enlarged on anatomical studies like chest computed tomography (CT), and/or have no increased uptake on a metabolic imaging modality like positron emission tomography (PET). Yet, how low should this prevalence be before mediastinoscopy no longer provides benefit? This chapter discusses the issue of whether routine cervical mediastinoscopy is of benefit when noninvasive studies have demonstrated clinical stage I disease. Because our recommendations in large part depend on the performance characteristics of chest CT scan and PET scan, data pertaining to their use in this patient population is included; however, we do not address the issue of whether PET should be included in the staging workup. Also, because PET is not part of the routine preoperative staging in many countries, we will discuss this topic with and without the availability of PET as clinical scenarios.

7.1. Limitations

The available literature on this specific topic is limited. Although there is a modest collection of data on mediastinoscopy in general, few focus narrowly on this topic. The majority of reporting series contain the clinical stage I subgroup of patients, but this data is not reported separately and is not extractable. In addition to heterogeneous populations, reports over the last two decades contain nonconsecutive patients and inconsistent screening criteria. The confusion is furthered by the varying qualities of the imaging equipment used for clinical staging. Because the present evidence has considerable faults and limitations, formulating a straightforward answer to this specific question is impossible. There is a greater volume of literature on chest CT and PET scanning, which has been summarized in a well-done meta-analysis,[6] and to which we refer to rather than quoting each study separately.

7.2. Definition of Benefit

When a procedure or test is said to be "of benefit," what is meant exactly, and how does this definition affect the conclusions drawn? There are a few possible measures of benefit from a strategy of routine mediastinoscopy. Survival, whether measured absolutely or by quality-adjusted life-years (QALYs) is the most obvious. These can be used to factor cost effectiveness or cost utility, while costs are very sensitive to local system issues and difficult to widely translate. Another possible measure of benefit that has been used in some studies is the rate of avoidance of "unnecessary" thoracotomy.[7] For example, some investigators might define this as situations where N2 disease is discovered at thoracotomy in a cN0 patient, in which case an outright lung resection is deemed of no survival advantage compared to no resection. We would contend that this definition and concept is at present being challenged by new evidence, such as large phase III trials of adjuvant chemotherapy.[8,9]

The decision to perform routine mediastinoscopy for clinical stage I lung cancer depends in large part on the treating physician's opinion of how N2 disease is best treated. Specifically, what is the best treatment for clinical T1-2 N0 non-small cell lung cancer that turns out to be pathologic N2? The options include routine surgical resection followed by adjuvant chemotherapy, neoadjuvant chemotherapy with or without radiation followed by surgery, or chemoradiation without surgery. Although mediastinoscopy does detect N3 disease and could contribute significantly by excluding stage IIIB patients from surgery, the incidence of mediastinoscopy-detected N3 disease in the clinical stage I group is sufficiently low – 0% to 1%[10–12] – that it will not impact on our recommendations.

The best treatment for this very specific subset of patients is unknown. For those who feel that N2 disease is best treated without surgery at all, routine mediastinoscopy would clearly have some advantages. However, there is very little specific literature available on this subset of patients who are treated with chemoradiation alone. Thus, it is difficult to work out the cost savings per patient with this approach. Our view is that surgery is appropriate in many patients and has the potential to offer some improvement in survival. For example, we may make some inferences based on how overall N2 disease is best treated, and answers to this question are now emerging. The North American Intergroup 0139 trial is a multicenter randomized, controlled trial that explored the utility of preoperative chemo-radiation followed by surgery versus chemoradiation alone for T1-3 N2 non-small cell lung cancer. A statistically significant 50% increase in median survival was found for those patients whose tumors were amenable to a lobectomy.[13] However, patients who required pneumonectomy had a high operative mortality, and, in this group, the addition of surgery had no advantage to chemo-radiation alone in terms of overall survival. The patient population in this trial consisted of all categories of N2, but the subset of lobectomy patients probably represents a group with a lower tumor burden and therefore more similar to our patients of interest.

A cost-effectiveness analysis has been done, addressing the question of whether thoracotomy-discovered N2 disease is best managed by outright resection or by aborting the lung resection, administering neoadjuvant chemotherapy, and subsequently re-operating and performing the lung resection should there be no progression.[14] The pertinence of this analysis is that the patient population is predominantly cN0-1 who were subsequently found out to be pN2, which is precisely the subset which routine mediastinoscopy hopes to pick up. Does picking up N2 preoperatively in this subset provide any advantage over outright resection and just giving chemotherapy postoperatively? The answer from this analysis is yes, in terms of better median survival, QALY, and cost-effectiveness (incremental cost-effectiveness ratio of $17,119 per QALY), even with a reoperation. In this context, then, routine mediastinoscopy would be beneficial in reducing the number of patients subjected to exploratory thoracotomy and ensures that the maximum number of patients will undergo the preferred treatment – neoadjuvant chemotherapy. The drawback of this 2003 analysis, though, is that it used survival estimates from the 1990s for the adjuvant chemotherapy group. We now have mature results of two large phase III trials[8,9] that demonstrate a larger survival benefit for adjuvant cisplatin-based chemotherapy for stage IIIA; however, these studies combined T3N0 with cN2, and many of the patients did not have mediastinoscopy before treatment, so the clinical staging was not rigorously done. A direct comparison between pre- and postoperative chemotherapy administration will only be available when a phase III

TABLE 7.1. Prevalence (false-negative rate) of N2 disease in clinical stage I non-small cell lung cancer.

Staging examinations	Reference	N	Prevalence after negative examinations	Level of evidence
After CT	CLOG[7]	183	23%	1b
	De Leyn[20]	235	20%	4
	Suzuki[22]	342	17%	4
	Pieterman[21]	54	18.5%	1b
	Gould[6]	1119	20%	2a
	Choi[12]	291	15.5%	4
	Average		19.2%	
After CT + mediastinoscopy	De Leyn[20]	235	10.6%	4
	Choi[12]	291	9.2%	4
	Kim[23]	343	6%	4
	Average		8.3%	
After CT + PET	Gould[6]	479	6%	2a
	Viney[10]	42	4.8%	1b
	Meyers[11]	248	5.6%	2b
	Gonzalez-Stawinski[18]	137	11.7%	4
	Average		6.7%	
After CT + PET + mediastinoscopy	Meyers[11]	178	4.5%	2b

trial comparing these two administration regimens matures in a few years (the NATCH trial – neoadjuvant taxol-carboplatin HOPE trial).

Our choice as to whether pre- or postoperative administration is better is central to our decision for choosing or rejecting a routine mediastinoscopy strategy. The survival advantages mentioned above are difficult to compare at present – however, it is a well-established fact that patients are far more compliant with preoperative (90% completion) rather than postoperative (25%–65% completion) chemotherapy,[13,15–17] which alone would sway the balance towards preoperative administration. Our own experience with a standardized regimen of induction chemoradiation followed by surgery for cN2 over the last 7 years resulted in a median survival of 40 months, which we consider very favorable compared to our previous experiences with adjuvant chemotherapy. This experience, along with a higher completion rate with preoperative chemotherapy, has firmly entrenched our belief that neoadjuvant is better than adjuvant administration for N2 disease.

If it is accepted that induction treatment is a beneficial management strategy for N2 disease, then it would be useful to discuss routine mediastinoscopy. The next issue then is the prevalence of N2 disease in CT with or without PET-determined N0 and the performance characteristics of mediastinoscopy. The prevalence of N2 disease after successive steps in the preoperative workup is listed in Table 7.1.

7.3. Routine Mediastinoscopy in Clinical Stage I after a Negative PET Scan

Postiron emission tomography for staging of lung cancer has become widely used, particularly in the United States. After a negative PET scan, the prevalence of involved mediastinal nodes in clinical stage I is 4.8% to 11.7% (Table 7.1). There have been only two studies to our knowledge that address the specific issue of mediastinoscopy after PET.[11,18] One study[18] has more than double the prevalence of the other, in part because this paper reflects a T2-3 population rather than T1-2 N0, and the paper did not clearly state the clinical N status so it is possible that there are some cN1 patients included in this series. The quoted prevalence of 11.7%, therefore, is the mediastinoscopy-detected prevalence of involved mediastinal nodes in patients with cT2-3 and a negative PET scan. The incidence of thoracotomy-discovered N2 was not stated, so the post-PET + mediastinoscopy prevalence is unknown. In the other paper,[11] which specifically considers our population of interest, the post–negative PET, premediastinoscopy prevalence of N2 disease was 5.6%, and mediastinoscopy was able to reduce this to 4.5%. The sensitivity of mediastinoscopy in this extensively screened population was thus 38%. This 1.1% reduction in prevalence was subjected to a cost-effectiveness analysis in the same paper, with two-way sensitivity analyses to examine the impact of changes in the prevalence of N2 and the benefit of induction over adjuvant chemotherapy. The results showed that routine mediastinoscopy would add an average 0.01 years (3.65 days) of life at a cost of $201,918 per life-year gained. Although cost is indeed relative, most payers (public or private) may find this rather high. Sensitivity analyses showed that the prevalence of N2 would have to exceed 10% to reduce the cost to below $100,000 per life-year gained. We cannot recommend routine mediastinoscopy after a negative PET if it only achieves a 1.1% reduction in N2 prevalence, with or without consideration of the high cost of this strategy (grade C recommendation). The issue is not yet settled, however, as the above data on the value of mediastinoscopy in the context of a negative PET scan is derived from only one case series. Although this analysis was performed in a center of excellence where the diagnostic accuracy of PET and mediastinoscopy is probably above average, the data cannot be considered of sufficiently high quantity and quality to resolve the issue, and the question of routine mediastinoscopy after negative PET scanning should be considered an unanswered one.

> Routine mediastinoscopy is not recommended in the context of a negative PET; current data suggest it only achieves a 1.1% reduction in N2 prevalence (level of evidence 1b to 4; recommendation grade C).

7.4. Routine Mediastinoscopy in Clinical Stage I after a Negative Chest CT Scan

In institutions where PET is not readily available, the argument for or against routine mediastinoscopy depends on the prevalence of N2 after a chest CT shows no enlarged hilar or mediastinal lymph nodes (N0). This prevalence has been reported to be 15.5% to 23%, in contrast to 4.8% to 11.7% after PET (Table 7.1). The specificity of mediastinoscopy has been repeatedly shown to be 100%, with a more variable sensitivity rate that averages 84%.[19] However, these values were computed based on large series of patients with and without enlarged mediastinal lymph nodes, and its sensitivity should decrease as the prevalence decreases. There are very few studies that specifically address the issue of routine mediastinoscopy in cT1-2N0.[12,23] The largest case series of 291 patients with this exact patient population found N2 disease in 9.2% of mediastinoscopy-negative patients.[12] The sensitivity of mediastinoscopy in this study was 44.4%, in an institution where mediastinoscopy was done for all surgical candidates, regardless of nodal status by imaging. Another retrospective study done for economic analysis purposes reported a postmediastinoscopy prevalence of 6% despite including some cN1 patients.[23]

A reduction in N2 prevalence from an average 19.2% to 8.3% is not large, but we contend it is enough for surgeons to decide to routinely perform mediastinoscopy (grade C recommendation). Routine mediastinoscopy in the post-CT setting is also cost effective. As mentioned in the cost-effectiveness analysis paper that studied post-PET routine mediastinoscopy,[11] a prevalence of N2 of 10% results in an expense of $100,000 per life-year gained. A 20% prevalence will reduce the cost per life-year gained even more.

> In the absence of PET and in the context of normal mediastinal lymph nodes on CT, routine mediastinoscopy is recommended because it reduces N2 prevalence from 19% to 8% (level of evidence 1b to 4; recommendation grade C).

7.5. Perspective

Surgeons who choose to do selective mediastinoscopy on post-CT clinical stage I patients usually base their decisions on histology, location of tumor (central versus peripheral), and tumor

TABLE 7.2. Prevalence of pN2 in clinical stage I lung cancer by tumor characteristics.

Reference	N	Primary tumor characteristics	
		Central	Peripheral
Daly[24]	501	9.2%	5.8%
Suzuki[22]	379	11.1%	18.5%
	Average	10.0%	11.3%
		Adenocarcinoma	Squamous cell
Vallieres[25]	35	15.8%	10%
Lewis[26]	418	7.3%	6.1%
Funatsu[27]	164	10.7%	7.1%
De Leyn[20]	235	21.5%	16.8%
Suzuki[22]	379	20%	12%
Choi[12]	291	11.5%	3.3%
	Average	14.0%	8.9%
		T2	T1
McKenna[28]	47	18%	
Vallieres[25]	35		13%
Lewis[26]	418	8.5%	7%
De Leyn[20]	235	17.7%	9.5%
Tahara[29]	30		11%
Choi[12]	291	6.1%	8.9%
	Average	10.4%	8.4%

size. Table 7.2 summarizes the prevalence of pN2 in papers that had data for clinical stage I patients. Although there is a trend towards a higher pN2 rate in T2 as opposed to T1 lesions, the two series comparing central and peripheral lesions had opposite findings, and none of the differences are significant enough to make a recommendation for selective mediastinoscopy in a particular group. Of note, a large, well-analyzed series[24] found a significant difference between central and peripheral tumor locations; but when the T3-T4 tumors were excluded, the difference became more modest (9.2% vs. 5.8%).

Histology, if it is available, provides a better discriminant of pN2 rates, with metastases found in an average 14% of non-bronchioloalveolar carcinoma adenocarcinomas versus 8.9% of squamous cell carcinomas. However, the surgeon still has to contend with the knowledge that there is an 8.9% chance of missing N2 disease if he/she does not perform mediastinoscopy in stage I squamous cell carcinoma. There is not much data for large cell carcinomas, but the suggested prevalence rates of 33% to 40%[25,27,30,31] mandate a mediastinoscopy if this diagnosis is obtained preoperatively.

At our institution, routine mediastinoscopy continues to be done on all patients, whether clinical stage I by chest CT only, or by chest CT with PET. Continuing this practice has a number of advantages at the present time. Routine mediastinoscopy provides the most precise staging, whether cost effective or not. Precision of staging, aside from benefiting the individual patient (and society, indirectly), adds to the worldwide fund of knowledge about lung cancer staging and treatment, which if collected properly will eventually generate enough data to answer questions like "should routine mediastinoscopy be done in clinical stage I lung cancer?" It maximizes opportunities to offer patients the chance to participate in neoadjuvant trials for N2 disease. We consider these trials important, and it is precisely the patients with microscopic N2 disease who we believe are most likely to benefit from an aggressive approach. Another advantage is the maintenance of expertise in this operator-dependent diagnostic modality, which has uses other than for staging lung cancer. Depending on an institution's patient population and mediastinoscopy policy, 5% to 20% of patients undergo mediastinoscopy for non-lung cancer indications, the most common of which is undiagnosed mediastinal lymphadenopathy. Greater than 90% of these lesions (half of which are benign) can be diagnosed by mediastinoscopy.[1,32,33] For most of these patients, mediastinoscopy obviates the need for a thoracoscopy or thoracotomy. Thus, training and maintenance of competence through frequent mediastinoscopy is another indirect benefit of a routine mediastinoscopy policy.

We believe that the data is sufficient for the recommendation of routine mediastinoscopy in patients staged as cT1-2 N0 after chest CT. However, the issue is unresolved in the increasing number of post-PET patients. A randomized trial of mediastinoscopy versus no mediastinoscopy in post-PET clinical stage I patients certainly could be done, though there will probably be little interest in pursuing this. In the absence of a randomized trial, prospective data collection in institutions implementing routine mediastinoscopy will probably be what will determine future practice. Of greatest usefulness would be an analysis of the prevalence of N2 disease in PET-negative patients according to histology, location of tumor, and T status. As in the discussion on selective mediastinoscopy for post-CT cN0, this information will refine the decision-making process. It should help thoracic surgeons decide which of their PET-negative stage I patients require mediastinoscopy, should they choose not to do it routinely. For now, however, it is suggested that thoracic surgeons perform routine mediastinoscopy on their patients until a sufficient body of evidence accumulates to better answer this question.

References

1. Hammoud ZT, Anderson RC, Meyers BF, et al. The current role of mediastinoscopy in the evaluation of thoracic disease. *J Thorac Cardiovasc Surg* 1999;118:894–899.
2. Luke WP, Pearson FG, Todd TR, et al. Prospective evaluation of mediastinoscopy for assessment of carcinoma of the lung. *J Thorac Cardiovasc Surg* 1986;91:53–56.
3. Cybulsky IJ, Bennett WF. Mediastinoscopy as a routine outpatient procedure. *Ann Thorac Surg* 1994;58:176–178.
4. Ginsberg RJ, Rice TW, Goldberg M, et al. Extended cervical mediastinoscopy: a single staging procedure for bronchogenic carcinoma of the left upper lobe. *J Thorac Cardiovasc Surg* 1987;94:673–678.
5. Coughlin M, Deslauriers J, Beaulieu M, et al. Role of mediastinoscopy in pretreatment staging of patients with primary lung cancer. *Ann Thorac Surg* 1985;40:556–560.
6. Gould MK, Kuschner WG, Rydzak CE, et al. Test performance of positron emission tomography and computed tomography for mediastinal staging in patients with non-small cell lung cancer. *Ann Int Med* 2003;139:879–892.
7. The Canadian Lung Oncology Group. Investigation for mediastinal disease in patients with apparently operable lung cancer. *Ann Thorac Surg* 1995;60:1382–1389.
8. Douillard JY, Rosell R, De Lena M, et al. ANITA: phase III adjuvant vinorelbine and cisplatin versus observation in completely resected non-small cell lung cancer patients: final results after 70-month median follow-up [abstract]. *Proc Am Soc Oncol* 2005; Abstract 7013.
9. The International Association for Lung Cancer Trial Collaborative Group. Cisplatin-based adjuvant chemotherapy in patients with completely resected non-small-cell lung cancer. *N Engl J Med* 2004;350:351–360.
10. Viney RC, Boyer MJ, King MT, et al. Randomized controlled trial of the role of positron emission tomography in the management of stage I and II non-small-cell lung cancer. *J Clin Oncol* 2004;22:2357–2362.
11. Meyers BF, Haddad FJ, Siegel BA, et al. Cost-effectiveness of routine mediastinoscopy in CT- and PET-screened patients with stage I lung cancer. J Thorac Cardiovasc Surg 2006;131:822–829.
12. Choi YS, Shim YM, Kim J, Kim K. Mediastinoscopy in patients with clinical stage I non-small-cell lung cancer. *Ann Thorac Surg* 2003;75:364–366.
13. Albain KS, Swann RS, Rusch VR, et al. Phase III study of concurrent chemotherapy and radiotherapy (CT/RT) vs CT/RT followed by surgical resection for stage IIIA (pN2) non-small cell lung cancer: outcomes update of north american intergroup 0139 (RTOG 9309) [abstract]. *Proc Am Soc Clin Oncol* 2005; Abstract 7014
14. Ferguson MK. Optimal management when unsuspected N2 nodal disease is identified during thoracotomy for lung cancer: cost-effectiveness analysis. *J Thorac Cardiovasc Surg* 2003;126:1935–1942.
15. Alam N, Shepherd F, Winton T, et al. Compliance with post-operative adjuvant chemotherapy in non-small-cell lung cancer. An analysis of national cancer institute of Canada and intergroup trial JBR10 and a review of the literature. *Lung Cancer* 2005;47:385–394.
16. Pisters KM, Ginsberg RJ, Giroux DJ, et al. Bimodality lung oncology team trial of induction paclitaxel/carboplatin in early-stage non-small cell lung cancer: long-term follow-up of a phase II trial. *Proc Am Soc Clin Oncol* 2003;22:633.
17. Depierre A, Milleron D, Moro-Sibilot D, et al. Preoperative chemotherapy followed by surgery compared with primary surgery in resectable stage I (except T1N0), II, and IIIA non-small cell lung cancer. *J Clin Oncol* 2002;20:247–253.
18. Gonzalez-Stawinski GV, Lemaire A, Merchant F, et al. A comparative analysis of positron emission tomography and mediastinoscopy in staging non-small cell lung cancer. *J Thorac Cardiovasc Surg* 2003;126:1900–1905.
19. Detterbeck FC, Jones DR, Parker LA. Intrathoracic staging. In: Detterbeck FC, Rivera MP, Socinski MA, eds. *Diagnosis and Treatment of Lung Cancer.* Philadelphia: Saunders; 2001:73–93.
20. De Leyn P, Vansteenkiste J, Cuypers P, et al. Role of cervical mediastinoscopy in staging of non-small cell lung cancer without enlarged mediastinal lymph nodes on CT scan. *Eur J Cardio-Thorac Surg* 1997;12:706–712.

21. Pieterman RM, Van Putten JW, Meuzelaar JJ, et al. Preoperative staging of non-small-cell lung cancer with positron-emission tomography. *N Engl J Med* 2000;343:254–261.

22. Suzuki K, Nagai K, Yoshida J, et al. Clinical predictors of N2 disease in the setting of a negative computed tomographic scan in patients with lung cancer. *J Thorac Cardiovasc Surg* 1999;117:593–598.

23. Kim K, Rice TW, Murthy SC, et al. Combined bronchoscopy, mediastinoscopy, and thoracotomy for lung cancer: who benefits? *J Thorac Cardiovasc Surg* 2004;127:850–856.

24. Daly BD, Mueller JD, Faling LJ, et al. N2 lung cancer: outcome in patients with false-negative computed tomographic scans of the chest. *J Thorac Cardiovasc Surg* 1993;105:904–910.

25. Vallieres E, Waters PF. Incidence of mediastinal node involvement in clinical T1 bronchogenic carcinomas. *Can J Surg* 1987;30:341–342.

26. Lewis JW, Pearlberg JL, Beute GH, et al. Can computed tomography of the chest stage lung cancer? – yes and no. *Ann Thorac Surg* 1990;49:591–596.

27. Funatsu T, Matsubara Y, Ikeda S, et al. Preoperative mediastinoscopic assessment of N factors and the need for mediastinal lymph node dissection in T1 lung cancer. *J Thorac Cardiovasc Surg* 1994;108:321–328.

28. Mckenna RJ, Libshitz HI, Mountain CE, et al. Roentgenographic evaluation of mediastinal nodes for preoperative assessment in lung cancer. *Chest* 1985;88:206–210.

29. Tahara RW, Lackner RP, Graver LM. Is there a role for routine mediastinoscopy in patients with peripheral T1 lung cancers? *Am J Surg* 2000;180:488–492.

30. Dillemans B, Deneffe G, Verschakelen J, et al. Value of computed tomography and mediastinoscopy in preoperative evaluation of mediastinal nodes in non-small cell lung cancer: a study of 569 patients. *Eur J Cardiothorac Surg* 1994;8:37–42.

31. Rhoads AC, Thomas JH, Hermreck AS, et al. Comparative studies of computed tomography and mediastinoscopy for the staging of bronchogenic carcinoma. *Am J Surg* 1986;152:587–591.

32. Forse RA, Dutton JW, Munro DD. Mediastinoscopy for diagnosing diseases of the lung other than primary carcinoma. *Can J Surg* 1978;21:438–440.

33. Porte H, Roumilhac D, Eraldi L, et al. The role of mediastinoscopy in the diagnosis of mediastinal lymphadenopathy. *Eur J Cardiothorac Surg* 1998;13:196–199.

8
Management of Unexpected N2 Disease Discovered at Thoracotomy

Hyde M. Russell and Mark K. Ferguson

The appropriate therapy for stage IIIa (N2) non-small cell lung cancer (NSCLC) is not clearly established. Recent randomized trials demonstrate that preoperative chemoradiotherapy followed by resection improves long-term and disease-free survival compared with surgery alone.[1,2] These results have bolstered the interest in multimodality treatment for patients with resectable N2 disease. Furthermore, the literature suggests that neoadjuvant therapy followed by surgery is superior to resection and subsequent adjuvant treatment, although such a comparison has not been definitively studied. Based on these results, patients who are found to have N2 nodal metastasis prior to thoracotomy, using methods such as mediastinoscopy, thoracoscopy, endoscopic ultrasonography, transbronchial needle aspiration, or possibly positron emission tomography (PET) scanning, should receive neoadjuvant treatment prior to resection.

A therapeutic dilemma arises when unsuspected N2 nodal disease is encountered intraoperatively during a planned formal lung resection for clinical stage I or II NSCLC. The management options include proceeding with resection or aborting the planned resection to allow for neoadjuvant treatment with possible subsequent reoperation and resection. The prevailing practice pattern favors initial resection for several reasons: the patient has already been subjected to the morbidity of a thoracotomy; intraoperative mediastinal nodal staging is time consuming and is unlikely to change the long-term outcome; and many surgeons perform only sampling of suspicious nodal stations at best, making nodal staging incomplete and often inaccurate. Arguments for aborting a planned resection when N2 nodal disease is discovered intraoperatively include: the morbidity of an exploratory thoracotomy is substantially less than that of a formal lung resection; preoperative systemic therapy is more effective in prolonging survival than is postoperative adjuvant therapy; and not all patients with N2 nodal disease should be subjected to resection. There is no direct comparison of outcomes of the two choices to guide decision making in this setting, and conclusions must be extrapolated from several different data sets.

8.1. Published Data

The current practice pattern among most thoracic surgeons who discover involved ipsilateral mediastinal nodes at the time of formal lung resection is to proceed with the planned resection.[3] Determining the optimal therapy for such patients requires examining all available options, including surgery alone, surgery with postoperative therapy, induction therapy followed by resection, and chemoradiotherapy alone. In order to obtain data for comparison of these four choices, published outcomes from a variety of studies were reviewed. A Medline search of English language publications from 1990 to 2005 using the criteria "lung resection" and "lung neoplasm" and "stage III" or "mediastinal adenopathy" or "N2" yielded 744 results. One hundred twenty abstracts were reviewed and an article search was performed on selected abstracts. Additional references from article bibliographies were included as appropriate.

8.1.1. Surgery Alone for N2 Disease

The reported outcomes of surgically resected N2 disease are uniformly poor, with 5-year survival ranging from 10% to 27%, with most articles reporting 20% survival at 5 years and median survival times of 18 to 24 months.[4-8] (Table 8.1). Despite these low numbers, surgery remains a common therapeutic option because the outcomes for resected patients are still significantly better than for those who do not undergo operation, in whom 5-year survival is 0%. While this difference may largely be due to a selection bias that eliminates patients with advanced age, poor performance status, and clinical N2 disease from consideration for resection, surgery clearly has an impact in some patients. A Japanese study[6] evaluated the prognosis of N2 NSCLC in 222 patients who had undergone resection. Overall, 5-year survival was 27%, but in subgroup analyses survival varied markedly from 0% to over 50%. Prognostic factors found to be particularly important were clinical N2 nodal status, multiple diseased N2 nodes, tumor size, and complete resectability. Patients with clinical N2 disease, often described as bulky stage IIIa disease, and multiple pathologic mediastinal nodes had a 5-year survival of 5%; in those who exhibited neither of those factors survival was 57% at 5 years. The site of N2 disease was also significant: patients with involved inferior N2 nodes fared worse (5-year survival 12%, $p < 0.05$) than others.

Miller and associates[7] at the Mayo Clinic performed a retrospective analysis of 167 patients who were found to have N2 disease at thoracotomy. Multivariate analysis revealed that younger age, negative inferior lymph nodes, fewer involved nodal stations, postoperative radiotherapy, and lobectomy rather than pneumonectomy all had a significant positive impact on survival. Their patients' 5-year survival rates following lobectomy and pneumonectomy were 31% and 17%. These outcomes demonstrate the heterogeneity of this population of patients and reveal that, while some patients clearly derive benefit from surgery, others are subjected to the risks of lung resection without an appreciable impact on the course of their disease.

8.1.2. Adjuvant Therapy

Postoperative (or adjuvant) chemotherapy has been the subject of many randomized, controlled trials, seven of which specifically address stage III disease (Table 8.2), and two of which focus solely on patients with N2 metastases.[9-15] The results of these studies as a whole have largely been disappointing, as six of seven studies failed to find an advantage to the use of adjuvant chemotherapy. A phase III trial conducted at Memorial Sloan-Kettering in 1994 randomized seventy-two patients with stage IIIa N2 disease to surgery with or without adjuvant chemotherapy. Median and 5-year survivals were 16.5 months and 17% in the treatment arm compared with 19.1 months and 30% in the control group, leading the investigators to conclude that there was no evidence of benefit from the postoperative chemotherapy that was administered.

The Japan Clinical Oncology Group reported results of a phase III study in 1993 in which they randomized 181 patients with completely resected stage III disease to receive postoperative chemotherapy (cisplatin + vindesine) or no further treatment. They also failed to demonstrate any benefit to the postoperative regimen. Three-year disease-free survival rates were 37% versus 42%, and median survivals were 31 months and 37 months for the treated and untreated group, respectively.

More recently in Japan, Tada and colleagues looked specifically at patients with N2 metastases. One hundred nineteen patients with completely resected N2 disease were randomized to

TABLE 8.1. Outcomes of surgery alone for N2 disease.

Reference	Year	No. patients	Median survival (months)	5-year survival (%)	EBM grade
Van Klaveren[3]	1993	44	12	10%	3
Ishida[4]	1990	115	n/a	18%	3
Suzuki[5]	1999	222	30	27%	3
Miller[6]	1994	167	18	21%	3
Nakanishi[7]	1997	53	25	21%	3

TABLE 8.2. Outcomes of randomized, controlled studies of adjuvant postoperative therapy.

Reference	Year	Stages included	No. patients (%N2)	Regimen	Median survical months: treatment vs. control	5-year overall survival: treatment vs. control	p value	EBM grade
Pisters[9]	1994	IIIa, N2	72 (100%)	CT/RT vs. RT	16.3 vs. 19.1	17% vs. 30%	0.42	1−
Tada[11]	2003	IIIa, N2	119 (100%)	CT vs. observation	18.3 vs. 16.1	28.2% vs. 36.1%	0.89	1+
Ohta[10]	1993	III	181 (66%)	CT vs. observation	31 vs. 37	35% vs. 41%	0.595	1+
Dautzenberg[13]	1995	I–IIIa	267 (51%)	CT/RT vs. RT	N2: 15.3 vs. 8	N2: 19% vs. 6%	0.003	1+
ECOG[14]	2000	II–III	488 (54%)	CT/RT vs. RT	38 vs. 39	33% vs. 39%	0.56	1++
IALT[12]	2000	I–IIIa	1867 (25%)	CT/RT vs. RT	na	N2: 32% vs. 28%	na	1++
Scagliotti[15]	2003	I–IIIa	1209 (25%)	CT vs. Obs w/wo RT (43% with)	55.2 vs. 48	Stage IIIa 20% vs. 19%	ns	1++

Abbreviations: na, not applicable; ns, not significant.

adjuvant chemotherapy versus no further treatment. Five-year survivals were 28% in the treatment group and 36% in the control arm. Median disease-free survivals were 18 months versus 16 months respectively, and no statistical difference was found between the two groups.

The International Adjuvant Lung Cancer Trial Collaborative Group produced the one study that did find a statistically significant survival advantage to postoperative chemotherapy. One thousand eight hundred sixty-seven patients with stage I-IIIa disease who underwent complete resection were randomized to chemotherapy versus observation. At five years, 45% of treatment arm patients were alive compared with 40% of the control group ($p < 0.03$). Patients with N2 disease constituted 26% of the study population. Among this subgroup, 32% of patients in the chemotherapy group were alive at the end of the study compared with 28% in the control group. No statistical information is given regarding the N2 subgroup, but the finding represents a marginal improvement at best.

The lack of benefit demonstrated by postoperative chemotherapy in patients with N2 nodal metastasis has made its application controversial among providers. With regard to the clinical problem of N2 nodal disease discovered at the time of surgery, there is no evidence that the availability of postoperative adjuvant therapy should alter the decision of whether or not to proceed with resection.

8.1.3. Induction Therapy

In contrast to the lack of benefit observed with adjuvant therapy in stage III N2 disease, preoperative or neoadjuvant chemotherapy shows more promise. Four prospective randomized studies comparing induction chemotherapy to surgery alone were published from 1992 to 2005 (Table 8.3).

Roth and colleagues[1] at MD Anderson randomized 60 patients with resectable stage IIIa NSCLC to either preoperative chemotherapy (PCT) followed by surgery or surgery alone (SA). Eighty-three percent of the patients had histologically confirmed N2 disease and they were equally distributed between the two groups. The operations (lobectomy, bi-lobectomy, and pneumonectomy) were similar between the two groups, as was the rate of resectability. The

TABLE 8.3. Outcomes of randomized studies of preoperative therapy.

Reference	Year	No. patients	Median survival (months): treatment vs. control	5-year overall survival: treatment vs. control	p value	EBM grade
Roselle[8]	1999	60	22 vs. 10	17% vs. 0%	<0.001	1−
Roth[7]	1998	60	64 vs. 11	36% vs. 15%	0.056	1−
Pass[19]	1992	27	28 vs. 15	nd	0.095	1−
Nagai[9]	2003	62	17 vs. 16	10% vs. 22%	0.53	1+

Abbreviation: nd, not determined.

median survival of preoperative chemotherapy group was 64 months compared to the surgery-only group's 11 months. A long-term follow-up to this study was published in 1998[16]: 5-year survival was 36% in the PCT group and 15% in the SA group. When analysis was limited to those patients who were able to be resected, the median survival in the PCT group had not yet been reached, and the median survival of the SA group was 18 months. Five-year survival rates among resected patients were 53% versus 24%, favoring the PCT group.

These impressive results were supported the following year by a Spanish study conducted by Roselle and others,[2] which randomized 60 patients to PCT + surgery or surgery alone. Both groups received postoperative radiotherapy. In the PCT group, 17% of patients were alive at 5 years compared with none in the surgery alone group.[17] Median survival was 26 months for PCT patients versus 8 months for the SA patients. This study was criticized on several issues: small size (60 patients), lack of biological equivalence between the two arms according to K-ras mutations and aneuploidy favoring the treatment arm, and unexpectedly low control group results. Those criticisms aside, the evidence remains compelling enough to recommend preoperative therapy to patients with documented N2 disease.

In contrast to the dramatic results of these two studies, two negative studies have been published more recently. Nagi and associates[18] with the Japan Clinical Oncology Group released data on 62 patients, all with N2 nodal metastasis, who were randomized to PCT or surgery alone with a median follow-up period of 6.2 years. Median survival was 17 months for the PCT group and 16 months for surgery alone. Five-year survival estimates were 10% [95% confidence interval (CI), 0%–20%] for the induction patients and 22% (95% CI, 7%–37%) for the surgery-alone group.

Pass and colleagues at the National Institutes of Health (NIH) published their data on a small randomized study comparing preoperative etoposide–platinum chemotherapy followed by surgery versus surgery with postoperative radiotherapy. Twenty-seven patients were randomized with a median follow-up of 30 months. Median survival for the preoperative chemotherapy group

was 29 months versus 16 months for the control group. Although the difference was remarkable, this result did not reach statistical significance ($p = 0.095$).[19]

Despite these conflicting results in studies of small sample sizes, the magnitude of benefit in the Roth and Roselle studies is compelling. In addition, a meta-analysis of four neoadjuvant studies was performed in 2004.[20] Quantitative analysis of the pooled survival curves found a nonsignificant hazard ratio (HR) of 0.65 (95% CI, 0.41–1.04) in favor of neoadjuvant chemotherapy in stage III disease.

8.1.4. Chemoradiotherapy Alone

Surgery has traditionally been the mainstay of potentially curative treatment for resectable disease. Given recent improvements in chemotherapy outcomes which rival those of surgery, the role of resection in the treatment of stage III N2 disease is increasingly a topic of debate. The North American Intergroup 0139 trial released interim data in abstract form at the 2005 American Society of Clinical Oncology (ASCO) meeting.[21] This trial included 484 patients with stage III N2 disease who were considered potentially resectable. Induction chemoradiotherapy was given to all patients followed by a re-evaluation and subsequent randomization of surgery eligible patients to either resection or observation. Both arms received consolidation chemotherapy (postoperatively in the surgery arm). There were 16 treatment-related deaths in the surgery arm, 14 of which occurred in pneumonectomy patients (26% of all pneumonectomies). In contrast, there were only four treatment-related deaths in the control group. The pattern of recurrence was significantly different between the two groups with 10% local relapse in the surgery group and 22% in the control arm. There was no difference in the development of distant metastasis between the two groups (37% vs. 42%). Tumor downstaging was evident with 46% of all resected specimens revealing N0 status. Five-year progression-free survival (PFS) was statistically different between the two groups favoring surgery (22% resected group vs. 11% observation group). There was a trend towards superior overall survival at 5 years in the surgery group (27% vs. 20%) but this difference did not reach statistical significance. Tumor downstaging appeared to affect overall survival: patients who were pN0 had a 41% 5-year survival compared with 24% in pN1–3 patients.

To clarify the effect of the pneumonectomy-related deaths on the study, an exploratory sub-group analysis was performed based on surgical procedure. Chemoradiotherapy followed by lobectomy had a statistically significant improvement in survival compared with matched controls in the non-operative arm (median, 34 vs. 22 months, 5-year, 36% vs. 18%). In contrast, neoadjuvant treatment followed by pneumonectomy resulted in no benefit over chemoradiotherapy alone (median, 19 vs. 29 months, 5-year, 22% vs. 24%).

This survival difference between pneumonectomy and lobectomy has been noted in previous studies of patients with N2 disease.[4,6,7] In one of these studies, the survival curves diverged even after the first year, suggesting that perioperative mortality may not be solely responsible for the long-term differences. Regardless of the cause, the finding raises the question of whether resection should be offered to a patient with N2 metastasis if a pneumonectomy is required.

8.2. Evidence Quality

The data discussed above come from multiple disparate sources of varying quality. The retrospective studies on surgery for N2 disease are case series and, as such, each receives a score of 3. The evidence regarding the effectiveness of adjuvant therapy is derived from prospective randomized, controlled trials and is graded between 1– and 1+. Likewise, the induction therapy studies also receive grades of 1– to 1+. The meta-analysis of these level 1 studies is graded as 1++. Because none of these studies deals specifically with the question at hand, data are extrapolated from them and applied to the problem. Finally, the Intergroup 0139 trial data has been released only in abstract form, which prevents assigning a formal grade. Given the study design and number of patients enrolled, it will likely meet criteria for a grade of 1+.

8.3. Discussion

Unsuspected N2 nodal metastasis found at the time of exploratory thoracotomy for intended resection is a problem that arises in approximately 15% of cases. There have been no phase III trials performed specifically addressing this clinical situation, and the clinical decision to proceed versus abort relies on the interpretation of a combination of studies. Although it is difficult to directly compare the studies investigating neoadjuvant therapy with those looking at adjuvant therapy because of the heterogeneity of the patient population, neoadjuvant therapy appears to offer a survival benefit that has not been matched with adjuvant treatment. Retrospective studies looking at this problem have attempted to identify factors that may help predict in which subgroup of patients it makes sense to continue with resection. Multivariate analyses have shown that tumor size, the number of involved nodes, and completeness of resection all statistically impact survival. However, fully evaluating lymph node status at the time of thoracotomy is generally not feasible. In addition, these same factors (smaller tumor size, number of nodal stations, extent of resection) are characteristic of the best subgroups in the neoadjuvant therapy studies and only strengthen the argument in favor of stopping the operation to intervene with chemoradiotherapy before returning for formal resection. We now know that there are clearly select patients with N2 disease who benefit from surgical resection. However, the current evidence suggests that providing this group with the best available cancer treatment requires preoperative chemoradiotherapy.

Given the oncologic superiority of induction therapy followed by subsequent resection, the clinician is then faced with the question of whether this approach makes sense for the individual patient from a quality-of-life and cost standpoint. A meta-analysis of survival data from published reports of patients undergoing resection with unsuspected N2 disease plus data from neoadjuvant therapy trials was performed by Ferguson in 2003.[22] Using decision analytic techniques, variables were weighted using a quality-of-life utility scale and costs of various treatment options calculated for a comparison of outcomes with the primary end points of median survival, QALY, and cost effectiveness. The results of this analysis favored aborting the initial resection to perform induction therapy followed by subsequent re-exploration and resection. As expected, median survival was higher in the induction therapy group (2.1 years vs. 1.7 years). Interestingly, despite prolonging the treatment time with induction therapy followed by a second operation and recovery, the QALY were greater (1.8 vs. 1.3) and the difference in cost per QALY was negligible. The author suggested that the survival advantage is a reflection of both the benefit of induction therapy combined with the exclusion of patients with more aggressive disease who progressed during therapy and did not return for resection. Given the importance of the weighted values assigned to the decision analysis variables, the results must be interpreted carefully. However, it is the first paper to quantify outcomes of the potential treatment choices in the setting of unsuspected N2 disease, and the conclusions are logical even if the inputs are subject to debate.

8.4. Recommendations

The accumulated data favor induction therapy over postoperative therapy for non-small cell lung cancer with N2 nodal involvement. When unsuspected N2 nodal disease is encountered during planned lung resection, our recommendation is to abort the operation to allow for neoadjuvant therapy. Provided the patient exhibits either a response to therapy or stable disease, subsequent redo thoracotomy and resection should be offered provided that the lesion is deemed completely resectable. Patients requiring pneumonectomy to achieve a complete resection should be selected with great care given the uncertainty of benefit in this population.

> The accumulated data favor induction therapy over postoperative adjuvant therapy for non-small cell lung cancer with N2 nodal involvement. When unsuspected N2 nodal disease is encountered during planned lung resection, our recommendation is to abort the operation to allow for neoadjuvant therapy (level of evidence 1++ to 3; recommendation grade B).

References

1. Roth JA, Fossella F, Komaki R, et al. A randomized trial comparing perioperative chemotherapy and surgery with surgery alone in resectable stage IIIA non-small-cell lung cancer. *J Natl Cancer Inst* 1994;86:673–680.
2. Rosell R, Gomez-Codina J, Camps C, et al. A randomized trial comparing preoperative chemotherapy pus surgery with surgery alone in patients with non-small-cell lung cancer. *N Engl J Med* 1994;330:153–158.
3. Goldstraw P, Mannam GC, Kaplan DK, et al. Surgical management of non-small cell lung cancer with ipsilateral mediastinal node metastasis (N2 disease). *J Thorac Cardiovasc Surg* 1994;107:19–27.
4. Van Klaveren RJ, Festen J, Otten HJ, et al. Prognosis of unsuspected but completely resectable N2 non-small cell lung cancer. *Ann Thorac Surg* 1993;56:300–304.
5. Ishida T, Tateishi M, Kaneko S, et al. Surgical treatment of patients with non-small-cell lung cancer and mediastinal lymph node involvement. *J Surg Oncol* 1990;43:161–166.
6. Suzuki K, Nagai K, Yoshida J, et al. The prognosis of surgically resected N2 non-small cell lung cancer: the importance of clinical N status. *J Thorac Cardiovasc Surg* 1999;118:145–153.
7. Miller DL, McManus KG, Allen MS, et al. Results of surgical resection in patients with N2 non-small cell lung cancer. *Ann Thorac Surg* 1994;57:1095–1101.
8. Nakanishi R, Osaki T, Nakanishi K, et al. Treatment strategy for patients with surgically discovered N2 stage IIIA non-small cell lung cancer. *Ann Thorac Surg* 1997;64:342–348.
9. Pisters KM, Kris MG, Gralla RJ, et al. Randomized trial comparing postoperative chemotherapy with vindesine and cisplatin plus thoracic irradiation with irradiation alone in stage III non-small cell lung cancer. *J Surg Oncol* 1994;56:236–241.
10. Ohta M, Tsuchiya R, Shimoyama M, et al. Adjuvant chemotherapy for completely resected stage III non-small-cell lung cancer. *J Thorac Cardiovasc Surg* 1993;106:703–708.
11. Tada H, Tsuchiya R, Ichinose Y, et al. A randomized trial comparing adjuvant chemotherapy versus surgery alone for completely resected pN2 non-small cell lung cancer. *Lung Cancer* 2004;43:167–173.
12. Arriagada R, Bergman B, Dunant A, et al. Cisplatin-based adjuvant chemotherapy in patients with completely resected non-small-cell lung cancer. *N Engl J Med* 2004;350:351–360.

13. Dautzenberg B, Chastang C, Arriagada R, et al. Adjuvant radiotherapy versus combined sequential chemotherapy followed by radiotherapy in the treatment of resected nonsmall cell lung carcinoma. A randomized trial of 267 patients. *Cancer* 1995;76:779–786.

14. Keller S, Adak S, Wagner H, et al. A randomized trial of postoperative adjuvant therapy in patients with completely resected stage II or IIIA non-small cell lung cancer. *N Engl J Med* 2000;343: 1217–1222.

15. Scagliotti G, Fossati R, Torri V, et al. Randomized study of adjuvant chemotherapy for completely resected stage I, II, or IIIA non-small-cell lung cancer. *J Natl Cancer Inst* 2003;95:1453–1461.

16. Roth JA, Atkinson N, Fossella F, et al. Long-term follow up of patients enrolled in a randomized trial comparing perioperative chemotherapy and surgery with surgery alone in resectable stage IIIA non-small-cell lung cancer. *Lung Cancer* 1998;21:1–6.

17. Rosell R, Gomez-Codina J, Camps C, et al. Preresectional chemotherapy in stage IIIA non-small-cell lung cancer: a 7-year assessment of a randomized controlled trial. *Lung Cancer* 1999;47:7–14.

18. Nagai K, Tsuchiya R, Mori T, et al. A randomized trial comparing induction chemotherapy followed by surgery with surgery alone for patients with stage IIIA N2 non-small cell lung cancer. *J Thorac Cardiovasc Surg* 2003;125:254–260.

19. Pass H, Pogrebniak H, Steinberg S, et al. Randomized trial of neoadjuvant therapy for lung cancer: interim analysis. *Ann Thorac Surg* 1992;53:992–998.

20. Berghmans T, Paesmans M, Meert AP, et al. Survival improvement in resectable non-small cell lung cancer with (neo)adjuvant chemotherapy: results of a meta-analysis of the literature. *Lung Cancer* 2005;49:13–23.

21. Albain K, Swann R, Rusch V, et al. Phase III study of concurrent chemotherapy and radiotherapy (CT/RT) vs CT/RT followed by surgical resection for stage IIIA(pN2) non-small cell lung cancer (NSCLC): outcomes update of North American Intergroup 0139 (RTOG 9309). *J Clin Oncol* 2005;23(suppl 16):624S.

22. Ferguson MK. Optimal management when unsuspected N2 nodal disease is identified during thoracotomy for lung cancer: cost-effectiveness analysis. *J Thorac Cardiovasc Surg* 2003;126:1935–1942.

9
Induction Therapy for Clinical Stage I Lung Cancer

David C. White and Thomas A. D'Amico

Non-small cell lung cancer (NSCLC) remains a leading cause of death and will cause approximately 163,500 deaths in the United States in 2005.[1] While patients presenting with localized disease have the best chance of being cured, they represent a minority of patients and unfortunately have a significant likelihood of developing recurrent disease after treatment and ultimately dying of their disease. The 5-year survival for patients presenting with clinical stage I lung cancer ranges from 38% to 61%; for those with pathological stage IA disease, the survival is 67%.[2]

Despite advances in staging, including the use of high-resolution computed tomography (CT) scanning, the advent of positron emission tomography (PET) scanning, and more widespread use of mediastinoscopy, the clinical staging of lung cancer remains inadequate. A recent multicenter trial of leading institutions demonstrated that only approximately 62% of patients with clinical stage I NSCLC retained that stage after full surgical staging.[3] Thus, a significant percentage of patients with clinical stage I NSCLC cancer may in fact have more advanced disease and could therefore potentially benefit from induction therapy. Of patients who are able to undergo complete resection for stage I NSCLC, approximately one-third will develop recurrent disease, and 70% of recurrences will be distant metastases.[4] In addition, retrospective studies have demonstrated that even within stage IA there is a worse prognosis with larger tumor size, suggesting a potential role for additional therapies in even the earliest stages of lung cancer.[5] Due to the poor overall prognosis for NSCLC, and the chance of recurrence even among

those with completely resected early-stage disease, great efforts have been focused on the development of effective adjuvant therapies.

While many trials have been performed in an attempt to demonstrate survival benefit with chemotherapy for NSCLC, only in the past decade has this been fruitful. Two small trials first demonstrated significant survival benefit for induction chemotherapy in stage IIIA NSCLC,[6,7] which has remained the standard of care.[8] In 1995, a meta-analysis of 52 randomized clinical trials suggested an absolute survival benefit of approximately 5% at 5 years with adjuvant chemotherapy and surgery compared to surgery alone for NSCLC.[9] More recently, three prospective, randomized clinical trials demonstrated the benefit of platinum-based adjuvant therapy in the treatment of stage I-IIIA NSCLC following complete surgical resection.[10-12] Based on the fact that adjuvant chemotherapy appears to improve survival in early-stage NSCLC, and the known occurrence of distant metastases in this patient population, it seems logical to ask whether induction therapy might prove beneficial in clinical stage I NSCLC, as it does for stage IIIA disease.

9.1. Induction Therapy for Non-Small Cell Lung Cancer

The potential advantages of induction therapy compared to adjuvant therapy are multiple. First, several trials of adjuvant chemotherapy have been hindered by poor compliance, as patients are either not able or not willing to undergo a full course of chemotherapy in the postoperative period, and this appears to hold true for patients with stage I and II NSCLC.[13] The compliance rates for induction therapy followed by surgery are higher[6,7] than for surgery followed by adjuvant chemotherapy.[9–12] In addition, preoperative therapy may have improved efficacy due to the intact vascular supply of the tumor, may aid in resectability by downsizing the primary tumor, and may provide a better chance of cure by treating micrometastatic disease earlier. Finally, it has been suggested that chemotherapy resistance may be related to genetic changes within the tumor itself, and thus chemotherapy may be more effective when given as early as possible after the disease is diagnosed, while the tumor burden is relatively smaller.[14] Potential disadvantages of induction therapy include impaired wound healing and increased risk of perioperative infections, such as empyema and bronchopleural fistula, although these potential disadvantages have not been demonstrated thus far.[15]

Several trials have been designed in an attempt to assess the risks and benefits of induction chemotherapy for resectable NSCLC, and some of these trials have included patients with clinical stage I disease. These trials have focused on chemotherapy, as the use of radiation therapy has been limited largely to an adjuvant role for patients at high risk of recurrence following resection. Trials of induction radiation therapy demonstrated no survival benefit in patients with NSCLC.[16]

9.2. Induction Therapy: Phase II Trials

A small phase II feasibility trial was reported in abstract form at the 2001 American Society of Clinical Oncology (ASCO) annual meeting. This North Central Cancer Treatment Group (NCCTG) study enrolled 52 patients for treatment with three cycles of preoperative carboplatin and paclitaxel.[17] The majority of patients in this trial were stage I, with 17% having T1 tumors, 71% having T2 tumors, and 12% having T3 tumors. Only 10% had nodal involvement, and mediastinoscopy was mandated to exclude N2 disease prior to enrollment in the trial. Forty-five of the 52 patients (87%) were able to receive all three cycles of preoperative therapy, and complete resection

was achieved in 36 of 46 patients (78%). Three patients died postoperatively, and 2-year survival was estimated at 73%. Grade 3 neutropenia occurred in 23 patients (44%), while grade 3 thrombocytopenia occurred in 9 (17%). Other complications included diarrhea (1), myalgia (4), hyperglycemia (2), vomiting (2), and dysrhythmia (1). The overall response rate to chemotherapy was 59%. These data appear to support the feasibility of induction chemotherapy, although the final results have not been published.

Another important trial was conducted by the Bimodality Lung Oncology Team between 1996 and 1998.[18] This was a phase II trial designed to assess the feasibility of preoperative chemotherapy consisting of carboplatin and paclitaxel in patients with early-stage NSCLC (stages IB–IIIA). Patients with stage IA disease were excluded. A total of 94 patients were enrolled in this multicenter trial and treated with two cycles of preoperative carboplatin and paclitaxel, followed by surgery, and an additional three cycles of adjuvant chemotherapy. Mediastinoscopy was required in patients with lymph nodes greater than 1 cm on chest CT. The primary end points of this trial were recurrence, long-term toxicities, and survival. Forty-two of the 94 patients (44.7%) enrolled were clinical stage IB (T2N0). Importantly, 90 of the 94 patients (96%) were able to receive both preoperative cycles of chemotherapy. Fifty-six percent of patients had a major radiographic response to preoperative therapy, while 34% of patients had stable disease and only 3% had progression of disease during preoperative chemotherapy. Also, 88 of 94 patients (94%) were able to undergo their planned surgery, and R0 resection was achieved in 81 patients (86%). Interestingly, despite aggressive preoperative staging with mediastinoscopy, 36% of patients were found to have more extensive disease at the time of surgery. Forty-three patients (46%) were not able to receive their planned postoperative chemotherapy for a variety of reasons, including perioperative complications and delayed recovery in 15 patients, again supporting the concept that preoperative chemotherapy is tolerated better than postoperative chemotherapy. Only 42 patients (45%) received all three planned postoperative cycles of chemotherapy. Toxicities in the preoperative chemotherapy group included severe

TABLE 9.1. Major trials of induction therapy for clinical stage I NSCLC.

Reference	No. patients	Stage	Chemotherapy	Control	Findings	Level of evidence
Marks[17] (NCCTG)	52	Ib–IIIa	Carboplatin, paclitaxel × 3	None	Preoperative chemotherapy feasible	2b
Pisters[18] (BLOT)	94	Ib–IIIa	Carboplatin, paclitaxel × 2 preop, × 3 postop	None	Preoperative chemotherapy feasible	2b
Depierre[20] (FTCG)	373	Ib–IIIa	Mitomycin, ifosfamide, cisplatin × 2 cycles	Surgery alone	Improved disease-free survival	2b
Pisters[21] (SWOG 9900)	354	Ib–IIIa	Carboplatin, paclitaxel × 3	Surgery alone	Nonsignificant trend towards improved overall and disease-free survival	2b

Abbreviations: BLOT, Bimodality Lung Oncology Team; FTCG, French Thoracic Cooperative Group; NCCTG, North Central Cancer Treatment Group; NSCLC, non-small cell lung cancer; SWOG, Southwest Oncology Group.

hypersensitivity to paclitaxel in three patients, severe anemia and thrombocytopenia in one patient each, and grade 3 neutropenia in 35% of patients. One patient died of a cerebrovascular accident after developing severe neutropenia and hyponatremia during induction therapy, and two deaths occurred in the postsurgical setting. Other surgical complications included arrhythmia, wound infection, hemorrhage, and respiratory infection.

In summary, this phase II trial demonstrated that preoperative chemotherapy is well tolerated and feasible prior to resection of early-stage NSCLC. It highlights, once again, the need for improved preoperative staging to better stratify patients. Because of the small number of patients and the variable stage presentations, it is impossible to comment specifically on the potential benefits of chemotherapy for stage I disease based on this trial. In addition, the omission of stage IA patients excludes a significant fraction of patients for whom the risks and benefits of induction therapy are unknown. Other phase II trials have evaluated the use of newer chemotherapeutic agents for induction regimens, including gemcitabine, and have found this to be a feasible approach as well.[19] (See Table 9.1.)

9.3. Phase III Trials

The most convincing data regarding the efficacy of induction chemotherapy in clinical stage I NSCLC comes from a randomized phase III trial conducted in France from 1991–1997 by the French Thoracic Cooperative Group.[20] This trial enrolled 373 patients with stage I (excluding T1N0), II, or IIIA NSCLC and randomized them to surgery alone or to induction chemotherapy (two cycles of mitomycin, ifosfamide and cisplatin given 3 weeks apart) followed by surgery 1 month later. Although this trial included patients with stage II and IIIA disease, 205 of the patients were clinical stage I. It should be noted that mediastinoscopy was not routinely performed prior to surgery, and treatment of the mediastinal lymph nodes at the time of surgery was left to the surgeon's discretion, although it was not different between groups.

Results of this trial demonstrated a nonsignificant trend towards improved survival in the induction therapy group. Specifically, there was a numerical absolute survival benefit of 3.8% at 1 year, 6.9% at 2 years, 10.4% at 3 years, and 8.6% at 4 years. Median survival improved from 26 months in the surgery arm to 37 months in the induction therapy arm, although this difference was also not statistically significant. ($p = 0.15$). Interestingly, the numerical survival benefit in the induction arm was limited to those patients with stage I or II disease. In addition, there was a statistically significant improvement in disease-free survival in the induction therapy arm. Disease-free survival increased from 12.9 months in the surgery arm to 26.7 months in the induction therapy arm, with 3-year disease-free survival rates of 44% and 33%, respectively.

However, the use of induction chemotherapy did result in a nonsignificant increase in the number of treatment-related deaths after surgery. In addition, there was a nonsignificant increase in perioperative morbidity in the induction therapy arm, including more empyemas and bronchopleural fistulas.

The correlation between clinical and pathological staging in this trial once again demonstrated the inadequacy of clinical staging. Of 82 patients with clinical N0 disease, only 47 (57%) proved to be pathological N0, while 18 were N1, 16 were N2, and 1 was N3. Thus, almost half the patients who were clinical stage I were upstaged at the time of complete surgical staging. Although the results of this trial are limited by the use of subset analysis, and the lack of a statistically significant overall survival benefit, the data is nevertheless intriguing and suggestive of a potential benefit of induction therapy in clinical stage I NSCLC.

A second phase III trial, a follow-up to the Bimodality Lung Oncology Team phase II study,[18] was recently closed. This trial, S9900, was a multigroup phase III trial comparing surgery alone to preoperative chemotherapy followed by surgery for early-stage NSCLC.[21] This trial stratified patients with early-stage disease, separating those with IB/IIA disease from those with IIB/IIIA disease (excluding superior sulcus tumors), and randomizing them to receive three preoperative cycles of chemotherapy with paclitaxel and carboplatin followed by surgery, or surgery alone. The trial was powered to detect a 33% increase over an expected 2.7-year median survival with surgery alone. The planned sample size was 600 patients; however, this study closed to new patient entry after positive results from adjuvant chemotherapy trials became available.[10,12]

At the time of closure, 354 patients had been accrued. Results were reported in abstract form at the American Society of Oncology (ASCO) 2005 meeting.[21] Seventy percent of the patients were stage IB/IIA. A major radiographic response was observed in 40% of patients, and a nonsignificant trend towards improved progression-free and overall survival was seen in the induction therapy group, with a 9-month improvement in median progression-free survival and a 5-month increase in median overall survival (42 vs. 37

months) with preoperative chemotherapy ($p = 0.26$). Overall 2-year survival was 68% in the treatment arm and 64% in the surgery arm ($p = 0.47$). There were four perioperative deaths in the surgery arm and six in the treatment arm. While the study closed early, this trial supports the feasibility of induction therapy, although no conclusions can be drawn regarding survival. The investigators concluded that further randomized trials are warranted comparing induction therapy to adjuvant therapy for early-stage NSCLC.

Several additional trials have been performed and are currently being evaluated. One of these was a phase III trial comparing surgery alone to surgery following preoperative gemcitabine–cisplatin in patients with stage IB-IIIA NSCLC.[22] Accrual to this trial was stopped early due to publication of data regarding adjuvant therapy;[10-12] however, early results suggest feasibility with the use of this regimen.

9.4. Meta-analysis

The evidence regarding induction therapy for early-stage NSCLC has been summarized in a meta-analysis presented at the ASCO meeting in 2005.[23] This included clinical trials between 1994 and 2004 on induction therapy for resectable NSCLC. Eight trials were identified, with a total of 1965 patients. The overall survival difference was statistically significant, with an odds ratio of 0.68 for induction therapy. However, when the highest quality trials were grouped separately, this difference was not statistically significant. Of importance, this meta-analysis included patients with a range of clinical stages, not just stage I NSCLC. The authors concluded that additional randomized trials are necessary to determine the efficacy of induction therapy for early-stage NSCLC.

9.5. Summary

Currently there exists insufficient published data to formulate an evidence-based recommendation regarding the use of induction therapy for clinical stage I NSCLC. The best evidence that suggests a survival benefit from induction therapy comes from subset analysis of one randomized, controlled trial that included patients with a range of stages of disease.[20] Furthermore, only disease-free survival, and not overall survival, was significantly improved in the induction therapy arm of this trial. Although this is a well-designed randomized, controlled trial, the evidence for improved survival is no higher than level 2b given the inclusion of multiple stages. The other randomized, controlled trial that was designed to assess the benefit of induction therapy, S9900, closed early due to publication of data demonstrating the benefit of adjuvant therapy, and this trial once again failed to demonstrate statistically significant improvements in overall survival with induction therapy, albeit possibly because of incomplete accrual.[21] Although well-intentioned, this trial is underpowered and therefore can only be considered level 2b evidence for the benefit of induction therapy. The two main cohort studies discussed above, while intriguing, provide at best level 2b evidence for a benefit from induction therapy. Furthermore, these trials did not evaluate patients with T1N0 disease, who make up a large portion of patients with clinical stage I disease, and for whom there is essentially no data regarding the utility of induction therapy. Thus, any benefit from induction therapy in clinical stage I NSCLC must be extrapolated from these trials, and therefore, a recommendation of grade C is the strongest one that can be made for the use of induction therapy in this population. While there is some hope of improved survival with induction therapy, higher grade evidence-based recommendations must await the results of randomized trials focused on clinical stage I disease. These trials must be designed to compare induction therapy followed by surgery with surgery plus adjuvant therapy for early-stage lung cancer. The current standard of care for patients with early stage (I and II) NSCLC is surgery, without induction therapy.[8] Patients with pathological stage IB-IIIA should be considered for adjuvant therapy.[10-12]

> There is insufficient published data to provide an evidence-based recommendation regarding the use of induction therapy for clinical stage I NSCLC.

References

1. Jemal A, Murray T, Ward E, et al. Cancer statistics, 2005. *CA Cancer J Clin* 2005;55:10–30.
2. Mountain CF. Revisions in the international system for staging lung cancer. *Chest* 1997;111:1710–1717.
3. D'Cunha J, Herndon II JE, Herzan DL, et al. Poor correspondence between clinical and pathologic staging in stage I non-small cell lung cancer: results from CALGB 9761, a prospective trial. *Lung Cancer* 2005;48:241–246.
4. Feld R, Rubinstein LV, Weisenberger TH. Sites of recurrence in resected stage I non-small cell lung cancer: a guide for future studies. *J Clin Oncol* 1984;2:1352–1358.
5. Port JL, Kent MS, Korst RJ, et al. Tumor size predicts survival within stage IA non-small cell lung cancer. *Chest* 2003;124:1828–1833.
6. Roth JA, Fossella F, Komaki R, et al. A randomized trial comparing perioperative chemotherapy and surgery with surgery alone in respectable stage IIIA MO non-small cell lung cancer. *J Natl Cancer Inst* 1994;86:673–680.
7. Rosell R, Gomez-Codina J, Camps C, et al. A randomized trial comparing preoperative chemotherapy plus surgery with surgery alone in patients with non-small cell lung cancer. *N Engl J Med* 1994;330:15308.
8. Non-small cell lung cancer clinical practice guidelines in oncology. *JNCCN* 2004;2:94–124.
9. Non-small Cell Lung Cancer Collaborative Group. Chemotherapy in non-small cell lung cancer: a meta-analysis using updated data on individual patients from 52 randomized clinical trials. *BMJ* 1995;311:899–909.
10. Arriagada R, Bergman B, Dunant A, et al. Cisplatin-based adjuvant chemotherapy in patients with completely resected non-small cell lung cancer. *N Engl J Med* 2004;350:351–360.
11. Winton TL, Livingston R, Johnson D, et al. Vinorelbine plus cisplatin vs. observation in resected non-small cell lung cancer. *N Engl J Med* 2005;352:2589–2597.
12. Strauss GM, Herndon J, Maddus A, et al. Randomized clinical trial of adjuvant chemotherapy with paclitaxel and carboplatin following resection in stage IB non-small cell lung cancer (NSCLC): report of cancer and leukemia group B (CALGB) protocol 9633 [abstract]. *Proc Am Soc Clin Oncol* 2004; abstract 7019.
13. Alam N, Shepherd FA, Winton T, et al. Compliance with post-operative adjuvant chemotherapy in non-small cell lung cancer: An analysis of National

Cancer Institute of Canada and intergroup trial JBR.10 and a review of the literature. *Lung Cancer* 2005;47:385–394.

14. Goldie D, Coldman A. A mathematic model for relating the drug sensitivity of tumors to their spontaneous mutation rate. *Cancer Treat Rep* 1979;63:1727–1733.

15. Siegenthaler MP, Pisters KM, Merriman KW, et al. Preoperative chemotherapy for lung cancer does not increase surgical morbidity. *Ann Thorac Surg* 2001;71:1105–1112.

16. Warram J. Preoperative irradiation of cancer of the lung: final report of a therapeutic trial collaborative study. *Cancer* 1975;36:914–925.

17. Marks R, Streitz J, Deschamps C, et al. Response rate and toxicity of pre-operative paclitaxel and carboplatin in patients with respectable non-small cell lung cancer: a north central cancer treatment group (NCCTG) study [abstract]. *Proc Am Soc Clin Oncol* 2001; abstract 1355.

18. Pisters K, Ginsberg RJ, Giroux DJ, et al. Induction chemotherapy before surgery for early-stage lung cancer: a novel approach. *J Thorac Cardiovasc Surg* 2000;119:429–439.

19. Aydiner A, Kiyik M, Cikrikcioglu S, et al. The combination of gemcitabine and cisplatin as neo-adjuvant chemotherapy for early stage non-small cell lung carcinoma (NSCLC): an interim analysis of a phase II trial [abstract]. *Proc Am Soc Clin Oncol* 2005; abstract 7303.

20. DePierre A, Milleron B, Moro-Sibilot D, et al. Preoperative chemotherapy followed by surgery compared with primary surgery in respectable stage I (except T1N0), II, and IIIa non-small cell lung cancer. *J Clin Oncol* 2001;20:247–253.

21. Pisters K, Vallieres E, Bunn P, et al. S9900: a phase III trial of surgery alone or surgery plus preoperative (preop) paclitaxel/carboplatin (PC) chemotherapy in early stage non-small cell lung cancer (NSCLC): Preliminary results [abstract]. *Proc Am Soc Clin Oncol* 2005; abstract 7012.

22. Scagliotti GV. Preliminary results of Ch.E.S.T: a phase III study of surgery alone or surgery plus preoperative gemcitabine-cisplatin in clinical early stages non-small cell lung cancer (NSCLC) [abstract]. *Proc Am Soc Clin Oncol* 2005; abstract 7023.

23. Huang Y, Wu Y, Yang X. A meta-analysis of neo-adjuvant chemotherapy for respectable stage 1–3A non-small cell lung cancer [abstract]. *Proc Am Soc Clin Oncol* 2005; abstract 7265.

10
Induction Therapy for Stage IIIA (N2) Lung Cancer

Shari L. Meyerson and David H. Harpole, Jr.

One of the major goals of the International Staging System for Lung Cancer, first introduced in 1986 and subsequently revised in 1997, was the separation of patients into potentially resectable and unresectable categories. This dividing line was set between stage IIIA and stage IIIB disease with contralateral lymph node metastases or local involvement of unresectable or marginally resectable structures defining the limits of surgical treatment. The advent of modern cancer therapy with multimodality approaches including surgery, chemotherapy, and radiation therapy has raised significant questions that are still not completely resolved as to the best approach for patients with potentially resectable stage IIIA (N2) disease at presentation. These questions were initially triggered in the early 1980s by the dismal survival, often less than 5% at 5 years, of stage IIIA (N2) patients treated with surgery alone, surgery plus radiotherapy, or radiotherapy alone, which were the common approaches at that time.[1,2] The recognition that stage IIIA non-small cell lung cancer (NSCLC) is a systemic disease with micrometastases present at the time of initial treatment in the vast majority of patients has changed the approach to treatment from one of local control with surgery and radiation to systemic control with the addition of chemotherapy. However, the optimum components, dosing, and timing of the treatment plan remain the subject of active investigation.

10.1. Development of Induction Therapy as Common Practice

The standard of care in the early 1980s included three options for the treatment of stage IIIA (N2) NSCLC: surgery alone, radiation therapy alone, or combined surgery and radiation therapy. With the new understanding of lung cancer as a systemic disease, several phase III studies comparing radiation alone with chemoradiation were published, including a meta-analysis of 14 trials involving 2589 patients.[3] This meta-analysis demonstrated a survival advantage in the combined chemoradiation group, reducing the risk of death by 12% at 1 year and 17% at 3 years. The most influential of the individual trials was the Cancer and Leukemia Group B (CALGB) 8433 trial published in the New England Journal of Medicine in 1990.[4] One hundred fifty-five patients were randomized to either chemoradiation (cisplatin and vinblastine followed by 60Gy radiation) or the same dose of radiation alone. Chemoradiation produced an increased response rate (56% vs. 43%) as well as statistically significant increases in median and long-term survival (median survival, 13.7 months vs. 9.6 months; long-term survival, 17% vs. 6% at 5 years). Encouraging results of adding chemotherapy to the local treatment of regionally advanced NSCLC led to a proliferation of studies on induction chemotherapy with or without radiation.

TABLE 10.1. Phase II trials of induction therapy for stage IIIA (N2) NSCLC.

Institution	Patients	Regimen	Resectability	Median survival	Long-term survival
		Induction chemotherapy only			
DFCI, Boston[5]	34	Cisplatin, 5-FU, leucovorin	62	18	18% (4 years)
CALGB 8935[6]	74	Cisplatin, vinblastine	62	15	23% (3 years)
MSK, NY[7]	136	Cisplatin, mitomycin, vindesine	65	19	17% (5 years)
Toronto[8]	39	Cisplatin, mitomycin, vindesine	56	19	26% (3 years)
		Induction chemotherapy and radiation therapy			
CALGB 8634[9]	41	Cisplatin, vinblastine, 5-FU	61	16	22% (9 years)
LCSG[10]	85	Cisplatin, 5-FU	52	13	20% (3 years)
Rush, Chicago[11]	85	Cisplatin, 5-FU, +/− etoposide	70	36	40% (3 years)

Abbreviations: CALGB, Cancer and Leukemia Group B; DFCI, Dana Farber Cancer Institute; LCSG, Lung Cancer Study Group; MSK, Memorial Sloan-Kettering; SWOG, Southwest Oncology Group.

From the mid-1980s to the mid-1990s, more than 30 phase II trials investigating induction therapy including over 1000 patients were published. Table 10.1 includes a representative sample of these studies. The first group investigated the effects of induction chemotherapy alone while the second group included radiotherapy in the regimen. Chemotherapy agents and doses as well as radiation doses and timing varied widely in these studies, making it somewhat difficult to draw uniform conclusions. However, these trials did identify several important overall concepts. First, clinical response to treatment is associated with increased resectability, most importantly an increased ability to achieve complete resection. Second, pathological complete resection leads to increased survival. Third, one subgroup of resected patients demonstrated improved survival, namely those with sterilization of mediastinal lymph nodes. Fourth, preoperative therapy shifts the pattern of recurrence from both local and distant disease to mostly distant disease.

These phase II studies paved the way for a series of small phase III studies that largely defined care for stage IIIA patients over the next decade. The first, published in 1992, came from the National Cancer Institute.[13] Twenty-seven patients with histologically confirmed stage IIIA (N2) NSCLC were prospectively randomized to either preoperative chemotherapy followed by surgery and postoperative chemotherapy or initial surgery followed by mediastinal radiation. Response to induction therapy was seen in 62% of the chemotherapy patients. Complete resection was able to be performed in 85% of patients

in each group. Results showed a trend towards increased disease-free survival (13 months vs. 6 months) and overall survival (29 months vs. 16 months) favoring the chemotherapy group; due to small sample size and limited follow-up, this did not reach statistical significance.

Two other prospective, randomized trials of induction therapy were both originally published in 1994. The first, from Barcelona, Spain, randomized 60 patients to either preoperative chemotherapy followed by surgery followed by mediastinal irradiation or initial surgery followed by mediastinal irradiation.[14] The response rate was 60% in the chemotherapy group. This study was stopped early when interim analysis identified a significant survival advantage for those patients receiving induction therapy. The median disease-free survival in the chemotherapy group was 20 months compared to 5 months in the surgery-alone group. Similarly, the overall survival was 26 months in the chemotherapy group compared to 8 months in the surgery-alone group. Updated results of this study were published in 1999 showing persistence of the survival advantage, with chemotherapy patients achieving 3- and 5-year survival rates of 20% and 17%, respectively, while in the primary surgical group only 5% survived 3 years and there were no 5-year survivors.[1]

The second study published in 1994 came from the MD Anderson Cancer Center in Texas.[15] Similar to the Barcelona study, 60 patients were randomized to receive induction chemotherapy plus surgery or surgery alone. Postoperative radiation therapy was performed as well in greater than 50% of patients in both arms of the study.

The induction therapy group had an estimated median survival of 64 months compared to 11 months in the surgery-alone group. An update of this study was published in 1998 demonstrating persistence of the survival benefit for induction therapy patients.[16] Median survival in the induction therapy group was 21 months compared to 14 months in the surgery-alone group. Three- and 5-year survival also significantly favored the induction therapy group (43% and 36% vs. 19% and 15%). Several criticisms of these trials have been advanced, including small sample sizes and early termination. Issues also have been raised that are specific to the Barcelona study: poorer than expected survival for the primary surgical arm, and possible imbalance in the two arms in terms of biochemical markers of disease virulence.

A decade later two additional trials challenged these conclusions. A French trial led by Depierre randomized 345 patients with stage IB-IIIA NSCLC to either primary surgery or chemotherapy before and after surgery.[17] Radiation therapy was given to all patients with either T3 or N2 disease. The trial demonstrated a trend towards improved survival in the chemotherapy arm (37 months vs. 26 months). However, subset analysis demonstrated improved survival in stage I and II but not stage IIIA patients. A second trial, JCOG 9209 from Japan, randomized 62 patients to receive induction chemotherapy followed by surgery or surgery alone.[18] Median and overall survival were not different between the two groups. This trial was, however, terminated early due to slow accrual that lowered its statistical power and could have affected the conclusions.

10.2. Risks of Surgery after Induction Therapy

As more reports of phase II and phase III trials of induction therapy appeared in the early 1990s, there was a simultaneous growth in reports of increased morbidity and mortality related to surgery after induction therapy. In 1993, the group from the Fox Chase Cancer Center in Philadelphia published a case series of 13 patients undergoing resection after combined chemotherapy and high-dose radiotherapy (60 Gy).[19] Of the six patients in whom lobectomy was performed,

there were no deaths and only one patient developed a culture-negative adult respiratory distress syndrome picture (ARDS). Of the seven patients undergoing pneumonectomy, five developed ARDS with two deaths and there was one additional death from bronchopleural fistula for a total mortality rate of 43%. Several other studies have also shown a high incidence of postoperative ARDS and bronchopleural fistula when pneumonectomy is required after induction therapy.[20,21]

More recently, with recognition of the potential problems specific to induction therapy, outcomes have improved, especially for patients requiring pneumonectomy.[22,23] Anesthesia techniques, such as careful attention to limiting barotrauma to the contralateral lung and limiting total fluid administration, as well as surgical techniques with routine use of muscle flaps to protect exposed bronchial stumps, have combined to decrease the incidence of high mortality complications such as ARDS and bronchopleural fistula.

10.3. Role of Surgery for Stage IIIA (N2) Non-Small Cell Lung Cancer

One conclusion that has become resoundingly clear from the past two decades of research is that response to induction therapy, specifically sterilization of mediastinal lymph nodes, is highly predictive of improved survival. A study from the Dana Farber Cancer Institute specifically investigated the impact of nodal stage after induction therapy on survival.[24] They showed that patients downstaged to N0 at the time of resection had a median survival of 21 months and a 5-year survival of 36%. This was significantly better than patients with residual N1 or N2 disease, for whom median survival was 16 months with only 9% 5-year survival. Interestingly, there was no difference between residual N1 and N2 disease in terms of survival. A second report from Switzerland studied a similar group of patients treated with induction therapy.[25] They concluded that the two most important factors for survival were the ability to achieve pathological complete resection and nodal downstaging. The Swiss group did report a benefit in patients downstaged to N1 that was intermediate between those with mediastinal clearance and residual N2 disease. These studies, as well as many others, have led many surgeons and oncologists to recommend resection only for patients with nodal downstaging after induction therapy.

The overwhelming importance of response to induction therapy leads to questions as to whether surgery itself adds to survival in patients responding to induction therapy. This is an important question given the potential added difficulty, morbidity, and mortality of resection after induction therapy. The North American Intergroup trial INT 0139 was designed to answer this question.[26] This trial enrolled 396 patients with stage IIIA (N2) NSCLC. Patients were initially randomized to either a surgical or nonsurgical arm. All patients received induction chemoradiotherapy with two cycles of cisplatin and etoposide concurrently with radiotherapy of 45 Gy. All patients were then restaged to evaluate response. Patients in the surgical arm without evidence of disease progression then underwent resection followed by two more cycles of chemotherapy. In the nonsurgical arm, radiation was continued without a treatment break to 61 Gy followed by the same two cycles of chemotherapy as the surgical arm. Sterilization of mediastinal nodes occurred in 46% of surgical patients with a 3-year overall survival of 53% in that subgroup. Progression-free survival significantly favored the surgical arm (median, 13 months vs. 10 months; 5-year survival, 22% vs. 11%). However, overall survival showed only a trend towards better outcomes in the surgical group. Overall survival did begin to separate in the latter part of the curve and may become significant over time. One reason for these results may be the higher percentage of treatment-related deaths in the surgical arm. Thirty-day mortality in surgical patients was 7.9%; the vast majority of these deaths were in patients undergoing postinduction pneumonectomy (14 of 16 deaths). Subgroup analysis was performed to investigate the effect of resection type on survival. Case-matched non–surgical arm patients were identified for the pneumonectomy and lobectomy patients. The analysis demonstrated a significant improved overall and disease-free survival for patients who underwent lobectomy, but the opposite was true if a pneumonectomy was required. These data suggested that induction chemotherapy plus lobectomy was the recommended treatment for patients with stage IIIA (N2) NSCLC, but patients who had larger tumors which may require a pneumonectomy should be treated with definitive chemoradiotherapy.

10.4. Optimal Induction Therapy for Stage IIIA (N2) Non-Small Cell Lung Cancer

Although together the three phase III studies comparing induction therapy with surgery alone only included 147 patients, the highly publicized beneficial results of chemotherapy led to a shift in the way stage IIIA NSCLC is treated. Induction therapy for stage IIIA (N2) NSCLC patients has become the standard approach, with most oncologists employing preoperative chemotherapy with or without the addition of radiotherapy. The optimal choice of chemotherapy regimen is less clear given the wide variety of regimens utilized in both the phase II and phase III trials. Many oncologists also include preoperative radiotherapy despite the fact that radiation use in all of the phase II and phase III trials was highly variable and has never been systematically evaluated.

The Radiation Therapy and Oncology Group (RTOG) and Southwest Oncology Group (SWOG) are sponsoring an ongoing trial (RTOG 0412/SWOG S0332) that opened to accrual in April 2005. The goal of this trial is to specifically investigate radiation as part of an induction therapy regimen for stage IIIA (N2) NSCLC. Five hundred seventy-four patients will be randomized to one of two arms. The first arm will receive induction therapy with cisplatin/docetaxel. The second arm will receive the same chemotherapy with the addition of radiation to 50 Gy. All patients without disease progression will then undergo resection followed by consolidation chemotherapy. Hopefully this trial will clarify the role of induction radiation therapy.

10.5. Summary of Current Evidence for Induction Therapy

The role of induction therapy for stage IIIA (N2) NSCLC has yet to be completely defined. Three generally concordant small randomized, controlled trials provide the evidentiary basis for the current generalized practice of induction therapy in some form for all patients with stage IIIA (N2) NSCLC thought to be resection candidates (recommendation grade A). Some evidence exists that patients who will still require pneumonectomy after induction therapy may be better served by definitive chemoradiotherapy (recommendation grade B). Evidence for what should constitute induction therapy is much less robust. There have been no systematic studies of what chemotherapeutic agents produce the best outcomes when used in induction therapy, and agent choice in any individual trial generally represents investigator and institutional bias as to preferred agents. The only overall theme in the majority of phase II and III is the inclusion of a platinum agent in the proscribed therapy, which is based on historical studies of agents with activity against NSCLC (recommendation grade C). As newer, potentially less toxic agents are developed, these should be studied systematically in comparison to current regimens using large multiinstitutional trials. Specific evidence for inclusion of radiation therapy in induction regimens is sparse, mostly based on the historical use of radiation as a primary mode of treatment for locally advanced lung cancer (recommendation grade D). However, an ongoing well-designed, randomized, controlled trial (RTOG 0412/SWOG S0332)

seeks to provide definitive evidence as to the importance of radiation. If radiation appears to be an important part of induction therapy, further studies will be needed to define dose and timing. If radiation does not contribute significantly to outcomes, perhaps induction with chemotherapy alone can be used as a strategy to reduce toxicity and allow more patients to undergo resection with decreased morbidity and mortality.

Induction therapy should be recommended for all patients with stage IIIA (N2) NSCLC thought to be resection candidates (level of evidence 1; recommendation grade A).

Patients who will still require pneumonectomy after induction therapy may be better served by definitive chemoradiotherapy (evidence level 1 to 2; recommendation grade B).

A platinum-based agent in the standard systemic therapy against NSCLC (evidence level 2 to 3; recommendation grade C).

Inclusion of radiation therapy in induction regimens is common but has not been adequately studied; its use is based on the historical role of radiation as a primary mode of treatment for locally advanced lung cancer (evidence level 4 to 5; recommendation grade D).

References

1. Rosell R, Gomez-Codina J, Camps C, et al. Preresectional chemotherapy in stage IIIA non-small-cell lung cancer: a 7-year assessment of a randomized controlled trial. *Lung Cancer* 1999;47:7–14.
2. Martini N, Flehinger BJ. The role of surgery in N2 lung cancer. *Surg Clin N Am* 1987;67:1037–1049.
3. Pritchard RS, Anthony SP. Chemotherapy plus radiotherapy compared with radiotherapy alone in the treatment of locally advanced, unresectable, non-small cell lung cancer. *Ann Intern Med* 1996;125:723–729.
4. Dillman RO, Seagren S, Propert K, et al. A randomized trial of induction chemotherapy plus high-dose radiation versus radiation alone in stage III non-small cell lung cancer. *N Engl J Med* 1990;323:940–945.
5. Elias AD, Skarin AT, Leong T, et al. Neoadjuvant therapy for surgically staged IIIA N2 non-small cell lung cancer (NSCLC). *Lung Cancer* 1997;17:147–161.
6. Sugarbaker DJ, Herndon J, Kohman LJ, et al. Results of Cancer and Leukemia Group B Protocol 8935: a multiinstitutional phase II trimodality trial for stage IIIA (N2) non-small cell lung cancer. *J Thorac Cardiovasc Surg* 1995;109:473–485.
7. Martini N, Kris MG, Flehinger BJ, et al. Preoperative chemotherapy for stage IIIA (N2) lung cancer: the Sloan Kettering experience with 136 patients. *Ann Thorac Surg* 1993;55:1365–1374.
8. Burkes RL, Ginsberg RJ, Shepard FA, et al. Induction chemotherapy with mitomycin, vindesine and cisplatin for stage III unresectable non-small cell lung cancer: results of a Toronto phase II trial. *J Clin Oncol* 1992;10:580–586.
9. Strauss GM, Herndon JE, Sherman DD, et al. Neoadjuvant chemotherapy and radiotherapy followed by surgery in stage IIIA non-small cell carcinoma of the lung: report of a Cancer and Leukemia Group B phase II study. *J Clin Oncol* 1992;10:1237–1244.

10. Weiden P, Piantadosi S. Preoperative chemotherapy (cisplatin and fluorouracil) and radiation therapy in stage III non-small cell lung cancer: a phase II study of the Lung Cancer Study Group. *J Natl Cancer Inst* 1991;83:266–272.

11. Faber LP, Kittle CF, Warren WH, et al. Preoperative chemotherapy and irradiation for stage III non-small cell lung cancer. *Ann Thorac Surg* 1989;47:669–675.

12. Albain KS, Rusch VW, Crowley JJ, et al. Concurrent cisplatin/etoposide plus chest radiotherapy followed by surgery for stages IIIA (N2) and IIIB non-small cell lung cancer: mature results of Southwest Oncology Group phase II study 8805. *J Clin Oncol* 1995;13:1880–1892.

13. Pass HI, Pogrebniak HW, Steinberg SM, et al. Randomized trial of neoadjuvant therapy for lung cancer: interim analysis. *Ann Thorac Surg* 1992;53:992–998.

14. Rosell R, Gomez-Codina J, Camps C, et al. A randomized trial comparing preoperative chemotherapy plus surgery with surgery alone in patients with non-small cell lung cancer. *N Engl J Med* 1994;330:153–158.

15. Roth JA, Fossella F, Komaki R, et al. A randomized trial comparing preoperative chemotherapy and surgery with surgery alone in resectable stage IIIA non-small cell lung cancer. *J Natl Cancer Inst* 1994;86:673–680.

16. Roth JA, Atkinson EN, Fossella F, et al. Long-term follow-up of patients enrolled in a randomized trial comparing perioperative chemotherapy and surgery with surgery alone in resectable stage IIIA non-small cell lung cancer. *Lung Cancer* 1998;21:1–6.

17. Depierre A, Milleron B, Moro-Sibilot D, et al. Preoperative chemotherapy followed by surgery compared with primary surgery in resectable stage I (except T1N0), II and IIIa non-small-cell lung cancer. *J Clin Oncol* 2002;20:247–253.

18. Nagai K, Tsuchiya R, Mori T, et al. A randomized trial comparing induction chemotherapy followed by surgery with surgery alone for patients with stage IIIA N2 non-small cell lung cancer (JCOG 9209). *J Thorac Cardiovasc Surg* 2003;125:254–260.

19. Fowler WC, Langer CJ, Curran WJ, et al. Postoperative complications after combined neoadjuvant treatment of lung cancer. *Ann Thorac Surg* 1993;55:986–989.

20. Deutsch M, Crawford J, Leopold K, et al. Phase II study of chemotherapy and radiation therapy with thoracotomy in the treatment of clinically staged IIIA non-small cell lung cancer. *Cancer* 1994;74:1243–1252.

21. Doddoli C, Thomas P, Thiron X, et al. Postoperative complications in relation with induction therapy for lung cancer. *Eur J Cardiothorac Surg* 2001;20:385–390.

22. Siegenthaler MP, Pisters KM, Merriman KW, et al. Preoperative chemotherapy for lung cancer does not increase surgical morbidity. *Ann Thorac Surg* 2001;71:1105–1112.

23. Sonett JR, Suntharalingam M, Edelman MJ, et al. Pulmonary resection after curative intent radiotherapy (>59 Gy) and concurrent chemotherapy in non-small-cell lung cancer. *Ann Thorac Surg* 2004;78:1200–1206.

24. Bueno R, Richards WG, Swanson SJ, et al. Nodal stage after induction therapy for stage IIIA lung cancer determines patient survival. *Ann Thorac Surg* 2000;70:1826–1831.

25. Betticher DC, Schmitz SH, Totsch M, et al. Mediastinal lymph node clearance after docetaxel-cisplatin neoadjuvant chemotherapy is prognostic of survival in patients with stage IIIA pN2 non-small-cell lung cancer: a multicenter phase II trial. *J Clin Oncol* 2003;21:1752–1759.

26. Albain KS, Swann RS, Rusch VR, et al. Phase III study of concurrent chemotherapy and radiotherapy (CT/RT) vs CT/RT followed by surgical resection for stage IIIA(pN2) non-small cell lung cancer (NSCLC): outcomes update of North American Intergroup 0139 (RTOG 93-09). *J Clin Oncol* 2005;23(suppl 16):624S.

11
Adjuvant Postoperative Therapy for Completely Resected Stage I Lung Cancer

Thomas A. D'Amato and Rodney J. Landreneau

Surgical resection is the standard of care for early-stage non-small cell lung cancer (NSCLC). A significant body of evidence from population-based observational studies shows that surgery offers patients the highest cure rate. Nevertheless, following lobectomy or pneumonectomy and mediastinal lymph node staging as standard therapy, only a 67% 5-year survival for stage IA (T1N0) and a 57% 5-year survival for stage IB (T2N0) is expected,[1,2] with most patients succumbing to metastatic disease. A subset of patients exists with clinical stage I disease and limited cardiopulmonary reserve where a sublobar resection is required and is associated with an increased frequency of local recurrence compared to lobectomy or pneumonectomy.[3] Traditionally, efforts to improve survival and decrease local recurrence following lung resection for NSCLC have consisted of adjuvant chemotherapy and radiation therapy alone or in combination.

To date, most randomized adjuvant therapy clinical trials for resected NSCLC have enrolled patients following complete surgical resection, yet the results were inconsistent. Heterogeneous patient populations, particularly with regard to stage and treatment modality, underpowered study design, and treatment-related toxicity, likely contributed to mixed results. Nevertheless, these early clinical trials did provide some evidence to support the use of postoperative therapy in selected patients with early-stage disease, and are the basis for more recently reported adjuvant trials.

This chapter will focus on adjuvant therapies following resection of early-stage NSCLC that

include mostly data from radiation therapy and chemotherapy trials. From a historical perspective, postoperative therapy for more advanced disease served as the background for contemporary clinical trials from which an evidence-based approach for adjuvant therapy in resected stage I NSCLC is formulated. Some laboratory data and observational clinical reports described in this chapter have not been validated by randomized trials, yet these studies may be helpful to stratify patients at high risk for recurrence and identify patients who may be resistant to adjuvant chemotherapy. These reports are included in this chapter to support evidence-based individualized patient treatment plans. Such laboratory and clinical findings may ultimately create a bridge towards the development of targeted therapeutics.

11.1. Adjuvant Radiation Therapy

For more than 20 years, postoperative radiation therapy was recommended to provide local control for residual disease following presumed R0 resection and particularly for occult mediastinal disease.[4-8] An analysis performed by the Post-Operative Radiation Therapy (PORT) Meta-analysis Trialist Group[9] reviewed nine randomized clinical trials that included 2128 patients, 562 of which were stage I. A significant adverse effect of adjuvant radiation therapy on survival {hazard ratio 1.21 [95% confidence interval (CI), 1.08–1.34]} corresponded to a 21% relative increase in the risk of death equivalent to an absolute decrement of 7% at 2 years, reducing overall survival from 55% to 48%. Subgroup analyses suggest that this adverse effect was greatest for patients with stage I-II, and N0-N1 disease (evidence level 1a). Controversy regarding the use of older ^{90}Co regimens in six of these studies prompted another meta-analysis that segregated ^{90}Co radiation delivery with linear accelerators (LINACs),[10] including three additional randomized trials[11-13] employing modern LINACs (evidence level 1b). Cobalt radiotherapy revealed no survival benefit [hazard ratio 1.22 (95% CI, 1.09–1.35)], whereas treatment with LINACs was associated with a marginal survival benefit in NSCLC patients receiving adjuvant radiation therapy [hazard ratio 0.86 (95% CI, 0.73–1.01)]. This latter meta-analysis[13] included one study restricted to patients with stage I disease (evidence level 1a).

Local recurrence in stage I NSCLC is noted in 19% of patients following sublobar resection, compared to 9% of patients following lobectomy.[14] In patients with impaired cardiopulmonary function in whom sublobar resection is required, local recurrence is reduced by applying "postage stamp" radiation therapy[15] to resection margins (evidence level 3). Difficulties with dose planning following resection, adjacent pulmonary toxicity from large treatment volumes, and patient compliance may compromise the suitability of postoperative radiotherapy for these patients,[16,17] (evidence level 2b).

Intraoperative brachytherapy with implantation of ^{125}I radiolabled beads, initially advocated for stage III disease,[18] was used on a small cohort of patients following video-assisted thoracoscopic wedge resection performed on stage I patients with poor pulmonary function.[19] This feasibility study was followed by a more comprehensive retrospective multicenter study of 291 patients in which sublobar resection was performed on 124 patients, 60 of whom had ^{125}I brachytherapy applied to resection margins with a prescribed dose of 10 to 12 Gy and a depth of 0.5 cm. Median follow-up was 34 months. Treatment with sublobar resection plus intraoperative brachytherapy[20] decreased the local recurrence rate significantly from 17% to 3%, compared to patients who only underwent sublobar resection [evidence level 3]. These findings subsequently prompted the recent development of a random-

ized phase III clinical trial, currently in the accrual phase, by the American College of Surgeons Oncology Group, ACOSOG Z4032, which will compare sublobar resection with brachytherapy to sublobar resection alone.[21]

There is little evidence supporting the use of postoperative external beam radiation therapy following lobectomy or pneumonectomy for resected stage I NSCLC (level of evidence 1a-1b; recommendation grade A). Postoperative external beam radiation therapy applied to resection margins following sublobar resection may decrease local recurrence rates (level of evidence 2b-3; recommendation grade B), but it is difficult to control the prescribed dose to the target volume and it may result in pulmonary toxicity. Intraoperative brachytherapy with implanted ^{125}I seeds may be a useful adjuvant radiation therapy modality to reduce the rate of local recurrence and attenuate adjacent lung injury following sublobar resection of early stage NSCLC that may benefit patients with impaired cardiopulmonary reserve (level of evidence 3; recommendation grade B).

> There is little evidence supporting the use of postoperative external beam radiation therapy following lobectomy or pneumonectomy for stage I NSCLC (level of evidence 1a to 1b; recommendation grade A).
>
> Postoperative external beam radiation therapy applied to resection margins following sublobar resection may decrease local recurrence rates (level of evidence 2b to 3; recommendation grade B).
>
> Intraoperative brachytherapy may be a useful adjunct to reduce the rate of local recurrence following sublobar resection of early stage NSCLC in patients with impaired cardiopulmonary reserve (level of evidence 3; recommendation grade B).

11.2. Adjuvant Chemotherapy

11.2.1. Platinum-Based Adjuvant Trials

Until recently, enthusiasm for adjuvant postoperative chemotherapy for early-stage NSCLC had diminished. Historically, studies performed over

30 years ago had mixed results and were underpowered. Patient populations were heterogeneous and perhaps ineffective agents were used. In 1995, a meta-analysis[22] by the Non-Small Cell Lung Cancer Collaborative Group (NSCLCCG) suggested that cisplatin-based chemotherapy without radiation improved the 5-year overall survival rate by 5% and reduced the risk of death by 13% as compared with no adjuvant therapy (level of evidence 1a). Interestingly, six cisplatin-based trials plus radiation therapy included in the meta-analysis showed a 6% lower risk of death [hazard ratio 0.94 (95% CI, 0.79–1.11); level of evidence 1b]. The results of the meta-analysis prompted several modern studies using platinum-based agents. The following interim randomized clinical trials kindled the debate over the efficacy of adjuvant chemotherapy for resected NSCLC.

The Italian IB Trial[23] enrolled 66 patients and compared postoperative cisplatin and etoposide to observation alone. Radiation therapy was not allowed. Seventy-five percent of patients received all six doses of cisplatin and etoposide in the chemotherapy arm. An 18% increase in overall survival was observed ($p = 0.04$), but the median survival in the chemotherapy arm was not reached. Disease-free survival was 77 months with chemotherapy and 22 months in the control group ($p = 0.02$; level of evidence 1b).

The North American Intergroup (INT 0115) trial comparing adjuvant cisplatin plus etoposide and radiation versus adjuvant radiation therapy alone in stage II and IIIA NSCLC[24] showed no benefit from adjuvant chemotherapy (level of evidence 1b).

The Adjuvant Lung Project Italy (ALPI) included 1209 stage I, II, or IIIA NSCLC patients, including 39% with stage I disease. Patients were treated with cisplatin, mitomycin, and vindesine. No statistically significant survival benefit was noted.[25] Toxicity from this adjuvant chemotherapy regimen likely contributed to the lack of benefit (level of evidence 1b).

Despite these negative results, and prompted in part by the results of the NSCLCCG meta-analysis,[22] the interest in adjuvant chemotherapy for resected NSCLC persisted and stimulated four prospective randomized clinical trials,[26–29] all of which included stage I patients.

The International Adjuvant Lung Cancer Trial (IALT) Collaborative Group evaluated cisplatin-based therapy in 1867 randomized stage IA-IIIA patients.[26] All but 22 had anatomical resections, 183 (10%) patients were stage IA and 498 (27%) were stage IB. All patients received a cisplatin doublet with either etoposide (57%), or a vinca alkaloid (43%) as a second agent. Radiation therapy with an average dose of 50 Gy was administered to 70% of the patients. An absolute 4% increase in overall survival was noted at 5 years ($p < 0.003$). Hazard ratios for stage-specific survival favoring adjuvant chemotherapy versus observation were significant only in patients with stage III disease (level of evidence 1b).

The Cancer and Leukemia Group B (CALGB) 9633 trial compared observation alone to adjuvant therapy with carboplatin plus paclitaxel in 344 randomized stage IB (T2N0) patients.[27] No patients received radiation therapy. At 4 years, a 12% increase in overall survival ($p < 0.028$) was observed with a median follow-up of 34 months. This is the only randomized adjuvant chemotherapy trial to demonstrate a survival advantage for patients with completely resected stage IB disease (level of evidence 1b).

The National Cancer Institute of Canada Clinical Trial Group JBR.10 trial limited enrollment to completely resected stage IB and II patients.[28] This study further confounded the role of adjuvant chemotherapy in resected NSCLC. Patients in the chemotherapy arm received cisplatin and vinorelbine. Of 482 patients randomized, 219 (45%) were stage IB. All patients were stratified based on *ras* mutation and nodal status. Radiation therapy was not permitted. Although an improvement in overall survival of 15% ($p < 0.012$) was observed in the adjuvant therapy group, upon further stratification, only patients with stage II disease had a statistically significant survival advantage (level of evidence 1b).

Results from the Adjuvant Navelbine International Trialist Association (ANITA) trial supported the findings of JBR.10 for stage IB NSCLC.[29] Cisplatin plus navelbline (vinorelbine) was used, similar to JBR.10. Randomization of 840 stage IB-IIIA patients included 301 (35%) with stage IB (T2N0) disease. Radiation therapy was permitted. Median follow-up was more than 70 months. Although chemotherapy significantly improved survival in patients with resected stage II and IIIA disease, no benefit was observed in stage IB patients (level of evidence 1b).

11.2.2. Uracil/Tegafur (UFT) Adjuvant Trials

Oral adjuvant therapy with uracil/tegafur has been studied only in Japan and results have not been confirmed by trails from other countries. Uracil/tegafur is not available in the United States and North American trials are lacking. The NSCLCCG included UFT in their 1995 meta-analysis[22] and although an absolute survival benefit of 4% was noted, it was not statically significant [hazard ratio 0.89 (95% CI, 0.72–1.11); $p = 0.30$; level of evidence 1a]. The largest trial utilizing adjuvant UFT for completely resected stage I NSCLC enrolled 979 patients with adenocarcinoma histology only and was stratified by tumor stage (T1 vs. T2), age, and sex.[30] A 3% improvement in overall 5-year survival ($p = 0.047$) was noted, particularly for stage IB disease, but disease-free survival was unaffected (level of evidence 1b).

Subsequently, a meta-analysis of individual patient data for 2003 patients from six studies including 1308 (T1N0) and 674 (T2N0) patients evaluated survival in patients receiving UFT plus surgery versus surgery alone.[31] Oral UFT significantly improved overall survival at 7 years by 7%

[hazard ratio 0.74 (95% CI, 0.61–0.88); $p = 0.001$; level of evidence 1a].

11.2.3. Chemotherapy Related Toxicity and Compliance with Planned Therapy

All anti-neoplastic drugs exhibit toxicity that often limits dosing or delays planned therapy in multicycle regimens. Toxicity data from the four most recently reported clinical trials described above are summarized in Table 11.1. In the IALT trial, 26% of the patients had incomplete treatment and more than half of the patients in these groups sustained adverse effects.[26] Lethal toxicity from platinum was not dose dependent and ranged from 0.6% to 2.4%.

Evaluation of the compliance with therapy for CALBG 9633 revealed that information on chemotherapy delivery was available on only 124/173 (72%), and even though 85% of these patients received four doses, 35% of this group required dose reductions and only 55% received four cycles at full dose.[27] Adverse event data were available for 149/173 (86%) of patients in the chemotherapy arm.

Vinorelbine dosing was reduced in the JBR.10 trial due the high rate of febrile neutropenia, and 19% of patients were hospitalized due to chemotherapy-related toxicity. Only 48% of patients completed four planned cycles of cisplatin-based therapy.[28]

TABLE 11.1. Stage response and toxicity in adjuvant chemotherapy trials for NSCLC.

Adjuvant trial	Regimen planned	Stage included	Patients completing therapy (%)	Stage response	Chemotherapy-related deaths	Grade 3 or 4 toxicity (%)
IALT	Cisplatin + VP-16 or vinca alkaloid	I, II, III	628/851 (74)	IIIA	7	23[a]
CALBG 9633	Carboplatin + paclitaxel	IB	68/124 (55)	IB	0	36[b]
JBR-10	Cisplatin + vinorelbine	IB, II	110/242 (48)[c,d]	II	2	73
ANITA[f]	Cisplatin + vinorelbine	IB, II, IIIA	368/407 (90)[e]	II, IIIA	5	86

[a]Only grade 4 toxicity reported.
[b]Toxicity data available for 149/173 (86%) of patients randomized, but data were available in only 124/173 (72%) of patients who received chemotherapy and only 55% received full dose.
[c]Dose reduction was required for 77%.
[d]Sixty-five percent completed three cycles.
[e]Percentage of patients receiving chemotherapy following randomization only 56% completed vinorelbine therapy, 76% completed cisplatin therapy.
[f]Thirty-nine percent received chemotherapy at relapse.

Only 56% of the planned doses for navelbine and 76% for cisplatin were given in the ANITA trial.[29] Grade 3 or 4 neutropenia occurred with 70% of doses prescribed in 80% of the patients receiving chemotherapy.

Based on these modern platinum-based adjuvant chemotherapy trials, patients with early-stage disease and good performance status, adjuvant chemotherapy for completely resected stage IB, IIA, IIB, and IIIA NSCLC became an accepted standard of care[31] even though only one clinical trial (CALGB 9633) showed improvement in stage IB disease[27] (level of evidence 1b). Yet in all adjuvant chemotherapy trials, anti-neoplastic regimens exhibited predictable toxicity. Although survival advantages were noted, the majority of patients treated did not benefit from adjuvant chemotherapy (level of evidence 1b).

There is evidence from only one randomized, controlled trial that patients with stage IB disease may benefit from postoperative platinum-based chemotherapy (level of evidence 1b; recommendation grade A). Chemotherapy toxicity, performance status, and patient preferences should be considered when recommending postoperative chemotherapy. There is some evidence to support the use of adjuvant UFT chemotherapy (where available) in selected patients with completely resected stage IA and IB NSCLC having adenocarcinoma histology (level of evidence 1b; recommendation grade A). Following sublobar resection, selected patients with early-stage disease and good performance status may benefit from adjuvant chemotherapy (stage IB), and intra-operative brachytherapy (stage IA, IB; level of evidence 1b-3; recommendation grade B). There is inconclusive evidence to support combined chemotherapy and external beam radiation therapy for stage I disease completely resected by lobectomy or pneumonectomy (level of evidence 1a; recommendation grade B).

> Patients with stage IB disease may benefit from postoperative platinum-based chemotherapy (level of evidence 1b; recommendation grade A).
> Adjuvant UFT chemotherapy may benefit patients with completely resected stage IA and IB NSCLC having adenocarcinoma histology (level of evidence 1b; recommendation grade A).

> Following sublobar resection, patients with early-stage disease and good performance status may benefit from adjuvant chemotherapy (stage IB), and intra-operative brachytherapy (stages IA, IB) (level of evidence 1b to 3; recommendation grade B).
> There is insufficient evidence to support combined chemotherapy and external beam radiation therapy for stage I disease completely resected by lobectomy or pneumonectomy (level of evidence 1a; recommendation grade B).

11.3. Laboratory Testing and Pharmacogenomics

11.3.1. In Vitro Drug Resistance Testing Assays

Tumor resistance to chemotherapy is multifactorial. Failure of clinical responsiveness may be related not only to an anti-neoplastic agent's ineffectiveness, but also to anatomical barriers, tumor vascularity, and to host factors of absorption, metabolism, and excretion. Drug-resistant assays obviate host factors and evaluate the in vitro tumor response to chemotherapy only.

In modern drug-resistant assays, human-tumor cell cultures are exposed to suprapharmacological doses of chemotherapeutic agents at concentrations several-fold higher than expected peak serum levels achieved in patients. Cellular proliferation is measured by ^{3}H-thymidine incorporation into DNA and compared to positive (lethal dose chemotherapy) and negative (media only) controls. Tumors are characterized as having either extreme, intermediate, or low resistance-based tumor cellular proliferation compared with controls and the entire population of tumors tested.

If a patient's tumor is resistant in vitro, then the probability of a clinical response is unlikely. In an analysis of 450 patient tumors of varied histology, only one of 127 patients with tumors showing extreme resistance [an assay result ≥1 standard deviation (SD) below the median] had a clinical response to chemotherapy.[32]

In NSCLC, only two of 20 patients' tumors exhibiting in vitro intermediate or extreme drug resistance had a clinical response to chemotherapy. Subset analysis comparing all tumor types expected to be sensitive and those expected to be resistant revealed that the proliferation assays ability to identify extreme drug resistance and to predict treatment failure (negative post-test probability of response), was independent of the expected (pretest) probability of response with a greater than 99% specificity (level of evidence 2a). Subsequent clinical application of the in vitro extreme drug resistance assay was correlative with clinical unresponsiveness to chemotherapy in breast,[33] ovarian[34,35] (level of evidence 2b), and brain[36] tumors (level of evidence 1b).

The prevalence of in vitro extreme chemotherapy resistance in 3042 resected NSCLC tumors was reported recently (level of evidence 3). For chemotherapeutic agents used as first-line therapy in the most recent adjuvant chemotherapy clinical trials, extreme or intermediate drug resistance of human NSCLC tumor cultures exposed to carboplatin was found in 1056/1565 (68%), to cisplatin in 1409/2227 (63%), to etoposide in 1581/2505 (63%), to navelbine in 603/1444 (42%), and to paclitaxel in 689/1706 (40%). Intermediate or extreme resistance to gemcitabine, an agent often administered as first-line therapy but not included in recent platinum-based adjuvant therapies, occurred in 594/823 (72%) and to doxorubicin, a drug essentially abandoned because of toxicity, occurred in 1101/1471 (75%) of tumors evaluated. Taxotere (docitaxel) extreme and intermediate resistance was noted in 273/521 (51%) of tumor cultures. Topotecan extreme or intermediate resistance occurred in 280/896 (31%) of tumors tested; yet, this agent is not considered a first-line therapy for resected NSCLC.[37]

Non-small cell lung cancer tumor culture in vitro resistance to anti-neoplastic agents is consistent with the marginal increased survival benefit (4% to 15%) in patients prescribed from adjuvant chemotherapy for completely resected NSCLC noted in recent studies.[26–30]

Chemoresistance testing for resected NSCLC may be applied clinically to "de-select" potentially ineffective agents thereby avoiding unnecessary toxicity and may encourage use of alternative targeted therapies. Clinical validation of in vitro chemotherapy resistance with respect to patient survival by randomized prospective trials is lacking and currently under development (level of evidence 4).

11.3.2. Prognostic Markers and Biological Staging

Following complete resection of stage I NSCLC, over one third of patients will develop metastatic cancer within 5 years and ultimately die following a "curative" resection. Adjuvant chemotherapy may only improve survival between 4% and 15%, such that the majority of patients endure unnecessary toxicity without a survival benefit. A priori, anatomical pathological staging is fallible.

Identification of patients at high risk for recurrence, those who are unlikely to respond to specific chemotherapeutic agents, and determining which patients may benefit from targeted therapeutics is the rationale for measuring specific biochemical markers.

Several molecular markers,[38–46] including growth factor receptors such as vascular endothelial growth factor (VEGF),[38,39] hepatocyte growth factor,[41] hormone receptors, CEA and cytokeratin isoforms,[42] metabolic enzymes,[45] proto-oncogenes, and suppressor genes[48] may portend poor prognosis (level of evidence 2a). High expression levels of ERCC1, a DNA repair enzyme, is associated with platinum drug resistance (level of evidence 1b), increased expression of ribonucleotide reductase is correlated with gemcitabine resistance,[46] and overexpression of B-tubulin III is associated with vinorelbine and paclitaxel resistance[47] (level of evidence 2a). Many of these assays are not readily available, yet may hold promise toward the development of targeted therapy and will lead to an understanding of chemotherapy unresponsiveness in future clinical trials.

Clinical application of routinely available molecular markers may also help segregate patients at high risk for recurrence. High VEGF expression and increased microvessel density in stage IB patients[43] is associated with decreased overall survival (level of evidence 3). Simultaneous expression of epidermal growth factor (EGFR) and HER2-neu in resected stage I NSCLC[44] is associated with poor survival (level of evidence 3). Phosphoglycerate kinase 1, an enzyme for glycolytic and gluconeogenic pathways, is strongly associated with poor prognosis in early-stage adenocarcinoma[45] and was validated with an independent tumor set for which clinical data were available (level of evidence 2a).

From an analysis of 275 resected stage I NSCLC patients, a retrospective analysis of histological characteristics and immunohistochemical assays showed that angiogenesis is one of the most important independent characteristic that predicts decreased disease-specific survival.[48] An additive effect for the expression of proto-oncogene erbB-2, tumor suppressor gene p53, and the proliferation marker KI-67 was seen, which correlated with decreased survival (level of evidence 2b).

Molecular staging and utilization of chemotherapy resistance testing of NSCLC tumor specimens with the cellular proliferation assay has not been clinically validated; however, based upon clinical correlation with in vitro drug-resistance testing for other solid tumors, such testing should be considered to avoid potentially ineffective agents, particularly when several different clinically equivalent regimens exist. This is probably most important for stage IB tumors (level of evidence 2a to 4; recommendation grade C). Tumor prognostic marker testing in patients with stage I NSCLC should be considered prior to recommending adjuvant chemotherapy for completely resected disease to avoid toxicity in patients with low risk for progression (level of evidence 2a; recommendation grade B). Such testing should be considered in resected stage I patients to select those patients that may be at high risk for recurrent disease (level of evidence 2b; recommendation grade B).

Based upon clinical correlation with in vitro drug-resistance testing for other solid tumors, molecular staging and utilization of chemotherapy-resistance testing of NSCLC tumor specimens should be considered for stage IB tumors (level of evidence 2a to 4; recommendation grade C).

Tumor prognostic marker testing in patients with stage I NSCLC should be considered prior to recommending adjuvant chemotherapy for completely resected disease to select those patients that may be at high risk for recurrent disease (level of evidence 2a; recommendation grade B).

Careful anatomical, histological, and particularly biological staging is necessary to develop adjuvant therapies with greater efficacy for patients with completely resected early-stage NSCLC. A new paradigm of laboratory testing prior to random treatment holds promise to increase survival for the majority of patients following adjuvant therapy.

References

1. Mountain CF. Revisions in the international system for staging lung cancer. *Chest* 1997;111: 1710–1717.
2. Ginsberg RJ, Rubinstein LV for the Lung Cancer Study Group. Randomized trial of lobectomy versus limited resection for T1 N0 non-small cell lung cancer. *Ann Thorac Surg* 1995;60:615–623.
3. Patel AN, Santos SS, De Hoyos A, et al. Clinical trials of peripheral stage I (T1N0M0) non-small cell lung cancer. *Semin Thorac Cardiovasc Surg* 2003;15:421–430.
4. Choi NC, Grillo HC, Gardiello M, et al. Basis for new strategies in postoperative radiotherapy of bronchgenic carcinoma. *Int J Radiat Oncol Biol Phys* 1980;6:31–35.
5. Kirsh MM, Sloan H. Mediastinal metastases in bronchgenic carcinoma: influence of postoperative irradiation, cell type, and location. *Ann Thorac Surg* 1982;33:459–463.
6. Sawyer TE, Bonner JA, Gould PM, et al. The impact of surgical adjuvant thoracic radiation therapy for patients with non-small cell lung carcinoma with ipsilateral mediastinal lymph node involvement. *Cancer* 1997;80:1339–1408.
7. Astudillo J, Conill C. Role of postoperative radiation therapy in stage IIIa non-small cell lung cancer. *Ann Thorac Surg* 1990;50:618–623.
8. Effects of postoperative mediastinal radiation on completely resected stage II and stage III squamous cell carcinoma of the lung. The Lung Cancer Study Group. *N Engl J Med* 1986;315:1377–1381.
9. Burdett S, Parmar MKB, Stewart LA. Postoperative radiotherapy in non-small cell lung cancer: systematic review and metaanalysis of individual patient data from nine randomized controlled trials. PORT Meta-analysis Trialists Group. *Lancet* 1998;352:257–263.
10. Sedrakyan A, Hunt I, Hill J. Multimodality treatment in non-small cell lung cancer surgery. In: Treasure T, Hunt I, Keogh B, Pagano D, eds. *The Evidence for Cardiothoracic Surgery*. tfm Publishing Ltd.; Harley, Shrewsberry, UK, 2005.

11. Mayer R, Smolle-Juettner FM, Szolar D, et al. Postoperative radiotherapy in radically resected non-small cell lung cancer. *Chest* 1997;112:954–959.

12. Feng QF, Wang M, Wang LJ, et al. A study of postoperative radiotherapy in patients with non-small cell lung cancer: a randomized trial. *Int J Radiat Oncol Biol Phys* 2000;47:925–929.

13. Trodella L, Granone P, Valente S, et al. Adjuvant radiotherapy in non-small cell lung cancer with pathological stage I: definitive results of a phase III randomized trial. *Radiother Oncol* 2002;62:11–19.

14. Landreneau RJ, Sugarbaker DJ, Mack MJ, et al. Wedge resection versus lobectomy for stage I (T1N0M0) non-small cell lung cancer. *J Thorac Cardiovasc Surg* 1997;113:691–700.

15. Miller JI, Hatcher CR. Limited resection of bronchogenic carcinoma in the patient with marked impairment of pulmonary function. *Ann Thorac Surg* 1987;44:340–343.

16. Shennib H, Bogart JA, Herndon J, et al. Thoracoscopic wedge resection and radiotherapy for T1N0 non-small cell lung cancer (NSCLC) in high risk patients: preliminary analysis of a Cancer and Leukemia Group B and Eastern Cooperative Oncology Group phase II trial [abstract]. *Int J Radiat Oncol Biol Phys* 2000;48(suppl 3): abstract 240.

17. Bogart, JA. Early stage medically inoperable non-small cell lung cancer. Current treatment. *Options Oncol* 2003;4:81–88.

18. Nori D, Li X, Pugkhem T. Intraoperative brachytherapy using Gelfoam radioactive plaque implants for resected stage III non-small cell lung cancer with positive margin: a pilot study. *J Surg Oncol* 1995;60:257–261.

19. d'Amato TA, Galloway M, Szydlowski G, et al. Intraoperative brachytherapy following thoracoscopic wedge resection of stage I lung cancer. *Chest* 1998;114:1112–1115.

20. Fernando HC, Santos RS, Benfield JR, et al. Lobar and sublobar resection with and without brachytherapy for small stage IA non-small cell lung cancer. *J Thorac Cardiovasc Surg* 2005;129:261–267.

21. American College of Surgeons Oncology Group (ACOSOG) trial Z4032. A randomized phase III study of sublobar resection versus sublobar resection plus brachytherapy in high risk patients with non-small cell lung cancer (NSCLC), 3cm or smaller. Availabe at https://www.acosog.org/studies/organ_site/thoracic/index.jsp. Accessed 8.29.06.

22. Non-Small Cell Lung Cancer Collaborative Group. Chemotherapy in non-small cell lung cancer: a meta-analysis using updated data on individual patients from 52 randomized clinical trials. *BMJ* 1995;311:899–909.

23. Mineo TC, Ambrogi V, Corsaro V, et al. Postoperative adjuvant therapy for stage IB nonsmall cell lung cancer. *Eur J Cardiothorac Surg* 2001;20:378–384.

24. Keller SM, Adak S, Wagner H, et al. A randomized trial of postoperative adjuvant therapy in patients with completely resected stage II or IIIA non-small cell lung cancer. *N Engl J Med* 2000;343:1217–1222.

25. Scagliotti GV, Fossati R, Torri V, et al. Randomized study of adjuvant chemotherapy for completely resected stage I, II, or IIIA non small-cell lung cancer. *J Natl Cancer Inst* 2003;95:1453–1461.

26. The International Adjuvant Lung Cancer Trial Collaborative Group. Cisplatin-based adjuvant chemotherapy in patients with completely resected non-small-cell lung cancer. *N Engl J Med* 2004;350:351–360.

27. Strauss GM, Herndon J, Maddaus, MA, et al. Randomized clinical trial of adjuvant chemotherapy with paclitaxel and carboplatin following resection in Stage IB non-small cell lung cancer (NSCLC): report of Cancer and Leukemia Group B (CALGB) Protocol 9633. ASCO Annual Meeting Proceedings, New Orleans, Louisiana, USA. *J Clin Oncol* 2004;22:7019.

28. Winton TL, Livingston R, Johnson D, et al. A prospective randomised trial of adjuvant vinorelbine (VIN) and cisplatin (CIS) in completely resected stage 1B and II non small cell lung cancer (NSCLC) Intergroup JBR.10. *N Engl J Med* 2005;352:2289–2297.

29. Douillard J, Rosell R, Delena M, et al. ANITA: phase III adjuvant vinorelbine (N) and cisplatin (P) versus observation (OBS) in completely resected (stage I-III) non-small-cell lung cancer (NSCLC) patients (pts): final results after 70-month median follow-up. On behalf of the Adjuvant Navelbine International Trialist Association. ASCO Annual Meeting Proceedings, Orlando, Florida, USA. *J Clin Oncol* 2005;23:7013.

30. Kato H, Ichinose Y, Ohta M, et al. A randomized trial of adjuvant chemotherapy with uracil-tegafur for adenocarcinoma of the lung. *N Engl J Med* 2004;350:1713–1721.

31. Pisters KMW. Adjuvant chemotherapy for non-small cell lung cancer – the smoke clears. *N Engl J Med* 2005;353:2640–2642.

32. Kern D, Weisenthal L. Highly specific prediction of antineoplastic drug resistance with an in vitro

assay using suprapharacologic drug exposures. *J Natl Cancer Inst* 1990;82:582–558.

33. Mehta R, Bomstein R, Yu I-R, et al. Breast cancer survival and in vitro tumor response in the extreme drug resistance assay. *Breast Cancer Res Treat* 2001;66:225–237.

34. Loizzi V, Chan JK, Osann K, et al. Survival outcomes in patients with recurrent ovarian cancer who were treated with chemoresistance assay-guided chemotherapy. *Am J Obstet Gynecol* 2003; 189:1301–1307.

35. Holloway R, Mehta R, Finkler N, et al. Association between in vitro platinum resistance in the EDR assay and clinical outcomes for ovarian cancer patients. *Gynecol Oncol* 2002;87:8–16.

36. Parker RJ, Fruehauf JP, Mehta R, et al. A prospective blinded study of predictive value of extreme drug resistance assay in patients receiving CPT-11 for recurrent glioma. *J Neurooncol* 2004;66:365–375.

37. D'amato TA, Landreneau RJ, McKenna RJ, et al. Prevalence of *in vitro* extreme chemotherapy resistance in resected non-small cell lung cancer. *Ann Thorac Surg.* 2006;81:440–447.

38. Huang C, Liu D, Masuya D, et al. Clinical application of biological markers for treatments of resectable non-small cell lung cancers. *Br J Cancer* 2005;92:1231–1239.

39. Han H, Silverman JF, Santucci TS, et al. Vascular endothelial growth factor expression in stage I non-small cell lung cancer correlates with neoangiogenesis and a poor prognosis. *Ann Surg Oncol* 2001;8:72–79.

40. Lu C, Soria J-C, Tang X, et al. Prognostic factors in resected stage I non-small cell lung cancer: a multivariate analysis of six molecular markers. *J Clin Oncol* 2004;22:4575–4583.

41. Siegfried JM, Weissfeld LA, Luketich JD, Weyant RJ, Gubish CT, Landreneau RJ. The clinical significance of hepatocyte growth factor for non-small cell lung cancer. *Ann Thorac Surg* 1998;66:1915–1918.

42. Muley T, Dienemann H, Ebert W. CYFRA 21-1 and CEA are independent prognostic factors in 153 operated stage I NSCLC patients. *Anticancer Res* 2004;24:1953–1956.

43. Mineo TC, Ambrogi V, Baldi A, et al. Prognostic impact of VEGF, CD31, CD34, and CD 105 expression and tumor vessel invasion after radical surgery for IB-IIA non-small cell lung cancer. *J Clin Pathol* 2004;57:591–597.

44. Onn A, Correa AM, Gilcrease M, et al. Synchronous overexpression of epidermal growth factor and HER2-*neu* protein is a predictor of poor outcome in patients with stage I non-small cell lung cancer. *Clin Cancer Res* 2004;10:236–243.

45. Chen G, Gharib TG, Wang H, et al. Protein profiles associated with survival in lung adenocarcinoma. *Proc Natl Acad Sci U S A* 2003;100: 13537–13532.

46. Rosell R, Fossella F, Milas L. Molecular markers and targeted therapy with novel agents: prospects in the treatment of non-small cell lung cancer. *Lung Cancer* 2002;38:S43–S49.

47. Rosell R, Cobo M, Isla D, et al. ERCC1 mRNA-based randomized phase III trial of docetaxel (doc) doublets with cisplatin (cis) or gemcitabine (gem) in stage IV non-small-cell lung cancer (NSCLC) patients (p). ASCO Annual Meeting Proceedings, Orlando, Florida, USA. *J Clin Oncol* 2005;23:7002.

48. D'Amico TA, Aloia TA, Moore M-BH, et al. Molecular biologic substaging of stage I lung cancer according to gender and histology. *Ann Thorac Surg* 2000;69:882–886.

12
Sleeve Lobectomy Versus Pneumonectomy for Lung Cancer Patients with Good Pulmonary Function

Lisa Spiguel and Mark K. Ferguson

Surgical resection of lung cancer is the mainstay for potentially curative cancer therapy. However, controversy exists regarding appropriate surgical management of centrally located tumors. Initially, surgical therapy of central tumors consisted of pneumonectomy as the only surgical option with favorable outcomes. However, parenchymal-sparing procedures, such as sleeve lobectomy, were subsequently described for patients unable to tolerate pneumonectomy because of poor pulmonary reserve. The favorable results in terms of operative morbidity and mortality after sleeve lobectomy in patients with inadequate cardiopulmonary function stimulated the use of parenchymal-sparing procedures for patients with adequate pulmonary function. Increasing clinical evidence suggests that short-term outcomes for sleeve lobectomy are similar to those for pneumonectomy, regardless of cardiopulmonary reserve.[1,2]

Thoracic surgeons face a challenge when posed with the decision of how much lung parenchyma to preserve in patients with central lung cancers. Many studies demonstrate similar, if not better, overall operative morbidity and mortality for parenchymal-sparing sleeve lobectomy as compared to pneumonectomy for the treatment of central lung cancers. The advantage results primarily from the reduced operative mortality associated with sleeve lobectomy.[2-5] Advocates of parenchymal conservation also present provocative evidence that, in patients with anatomically suitable lung tumors, sleeve lobectomy not only has similar long-term survival, but also provides a better postoperative quality of life than does pneumonectomy.[4,6-8] Furthermore, by preserving

pulmonary parenchyma, the ability to perform additional parenchymal resections is maintained should a second primary lung cancer occur.[5,8-11]

Parenchymal preservation is not without its drawbacks. Concerns include the impact of increased rates of local recurrence associated with parenchymal conservation, the potential for anastomotic complications, and the effect of N2 nodal involvement on survival. These concerns suggest that pneumonectomy may be the procedure of choice in selected patient populations. This chapter addresses the challenging question of sleeve lobectomy versus pneumonectomy for centrally located lung cancers in patients with good pulmonary function through an evidence-based investigation of the current literature.

12.1. Approach to the Question

To obtain information regarding outcomes after sleeve lobectomy and pneumonectomy, a Medline search was performed of reports published in English between January 1, 1996 and June 1, 2005 using the search terms ["sleeve lobectomy" OR "pneumonectomy"] AND "non-small cell lung cancer." The search yielded 628 abstracts, each of which was reviewed. Articles were selected based on the following criteria: a minimum of 40 patients per study population; outcomes classified according to stage or nodal status; documentation of operative mortality; and calculation of 5-year survival according to stage (or nodal status as a respective surrogate for stage). Papers that were not selected included those integrating malignant and nonmalignant lung disease in the calculation of postoperative morbidity and mortality and those combining outcomes of isolated bronchial sleeve resection with sleeve lobectomy. In addition, the abstracts selected were published during the same time period that studied postoperative pulmonary function and postoperative quality of life. Each article was assigned a level of evidence (1, 2, 3, 4, or 5), calculated based on the study type, risk of bias, and attempts to minimize bias. An overall grade (A, B, C, or D) was then assigned to categorize the level of data as a whole. A meta-analysis of operative mortality, survival, postoperative complications, and postoperative recurrence was performed by calculating weighted means based on the number of patients composing each stage or nodal status. In addition, the prognostic impacts of nodal status, preservation of lung function, and postoperative quality of life were assessed. Twelve articles met the defined criteria and were used for data abstraction for 1144 sleeve lobectomy patients and 1623 pneumonectomy patients.[1–5,7–9,12–15]

12.2. Overall Survival

The decision to perform pneumonectomy or sleeve lobectomy is based on both oncological and physiological considerations. Some believe

that pneumonectomy, especially right pneumonectomy, is a disease in itself, with severe breathlessness and impaired quality of life affecting many patients for the rest of their lives. Alexiou and coworkers argue in favor of sleeve lobectomy, stating that pneumonectomy is an independent predictor of poorer survival for patients with non-small cell lung cancer.[14] In contrast, Ferguson and Karrison suggest that the type of operation is not a predictor of long-term outcomes, after adjusting for covariates such as age, T status, N status, performance status, and $FEV_1\%$.[16] Kim and others also illustrate the lack of significance of the operative procedure on long-term survival through a multivariate analysis.[1]

We analyzed survival based on 5-year survival data, and stratified survival according to stage and nodal status (Table 12.1). According to the meta-analysis, sleeve lobectomy results in higher survival rates for stages I, II, and III, although the survival advantage for sleeve lobectomy in stage III patients appears to be small. This general survival advantage following sleeve lobectomy accounts for the increasing use of parenchymal preservation in patients with good cardiopulmonary function, provided a complete surgical resection is accomplished.[2,3,5,9] In a multivariate analysis, Ludwig and colleagues revealed sleeve lobectomy to be a statistically significant positive

TABLE 12.1. Patient demographics.

Reference	Year	Period	Procedure	Patients	Age (years)	Men (%)	Stage I (%)	Stage II (%)	Stage III (%)	N0 (%)	N1 (%)	N2 (%)
Gaissert[4]	1996	1962–1991	SL	72	63	78	40	43	17	43	47	10
Icard[9]	1999	1981–1995	SL	110	61	95	29	52	15	33	59	8
Okada[5]	2000	1984–1998	SL	60	61	87	23	27	50	23	27	50
Tronc[8]	2000	1972–1998	SL	184	60	83	45	39	14	53	37	10
Fadel[12]	2002	1981–2001	SL	139	59	80	39	34	26	47	36	17
Mezzetti[13]	2002	1997–1999	SL	83	60	na	41	39	20	48	31	20
Terzi[7]	2002	1965–1999	SL	151	61	97	38	34	33	38	34	33
Deslauriers[3]	2004	1972–2000	SL	184	60	83	45	39	16	53	37	10
Kim[1]	2005	1989–1998	SL	49	59	90	28	41	31	37	37	26
Ludwig[2]	2005	1987–1997	SL	116	62*	88*	27	35	38	40	28	32
Gaissert[4]	1996	1986–1990	PN	56	61	75	16	45	37	26	57	17
Mizushima[15]	1997	1985–1996	PN	107	na	91	7	14	79	24	29	41
Okada[5]	2000	1984–1998	PN	60	61	88	20	28	52	20	28	52
Alexiou[14]	2003	1991–2000	PN	111	63	74	100	0	0	100	0	0
Deslauriers[3]	2004	1972–2000	PN	1046	61	79	16	35	45	25	42	30
Kim[1]	2005	1989–1998	PN	49	58	94	49	26	22	57	22	21
Ludwig[2]	2005	1987–1997	PN	194	59*	88*	16	27	57	30	25	44

Abbreviations: Age, median age; Men, overall study percentage; na, not applicable; PN, pneumonectomy; SL, sleeve lobectomy.

prognostic factor for long-term survival, with a survival advantage for sleeve lobectomy patients over pneumonectomy patients with N0, N1, and N2 disease.[2] As shown by the data in our meta-analysis, the modest advantage for sleeve lobectomy in both overall and stage-adjusted outcomes reinforces the use of sleeve lobectomy in the surgical management of non-small cell lung cancer patients with good cardiopulmonary function. Whether sleeve lobectomy is an oncologically acceptable procedure for patients with N2 nodal involvement is unclear.

12.3. Effect of Nodal Status

One of the strongest determinants of survival is nodal status. Some authors argue that sleeve lobectomy is only applicable to N0 tumors, concluding that pneumonectomy may be the best option for N1 and N2 involvement.[1,3,7-9,13] In contrast, other studies reveal only N2 involvement as a significant negative predictor for diminished 5-year survival in patients undergoing sleeve lobectomy, showing significant survival decrease with N2 tumors compared to N0 or N1 cancers.[2,12]

Our meta-analysis demonstrates that worsening nodal status is associated with substantial decrements in 5-year survival rates in patients undergoing sleeve lobectomy for increasing degrees of nodal involvement, with N2 status producing the largest negative effect (Table 12.2). However, N2 disease has a substantial adverse effect on survival for both sleeve lobectomy and pneumonectomy patients, albeit with a more profound effect in patients undergoing sleeve lobectomy.

There is recent focus on the role of complete mediastinal node dissection in non-small cell lung cancer patients with N2 nodal involvement. A study by Keller and colleagues suggested that a complete mediastinal nodal dissection is associated with improved long-term survival in patients with N2 disease.[17] However, some studies report that mortality in patients with N2 involvement is not from local tumor causes but most often secondary to distant disease.[1,6-10,12] Given our current level of understanding, it is unclear exactly whether or how the operative procedure impacts overall survival. According to the data in our meta-analysis, nodal status does not appear to be a strong contraindication for sleeve lobectomy as long as complete nodal resection can be

TABLE 12.2. Five-year survival related to stage and nodal status.

Reference	Stage I 5-year survival (%)	Stage II 5-year survival (%)	Stage III 5-year survival (%)	N0 5-year survival (%)	N1 5-year survival (%)	N2 5-year survival (%)
Sleeve lobectomy						
Gaissert[4]	42	53	43	57	38	43
Icard[9]	60	30	27	57	29	33
Okada[5]	70	70	21	70	70	21
Tronc[8]	63	48	8	63	48	8
Fadel[12]	55	62	21	55	68	0
Mezzetti[13]	61	39	9	61	39	9
Terzi[7]	62	34	22	57	33	19
Deslauriers[3]	66	50	19	63	48	8
Kim[1]	88	52	8	88	52	8
Ludwig[2]	57	40	28	56	38	24
Weighted mean	61	46	21	61	44	15
Pneumonectomy						
Gaissert[4]	na	43	na	na	43	na
Mizushima[15]	58	42	13	58	42	13
Okada[5]	42	42	16	42	42	16
Alexiou[14]	43	na	na	43	na	na
Deslauriers[3]	50	34	22	43	30	21
Kim[1]	75	36	38	75	36	38
Ludwig[2]	45	42	13	47	30	12
Weighted mean	49	36	19	46	32	19

Abbreviation: na, not applicable.

achieved; nevertheless, the potential negative impact of N2 involvement must be considered, and remains a controversial issue.

12.4. Postoperative Complications

Postoperative morbidity and mortality data reveal an overall lower mortality for patients undergoing sleeve lobectomy, in addition to a lower overall incidence of postoperative complications (Table 12.3). However, when postoperative complication rates are categorized according to airway complications, pulmonary complications, and cardiac complications, sleeve lobectomy patients appear to experience a higher incidence of airway and pulmonary complications. These results persist despite multiple techniques utilized to decrease the anastomotic complications, such as preservation of bronchial blood supply, creation of a tension-free bronchial anastomosis, improved suture materials, and utilization of pleural, pericardial, or mediastinal flaps to prevent bronchovascular fistulas.[2,12] The incidence of microscopically positive margins becomes important when evaluating the incidence of both anastomotic complications and local recurrence. Kim and others reported a high incidence of anastomotic disruption in their sleeve lobectomy patients; however they also

revealed a high incidence of microscopically positive margins in their sleeve lobectomy patients on frozen section.[1] On the other hand, sleeve lobectomy patients appear to have a lower cardiac complication rate compared to pneumonectomy patients. Therefore, when evaluating overall morbidity and mortality, sleeve lobectomy appears to be a safer operative procedure. However, important airway complications do arise more often in patients undergoing sleeve lobectomy.

12.5. Recurrence Patterns

Lung cancer recurrences are categorized into three patterns: local/regional, distant, and combined recurrence. Sleeve lobectomy preserves lung parenchyma, posing a theoretical risk of increased local/regional cancer recurrence. A recent study published by Terzi and others reported similar local/regional recurrence rates for stage I and II patients undergoing sleeve lobectomy, but there was a large increase in distant recurrence rates associated with stage III disease.[7] Kim and coworkers suggested that N1 involvement and adjuvant radiotherapy were independent risk factors for local/regional recurrence in patients undergoing sleeve lobectomy for non-small cell lung cancer.[1] Fadel and others also reported an increase in local/regional recurrence

TABLE 12.3. Postoperative complication rates.

Reference	Operative mortality (%)	Postoperative complications (%)	Stump/anastomotic (%)	Pulmonary (%)	Cardiac (%)
Sleeve lobectomy					
Gaissert[4]	4	11	1	10	0
Icard[9]	2.8	44	18	42	7
Okada[5]	0	13	3	8	1
Tronc[8]	1.6	16	3	9	0
Fadel[12]	2.9	16	4	12	1
Mezzetti[13]	3.6	10.8	4	7	0
Terzi[7]	12	14.5	3	5	4
Kim[1]	6.1	74.9	35	35	4
Ludwig[2]	4.3	38	18	13	3
Weighted mean	4.4	23.6	8.2	14.2	2.2
Pneumonectomy					
Gaissert[4]	9	16	1	7	1
Okada[5]	2	22	7	12	3
Kim[1]	4.1	44	0	12	8
Ludwig[2]	4.6	26	4	7	4
Weighted mean	4.8	26.2	2.8	8.5	3.7

TABLE 12.4. Postoperative recurrence rates.

Reference	Local/regional recurrence only (%)	Distant recurrence only (%)
Sleeve lobectomy		
Gaissert[4]	14	na
Icard[9]	17	24
Okada[5]	8	na
Tronc[8]	22	11
Fadel[12]	15	11
Mezzetti[13]	20	na
Terzi[7]	5	18
Deslauriers[3]	22	na
Kim[1]	22	22
Weighted mean	17	16
Pneumonectomy		
Okada[5]	10	na
Deslauriers[3]	35	na
Kim[1]	6	20
Weighted mean	32	20

Abbreviation: na, not applicable.

rates with advancing nodal status in patients undergoing sleeve lobectomy, with the rate increasing from 11% in patients with N0 disease to 40% in patients with N2 disease.[12]

Surprisingly, our analysis (Table 12.4) suggests that the incidences of both local/regional and distant recurrences are higher in patients undergoing pneumonectomy as compared to patients undergoing sleeve lobectomy. However, few of the studies included in the meta-analysis evaluated the relationship between nodal status or stage and recurrence patterns and rates. Without this information, it is difficult to assess whether the operative procedure or the stage and nodal status of the patient are the significant factors in determining recurrence. The few studies evaluating risk factors for recurrence illustrate stage and nodal status as the negative predictive factors, rather than the procedure performed.[1,7,12]

12.6. Quality of Life

Postoperative quality of life is an important factor when deciding between sleeve lobectomy and pneumonectomy as the treatment for centrally located lung cancers. Many studies suggest that lung tissue preservation benefits postoperative quality of life in terms of greater cardiopulmonary reserve, less postoperative pulmonary edema, and less right ventricular dysfunction due to a lower pulmonary vascular resistance.[6,7] Handy and others reported that postoperative quality of life is strongly dependent on the amount of lung resected, and that only pneumonectomy causes a decreased postoperative cardiopulmonary function and exercise capacity.[18] Ferguson and Lehman investigated postoperative quality of life in a decision analytic model comparing sleeve lobectomy and pneumonectomy for patients with non-small cell lung cancer. When analyzed using quality-adjusted life-years (QALY) as the outcome, the model strongly favored sleeve lobectomy over pneumonectomy, regardless of underlying cardiopulmonary status. These results are most likely related to the relatively low overall risk of isolated local/regional recurrence and the improved postoperative cardiopulmonary status associated with parenchymal preservation.[19] In addition to preserving cardiopulmonary function, lung preservation allows for patients who develop a second lung cancer to undergo a second lung resection safely, an incidence occurring as high as 12% in our studies.[9]

12.7. Levels of Evidence

Determining the validity of a study's results is essential when assessing its potential impact on surgical intervention. The studies included in the meta-analysis were assigned a score based on the quality of evidence. All of the studies cited in the meta-analysis were rated a level 4. Although ranked lower on the grading scale, research evaluating operative techniques is rarely categorized as level 1 because few procedural-based studies can be designed as randomized, controlled trials because of obvious ethical, scientific, and practical considerations.[20] The current evidence is adequate to impact decision making for surgical treatment of non-small cell lung cancer.

12.8. Recommendations

Survival rates, postoperative complication rates, recurrence rates, and postoperative quality of life are all important topics to assess in the decision making for surgical intervention in patients with lung cancer. Five-year survival rates reveal an advantage for patients undergoing sleeve lobectomy across all three stages (I, II, and III). Furthermore, overall operative mortality rates and postoperative complication rates are lower in sleeve lobectomy patients, suggesting that sleeve lobectomy is a safer procedure. Postoperative quality of life also appears to be superior in patients undergoing sleeve lobectomy, which is most likely related to the greater amount of residual functioning lung tissue and perhaps to the lower incidence of local/regional recurrence in patients undergoing sleeve lobectomy. However, recurrence rates in our meta-analysis are inadequately assessed owing to the lack of data on outcomes stratified by stage and nodal status. Based on the overall outcomes, sleeve lobectomy should be used whenever possible for resection of anatomically suitable lung cancers in order to avoid the adverse effects of pneumonectomy, particularly the impact on postoperative quality of life (level of evidence 3 to 4; recommendation grade C).

In the absence of N2 disease, sleeve lobectomy should be used whenever possible for resection of anatomically suitable lung cancers in order to avoid the adverse effects of pneumonectomy, particularly the impact on postoperative quality of life (level of evidence 3 to 4; recommendation grade C).

In patients with N2 disease there is inadequate information available at present to determine whether the risk of local/regional or distant recurrence is increased when parenchymal sparing procedures are used instead of pneumonectomy.

The use of parenchymal-sparing procedures in patients with N2 disease remains controversial. There is inadequate information available at present to determine whether the risk of local/regional or distant recurrence is increased when parenchymal-sparing procedures are used instead of pneumonectomy. A growing body of information suggesting that complete mediastinal nodal dissection limits recurrence and improves long-term survival may ultimately impact decisions regarding indications for parenchymal-sparing operations.

References

1. Kim YT, Kang CH, Sung SW, et al. Local control of disease related to lymph node involvement in non-small cell lung cancer after sleeve lobectomy compared with pneumonectomy. Ann Thorac Surg 2005;79:1153–1161.
2. Ludwig C, Stoelben E, Olschewski M, et al. Comparison of morbidity, 30-day mortality, and long-term survival after pneumonectomy and sleeve lobectomy for non-small cell lung carcinoma. Ann Thorac Surg 2005;79:968–973.
3. Deslauriers J, Gregoire J, Jacques L, et al. Sleeve lobectomy versus pneumonectomy for lung cancer: a comparative analysis of survival and sites or recurrences. Ann Thorac Surg 2004;77:1152–1156.
4. Gaissert H, Mathisen D, Moncure A, et al. Survival and function after sleeve lobectomy for lung cancer. J Thorac Cardiovasc Surg 1996;111:948–953.
5. Okada M, Yamagishi H, Satake S, et al. Survival related to lymph node involvement in lung cancer after sleeve lobectomy compared with pneumonectomy. J Thorac Cardiovasc Surg 2000;119:814–819.
6. Martin-Ucar AE, Chaudhuri N, Edwards JG, et al. Can pneumonectomy for non-small cell lung cancer be avoided? An audit of parenchymal sparing lung surgery. Eur J Cardiothorac Surg 2002;21:601–605.
7. Terzi A, Lonardoni A, Falezza G, et al. Sleeve lobectomy for non-small cell lung cancer and carcinoids: results in 160 cases. Eur J Cardiothorac Surg 2002;21:888–893.
8. Tronc F, Gregoire J, Rouleau J, et al. Long-term results of sleeve lobectomy for lung cancer. Eur J Cardiothorac Surg 2000;17:550–556.
9. Icard Ph, Regnard JF, Guibert L, et al. Survival and prognostic factors in patients undergoing parenchymal saving bronchoplastic operation for primary lung cancer: a series of 110 consecutive cases. Eur J Cardiothorac Surg 1999;15:426–432.
10. Massard G, Kessler R, Gasser B, et al. Local control of disease and survival following bronchoplastic lobectomy for non-small cell lung cancer. Eur J Cardiothorac Surg 1999;16:276–282.
11. Mehran RJ, Deslauriers J, Piraux M, et al. Survival related to nodal status after sleeve resection for lung cancer. J Thorac Cardiovasc Surg 1994;107:576–583.
12. Fadel E, Yildizeli B, Chapelier A, et al. Sleeve lobectomy for bronchogenic cancers: factors affecting survival. Ann Thorac Surg 2002;74:851–859.
13. Mezzetti M, Panigalli T, Giuliani L, et al. Personal experience in lung cancer sleeve lobectomy and

sleeve pneumonectomy. *Ann Thorac Surg* 2002; 73:1736–1739.

14. Alexiou C, Beggs D, Onyeaka P, et al. Pneumonectomy for stage I (T1N0 and T2N0) nonsmall cell lung cancer has potent, adverse impact on survival. *Ann Thorac Surg* 2003;76:1023–1028.

15. Mizushima Y, Noto H, Kusajima Y, et al. Results of pneumonectomy for non-small cell lung cancer. *Acta Oncologica* 1997;36:493–497.

16. Ferguson MK, Karrison T. Does pneumonectomy for lung cancer adversely influence long-term survival? *J Thorac Cardiovasc Surg* 2000;119:440–448.

17. Keller SM, Adak S, Wagner H, et al. Mediastinal lymph node dissection improves survival in patients with stages II and IIIa non-small cell lung cancer. Eastern Cooperative Oncology Group. *Ann Thorac Surg* 2000;70:358–365.

18. Handy J, Asaph J, Skokan L, et al. What happens to patients undergoing lung cancer surgery? Outcomes and quality of life before and after surgery. *Chest* 2002;122:21–30.

19. Ferguson MK, Lehman AG. Sleeve lobectomy or pneumonectomy: optimal management strategy using decision analysis techniques. *Ann Thorac Surg* 2003;76:1782–1788.

20. Kral JG, Dixon JB, Horber FF, et al. Flaws in methods of evidence-based medicine may adversely affect public health directives. *Surgery* 2005;137:279–284.

13
Lesser Resection Versus Lobectomy for Stage I Lung Cancer in Patients with Good Pulmonary Function

Anthony W. Kim and William H. Warren

Historically, the surgical procedure of choice for curative resection of lung cancer, even in its early stages, has been a lobectomy or pneumonectomy. The role of a more conservative resection, such as a segmentectomy or wedge resection, has been explored by many, paralleling the interest in conservative resection of breast cancer, where studies determined that clinical results of lumpectomy compared favorably with modified radical mastectomy.

Although segmentectomy was first described as a surgical procedure for bronchiectasis, the role of segmental resections in the management of lung cancer dates back more than 30 years.[1] Since the original description, many authors have examined the role of lobectomy over a more limited resection.[2-7] These were often retrospective studies, examining the outcomes of patients who underwent a limited resection having been determined to be a poor surgical risk for lobectomy.

In 1995, Ginsberg and Rubinstein published the results of a Lung Cancer Study Group (LCSG) randomized, controlled trial evaluating the role of limited pulmonary resection versus lobectomy in the surgical management of early-stage lung cancer.[8] All patients entered in this trial were good-risk patients and were able to undergo either a lobectomy or limited resection. This sentinel report concluded that, based on the higher incidence of local recurrence and decreased 5-year survival in patients undergoing a limited pulmonary resection, lobectomy remained the procedure of choice for patients with T1N0 non-small cell lung carcinoma.

These findings were essentially the same as those reached by Warren and colleagues, who re-assessed a series of patients having undergone lobectomy or segmental resection for stage I lung cancer.[7] Of note, those patients had been reported previously in papers advocating limited resections. Interestingly, some of these patients were used as the case material of reports about second and third primary tumors,[9] suggesting that an unfavorable outcome after limited resection might have been related to a prior lung cancer.

A number of other papers have emerged supporting the conclusion that limited resection should be reserved for poor pulmonary risk patients.[10-12] To a lesser degree, papers have also emerged arguing for wider adoption of limited pulmonary resections, even in good-risk patients, particularly for small peripheral adenocarcinomas with bronchoalveolar features. In this chapter, we will review data published since the LCSG findings were released. In particular, we will attempt to reassess the value of limited pulmonary resections in patients considered to be able to tolerate a lobectomy (i.e., good-risk patient).

13.1. Nomenclature and Definitions

A *segmentectomy* is an anatomical resection whereby one or more segments are resected by dissecting out, ligating, and dividing the segmental arteries and veins and dividing the segmental bronchus or bronchi. A *wedge resection* is a non-anatomical resection of lung without hilar dissection and therefore, does not identify pulmonary vessels or segmental bronchi. *"Limited" or "lesser resections"* have been defined in the literature as anything less than a standard lobectomy. As such, an anatomical segmentectomy (involving one or more segments) and a wedge resection have both fallen into this umbrella term of "limited pulmonary resection." Whenever possible, we will attempt to distinguish between these two procedures. A lobar and mediastinal lymph node dissection is an integral part of the procedure whenever a carcinoma is resected, even when the pulmonary resection is limited. *Early-stage lung cancer* is defined as tumor limited to the lung parenchyma (i.e., not invading surrounding structures and the absence of nodal or systemic metastatic disease).

According to the most recent TNM classification, T1 disease is defined as carcinoma that is 3 cm or less is maximal diameter, not invading visceral pleura and more than 2 cm from the carina. T2 disease is defined as primary lung carcinoma either measuring greater than 3 cm in maximal diameter, or invading the visceral pleura (but not the parietal pleura), or involving a lobar bronchus (with/without lobar obstructive pneumonia or atelectasis) but more than 2 cm from the carina. Stage I is comprised of T1N0M0 (stage IA) or T2N0M0 (stage IB) carcinoma. The publications from North America and Europe western concentrate on the role of limited resections for stage IA disease.

There is no universally accepted definition of what comprises poor pulmonary function, especially as it pertains to selection of patients for lobectomy versus lesser pulmonary resections. A patient is deemed at high operative risk for complications after lobectomy if he/she: presents with a Pco_2 greater than 45 mmHg, Po_2 less than 50 mmHg (without supplimental O_2), has a predicted postoperative forced expiratory volume in 1 s (FEV_1) less than 0.8 L or less than 40% predicted, or has poor exercise performance status (unable to climb a flight of stairs without resting). In addition, cardiac function must be considered. An ejection fraction of under 15%, and Pa pressure of over 45 mmHg and angina or systemic hypertension refractory to medical management would also qualify a patient to be a high surgical risk. Inevitably, patient compliance and overall

state of health must also be considered. Although most thoracic surgeons can agree that a given patient is at high risk for complications after lobectomy (and therefore more likely to be considered for a limited resection), the designation of a patient as high risk must remain, for the time being, to a large degree, a matter of clinical judgment.

Upon reviewing the literature, one must attempt to distinguish the experience of those patients deemed by the surgeon to have been able to tolerate a lobectomy from those who could not on the basis of the above-stated criteria. A surrogate indicator of good pulmonary function, other than the obvious declaration of such in the literature, has been the description of intentional limited resection in patients who would otherwise tolerate a more extensive formal resection.

Of the many outcomes reported in the literature on the role of limited pulmonary resection, survival and local recurrence are the most objective and common to virtually all the recent publications. Typically, survival has been reported as 5-year Kaplan Meier survival curves, although 2-year and 3-year survival is also occasionally reported. This study has proposed *local recurrence* to be defined as the presence of lung cancer in the ipsilateral hemithorax (including mediastinum) following resection. This study and others have adopted this definition to avoid potential confusion distinguishing recurrence from incomplete resections versus a second primary tumors. As such, for the purposes of this analysis, the development of carcinoma in the ipsilateral lung after a resection is reported as a local/regional recurrence regardless of the exact location within the hemithorax, histology, or time interval since the resection. According to this definition, there is no exception or allowance for a second primary tumor. While the foregoing definition may be overly broad from a tumor biology point of view, if adopted, it is unambiguous and therefore serves as a statistic by which diverse clinical series can be compared.

13.2. Evidence-Based Medicine

In keeping with the theme of this book, this chapter will attempt to focus on a review of papers filling the following criteria: (1) patients with

TABLE 13.1. Local/regional recurrence after lobectomy, segmentectomy, and wedge resection for stage 1 NSCLC.

| Reference | Year | Lobectomy | Limited resections | | | p Value |
			Combined	Segment	Wedge	
Warren[7]	1994	4.9%		22.7%		0.004
Ginsberg[8]	1995	6.4%	17.2%			0.008
Landreneau[13]	1997	7.7%			Open 57.1%	0.07
					VATS 26.7%	
Miller[15]	2002	13.32%		8.3%	30.8%	ns
Koike[21]	2003	0.6%		2.7%		ns
Campione[11]	2004	2.0%		19%		Significant

Abbreviation: ns, not significant.

stage I lung carcinoma, (2) patients undergoing a limited but complete pulmonary resection, (3) at a minimum, survival data is reported, (4) the series was comprised of at least 40 patients. As is expected with any controversial topic, significant clinical data exist that refute or support the advantages of limited resections over lobectomy.

13.2.1. Literature Critical of the Use of Limited Pulmonary Resection

After an extensive review of the literature, the publication by the LCSG[8] is the only report that can be categorized as level 1 evidence reporting the role of limited resection versus lobectomy for stage IA non-small cell lung cancer (NSCLC) in good-risk patients. In their report of this prospective and randomized trial, there was a statistically significant increase in the incidence of local recurrence in the limited resection group

(even after the authors attempted to exclude second primary lesions). Among patients undergoing a segmentectomy, there was a 2.0-fold increase, and among those undergoing a wedge resection, there was a 3.9-fold increase over the incidence after lobectomy (Table 13.1). Furthermore, the 5-year survival of patients undergoing a limited resection was worse than those who undergoing a lobectomy, a difference that reached statistical significance (Table 13.2). The only beneficial effect noted was in pulmonary function tests at 6-month follow-up, where virtually every parameter was observed to be better preserved in the limited resection compared to the lobectomy group. However, this benefit was not sustained when patients were studied 12 or 18 months postoperatively. Ginsberg and Rubinstein concluded that there were no statistically significant differences in the perioperative morbidity and mortality.[8] On the basis of the increased incidence of

TABLE 13.2. Overall 5-year survival after lobectomy, segmentectomy, and wedge resection for stage 1 NSCLC.

| Reference | Year | Lobectomy | Limited resections | | | p Value |
			Combined	Segment	Wedge	
Warren[7]	1994	68%		44%		0.035
Ginsberg[8]	1995	68%	48%			0.088
Kodama[17]	1997	88%	93% good risk			ns
			48% poor risk			0.003
Landreneau[13]	1997	70%			Open = 58%	ns
					VATS = 65%	
Sugarbaker[14]	2000	74%	48%			0.0014
Okada[20]	2001	88%		87%		ns
Koike[21]	2003	90%		89%		ns
Keenan[22a]	2004	67%		62%		ns

Abbreviation: ns, not significant.
[a]Four-year survival data.

local/regional recurrence and 5-year survival, they concluded that limited resections should not be considered the oncological equivalent of a lobectomy, discouraging the use of a limited resection when the patient is deemed to be able to tolerate either resection.

Landreneau and colleagues published their multi-institutional retrospective review of wedge resections, either by VATS (60 patients) or open (42 patients) versus lobectomy (117 patients) for the surgical management of stage IA lung cancer.[13] They observed that, although postoperative morbidity was significantly less after wedge resection than after lobectomy, local recurrence following wedge resection was higher than lobectomy. Their analysis, however, showed that although this incidence approached, it did not reach statistical significance ($p = 0.07$). Of concern was the fact that local recurrence seemed to occur earlier after wedge resection (median time to recurrence of 10 months) than in the lobectomy group (median time to recurrence of 19 months). Based on their findings, the authors concluded that, in the face of the increased risk of local recurrence and poorer survival, lobectomy was the procedure of choice for the good-risk pulmonary patient. They agreed that wedge resections should be reserved for those patients deemed to be poor-risk patients.

In another retrospective study, Sugarbaker and Strauss compared the clinical courses of 58 patients undergoing a limited resection and 186 patients undergoing lobectomy or pneumonectomy for clinical stage I lung cancer.[14] They observed that patients undergoing a limited resection (90% of whom had T1N0 tumors) had a worse survival than patients undergoing lobectomy/pneumonectomy (57% of whom had T1N0 tumors). Thus, patients undergoing a limited pulmonary resection had with a worse 5-year survival than patients undergoing a lobectomy/pneumonectomy despite the earlier stage in the limited resection group. On the basis of these findings, Sugarbaker and Strauss also endorsed the concept that a lobectomy is the operation of choice for stage I lung cancer.

Miller and associates analyzed a subset of patients with NSCLC less than 1.0cm in diameter.[15] In their retrospective analysis of 100 patients (stage I, 93; stage II, 6; stage IIIA, 2), the incidence

of local recurrence (wedge resection, 30.8%; segmentectomy, 8.3%; lobectomy, 13.3%), approached, but did not reach, statistical significance (probably due to the low number of patients). There was, however, a decreased 5-year overall and lung cancer–free survival in patients undergoing a limited resection (33% and 47%, respectively) when compared to lobectomy (71% and 92%, respectively). In addition, as Ginsberg and Rubinstein had observed, upon further subdividing limited resection into wedge resection and segmentectomy, patients undergoing segmentectomy had a statistically significant better 5-year survival (57%) than those undergoing wedge resection (27%). Based on their results, the authors concluded that a lobectomy is the resection of choice, even for tumors 1.0cm or less in diameter.

In 1999, Takizawa and colleagues published their results comparing the pulmonary function of 40 patients before and after undergoing a segmental resection versus 40 patients undergoing a lobar resection for T1 peripheral lung carcinomas.[16] All patients undergoing segmentectomy were deemed able to tolerate either a limited resection or a lobectomy. Patients were studied 2 weeks and again at 12 months after surgery. Despite the tendency toward improved pulmonary function in the patients undergoing the more conservative resections, analysis showed that this difference was not statistically significant. The authors concluded that suspected improvement in performance status did not merit advocating limited pulmonary resections in good-risk patients after considering adequacy of lymph node dissection, higher incidence of local recurrence, and decreased 5-year survival.

13.2.2. Literature Supporting the Use of Limited Pulmonary Resection

Despite the studies that have concluded that limited pulmonary resections are not the oncological equivalent of lobectomy, numerous studies have been supportive of the use of limited pulmonary resection, even in patients judged to be able to tolerate a lobectomy. Shortly after the LCSG publication, literature from Japan emerged advocating limited pulmonary resections. Kodama and associates evaluated their clinical experience with limited resections in 63 good-risk and 17 poor-risk patients with stage IA NSCLC, comparing the results with 77 patients undergoing a lobectomy.[17] The average diameter for pulmonary lesions in the limited resection group was 1.67 cm versus 2.29 cm in the lobectomy group. The authors did not observe a significant difference in rates of local recurrence comparing the good-risk patients undergoing a limited resection versus lobectomy. However, there was a statistically significant higher incidence in local/regional recurrence in poor-risk patients undergoing limited resection compared to lobectomy patients. This was thought to be due, at least in part, to two factors. Patients with larger tumors tended to undergo a lobectomy if they were good risk, but underwent a limited resection if they were deemed poor risk. Good-risk patients tended to undergo a limited resection only if their tumors were small. Furthermore, none of the 17 poor-risk (and only 13 of the 46 good-risk) patients undergoing a limited resection underwent a complete lobar and mediastinal node dissection. Six patients having undergone a limited pulmonary resection had recurrence in the mediastinum. There was no statistically significant difference in 5-year survival comparing good-risk segmentectomy patients with lobectomy patients (88% vs. 93%). The authors concluded that a complete mediastinal lymph node dissection was indicated in patients undergoing a limited pulmonary resection, even in poor-risk patients. Based on their findings, however, citing the fact that there was no difference in survival in good-risk patients, the authors concluded that segmentectomy combined with mediastinal lymph node dissection could be adequate therapy for stage IA disease.

Several reports have appeared from the Study Group of Extended Segmentectomy for Small Lung Tumors. The authors define extended segmentectomy as segmentectomy and complete lobar/mediastinal lymph node dissection. This study group has examined the role of such resections on patients with tumors less than 2 cm in diameter and have produced several reports.[18,19] In this prospective multi-institutional trial, they reported on 70 patients undergoing a segmentectomy with mediastinal lymph node dissection and 107 patients undergoing lobectomy for path-

ological stage IA carcinoma. The 5-year survival rates were 87.3% for patients undergoing segmentectomy versus 72.7% for patients undergoing lobectomy for stage IA disease. In patients with T1 (T less than 2.0 cm) tumors, the 5-year survival rate was 87.1% for segmentectomy versus 87.8% for the lobectomy population. This difference was not statistically significant. The authors emphasized the value of frozen section to help stage the patient intra-operatively when considering limited resection. As long as preoperative selection criteria were stringently adhered to, and a concerted effort was made to eliminate patients with more advanced stage, the authors advocated segmentectomy with good pulmonary margins and mediastinal node dissection as a good alternative to lobectomy. The major disadvantage of the work of this group, however, is that the segmentectomy patients were studied prospectively and compared retrospectively with patients having undergone a lobectomy at the same institutions. Nevertheless, Okada and colleagues[20] have achieved enviable 5-year survival in this subset of patients. Not surprisingly, they advocate segmentectomy with mediastinal node dissection in the management of stage IA lesions (especially when the tumor is less than 2 cm in diameter), even in patients considered to be a good risk for lobectomy.

In 2003, Koike and colleagues reported retrospectively on results of limited resection for good-risk patents with tumors less than 2 cm,[21] and compared them to patients undergoing a standard lobectomy for T1N0M0 (T less than 2 cm) disease. Of this group, 74 patients had a limited resection (segmentectomy in 60 patients, wedge resection in 14 patients). Only 48 patients underwent a complete hilar and mediastinal node dissection. Segmentectomy was only performed if the surgeon felt that a 2-cm surgical margin could be obtained. Lobectomy was performed in 159 patients meeting the same criteria. There was no significant difference in the perioperative morbidity and mortality. Nor was there any significant difference in local recurrence. Both the 3-year and 5-year survival data showed no important difference between patients undergoing lobectomy versus limited resection (97.0% vs. 94.0%, and 90.1% vs. 89.1%, respectively). The authors concluded that patients with tumors less than 2cm in diameter may be candidates for a limited resection, but admitted that more controlled studies exploring this option are warranted.

In the United States, Keenan and colleagues retrospectively analyzed 201 patients with T1N0 NSCLC who underwent surgical resections over a 5-year period.[22] In addition to studying local recurrence and survival, the authors used preoperative and 12-month postoperative pulmonary function tests to determine if there was any functional advantage of a segmentectomy (54 patients) versus a lobectomy (147 patients). Mediastinal lymph node dissection was performed routinely in the lobectomy patients, but not in the segmentectomy patients. There was no observed statistically significant difference in local/regional recurrence (but the trend was in favor of lobectomy). Likewise, there was no statistically significant difference in the 1-year and 4-year survival between the two groups (but once again, the trend was in favor of lobectomy). Preoperatively, the patients undergoing segmentectomies had significantly greater pulmonary compromise when compared those undergoing lobectomy. These differences in forced vital capacity (FVC), FEV_1, maximum voluntary ventilation (MVV), and diffusing capacity for carbon monoxide (DCCO), were all significant. When compared to the preoperative status, the segmentectomy patients experienced a postoperative decrease in FVC, FEV_1, MCC, and DLCO at 12 months, but only the DLCO change was statistically significant. On the other hand, patients undergoing lobectomy demonstrated statistically significant decreases in all these same parameters. Based on their findings, the authors supported the notion that segmental resection be performed in peripheral carcinomas less than 3.0cm when completely within anatomical boundaries of the segment, and in all lesions 2.0cm or less.

13.3. Impact of Evidence

13.3.1. Age

In 2005, Mery and coworkers published their findings on the role of limited resection in the elderly.[23] Patient information was accessed through SEER (Surveillance, Epidemiology, and End Results) database from 1992 to 1997. Patients were divided into three groups based upon their age: group 1, ≤65 years; group 2, from 65 and 74 years; and group 3, ≥75 years of age. Stages I and II disease were included in this analysis (stage I, 83%; stage II, 17%). Limited resections were performed with increasing frequency among the three groups: group 1 (8.1%), group 2 (12%), and group 3 (17%). The authors assumed the decision to perform limited resections was based on perceived greater surgical risk (i.e., comorbidities and poorer pulmonary reserve), although the exact criteria by which selection was made were not stated. Not surprisingly, the authors found that overall survival decreased as a function of age. Furthermore, the overall survival benefit of lobectomy over limited pulmonary resection proved to be a function of age. A survival benefit for patients undergoing lobectomy versus limited resection was seen in groups 1 and 2, but was not apparent in group 3 (patients 75 years or older). By post hoc statistical analysis, it was determined that patients beyond age 71 undergoing lobectomy were not likely to see a survival advantage (beyond 25 months) when compared to patients undergoing segmentectomy. The authors concluded that limited resections could be a feasible alternative in patients greater than 71 years without impacting long-term survival.

13.3.2. Tumor Size

Although stage IA disease has been described typically as early-stage disease, several authors have made attempts to subclassify T1N0 tumors according to the tumor diameter (such as <1.0cm or <2.0cm.). Tumor size within the T1N0 classification has been shown to correlate with survival. Several authors have concluded that patients with tumors ≤2.0cm. have a statistically significant 5-year survival advantage over patients with tumors 2.1 to 3.0cm, regardless of the extent of the surgical resection, provided a complete resection was performed, including a mediastinal lymph node dissection.[3,20] Port and colleagues reached the same conclusion with respect to the disease-specific 5-year survival.[24] It is important to take this observation into account, whenever analyzing these retrospective papers, many of which reserved limited pulmonary resections to patients with tumors <2.0cm.

13.3.3. Tumor Biology

In addition to tumor size, histopathology has been the subject of studies to determine when to consider performing a limited pulmonary resection. Yamato and colleagues review their 4-year experience of 42 patients undergoing limited resection for a bronchioloalveolar carcinoma less than 2.0 cm.[25] Thirty-four of these patients underwent a nonanatomical wedge resection, 2 underwent segmentectomy, and 6 were converted to a lobectomy. All patients underwent a mediastinal lymph node dissection. In addition to using frozen section analysis to evaluate the presence of nodal metastases, frozen section analysis was used to confirm the absence of active fibroblastic proliferation, which has been shown to portend a worse prognosis.[26] Patients with nodal metastases or invasion of the pleura or stroma, or who had demonstrable active fibroblastic proliferation, were converted to a lobectomy. During the follow-up period, ranging from 12 to 47 months, all patients were alive without signs of local recurrence. Based on their careful selection criteria (including tumor size and histological features), the authors concluded that a limited pulmonary resection is a viable option for this subgroup of patients with T1N0 bronchioloalveolar carcinoma meeting their size and histological criteria. They also rationalized that a wedge resection had an advantage over a segmentectomy by alluding to the theoretical advantage of preserving as much pulmonary volume. However, their study was single armed, the clinical follow-up was short, and these tumors are known to be biologically more indolent than other non-small cell carcinomas. In addition, no data was given on the incidence of local/regional recurrence in these notoriously soft and ill-defined tumors, making it difficult to determine the appropriate resection margin clinically. In addition, bronchioloalveolar carcinoma is known for its multifocal nature, which is presumably spread directly through regional airways.

13.3.4. Meta-analysis

Recently, Nakamura and colleagues analyzed 14 articles published in the period 1980 to 2004 containing postoperative survival data on patients undergoing limited pulmonary resections.[27] Care was taken to select independent authors and study groups, and that patients had early-stage disease. Of the 14 publications cited, in only 4 papers were limited resections performed on patients assessed to be able to tolerate a lobectomy. Although the authors performed an extensive search of the literature, publication bias may have been a factor because potentially important studies, such as those of Porrello and colleagues and Yamato and colleagues, were not included. The authors did acknowledge limitations of performing meta-analysis on retrospective studies. Other expressed limitations included heterogeneity of the patient populations (ability or inability to tolerate a lobectomy, age differences), heterogeneity in the carcinomas (size, histology, and pathological stage), and variability in surgical technique (wedge vs. segmentectomy, presence or absence of a mediastinal node dissection).

Upon performing a meta-analysis, the authors concluded, once again, that while there was an apparent overall survival advantage at 1-, 3-, and 5-year mark in favor of patients undergoing a lobectomy over patients undergoing a limited pulmonary resection; this advantage did not reach statistical significance.

13.4. Conclusions

Based on an extensive review of the currently available English language literature, and in accordance with the Oxford Centre for Evidence-Based Medicine,[28] it is our recommendation that (1) a pulmonary wedge resection not be performed on any patient with stage I NCSLC. This recommendation is based upon level 1 and 2 evidence. The grade of recommendation for this is A. (2) In the good-risk pulmonary patient with T1N0 NSCLC, our recommendation is for a lobectomy and complete nodal dissection to achieve the maximum survival benefit. While several studies failed to demonstrate a statistically significant survival advantage in small T1N0 tumors, no study proved that these operations were equivalents. In fact, in every study, there was a survival advantage for patients undergoing lobectomy, but in no single study did this reach statistical significance. This recommendation is based upon level of evidence that is classified as 2. The grade of recommendation for this is B. In the case of the extremely small stage IA lesions, a segmentectomy may be a reasonable option, but should be approached with caution and close follow-up. There is a need for a more thorough prospective randomized, controlled trial to elucidate the true benefit of segmentectomy (in contradistinction to a wedge resection), in this subset of patients with T1N0 tumors (T1 < 2.0 cm). (3) Patients with T2N0 tumors should undergo lobectomy. There is an extreme paucity of literature regarding limited resection in this subset of stage I patients. Furthermore, use of a lesser resection is counterintuitive, leaving the patient with a narrow margin of resection. Therefore, although level of evidence is at best classified as 2, the grade of recommendation for this is A. (4) Patients T1N0 tumors and deemed to be at high risk for postoperative morbidity and mortality after lobectomy should be considered for anatomical segmentectomy together with hilar and mediastinal node dissection. However, the exact criteria by which patients are deemed to be high-risk remains an open question and worthy of additional studies.

Pulmonary wedge resection not be performed on patients with stage I NCSLC (level of evidence 1 and 2; grade of recommendation A).

In the good-risk patient with T1N0 NSCLC, lobectomy and complete nodal dissection achieve the maximum survival benefit. Segmentectomy may be a reasonable for small stage IA lesions, but should be approached with caution and close follow-up (level of evidence 2; grade of recommendation B).

Patients with T2N0 tumors should undergo lobectomy (level of evidence 2; grade of recommendation A).

High-risk patients with T1N0 tumors should be considered for anatomical segmentectomy together with hilar and mediastinal node dissection (level of evidence 2; grade of recommendation B).

References

1. Jensik RJ, Faber LP, Milloy FJ, Monson DO. Segmental resection for lung cancer. A fifteen-year experience. *J Thorac Cardiovasc Surg* 1973;66:563–572.
2. Hoffmann TH, Ransdell HT. Comparison of lobectomy and wedge resection for carcinoma of the lung. *J Thorac Cardiovasc Surg* 1980;79:211–217.
3. Read RC, Yoder G, Schaeffer RC. Survival after conservative resection for T1 N0 M0 non-small cell lung cancer. *Ann Thorac Surg* 1990;49:391–398.
4. Harpole DH Jr, Herndon JE 2nd, Young WG Jr, Wolfe WG, Sabiston DC Jr. Stage I nonsmall cell lung cancer. A multivariate analysis of treatment methods and patterns of recurrence. *Cancer* 1995;76:787–796.
5. Cerfolio RJ, Allen MS, Trastek VF, Deschamps C, Scanlon PD, Pairolero PC. Lung resection in patients with compromised pulmonary function. *Ann Thorac Surg* 1996;62:348–351.
6. Lederle FA. Lobectomy versus limited resection in T1 N0 lung cancer. *Ann Thorac Surg* 1996;62:1249–1250.
7. Warren WH, Faber LP. Segmentectomy versus lobectomy in patients with stage I pulmonary carcinoma. Five-year survival and patterns of intrathoracic recurrence. *J Thorac Cardiovasc Surg* 1994;107:1087–1093.
8. Ginsberg RJ, Rubinstein LV. Randomized trial of lobectomy versus limited resection for T1 N0 non-small cell lung cancer. Lung Cancer Study Group. *Ann Thorac Surg* 1995;60:615–62.
9. Mathisen DJ, Jensik RJ, Faber LP, Kittle CF. Survival following sequential resections for second and third primary lung cancers. *J Thorac Cardiovasc Surg* 1984;88:502–510.
10. Jones DR, Stiles BM, Denlinger CE, Antippa P, Daniel TM. Pulmonary segmentectomy: results and complications. *Ann Thorac Surg* 2003;76:343–348.
11. Campione A, Ligabue T, Luzzi L, et al. Comparison between segmentectomy and larger resection of stage IA non-small cell lung carcinoma. *J Cardiovasc Surg* 2004;45:67–70.
12. Porrello C, Alifano M, Forti Parri SN, et al. Surgical treatment of stage I lung cancer. Results and prognostic factors. *J Cardiovasc Surg* 2002;43:723–727.
13. Landreneau RJ, Sugarbaker DJ, Mack MJ, et al. Wedge resection versus lobectomy for stage I (T1

N0 M0) non-small-cell lung cancer. *J Thorac Car-diovasc Surg* 1997;113:691–698.

14. Sugarbaker DJ, Strauss GM. Extent of surgery and survival in early lung carcinoma: implications for overdiagnosis in stage IA nonsmall cell lung carcinoma. *Cancer* 2000;89:2432–2437.

15. Miller DL, Rowland CM, Deschamps C, Allen MS, Trastek VF, Pairolero PC. Surgical treatment of non-small cell lung cancer 1 cm or less in diameter. *Ann Thorac Surg* 2002;73:1545–1550.

16. Takizawa T, Haga M, Yagi N, et al. Pulmonary function after segmentectomy for small peripheral carcinoma of the lung. *J Thorac Cardiovasc Surg* 1999;118:536–541.

17. Kodama K, Doi O, Higashiyama M, Yokouchi H. Intentional limited resection for selected patients with T1 N0 M0 non-small-cell lung cancer: a single-institution study. *J Thorac Cardiovasc Surg* 1997;114:347–353.

18. Tsubota N, Ayabe K, Doi O, et al. Ongoing prospective study of segmentectomy for small lung tumors. *Ann Thorac Surg* 1998;66:1787–1790.

19. Yoshikawa K, Tsubota N, Kodama K, Ayabe H, Taki T, Mori T. Prospective study of extended segmentectomy for small lung tumors: the final report. *Ann Thorac Surg* 2002;73:1055–1058.

20. Okada M, Yoshikawa K, Hatta T, Tsubota N. Is segmentectomy with lymph node assessment an alternative to lobectomy for non-small cell lung cancer of 2 cm or smaller? *Ann Thorac Surg* 2001;71:956–960.

21. Koike T, Yamato Y, Yoshiya K, Shimoyama T, Suzuki R. Intentional limited pulmonary resection for peripheral T1 N0 M0 small-sized lung cancer. *J Thorac Cardiovasc Surg* 2003;125:924–928.

22. Keenan RJ, Landreneau RJ, Maley RH Jr, et al. Segmental resection spares pulmonary function in patients with stage I lung cancer. *Ann Thorac Surg* 2004;78:228–233.

23. Mery CM, Pappas AN, Bueno R, et al. Similar long-term survival of elderly patients with non-small cell lung cancer treated with lobectomy or wedge resection within the surveillance, epidemiology, and end results database. *Chest* 2005;128:237–245.

24. Port JL, Kent MS, Korst RJ, Libby D, Pasmantier M, Altorki NK. Tumor size predicts survival within stage IA non-small cell lung cancer. *Chest* 2003;124:1828–1833.

25. Yamato Y, Tsuchida M, Watanabe T, et al. Early results of a prospective study of limited resection for bronchioloalveolar adenocarcinoma of the lung. *Ann Thorac Surg* 2001;71:971–974.

26. Noguchi M, Morikawa A, Kawasaki M, et al. Small adenocarcinoma of the lung. Histologic characteristics and prognosis. *Cancer* 1995;75:2844–2852.

27. Nakamura H, Kawasaki N, Taguchi M, Kabasawa K. Survival following lobectomy vs limited resection for stage I lung cancer: a meta-analysis. *Br J Cancer* 2005;92:1033–1037.

28. Harbour R, Miller J. A new system for grading recommendations in evidence-based guidelines. *BMJ* 2001;323:334–336.

14

Lesser Resection Versus Radiotherapy for Patients with Compromised Lung Function and Stage I Lung Cancer

Jeffrey A. Bogart and Leslie J. Kohman

The prospect for cure is excellent for fit patients treated with anatomical resection for pathological stage IA non-small cell lung cancer (NSCLC).[1] Unfortunately, a substantial subset of patients diagnosed with early-stage NSCLC suffer from cardiopulmonary disease and/or other underlying medical comorbidities, and therefore are not suitable candidates for standard therapy.[2] Treatment options for patients unable to tolerate lobectomy are typically guided by the severity of comorbid disease and traditionally have included limited resection (via open thoracotomy or a thoracoscopic approach) and external beam radiotherapy. Newer approaches including stereotactic radiosurgery and radiofrequency ablation are now utilized with increasing frequency. Recently, brachytherapy has been introduced as an adjuvant to wedge resection.[3,4] Although high-risk patients have been relatively neglected with regards to clinical research, this population is expected to increase in the future given factors such as the aging of the U.S. population and the increasing utilization of lung cancer screening.[5,6] In this chapter, we explore the data (retrospective and prospective) regarding these choices of therapy and describe the rationale and hypotheses of current ongoing clinical trials. The baseline management option is observation: the expected outcome of patients not eligible for standard surgical therapy (lobectomy) due to concurrent medical conditions.

By far the major reason that patients are turned down for lung cancer surgery is compromised pulmonary function, although a proportion has severe cardiac illness or overall poor performance status. Various algorithms are available for assessing whether or not a patient will tolerate a lobectomy. There is no commonly accepted absolute for which patients with significant pulmonary disease will and which will not tolerate surgical resection of their lung cancer. Few of the published articles give specifics on how the patients were chosen for alternative therapies. There is no high level evidence available on this topic.

14.1. Published Data

14.1.1. Observation

Prospective data are not available regarding the role of observation for high-risk patients with early-stage NSCLC. The poor outcome for patients with early-stage NSCLC who do not receive any treatment is illustrated by recent retrospective experiences. Of 128 patients identified with stage I and II NSCLC at the Veterans Administration Medical Center in Indianapolis between 1994 and 1999, 49 (38%) patients did not receive treatment due to either refusal of therapy or comorbid medical problems.[7] The median survival for this cohort of patients was 14.2 months and the majority of patients died from lung cancer. A separate report from the University of Arkansas included 97 patients who did not undergo resection for stage I and II NSCLC.[8] Seventy of 97 (72%) of patients did not receive cancer-specific therapy. The median survival was 11 months for these patients compared with 22 months for treated patients. Given the retrospective nature of these experiences, the impact of patient selection on outcomes cannot be ascertained. Evidence from prospectively collected data in a screening context[9] shows that even small lung cancers, left untreated, have a very poor outcome: The 8-year fatality rate for the diagnosed but untreated cases of lung cancer 6 to 15 mm in diameter was 87%, for 16 to 25 mm it was 94%, and for 26 to 30 mm it was 88%. The corresponding estimates of cure rates with resection were 71%, 67%, and 55%, respectively. These results for untreated patients come from a group of patients who were eligible for the screening because they were felt on general clinical evaluation to be fit enough to tolerate lobectomy. Results in a group of patients medically unfit for surgery would be worse because they would include deaths from comorbid conditions.

14.1.2. Comparisons of Surgery with Radiotherapy in Patients with Compromised Lung Function (Evidence Level 2 to 3)

A prospective comparison of surgery and radiotherapy conducted during the 1960s is limited by the use of antiquated staging and radiotherapy technology and the inclusion of patients with small cell lung cancer, and thus does not provide relevant data for modern-day treatment decisions.[10] There are no randomized, controlled studies on this topic.

Retrospective reports comparing surgery and radiotherapy for high-risk and/or elderly patients have reached differing conclusions. Yano and colleagues, from the National Kyushu Cancer Center in Fukuoka, Japan, retrospectively reviewed treatment results in compromised or poor-risk patients with clinical stage I NSCLC.[11] Seventeen patients underwent a limited resection (9 wedge resections and 8 segmentectomies), while 18 patients received radiation therapy. The 5-year survival rates for patients in the limited resection group and the radiation treatment group were 55.0% and 14.4%, respectively. Moreover, the reported incidence of severe treatment-related complications was not different between the limited operation group and the radiotherapy group (11.8% vs. 11.1%). Alternatively, Noordijk and colleagues, from Leiden, The Netherlands, described outcomes for patients irradiated for

peripherally located T1-2 N0M0 NSCLC.[12] Patients included did not have surgery because of poor medical condition, advanced age, or patient refusal. These results were compared to a group of 86 patients over 70 years of age treated surgically in the same hospital. The median survivals for patients treated with surgery and radiotherapy were 23 months and 27 months, respectively.

14.1.3. Retrospective Studies Assessing Surgery in Patients with Compromised Lung Function (Evidence Level 2 to 3)

Outcomes for high-risk patients treated with surgical resection vary greatly in retrospective studies. In a report of 116 patients with T1N0 NSCLC, 5-year survival was reduced for patients with chronic cardiopulmonary disease after standard surgery compared with patients without cardiopulmonary disease, 35% versus 53%, respectively.[13] Higher operative mortality was the main reason for the lower observed survival. Trials employing limited resection for patients with well-defined pulmonary dysfunction report lower operative mortality but similar survival. Five-year survival was 29% for 73 high-risk patients [mean ASA class II and mean forced expiratory volume in 1s (FEV$_1$) of 1.25] following wedge resection in a report from the Veterans Hospital in Washington, D.C.[14] In a separate study from Emory University, 5-year survival was 31% (excluding one postoperative death) following segmental or wedge resection for 32 patients with an FEV$_1$ less than 1.0.[15] All patients had clinical T1N0 NSCLC, and 31/32 patients had pathological T1N0 tumors.

Retrospective trials that appear to employ more liberal criteria for performing limited surgery report better outcomes. A report from the Arkansas Veterans Administration included 244 patients with T1N0 NSCLC. Five-year survival for the 113 patients treated with limited resection was 51%, and exceeded the outcomes for patients treated with lobectomy.[16] Similarly, Errett and colleagues reported 75% 6-year overall survival with wedge resection compared with 69% 6-year survival following lobectomy.[17] The median FEV$_1$ prior to wedge resection was 1.56L and wedge resection was more frequently employed than lobectomy in their series. A large retrospective analysis from Allegheny General Hospital compared segmental resection and lobectomy for stage I NSCLC (18). Four-year survival was comparable in both groups (67 % vs. 62%) and pulmonary function was more likely to be spared following segmental resection, as a decline in diffusing capacity was the only significant change observed in this group. A recent report supports the feasibility of safely performing limited resection in patients with pulmonary dysfunction.[19] In a study of 219 patients with stage IA NSCLC, there was no operative mortality with wedge resection (via either an open or thoracoscopic approach), compared with 3% mortality following lobectomy. Five-year survival was 58% for following open wedge resection, 65% following video-assisted wedge resection, and 70% after lobectomy.

An increased risk of local tumor relapse has been reported for limited resection compared with lobectomy. The local recurrence rate was 22.7% (15/66) with segmentectomy versus 4.9% (5/103) with lobectomy in a study from Rush Medical Center.[20] Miller reported the potential for adjuvant external beam radiotherapy to reduce the risk of local relapse after limited resection for stage I NSCLC, particularly when the lesion crossed an intersegmental plane.[15] In their series, local tumor relapse was reduced from 33% to 11% (2/18) with the addition of adjuvant external beam radiotherapy.

In an effort to address the risk of local tumor relapse, two retrospective studies have addressed a combined approach of limited resection and permanent ^{125}I brachytherapy. D'Amato reported a series of 14 patients, with an average FEV_1 of 0.59L (23% predicted) and an average diffusion of carbon monoxide was 6.8mL/min/mmHg (30% predicted), with peripheral pathological T1N0 NSCLC.[3] Surgical margins were pathologically clear and mediastinal nodes were sampled in all patients. Treatment included video-assisted thoracoscopic wedge resection with a polyglyconate mesh containing ^{125}I seeds applied to pulmonary resection margins. The short follow-up time (average 7 months and maximum 12 months) precluded an assessment of outcome, but no significant operative morbidity or radiation related toxicity was observed. A larger experience was reported from the New England Medical Center.[4] Thirty-three patients underwent a limited resection with ^{125}I brachytherapy seeds implanted along the resection margin. With a median follow-up of 51 months, the 5-year survival was 47%, 67% for patients with T1N0 tumors, and 39% for patients with T2N0 tumors. Two local and six regional recurrences were observed.

14.1.4. Prospective Trials Assessing Limited Resection in Patients with Compromised Lung Function (Level of Evidence 2++)

The Lung Cancer Study Group conducted a prospective, randomized phase III trial comparing limited resection with lobectomy for patients with peripheral, pathologically documented T1N0 NSCLC. Patients were required to have adequate pulmonary reserve for lobectomy.[21] Limited resection was associated with a 30% increase in the overall death rate, a 50% increase in the observed death with cancer rate, and a tripling of local recurrence compared to lobectomy. Local recurrence was, likewise, increased following wedge resection compared with segmentectomy. Moreover, limited pulmonary resection did not reduce perioperative morbidity or mortality, or improve postoperative pulmonary function.

The results of a prospective phase II trial limited to patients with pulmonary dysfunction were recently published.[22] The Cancer and Leukemia Group B (CALGB) 9335 enrolled high-risk patients with one or more of the following risk factors: FEV_1 less than 40%, carbon monoxide diffusing capacity in lung (DLCO) less than 50%, and maximum oxygen consumption (VO_2max) less than 45mmHg. Patients underwent video-assisted wedge resection followed by local (56Gy) radiotherapy if they were found to have pathological T1N0 NSCLC. The primary end point was the proportion of patients whose disease could be completely resected and who received radiotherapy without treatment complications. Overall, video-assisted wedge resection was not technically feasible in 29% of patients. Of 58 eligible patients registered in the study, 32 patients were found to have pathologically staged T1 NSCLC. The median survival of patients with pathological T1 disease (excluding one postoperative death) was 32 months and 5-year survival was

TABLE 14.1. Selected reports of surgery for high-risk early-stage NSCLC.

Reference	Method	n	Stage	Surgery	OS	Level of evidence
Pastorino[13]	R	116	IA	Lobe/Pn	35% (5 years)	3
Miller[15]	R	31	IA	Wed (21)/Seg (10)	31% (5 years)	3
Errett[17]	R	100	I	Wedge	69% (6 years)	3
Read[16]	R	113	IA	Seg (106)/Weg (7)	51% (5 years)	3
Landreneau[19]	R	102	IA	Wed (42)/VATS (60)	58%/65% (5 years)	3
Shennib[22]	P	31	IA	VATS[a]	29% (5 years)	2++

Abbreviations: Lobe, lobectomy; OS, overall survival; P, prospective; Pn, pneumonectomy; R, retrospective; Seg, segmental resection; VATS, video-assisted thorascopic resection; Wed, wedge.
[a]Postoperative radiotherapy planned.

29%. Detailed patterns of failure have not been published, although a 29% local relapse rate was observed: 36% for narrowly resected (e.g., margin <1 cm) lesions and 21% for widely resected lesions. The influence of adjuvant radiotherapy on survival and local tumor control is not discernable.

A recently activated prospective phase III trial, headed by the American College of Surgeons Oncology Group, seeks to confirm the provocative retrospective experience of combined wedge resection and ^{125}I brachytherapy. Patients with NSCLC less than 3 cm are randomized to treatment with sublobar resection or sublobar resection and intraoperative ^{125}I brachytherapy (100 Gy). Eligibility criteria are more liberal than the CALGB prospective trial, and advanced age is included in the criteria for protocol entry. The primary end point of the study is 2-year local tumor relapse, and approximately 225 patients will be accrued. Table 14.1 summarizes the results of select surgery series.

14.1.5. Retrospective Trials of Radiotherapy in Patients with Compromised Lung Function (Level of Evidence 2– to 3)

Published reviews summarize the results of early NSCLC following radiotherapy in retrospective reports. Sibley reviewed the results of 10 studies utilizing megavoltage irradiation to doses of more than 55 Gy for medically inoperable stage I NSCLC.[23] Although there was a substantial rate of death from intercurrent disease, the main cause of death in this patient population was lung cancer progression. Overall, 15% of patients were long-term survivors, 30% died from progression of local disease, 30% died from distant metasta-

ses, and 25% died from other causes. Prognostic factors for survival included tumor size and age, and 5-year overall survival ranged from 26% to 67% for T1 lesions and from 4% to 24% for T2 lesions. A correlation between radiation dose and local tumor failure and/or improved survival was suggested in several studies. Toxicity was minimal and 8 of 10 studies reported grade 3+ complication rates less than 2%.

More recently, Rowell and Williams reviewed all published trials of radiotherapy for stage I/IIA NSCLC delivering more than 4000 cGy.[24] Twenty-seven trials were identified with greater than 2000 patients, including one prospective randomized trial for which a subset analysis was available for patients with clinical stage I/II A NSCLC.[5] It was noted that the population included in these trials is poorly defined: the rationale for nonoperative therapy was stated for only approximately 50% of patients, pretreatment pulmonary function testing was reported in only one trial, CT staging was utilized haphazardly in many studies, and mediastinoscopy was rarely employed. Overall, observations were similar to those of Sibley, in that most patients died from their cancer despite a presumed high rate of comorbid illness, improved survival was observed with smaller tumors, and better results (i.e., response rates) were suggested with higher doses of radiotherapy. In fact, more than one third of patients with T1 tumors survived 5 years. Treatment outcome was related to pretreatment weight loss, but in contrast to the findings of Sibley, age was not a prognostic factor. Only one fatal pneumonitis was reported, although morbidity was likely underreported due to the retrospective nature of these studies.

The largest reported retrospective radiotherapy series employing conventional radiotherapy planning, from Queensland Radium Institute, consists of 347 patients with T1N0 and T2N0 tumors.[25] The median age for the group was 70 years, and all patients were treated to 50 Gy in 20 fractions over 4 weeks. Survival correlated with tumor size with 5-year survival rates of 32% and 21% for T1 and T2 tumors, respectively. Despite the use of clinical staging, results from this large series are similar to those reported for patients with cardiopulmonary dysfunction undergoing limited surgery for comparably sized tumors.

14.1.6. Prospective Trials of Radiotherapy in Patients with Compromised Lung Function (Level of Evidence 2+)

The advent of three-dimensional conformal therapy helps to ensure appropriate coverage of the intended target, while at the same time limiting radiation exposure to the surrounding normal structures. Few trials have been designed exclusively for high-risk stage I NSCLC, but recently reported prospective dose escalation trials have included this population. A phase I/II Radiation Therapy Oncology Group (RTOG) study administered escalating radiation doses with conformal techniques depending on the percentage of lung volume irradiated. In the small volume bin (i.e., 20 Gy to <25% total lung volume), dose was sequentially increased from 70.9 Gy to 90.3 Gy.[26] Clinical stage I NSCLC composed 44% (77/177) of the study population. Median follow-up ranged from 13.4 months to 18 months, with an estimated median survival approaching 27 months for patients with clinical stage I NSCLC. A dose escalation study at the University of Michigan demonstrated that doses as great as 102.9 Gy could be delivered with conventional fractionation when the volume of irradiated lung was restricted.[27] The median survival for patients with stage I /II NSCLC was 20 months and local tumor control was 61% if doses greater than or equal to 92 Gy were applied.

Radiotherapy treatment schemes that accelerate completion of the treatment course may be more effective than conventionally fractionated (e.g., protracted) regimens. A randomized trial in the United Kingdom compared continuous hyperfractionated accelerated radiotherapy (CHART), 54 Gy in 36 fractions of 1.5 Gy over 12 days, to conventional radiotherapy, 60 Gy over 6 weeks.[28] While the majority of patients had stage III disease, 169 patients with stage I/IIA NSCLC were included. However, only a small subset of patients with early stage disease (~20%) had clinical T1N0 lesions. Two-year survival was significantly improved with CHART for patients with stage I/II disease, 37% versus 24%, and the difference remained at 4 years (18% vs. 12%).

Accelerated once-daily (e.g., hypofractionated) conformal radiotherapy is currently being explored in a phase I prospective clinical trial conducted by the Cancer and Leukemia Group B (CALGB). Eligibility is limited to high-risk patients with stage I NSCLC (i.e., <4 cm). The radiation fraction size is progressively increased from 2.41 Gy to 4.11 Gy while the total nominal dose is kept at 70 Gy and the total treatment time is reduced to 3.5 weeks. This schedule yields a stepwise reduction in the treatment time, with a corresponding potential increased biological effect.

Hypofractionated therapy with charged particles has also been evaluated prospectively for early-stage NSCLC. Protons and carbon ions have physical advantages over conventional X-ray beams and may be shaped to deliver a high dose of radiation to a central lung tumor with relative sparing of the surrounding functioning lung tissue. Accordingly, these treatments should help minimize the extent and severity of pulmonary injury and may benefit patients with severe underlying pulmonary disease. A phase II trial from Loma Linda enrolled 68 patients with stage I NSCLC.[29] Proton therapy at doses ranging from 51 to 60 cobalt Gy equivalent (CGE) in 10 fractions/2 weeks was utilized. With a median follow-up of 30 months, 3-year local tumor control and disease-specific survival were 74% and 73%, respectively, and symptomatic radiation pneumonitis was not observed. Superior local tumor control was obtained for clinical T1N0 lesions (87%), compared with T2N0 disease (49%). A phase I/II study evaluating hypofractionated delivery of carbon ion particles included 81 patients treated to a dose of 59 to 94 CGE in 9 to 18 fractions.[30] Thirty-seven of 81 patients remain alive after a median follow-up of 40 months, and

TABLE 14.2. Selected reports of radiotherapy for early-stage NSCLC.

Reference	Method	n	Stage	Dose/Fx size	LC	OS	Level of evidence
Gauden[25]	R	167	IA	50/2.5	–	32% (5 years)	3
Henning[27]	3D/P	11	I	92.4–102.9/2.1	76% (2 years)	–	2+
Bradley[26]	3D/P	77	I	70.9–90.3/2.15	65% (3 years)[a]	36% (3 years)[a]	2++
Bush[29]	Proton	27	I	50.1–73.8 CGE/5.1	87% (2 years)	86%	2+
Timmerman[31]	SRS/P	37	I	24–60/8–20	31/37	–	2+

Abbreviations: 3D, conformal radiotherapy; CGE, cobalt GY equivalent; LC, local tumor control; OS, overall survival; P, prospective; R, retrospective; SRS sterotactic radiosurgery.
[a]Estimated from survival curve.

23% absolute local tumor relapse was noted. Whether charged particle therapy is more efficacious than photon irradiation delivered with advanced technologies (e.g., three-dimensional conformal therapy) has not been assessed and charged particle therapy is not widely available given the prohibitive cast of such facilities.

14.1.7. Body Stereotactic Radiosurgery (Level of Evidence 2+)

The preliminary results of prospective studies exploring stereotactic radiosurgery have recently been reported. A phase I dose escalation trial assessing stereotactic radiosurgery was conducted at Indiana University.[31] Eligible patients included those with clinically staged T1 or T2 (tumor size <7cm) N0M0 biopsy-confirmed NSCLC. All patients had comorbid medical problems that precluded thoracotomy. The median age was 75 years. Radiosurgery was administered in three separate fractions over 2 weeks. The dose was safely increased from 800cGy per fraction (2400cGy total) to 2000cGy per fraction (6000cGy total) for patients with both T1 and T2 lesions. The overall response rate (n = 37) was 87% (complete response, 27%). Six local tumor recurrences were observed after a median follow-up 15.2 months. A phase II multi-institutional trial based on the Indiana University experience was recently activated by the RTOG. Single fraction radiosurgery has been explored in Europe, and Hof and colleagues conducted a phase I/II study of stereotactic radiosurgery in 10 patients with stage I NSCLC.[32] Total doses applied ranged from 19 to 26Gy. Local tumor control was obtained in 8 of 10 lesions with a median follow-up period of 14.9 months and actuarial overall survival was 64% at

24 months. Distant metastases developed in five patients and mediastinal lymph node relapse was found in an additional patient. Table 14.2 summarizes the results of select radiotherapy series.

14.2. Summary of Published Data and Their Impact on Clinical Practice

The available published clinical data are not of sufficient quality to provide definitive guidance for patients with early stage NSCLC. Trials of surgery and radiotherapy vary greatly regarding patient selection, thoroughness of staging [e.g., mediastinoscopy, positron emission tomography (PET) scan], tumor location, and tumor burden. The published evidence is generally of level 2 to 3, the results are conflicting, and no recommendation can be made. The choice of therapy should be individualized by patient and the experience of the institution.

The results of the LCSG phase III trial clearly indicate lobectomy should be considered the optimal surgical procedure for stage I NSCLC. Therefore, patients should be thoroughly evaluated and pulmonary rehabilitation should be considered for patients with marginal pulmonary function. The level of evidence is 1– and the grade of recommendation is A.

Lobectomy should be considered the optimal surgical procedure for stage I NSCLC; preoperative pulmonary rehabilitation should be considered for patients with marginal pulmonary function (level of evidence 1–; grade of recommendation A).

The outcome of limited surgical resection and radiotherapy are greatly dependent on patient selection. Stage IA patients with defined poor lung function and/or medical comorbidity precluding anatomical resection appear to have an approximate 30% expectation for long-term survival with either limited resection or aggressive radiotherapy delivered with modern techniques. Segmental resection with wide surgical margins results in a lower risk of local tumor relapse compared with wedge resection and may reduce the risk of local tumor failure compared with conventionally fractionated radiotherapy. Moreover, local tumor control following radiotherapy relates directly with tumor volume, and a surgical approach may be advantageous for larger tumors (e.g., >3.5–4 cm) if adequate margins can be obtained. Newer radiotherapy approaches, including accelerated conformal treatment and stereotactic body radiosurgery, may improve results compared with traditional radiotherapy. The quality of evidence is 2 to 3, and the grade of recommendation is C. Large-scale multi-institutional trials are necessary for confirmation. The treatment decision should be based on the experience of the center and patient preference, guided by estimates of relative toxicity.

Whether adjuvant radiotherapy reduces local tumor failure and improves outcomes after limited surgery remains to be determined. While local tumor relapse is clearly increased following limited resection compared with lobectomy, CALGB 9335 did not establish the value of external beam radiotherapy. The concerns raised regarding the potential detrimental effects of postoperative radiotherapy in the PORT meta-analysis (particularly for N0 disease) may be germane, particularly if large radiotherapy portals are utilized.[33] Initial retrospective trials of adjuvant brachytherapy report promising results, but prospective data from the recently activated ACOSOG trial will not be available for several years. No recommendation can be made regarding the role of adjuvant radiotherapy at this time.

> The value of adjuvant radiotherapy on local tumor control and improved survival after limited surgery remains to be determined.

14.2.1. Our Personal View of the Data and Future Trends

All patients with potentially resectable lung cancer and compromised pulmonary function should be evaluated in a multidisciplinary lung cancer clinic, with input by an experienced chest radiologist, thoracic surgeon, radiation oncologist, pulmonologist, and medical oncologist. All continuing smokers should have intense and ongoing smoking cessation counseling beginning with their first visit. High-risk patients should be immediately enrolled in a pulmonary rehabilitation program. Sometimes the combination of smoking cessation and pulmonary rehabilitation will render a patient fit enough for lobectomy or at least segmentectomy. If not, thorough staging (PET scan, sometimes mediastinoscopy) will determine the clinical stage as accurately as possible.

Options for patients who cannot undergo standard resection include wedge resection (open or thoracoscopic), wedge resection with adjuvant radiotherapy, wedge resection with brachytherapy, primary radiotherapy (hypofractionation, intensity–modulated radiation therapy (IMRT), respiratory gating, stereotactic radiosurgery), radiofrequency ablation (experimental), and any of the preceding combined with chemotherapy, including radiosensitizing chemotherapy. All patients should be considered for inclusion in one of several current and upcoming clinical trials evaluating these modalities in a prospective and occasionally randomized fashion.

Patients at high-risk for receiving anesthesia and patients with extremely limited pulmonary reserve will generally be treated nonsurgically. Central lesions that are not amenable to limited resection are also generally treated nonsurgically. Modestly hypofractionated three-dimensional conformal radiotherapy is generally employed outside of the clinical trial setting. The extent of hypofractionation/acceleration is guided by the volume of irradiated lung. Patients treated with radiotherapy are also evaluated for respiratory gating in order to limit the effect of tumor motion.

Patients who have potential for surgical resection should have smoking cessation and pulmonary rehabilitation and a complete cardiac evaluation. At the time of wedge resection, placement of large hemoclips at the apex of the wedge or the area of closest margin will facilitate postoperative radiotherapy.

Given the heterogeneous nature of the high-risk patient population, comparative prospective, randomized trials of surgery and radiotherapy may not be feasible. The mature results of ongoing trials exploring accelerated conformal radiotherapy, stereotactic radiosurgery, and wedge resection and brachytherapy will provide important information to help guide local therapy. Whether systemic chemotherapy may be of benefit has not been addressed, but this issue is of increasing consideration particularly given the results of recent trials demonstrating a survival benefit for the addition of chemotherapy to surgical resection for early-stage NSCLC.[34,35]

References

1. Williams DE, Pairolero PC, Davis CS, et al. Survival of patients surgically treated for stage I lung cancer. *J Thorac Cardiovasc Surg* 1981;82:70–76.
2. Mettlin CJ, Menck HR, Murphy GP, et al. A comparison of breast, colorectal, lung, and prostate cancers reported to the National Cancer Data Base and the Surveillance, Epidemiology, and End Results Program. *Cancer* 1997;79:2052–2061.
3. d'Amato TA, Galloway M, Szydlowski G, et al. Intraoperative brachytherapy following thoracoscopic wedge resection of stage I lung cancer. *Chest* 1998;4:1112–1115.
4. Lee W, Daly DB, Dipetrillo TA, et al. Limited resection for non-small cell lung cancer: observed local control with implantation of I-125 brachytherapy seeds. *Ann Thorac Surg* 2003;75:237–242; discussion 242–243.
5. Havlik RJ, Yancik R, Long S, et al. The National Institute on Aging and the National Cancer Institute SEER collaborative study on comorbidity and early diagnosis of cancer in the elderly. *Cancer* 1994;74(suppl 1):2102–2106.
6. Henschke CI, McCauley DI, Yankelevitz DF, et al. Early Lung Cancer Action Project: overall design and findings from baseline screening. *Lancet* 1999;354:99–105.
7. McGarry RC, Song G, des Rosiers P, et al. Observation-only management of early stage, medically inoperable lung cancer. *Chest* 2002;121:1155–1158.
8. Kyasa MJ, Jazieh AR. Characteristics and outcomes of patients with unresected earlystage non-

small cell lung cancer. *South Med J* 2002;95:1149–1152.
9. Henschke CI, Wisnevsky JP, Yankelevitz DF, et al. Small stage I cancers of the lung: genuineness and curability. *Lung Cancer* 2003;39:327–339.
10. Morrison R, Deeley TJ, Cleland WP. The treatment of carcinoma of the bronchus: a clinical trial to compare surgery and supervoltage radiotherapy. *Lancet* 1963;1:683–684.
11. Yano T, Yokoyama H, Yoshino I, et al. Results of limited resection for compromised or poor-risk patients with clinical stage I non-small cell carcinoma of the lung. *J Am Coll Surg* 1995;181:33–37.
12. Noordijk EM, Clement E, Hermans J, et al. Radiotherapy as an alternative to surgery in elderly patients with resectable lung cancer. *Radiother Oncol* 1988;13:83–89.
13. Pastorino U, Valente M. Bendini V, et al. Effect of chronic cardiopulmonary disease on survival after resection for stage Ia lung cancer. *Thorax* 1982;37:680–683.
14. Temeck BK, Schafer PW, Saini N. Wedge resection for bronchogenic carcinoma in high-risk patients. *South Med J* 1992;85:1081–1083.
15. Miller JI, Hatcher CR. Limited resection of bronchogenic carcinoma in the patient with marked impairment of pulmonary function. *Ann Thorac Surg* 1987;44:340–343.
16. Read RC, Yoder G, Schaeffer RC. Survival after conservative resection for T1N0M0 non-small cell lung cancer. *Ann Thorac Surg* 1990;49:391–398; discussion 399–400.
17. Errett LE, Wilson J, Chiu RC, et al. Wedge resection as an alternative procedure for peripheral bronchogenic carcinoma in poor-risk patients. *J Thorac Cardiovasc Surg* 1985;90:656–661.
18. Keenan RJ, Landreneau RJ, Maley RH Jr, et al. Segmental resection spares pulmonary function in patients with stage I lung cancer. *Ann Thorac Surg* 2004;78:228–233; discussion 228–223.
19. Landreneau RJ, Sugarbaker DJ, Mack MJ, et al. Wedge resection versus lobectomy for stage I (T1 N0 M0) non-small-cell lung cancer. *J Thorac Cardiovasc Surg* 1997;113:691–698; discussion 698–700.
20. Warren WH, Faber LP. Segmentectomy versus lobectomy in patients with stage I pulmonary carcinoma. Five-year survival and patterns of intrathoracic recurrence. *J Thorac Cardiovas Surg* 1994;107:1087–1093; discussion 1093–1094.
21. Ginsberg RJ, Rubinstein LV. Randomized trial of lobectomy versus limited resection for T1N0 non-small cell lung cancer. Lung Cancer Study Group. *Ann Thorac Surg* 1995;60:615–622; discussion 622–623.

22. Shennib H, Bogart J, Herndon JE, et al. Video-assisted wedge resection and local radiotherapy for peripheral lung cancer in high-risk patients: The Cancer and Leukemia Group B (CALGB) 9335, a phase II, multi-institutional cooperative group study. *J Thorac Cardiovasc Surg* 2005;129:813–818.

23. Sibley GS. Radiotherapy for patients with medically inoperable stage I nonsmall cell lung carcinoma: smaller volumed and higher doses – a review. *Cancer* 1998;82:433–438.

24. Rowell NP, Williams CJ. Radical radiotherapy for stage I/II non-small cell lung cancer in patients not sufficiently fit for or declining surgery (medically inoperable): a systematic review. *Thorax* 2001;56:628–638.

25. Gauden S, Ramsay J, Tripcony L. The curative treatment by radiotherapy alone of stage I non-small cell carcinoma of the lung. *Chest* 1995;108:1278–1282.

26. Bradley J, Graham MV, Winter K, et al. Toxicity and outcome results of RTOG 9311: a phase I-II dose-escalation study using three-dimensional conformal radiotherapy in patients with inoperable non-small-cell lung carcinoma. *Int J Radiat Oncol Biol Phys* 2005;61:318–328.

27. Henning GT, Littles JF, Martel ML, et al. Preliminary results of 92.4Gy or more for non-small cell lung cancer. *Int J Radiat Oncol Biol Phys* 2002;48(suppl 1):233.

28. Saunders M, Dische S, Barrett A, et al. Continuous hyperfractionated accelerated radiotherapy (CHART) versus conventional radiotherapy in non-small cell lung cancer: a randomised multi-centre trial. CHART Steering Committee. *Lancet* 1997;350:161–165.

29. Bush DA, Slater, Shin, et al. Hypofractionated proton beam radiotherapy for stage I lung cancer. *Chest* 2004;126:1198–1203.

30. Koto M, Miyamoto T, Yamamoto N, et al. Local control and recurrence of stage I non-small cell lung cancer after carbon ion radiotherapy. *Radiother Oncol* 2004;71:147–156.

31. Timmerman R, Papiez L, McGarry R, et al. Extra-cranial stereotactic radioablation: results of a phase I study in medically inoperable stage I non-small cell lung cancer. *Chest* 2003;124:1946–1955.

32. Hof H, Herfarth K, Debus J. Stereotactic irradiation of lung tumors [review]. *Radiologe* 2004;44:484–490.

33. Postoperative radiotherapy in non-small-cell lung cancer: systemic review and meta-analysis of individual patient data from nine randomized controlled trials. PORT Meta-analysis Trialists Group. *Lancet* 1998;352:257–263.

34. Winton TL, Livingston R, Johnson D, et al. A prospective, randomised trial of adjuvant vinorelbine (VIN) and cisplatin (CIS) in completely resected stage IB and II non small cell lung cancer (NSCLC) Intergroup JBR.10 [abstract]. *J Clin Oncol* 2004;22:7018.

35. Strauss GM, Herndon J, Maddaus MA, et al. Randomized clinical trial of adjuvant chemotherapy with paclitaxel and carboplatin following resection in Stage IB non-small cell lung cancer (NSCLC): report of Cancer and Leukemia Group B (CALGB) Protocol 9633 [abstract]. *J Clin Oncol* 2004;22:7019.

15
Resection for Patients Initially Diagnosed with N3 Lung Cancer after Response to Induction Therapy

Antonio D'Andrilli, Federico Venuta, and Erino A. Rendina

Lung cancer is classified as N3 when metastases to the contralateral mediastinal and hilar lymph nodes, the supraclavicular nodes, and the scalene nodes are present at the time of diagnosis. N3 lung tumors have been included in stage IIIB since 1986, when it appeared clear that such locally advanced disease needs to be grouped in a separate stage III category because of the extremely poor prognosis. In the large series reported by Mountain, 5-year survival for N3 patients was 3%.[1] These tumors have always been considered inoperable due to the difficulties in eradicating all the detectable disease that markedly limits the applicability of primary surgery in this setting.

N3 lung cancer has been approached aggressively with initial surgery in a few centers, mainly by Japanese groups.[2,3] The pulmonary resection is carried out through a median sternotomy, and complete bilateral lymphadenectomy is accomplished. The limited survival benefit observed with such an aggressive approach has, however, strongly discouraged the choice of primary operation.

Bimodality protocols of chemotherapy combined with definitive thoracic irradiation represents, at the moment, the standard treatment of care for N3 and all stage IIIB patients.[4-6] Recently, concurrent administration of these two therapeutic options has been recommended because it provides improved survival in comparison to sequential chemoradiotherapy, although it is frequently associated with increased toxicity.[4,7-9] With this combined modality therapy, the expected 5-year survival ranges between 10% and 15%.[4] However, this treatment achieves tumor sterilization in only 5% to 20% of the patients,[10,11] and locoregional failure is almost the rule with a local control of 17% at 1 year in randomized studies.[12] This argument strongly supports the search for an alternative strategy of treatment in the attempt to achieve a more complete oncologic control.

Neoadjuvant chemotherapy or chemoradiotherapy followed by surgical resection has been used in patients with stage IIIA-N2 disease since the end of 1980s, showing significant survival advantage in small randomized studies. In some of these studies, carefully selected IIIB patients have been enrolled and their survival results, in initial experiences, did not differ markedly from the IIIA group.

The analysis of data concerning complex and aggressive therapeutic options including surgery in poor-prognosis groups of patients, such as N3, has to necessarily undergo a meticulous evaluation of the methods employed and, in particular, of the staging and restaging modalities, inclusion criteria, induction protocols, and surgical technique.

15.1. Staging Modalities

Staging modalities should be rigorously evaluated and verified when comparing results by different centers, including heterogeneous protocols. Inaccurate clinical staging invariably limits the significance of reported clinical results. In particular, trials not including surgery usually enroll patients without positive histological staging. Even in the most recent studies with chemotherapy or radiochemotherapy followed by surgery, pretreatment staging accuracy is often questionable and varies from one investigator to another.

Diagnostic imaging of the mediastinum with purpose of lymph nodal staging before treatment is still most commonly based on computed tomography (CT). The use of dimensional criteria (lymph node size >1 cm) as the sole parameter to assess the presence of nodal metastases strongly limits the efficacy of the technique in this setting. Computed tomography alone has been found to have low sensitivity (56%–63%) and specificity (60%–90%), with an accuracy ranging from 61% to 85% for identification of malignant N2 and N3 lymph nodes.[13–15] The false-negative rate has been registered as high as 30% in several experiences.[16] Moreover, the sensitivity and the accuracy of CT scan for detecting lymph nodal metastases are lower after induction therapy.[17] Therefore, surgical exploration of the mediastinum, principally by means of mediastinoscopy, has often been advocated for histological confirmation of staging.

In experienced hands mediastinoscopy is extremely accurate, showing an average sensitivity of 84%, a specificity of 100%, and a false-negative rate averaging 9% in 10 large series[18–27] published over a 15-year period. Some authors[17] have recently hypothesized that the use of a video-assisted approach (videomediastinoscopy) has contributed an increased efficacy of mediastinoscopy, including after induction therapy. The accuracy of video-assisted mediastinoscopy after neoadjuvant chemotherapy has been reported as high as 91%, with results similar to those observed in patients without preoperative treatment.

Currently employed alternative tools for invasive mediastinal staging of lung cancer, including anterior mediastinotomy, videothoracoscopy, and extended mediastinoscopy, play a lesser role in the preoperative histological diagnosis of N3 disease. Extended cervical mediastinoscopy has been proven an effective technique for sampling enlarged lymph nodes in stations 5 and 6 that are not reachable by conventional mediastinoscopy. Ginsberg[28–30] reported a sensitivity of 69%, a specificity of 100%, and an accuracy of 91% in a series of 300 cases. However, concern about the technical complexity of this approach has limited its use to a few experienced centers and generally for confirmation of N2 disease in left lung cancer. There are sporadic experiences in the literature reporting the adoption of this procedure for staging of N3 disease. Similarly, videothoracoscopy, which has been proposed as an effective method for surgical exploration of the aortopulmonary window and the para-aortic lymph nodal station, has achieved a limited application in the diagnosis of the N3 disease. In clinical practice, it has been more frequently used for staging suspected T4 lung cancer. Direct biopsy of the supraclavicular nodes and the scalene nodes can be accomplished without particular technical difficulties, but the presence of tumor in these sites is considered an exclusion criteria in many trials including N3 patients.[6,31–33] More recently, fiber-optic transbronchial needle aspiration, by either cytological or histological needle, has been reported as a safe and effective alternative to mediastinoscopy in suspected N2 and N3 lung cancer.[34–36] Although sensitivity and accuracy of this technique in this setting have been reported as high as 71% and 73%, respectively (84% and 86% for the right paratracheal nodes),[35] these procedures are still not widely performed and only selected centers have reached adequate experience.

All the above-mentioned data have justified a general affirmation of invasive procedures for mediastinal staging. In the literature, almost all phase II trials including N3 patients have employed mediastinoscopy to confirm lymph nodal involvement.[6,9,10,32,33,37]

15.2. Restaging Tools

A number of considerations should be made when analyzing data from different studies administering induction therapy in order to evaluate the appropriateness of the restaging tools employed and the scientific accuracy of the results obtained. First, there is evidence in literature that pathological mediastinal downstaging is one of the most powerful predictors of survival after resection following induction therapy. This has been principally proven in series of N2 patients, but has been also verified in few selected experiences including N3 patients. Second, currently employed imaging methods have shown disappointing efficacy in mediastinal restaging after neoadjuvant treatment. Computed tomography can be very misleading in this setting because the presence of lymph nodes appearing with pathological size (more than 1 cm in diameter) has been proven to be unrelated to the neoplastic disease in up to 40% of patients.[38] This is due to the scarring and inflammatory changes induced by the treatment of the initially neoplastic lymphadenopathy, which may explain the persistence of radiologically anomalous tissue in the site of the previously detected pathologic nodes. Finally, fluorodeoxyglucose (FDG)-positron emission tomography (PET) has shown a significantly lower accuracy in mediastinal staging after induction therapy because chemotherapy and radiotherapy induce reactions in lymph nodes that may lead to increased FDG uptake.[39]

As a consequence, a number of authors have advocated surgical re-exploration of the mediastinum as the only effective means to achieve a proper selection of patients likely to benefit from surgical resection after induction therapy. Repeat mediastinoscopy has been routinely performed in this field only in selected centers with considerable experience.[33,38,40] Despite technical difficulties due to mediastinal fibrosis and peritracheal adhesions, this procedure can be done without increased morbidity and with satisfactory results. Sensitivity, specificity, and accuracy of repeated medistinoscopy after induction treatment have been reported as high as 73% to 75%, 100%, and 80% to 85% in the two larger series in the literature.[38,40] Although slightly lower than that of initial mediastinoscopy, the accuracy of this procedure allows adequate pathological restaging of the mediastinum in lung cancer. The only contrasting experience, in terms of results, is the one published by Pitz.[33] However, the lower diagnostic value of the technique in this series can be explained by the high number of incomplete procedures.

Lardinois[17] has recently investigated the role of videomediastinoscopy in patients submitted to induction therapy without previous exploration of the mediastinum, and who showed radiological response to treatment. Results were compared with those of the same technique in potentially operable patients without preoperative treatment. Safety (0% vs. 4% morbidity) and accuracy (91% vs. 95%) were similar with and without induction therapy. Videomediastinoscopy revealed the presence of N2 or N3 disease in 17% of patients with mediastinal lymph nodes smaller than 1 cm at CT scan after neoadjuvant therapy.

Thoracotomy is hardly acceptable as a staging or restaging method in a setting where the real benefit of surgery is still to be quantified. Therefore, thoracotomy might be employed only after other staging methods proved inconclusive. The introduction of FDG-PET scan has partially modified the diagnostic strategies for the selection of patients to either primary surgery or after induction therapy. In a recent prospective study, the integrated use of FDG-PET with CT has significantly improved the nodal staging accuracy if compared with CT alone, but also with FDG-PET alone.[41]

However, the combination of mediastinoscopy and PET has proved to considerably improve the efficacy of mediastinal staging of lung cancer.[42] In the study from Kernstine,[42] if PET is negative in either N2 or N3 nodes there is little probability of mediastinal disease (1%–8%), but when PET is positive in N2 or N3 sites, the metastatic tumor is not histologically confirmed in 40% to 60% of the cases, so that mediastinoscopy is recommended. Moreover, PET has shown a significantly lower accuracy for mediastinal staging in patients who underwent induction therapy than in patients without preoperative treatment, with a sensitivity of 67% and a specificity of 61%.[39] Among the possible explanation of this phenomenon, it has been hypothesized the release of metabolically active phagocytes and cytokines by nonpathological tissue as a reaction to the treatment, that may lead to increased FDG uptake in the site of original tumor producing false-positive results.

In conclusion, mediastinoscopy has increased accuracy in mediastinal staging compared with noninvasive methods, and is also effective in clinical re-evaluation after preoperative treatment. However, the increased technical complexity of re-operative mediastinoscopy often discourages surgeons to routinely repeat this procedure and only few trials in the literature[6,33] report its inclusion in the postinduction restaging.

15.3. Role of Surgery

15.3.1. Therapeutic Protocols, Surgical Techniques

There is general consensus about the principle that lung cancer cannot be cured unless all detectable disease is eradicated. All the integrated strategies of cure proposed in the last decades for patients with unresectable lung cancer, such as stage IIIB disease, have invariably failed in achieving adequate tumor sterilization. In addition, the disappointing results reported when surgery alone is employed suggest that the efficacy of this option should be reconsidered with a different strategy.

Selected N3 patients have been included in a number of phase II studies exploring the potential benefits of surgery after neoadjuvant treatment in stage IIIB. Data available in the literature usually do not report separate analysis for N3 and T4 patients, so that it is difficult to acquire specific prognostic indications for each of these subgroups. Moreover, published experiences in this field generally differ for restaging methods employed, because pathological re-evaluation of lymph nodal status is performed only in a few series, and for dishomogeneity of surgical technique, because the exploration of the contralateral mediastinum is only rarely carried out.

The Southwest Oncology Group has reported an induction chemoradiotherapy trial (SWOG 8805) that included a large group of patients with stage IIIB disease.[10] An effort was made to adhere to strict staging criteria prior to inclusion in the study: all N3 patients had histological confirmation by means of mediastinoscopy. The induction treatment consisted of concurrent chemotherapy and radiotherapy. Two cycles of cisplatin (50mg/m^2) were administered concurrently with 45Gy radiotherapy. Major toxicity was registered in 4% of patients. Fourteen of 27 patients with N3 disease (52%) underwent surgery after response to therapy. Repeat mediastinoscopy was not performed in the postinduction selection for thoracotomy. N3 patients were approached by standard thoracotomy and no attempt was made to resect the previously involved contralateral or supraclavicular lymph nodes. The decision apparently was based on the assumption that surgery was regarded only as an adjuvant for primary tumor control.

The last update of SWOG 8805 was issued in 1999[37] with 6-year survival data: the overall (all N3 and T4) survival was 22% with definitively more favorable prognosis (6-year survival, 49%) in the substage of T4 without mediastinal lymphadenectomy (N0-1). N2-3 patients showed markedly improved prognosis (6-year survival, 33%) when pathological downstaging to N0 was present if compared with patients presenting with unmodified lymph nodal status (6-year survival, 11%). Sites of relapses resulting in death were predominantly extrathoracic. Brain metastases were observed in 25 of 51 patients, being the sole site of recurrence in 18.

A second important phase II trial appearing in 1999 by Stamatis and colleagues[6] employed three cycles of cisplatin (60mg/m^2) and etoposide (150mg/m^2) followed by one cycle of concurrent hyperfractionated accelerated radiotherapy (45Gy) and chemotherapy with the same agents at lower doses. Among the N3 histologically proven patients, only those[32] without supraclavicular or scalene adenopathy were enrolled. The authors' purpose was to identify stage IIIB subgroup with better long-term prognosis. Repeat mediastinoscopy was performed after induction therapy and only patients with negative results proceeded to surgery. Major overall toxicity after the induction protocol was seen in 19.6% of patients with a 1.7% mortality rate. The complete resection rate was 48%.

As in the SWOG study, Stamatis and coworkers approached these patients by standard thoracotomy without any surgical exploration of the contralateral mediastinum. However, all former N3 patients had negative mediastinoscopy prior to surgery. The complex induction treatment protocol may have influenced the high postoperative complications rate (47%) observed, but it didn't strongly modify surgical mortality (2.9%). Survival rate of N3 patients at 5 years after operation was 28%. Long-term survival appeared possible in originally N3 patients with limited extension of the primary tumor (T1-2). As in the SWOG study, in the first part of this experience, a significant number of early brain metastases was noted. The addition of prophylactic cranial irradiation to the protocol reduced the incidence of cerebral metastases from 46% to 9%.

Another German trial[43] was published in 1999 including 15 N3 patients submitted to a complex and aggressive regimen. Chemotherapy (two cycles of ifosfamide, carboplatin, and etoposide) and subsequent radiotherapy (45Gy, twice daily 1.5Gy) concurrent with chemotherapy (carboplatin and vindesine) were administered. The intensive chemoradiotherapy regimen in this study significantly increased tumor regression rate (41% after chemotherapy alone and 69% after the complete chemoradiotherapy course), but critical toxicity was registered with a 9% mortality rate. Results for the sole N3 group were not reported in detail, but the overall median survival after surgery for stage IIIB (20 patients) of 17 months did not show significant differences with that of stage IIIA (25 months). Patients experiencing a 90% degree of pathologic tumor regression were most likely to achieve long-term survival.

A phase II study by Grunenwald and associates[32] has reported some innovative aspects, especially for the surgical approach to N3 disease. Induction regimen included two cycles of cisplatin, 5-fluoruracil (5-FU), and vinblastine combined with 42Gy of concurrent accelerated twice-daily radiotherapy. Nineteen mediastinoscopy proven N3 patients were enrolled. Complete disappearance of mediastinal lymph node involvement (N2/N3) was observed in 30% of patients. The operation was performed through a median sternotomy, and a complete bilateral mediastinal lymphadenectomy was carried out. Pneumonectomy was performed in 60% (18/29) of the patients with systematic bronchial stump protection by the omentum harvested using a small downwards extension of the midline skin incision. The reported complication rate was 24%, there was a 7% mortality rate, and the mean postoperative in-hospital stay was 20 days. Survival at 5 years was 17% for all N3 patients, including nonsurgically treated patients. However, significant survival improvement was observed when considering, in the whole study population (all stage IIIB), the partial responders with postinduction N0-1 status who were submitted to surgery (47% at 5 years). In this series, all 4 patients with histological complete response to treatment were not alive at the time of publication, suggesting also that adequate locoregional control may be not sufficient in achieving complete tumor sterilization.

The Massachusetts General Hospital group[44] focused on another aspect of induction therapy: the search of the best way of delivering radiotherapy. In association with cisplatin, vinblastine, and 5-FU, preoperative radiotherapy was administered with two levels of radiation doses: 45Gy in 25 fractions for 5 weeks to the initial volume (gross tumor plus adjacent lymph node–bearing region) and 44 to 60Gy to the gross tumor including involved lymph nodes by using boost radiation for a dose of 9 to 15Gy during chemotherapy. This algorithm was employed in 20 N3 and 5 T4 patients, 13 of whom (52%) underwent resection. No mention was made about surgical exploration of the contralateral mediastinum. The reported 3-year survival reached 54%.

Recently, a Dutch prospective phase II multicenter trial[33] has appeared investigating the role of surgery as a part of combined modality treatment in association with chemotherapy. Surgery plus chemotherapy was compared with radiotherapy plus chemotherapy, and the diagnostic value of postinduction repeated mediastinoscopy was analyzed. Histologically proven N3 patients were included in an overall study population of 41 patients and submitted to three courses of neoadjuvant gemcitabine/cisplatin chemotherapy. Four patients stopped the treatment after the first two cycles. Forty-eight percent of the N3 patients underwent resection after response to therapy. Survival in the whole study population did not show a significant advantage with a 15% survival rate at 3 years. Median survival of patients experiencing partial or complete response who were submitted to surgery was 21.5 months. There were equal incidences of local and distant recurrences as cause of death. Postinduction repeat mediastinoscopy proved to be an ineffective restaging tool because of the high number of incomplete procedures (40%) and the false-negative rate (28.6%).

Other interesting studies have dealt with the issue of induction therapy in stage IIIB[9,31,45] in the last years, but each of them includes a limited number of N3 surgically treated patients, so that data emerging by these experiences do not still provide meaningful indications in this setting. The results of phase II trials including operated N3 patients after induction therapy are reported in Table 15.1.

TABLE 15.1. Phase II trials of induction therapy plus surgery including N3 NSCLC patients.

Reference	Patients (Overall)	N3 Patients	Inclusion criteria	Induction therapy	Response rate	Resection rate	Complete resection	Perioperative mortality	Operative mortality	Survival (overall IIIB)	N3 survival
Choi[45]	25	16	N3 T4	Cisplatin + 5-FU + velban + RT (60 Gy)	65%	56%	52%	–	–	61% (2 year)	–
Rice[46]	45 (10 IIIB)	8	N2, N3 T4 (except pleural effusion)	Cisplatin + paclitaxel + RT (30 Gy)	53%	89%[a]	71%	20%	5%	17% (2 year)	–
Stamatis[6]	58	32	Mediastinal N3 T4	(Cisplatin + VP-16) × 3 + (Cisplatin + VP-16) × 1 + RT 45 Gy	61%	59%	48%	47%	5.8%	26% (5 year) C.R.: 43%	28% (5 year)
SWOG[10]	51	27	N3 T4 (except pleural effusion)	(Cisplatin + VP-16) × 2 + RT (45 Gy)	78%	63%	52% (N3)	26%	(5-sp) 5.2%	22% (8 year)	–
Thomas[45]	54 (29 IIIB)	15	N2, N3 T4	Ifost + carbopl. + VP-16 × 3 + (Carb + Vindesin) + 45 Gy RT	69%	74%[a]	63%	17.5%	7.5%	26% (3 year) 17 m (median)	–
Grunenwald[32]	40	19	Mediastinal N3 T4	(Cisplatin + 5-FU + Vinblastine) × 2 + RT (42 Gy)	73%	58%	50%	24%	7%	Res: 28% C.R.: 35%	17% (5 sp)
Pltz[33]	41	21	N3 T4	(Cisplatin + Gemcitabine) × 3	88%	50%	25%	30%	5%	15% (3 year) Res: 21.5 m (median)	Res N2-3: 17.5 m (median)
Ichinose[9]	27	7	N3 T4	LFT + Cisplatin + RT (40 Gy)	93%	81%	77%	36%	4%	58% (3 year) Res: 67% (3 year)	–

Abbreviations: C.R., completely resected; Res: responders.
[a] IIIA and IIIB.

Because investigation in this field is currently active, progressive adjustments and refinements have been proposed in the choice of the most effective drugs and the best way of delivering radiotherapy. Therefore, the optimal induction regimen has yet to be identified. Most of the published phase II trials utilized second generation chemotherapy generally based on cisplatin, a vinca alkaloid, and etoposide. Meta-analysis have indicated that the chance of survival increases when a platinum-based regimen is used.[46,47]

15.3.2. New Multimodality Regimens

A number of new agents, tested in clinical trials not including surgical resection, more recently have been introduced in neoadjuvant protocols. In particular, paclitaxel has shown a potent radiosensitizer effect. Gemcitabine, an antimetabolite that functions as an inhibitor of ribonucleoside reductase, has been shown to yield response rates of 20% to 30% when used as a single agent and of 58% to 60% when employed in combination with cisplatin.[5] A synergistic anti-tumor activity of the cisplatin has been shown also in combination with other drugs, such as 5-FU, with a response rate up to 74%, although 5-FU alone is thought to be inactive against non-small cell lung cancer (NSCLC).[31]

Concerning the choice of the best way of administering irradiation, indications have to be determined by phase III trials not including surgery. There are still no convincing data supporting the clinical benefits of altered fractionation modalities, such as hyperfractionated (two or more fractions daily) or continuous hyperfractionated accelerated radiotherapy (CHART), in combination with chemotherapy if compared with standard radiotherapy.[4,48] There is only one phase III trial showing superior results for CHART without chemotherapy with respect to standard radiotherapy, but the logistics of three treatments daily have not proven to be acceptable.[49,50]

Results of phase II trials have pointed out that the administration of multidrug chemotherapy and multimodality protocols, including radiotherapy preoperatively, is able to achieve higher clinical and pathological response rates.[6,32,33]

Response rates (reported for all stage IIIB patients) seem to be similar in almost all the studies reported, and range between 61% and 78%. The 93% rate registered by Ichinose and collegues[9] is justified, as explained by the authors, by the more restrictive inclusion criteria adopted. The complete response rate for N3 is specifically mentioned only in the SWOG study (52%). The complete histological response generally varies between 10 % and 15%; however, in the Stamatis trial,[6] based on a heavy chemoradioterapy regimen, the complete histological response rate increased up to 30%.

15.3.3. Effects of Nodal Downstaging

Maximal downstaging after induction therapy has been advocated in main experiences as the strongest predictor of survival in N3 and all stage IIIB patients undergoing surgical resection. Several authors have reported, as expected, a prominent prognostic significance of lymph node status after induction treatment. In the study by Choi and collegues,[51] the degree of lymph node downstaging showed a direct relation to survival benefit because the 5-year survivals were 79%, 42%, and 18% for postoperative tumor stages 0/I, II, and III, respectively. In the SWOG experience,[10] the most significant predictor of long-term survival after thoracotomy was the absence of tumor in the mediastinal nodes (3-year survival, 44% vs. 18%). Stamatis[6] reported a 4-year survival of 38% and 15% in postinduction N0/N1 and N2/N3 patients, respectively. Also in the French study,[32] postinduction completely resected N0-1 patients showed a 5-year survival of 42%, while postinduction N2-3 patients who underwent complete resection reached only a 12% survival rate at 5 years.

Altogether, all these prognostic evidences support the principle that admission to surgery after neoadjuvant therapy in advanced stage lung cancer, such as N3, has to be strictly limited to those patients who show a major clinical response. In the German trial,[6] only those N3 patients were operated in whom initially involved nodes were without evidence of residual cancer at repeat mediastinoscopy or if not more than one initially involved ipsilateral node remained positive.

15.3.4. Effects of Tumor Sterilization

The impact on prognosis of residual viable neoplastic cells in the primary tumor has not been completely clarified. In German Lung Cancer Cooperative Group study,[43] tumor regression of more than 90% appeared related to a significantly improved survival in the completely resected (R0) group of patients (3-year survival, 56% vs. 11%). Conversely, in the other German trial,[6,52] no difference in survival was found between resected patients assessed to have pathological complete response versus those with persistent viable tumor. It is still object of controversy whether pathological complete disappearence of tumor at the primary site has to be interpreted also as a predictor of responsiveness of distant micrometastases, determining an impact on long-term survival. In some authors' opinion,[6,52] especially when radiotherapy is added to preoperative chemotherapy, pathological complete regression at thoracotomy has only to be seen as the effect of the aggressive local treatment on the primary tumor and may no longer indicate superior efficacy in systemic control of the disease.

15.3.5. Treatment-related Morbidity and Mortality

Increasing complexity and aggressiveness of the induction regimens with the aim of maximal loco-regional control may have played a role in treatment-related morbidity. Although overall toxicity is generally acceptable with rates ranging between 4%[10,37] and 10%,[33] in some heavy multimodality regimens this incidence has proven definitely higher. In the Stamatis trial,[6] 19% of the patients had major toxicity that precluded further treatment and 9% refused to follow the protocol.

Furthermore, in many reports, the use of neoadjuvant therapies has produced increased postoperative complications and mortality rates. High rates of non–cancer-related deaths (20%–26%) have been reported by Grunenwald,[32] Albain,[10] and Eberhardt,[52] often associated with a critical incidence of acute distress syndrome or pneumonitis, if compared with standard resections without preoperative treatment. In particular, when also radiotherapy is administered, it has been frequently documented as a more evident impact on surgical morbidity, often associated with considerable intraoperative technical problems. Several studies have suggested that preoperative chemoradiotherapy may strongly promote bronchial stump insufficiency with a consequent increased incidence of bronchopleural fistulas up to 23%.[53] Postoperative mortality in Fowler's experience[53] has exceeded 20%.

Pneumonectomy, and especially right-side pneumonectomy, have produced more significant worsening of morbidity and mortality rates in several postinduction surgical series.[53,54] Moreover, also the occurence of a bronchial stump dehiscence has been more frequently observed after right pneumonectomy.[53] A significant reduction of broncho-pleural fistulas rates has been shown in some recent issues[32,55] performing bronchial reinforcement by viable tissue, principally with muscle or omentum. However, in other experiences[56,57] the appearance of fistulas in spite of bronchial stump coverage, especially when intercostal muscle is used, provides no complete evidence of efficacy to these procedures after induction therapy. Mainly when radiotherapy is performed, the tissues employed for the flap may be deteriorated by the oncological therapy, especially if included in the irradiation field. In some authors' opinion,[6] the introduction of twice-daily radiotherapy is a possible mean to shorten radiation duration, and, thus, leads to reduced development of fibrosis at the moment of surgery.

The strong impact on toxicity and surgical complication of the aggressive currently employed three modality treatments has indicated that enrolment in these protocols should be strictly limited to patients with good performance status (0–1) and minimal weight loss.

15.3.6. Impact of Extended Resections

It is now evident that major clinical response to therapy is mandatory to select patients with original N3 disease suitable for surgical resection. However, the slender data present in literature have still not clarified whether, after an intensive preoperative downstaging, the extension of the surgical resection can be confined to the primary lung tumor and the ipsilateral mediastinum or has to include the contralateral mediastinal nodes.

In the Grunenwald trial,[32] the authors advocated the need for extended procedures, including routine bilateral lymphadenectomy, for postinduction surgery. This choice was based on the principle that all the originally involved tissue should be removed despite restaging that showed complete disappearance of disease in mediastinal lymph nodes. In the Essen group experience,[6] employement of invasive mediastinal restaging by repeat mediastinoscopy was indicated as an effective method to avoid such extended resections. In the latter study, the low mediastinal relapse pattern observed in initially N3 patients, proved, in the authors' opinion, that standard procedures without bilateral lymphadenectomy may be sufficient after negative preoperative rebiopsy of the contralateral nodes.

Pneumonectomy is reported to be necessary to achieve complete tumor clearance in a high rate of patients, exceeding 40% in several series,[6,9,32,43] and this requirement further increases the risk for morbidity. In our previous experience,[58] we have shown that operations such as bronchovascular reconstruction not only are technically feasible after induction therapy, but also carry a lower morbidity and comparable long-term survival when compared with pneumonectomy in this setting. Complex surgical interventions, including sleeve resections or extended resections to the carina, the superior vena cava, the left atrium, the esophagus, and the vertebral bodies, have been performed in many of the series reported in this chapter[6,9,32,43] with a high incidence ranging from 40% to 88%, and the related surgical mortality did not show a significant worsening.

15.4. Conclusions

The results of the phase II studies suggest that therapeutic nihilism when confronted by N3 and stage IIIB NSCLC may partially be overcome. Investigators have to consider that, in selected series, surgery associated with currently available chemoradiotherapy may prove able to cure a meaningful rate of patients, which is a better rate than that obtained without surgery (level of evidence 2−; grade of recommendation D). This could be partially explained by the more restrictive selection criteria applied by these aggressive

protocols. Because the long-term survival improvement may average about 10% if compared with historical controls without surgery, future comparative analyses are awaited to assess whether this advantage could be confirmed in a randomized study.

> Resection in combination with currently available chemoradiotherapy may prove able to cure a meaningful number of patients with N3 NSCLC, which is a better rate than that obtained without surgery (level of evidence 2−; grade of recommendation D).

Although prospective, randomized trials have not yet reported and surgery cannot be recommended at the moment as a standard of care, some convincing indications can be acquired by the published experiences, and the data actually available may help to define precise guidelines for future phase III trials. The first evidence is that accurate preoperative staging and restaging is mandatory. Direct biopsy procedures, mainly by means of mediastinoscopy, have proved superior to all other conventional diagnostic methods in assessing the presence of N2/3 disease, both in the staging and in the restaging setting. Therefore, at the present time, invasive preoperative explorations can be recommended in order to achieve a more accurate selection of patients for such heavy therapeutic protocols (level of evidence 2++; grade of recommendation B). The second is that in well-identified subgroups, such as completely resected patients showing a mediastinal downstaging to N0-1 status, the benefits of surgery are more significant (level of evidence 2+; grade of recommendation C).

> Invasive preoperative explorations are recommended in order to achieve a more accurate selection of patients for resection after induction therapy (level of evidence 2++; grade of recommendation B).
>
> In well-identified subgroups, such as patients with mediastinal downstaging to N0-1 status, the benefits of surgery are more significant (level of evidence 2+; grade of recommendation C).

Multi-institutional studies appear necessary to confirm in larger series the clinical evidences observed. Moreover, there are other questions that still remain open: they regard the need of extending the surgical resection to the contralateral mediastinum after high response to treatment, and the choice of the most appropriate induction regimen. Both questions can only be clarified by further controlled studies.

References

1. Mountain CF. A new international staging system for lung cancer. *Chest* 1986;89:225–233.
2. Hata E, Hayakawa H, Miyamoto H, et al. The incidence and prognosis of the controlateral mediastinal node involvement of the left lung cancer patients who underwent bilateral mediastinal dissection and pulmonary resection through the median sternotomy. *Lung Cancer* 1998;4(suppl): A87.
3. Watanabe Y, Ichihashi T, Iwa T. Median sternotomy as an approach for pulmonary surgery. *Thorac Cardiovasc Surg* 1988;36:227–231.
4. Jett JR, Scott WJ, Rivera MP, Sause WT. Guidelines on treatment of stage IIIB non-small cell lung cancer. *Chest* 2003;123(suppl 1):221S–225S,
5. Rendina EA, Venuta F, GeGiacomo T, Coloni GF. Stage IIIB non-small-cell lung cancer. *Chest Surg Clin N Am* 2001;11:101–119.
6. Stamatis G, Eberhardt W, Stüben G, Bildat S, Dahler O, Hillejan L. Preoperative chemoradiotherapy and surgery for selected non-small cell lung cancer IIIB subgroups: long-term results. *Ann Thorac Surg* 1999;68:1144–1149.
7. Curran W, Scott C, Langer C, et al. Phase III comparison of sequential vs concurrent chemoradiation for pts with unresected stage III non-small cell lung cancer (NSCLC): report of Radiation Therapy Oncology Group (RTOG). *Proc World Conf Lung Cancer* 2000;29:303.
8. Furuse K, Fukuoka M, Kawahara M, et al. Phase III study of concurrent versus sequential thoracic radiotherapy in combination with mitomycin, vindesine, and cisplatin in unresectable stage III non-small cell lung cancer. *J Clin Oncol* 1999; 17:2692–2699.
9. Ichinose Y, Fukuyama Y, Asoh H, et al. Induction chemoradiotherapy and surgical resection for selected stage IIIB non-small-cell lung cancer. *Ann Thorac Surg* 2003;76:1810–1814.
10. Albain KS, Rusch VW, Crowley JJ, et al. Concurrent cisplatin/etoposide plus chest radiotherapy followed by surgery for stages IIIA (N2) and IIIB non–small cell lung cancer: mature results of Southwest Oncology Group phase II study 88-05. *J Clin Oncol* 1995;13:1880–1892.
11. Faber LP, Kittle CF, Warren WH, et al. Preoperative chemotherapy and irradiation for stage III non-small cell lung cancer. *Ann Thorac Surg* 1989;47:669–675.
12. Arriagada R, Le Chevalier T, Quoix E, et al. ASTRO plenary: effect of chemotherapy on locally advanced non-small cell lung carcinoma: a randomized study of 353 patients. GETCB, FLNCC and the CEBI trialists. *Int J Radiat Oncol Biol Physiol* 1991;20:1183–1190.
13. Bury T, Corhay JL, Paulus P, et al. Positron emission tomography in the evaluation of intrathoracic lymphatic extension of non-small cell bronchial cancer: a preliminary study of 30 patients. *Rev Mal Respir* 1996;13:281–286.
14. Gupta NC, Graeber GM, Rogers JS, et al. Comparative efficacy of FDG-PET and CT scanning in the preoperative staging of NSCLC. *Ann Thorac Surg* 1999;229:286–291.
15. Steinert HC, Hauser M, Alleman F, et al. Non-small cell lung cancer: nodal staging with FDG PET versus CT with correlative lymph node mapping and sampling. *Radiology* 1997;202:441–446.
16. Patterson GA, Ginsberg RJ, Poon PY, et al. A prospective evaluation of magnetic resonance imaging, computed tomography and mediastinoscopy in the preoperative assessment of mediastinal node status in bronchogenic carcinoma. *J Thorac Cardiovasc Surg* 1987;89:679–684.
17. Lardinois D, Schallberger A, Betticher D, Ris HB. Postinduction video-mediastinoscopy is as accurate and safe as video-mediastinoscopy in patients without pretreatment for potentially operable non-small cell lung cancer. *Ann Thorac Surg* 2003;75:1102–1106.
18. Brion JP, Depauw L, Kuhn G, et al. Role of computed tomography and mediastinoscopy in preoperative staging of lung carcinoma. *J Comput Assist Tomogr* 1985;9:480–484.
19. Coughlin M, Deslauriers J, Beaulieu M, et al. Role of mediastinoscopy in pretreatment staging of patients with primary lung cancer. *Ann Thorac Surg* 1985;40:556–560.
20. De Leyn P, Schoonooghe P, Deneffe G, et al. Surgery for non-small cell lung cancer with unsuspected metastasis to ipsilateral mediastinal or subcarinal nodes (N2 disease). *Eur J Cardiothorac Surg* 1996; 10:649–654.
21. Dillman RO, Herndon J, Seagren SL, Eaton WL Jr, Green MR. Improved survival in stage III non

small cell lung cancer: seven year follow-up of cancer and leukemia group B (CALGB) 8433 trial. *J Natl Cancer Inst* 1996;88:1210–1215.

22. Gdeedo A, Van Schil P, Corthouts B, Van Mieghem F, Van Meerbeck J, Van Marck E. Prospective evaluation of computed tomography and mediastinoscopy in mediastinal lymph node staging. *Eur Resp J* 1997;10:1547–1551.

23. Hammoud ZT, Anderson RC, Meyers BF, et al. The current role of mediastinoscopy in the evaluation of thoracic disease. *J Thorac Cardiovasc Surg* 1999; 118:894–899.

24. Jolly P, Hutchinson C, Detterbeck F, Guyton S, Hofer B, Anderson R. Routine computed tomographic scans, selective mediastinoscopy, and other factors in evaluation of lung cancer. *J Thorac Cardiovasc Surg* 1991;102:270–271.

25. Ratto GB, Mereu C, Motta G. The prognostic significance of preoperative assessment of mediastinal lymph nodes in patients with lung cancer. *Chest* 1988;93:807–813.

26. Staples CA, Muller NL, Miller RR, Evans KG, Nelems B. Mediastinal nodes in bronchogenic carcinoma: comparison between CT and mediastinoscopy. *Radiology* 1991;167:367–372.

27. Whittlesey D. Prospective computed thomographic scanning in the staging of bronchogenic cancer. *J Thorac Cardiovasc Surg* 1988;95:876–882.

28. Ginsberg RJ. The role of preoperative surgical staging in left upper lobe tumors. *Ann Thorac Surg* 1994;57:526–527.

29. Ginsberg RJ, Rice TW, Goldberg M, Waters PF, Schmoker BJ. Extended cervical mediastinoscopy. A single staging procedure for bronchogenic carcinoma of the left upper lobe. *J Thorac Cardiovasc Surg* 1987;94:673–678.

30. Ginsberg RJ. Extended cervical mediastinoscopy. *Chest Surg Clin N Am* 1996;6:21–30.

31. Galetta D, Cesario A, Margaritora S, et al. Enduring challenge in the treatment of nonsmall cell lung cancer with clinical stage IIIB: results of a trimodality approach. *Ann Thorac Surg* 2003;76:1802–1809.

32. Grunenwald DH, André F, Le Péchoux C, et al. Benefit of surgery after chemoradiotherapy in stage IIIB (T4 and/or N3) non–small cell lung cancer. *J Thorac Cardiovasc Surg* 2001;12:796–802.

33. Pitz CM, Maas KW, Van Swieten HA, Brutel de la Rivière A, Hofman P, Schramel F. Surgery as part of combined modality treatment in stage IIIB non-small cell lung cancer. *Ann Thorac Surg* 2002:74; 164–169.

34. Garpestad E, Goldberg SN, Hert F, et al. CT fluoroscopy guidance for transbronchial needle aspiration. *Chest* 2001;119:329–332.

35. Patelli M, Lazzari Agli L, Poletti V, et al. Role of fiberscopic transbronchial needle aspiration in the staging of N2 disease due to non–small cell lung cancer. *Ann Thorac Surg* 2002:73;407–411.

36. White CS, Weiner EA, Patel P, James BE. Transbronchial needle aspiration: guidance with CT fluoroscopy. *Chest* 2000;118:1630–1638.

37. Albain K, Rush V, Crowley J, et al. Long term survival after concurrent cisplatin/etoposide (PE) plus chest radiotherapy (RT) followed by surgery in bulky, stage IIIA(N2) and IIIB non-small cell lung cancer (NSCLC): 6-year outcome from Southwest Oncology Group Study 8805. *Proc Am Soc Clin Oncol* 1999;18:1801.

38. Mateu-Navarro M, Rami-Porta R, Bastus-Piulats R, Cirera-Nogueras L, Gonzalez-Pont G. Remediastinoscopy after induction chemotherapy in non-small cell lung cancer. *Ann Thorac Surg* 2000;70: 391–395.

39. Akhurst T, Downey RJ, Ginsberg MS, et al. An initial experience with FDG-PET in the imaging of residual disease after induction therapy for lung cancer. *Ann Thorac Surg* 2002;73:259–266.

40. Van Schil PE, Van Hee RH, Schoofs RL. The value of mediastinoscopy in preoperative staging of bronchogenic carcinoma. *J Thorac Cardiovasc Surg* 1989;97:240–244.

41. Lardinois D, Weder W, Hany TF, et al. *N Engl J Med* 2003;348:2500–2507.

42. Kernstine KH, Mclaughin KA, Menda Y, et al. Can FDG-PET reduce the need for mediastinoscopy in potentially resectable non-small cell lung cancer? *Ann Thorac Surg* 2002;73:394–402.

43. Thomas M, Rube C, Semik M, et al. Impact of preoperative bimodality induction including twice daily radiation on tumor regression and survival in stage III non–small cell lung cancer. *J Clin Oncol* 1999;17:1185–1193.

44. Choi NC, Carey RW, Myojin M, et al. Preoperative chemo-radiotherapy using concurrent boost radiation and resection for good responders in stage IIIB (T4 or N3) non-small cell lung cancer: a feasibility study [abstract]. *Lung Cancer* 1997;18: 76.

45. Rice TW, Adelstein DJ, Ciezki JP, et al. Short-course induction chemoradiotherapy with paclitaxel for stage III non-small-cell lung cancer. *Ann Thorac Surg* 1998;66:1909–1914.

46. Johnson DH, Turrisi AT, Pass HI. Combined modality treatment for locally advanced non-

small cell lung cancer. In: Pass HI, Mitchell JB, Johnson DH, Turrisi AT, eds. *Lung Cancer: Principles and Practice*. Philadelphia: Lippincott-Raven; 1996:863–873.

47. Non-small Cell Lung Cancer Collaborative Group. Chemotherapy in non-small cell lung cancer: a meta-analysis using updated data on individual patients from 52 randomised clinical trials. *BMJ* 1995;311:899–909.

48. Stella P, Marks R, Schild S, et al. Phase III trial of chemotherapy either standard radiotherapy or accelerated hyperfractionated thoracic radiotherapy for stage III non-small cell lung cancer [abstract]. *Proc Amer Soc Clin Oncol* 2001;20: 312.

49. Saunders M, Dische S, Barrett A, et al. Continuous hyperfractionated accelerated radiotherapy (CHART) vs conventional radiotherapy in non-small cell lung cancer: a randomized multicentre trial. *Lancet* 1997;350:161–165.

50. Saunders M, Dische S, Barrett A, et al. Continuous, hyperfractionated, accelerated radiotherapy (CHART) vs conventional radiotherapy in non-small cell lung cancer: mature data from the randomized multicentre trial. *Radiother Oncol* 1999;52:137–148.

51. Choi NC, Carey RW, Daly W, et al. Potential impact on survival of improved tumor down staging and resection rate by preoperative twice-daily radiation and concurrent chemotherapy in stage IIIA non-small cell lung cancer. *J Clin Oncol* 1977;15:712–722.

52. Eberhardt W, Wilke H, Stamatis G, et al. Preoperative chemotherapy followed by concurrent chemo-radiation therapy based on hyperfractionated accelerated radiotherapy and definitive surgery in locally advanced non-small cell lung cancer: mature results of a phase II trial. *J Clin Oncol* 1998;16:622–634.

53. Fowler WC, Langer CJ, Curran WJ, et al. Postoperative complications after combined neoadjuvant treatment of lung cancer. *Ann Thorac Surg* 1997;55:986–989.

54. Deutsch M, Crawford J, Leopold K, et al. Phase II study of neoadjuvant chemotherapy and radiation therapy with thoracotomy in the treatment of staged IIIA non-small cell lung cancer. *Cancer* 1994;74:1243–1252.

55. Stamatis G, Djuric D, Eberhardt W, et al. Postoperative morbidity and mortality after induction chemoradiotherapy for locally advanced lung cancer: ananalysis of 350 operated patients. *Eur J Cardiothorac Surg* 2002;22:292–297.

56. Doddoli C, Thomas P, Thirion X, Seree Y, Giudicelli E, Fuentes P. Postoperative complications in relation with induction therapy for lung cancer. *Eur J Cardiothorac Surg* 2001;20:385–390.

57. Regnard JF, Icard P, Deneuville M, et al. Lung resection after high doses of mediastinal radiotherapy (sixty grays or more). Reinforcement of bronchial healing with thoracic muscle flaps in nine cases. *J Thorac Cardiovasc Surg* 1994;107:607–610.

58. Rendina EA, Venuta F, DeGiacomo T, Flaishman I, Fazi P, Ricci C. Safety and efficacy of bronchovascular reconstruction after induction chemotherapy for lung cancer. *J Thorac Cardiovasc Surg* 1997;114:830–837.

16
Video-Assisted Thorascopic Surgery Major Lung Resections

Raja M. Flores and Naveed Z. Alam

The earliest reports of minimally invasive lobectomies were published more than a decade ago.[1,2] The reaction to this development was summarized by the results of an opinion survey conducted of members of the General Thoracic Surgery Club in 1997.[3] The results showed that 4% of surgeons deemed video-assisted thorascopic suegery (VATS) major lung resections preferable to thoracotomy, 15% deemed it acceptable, 45% viewed it as an investigational procedure, and 36% thought it was unacceptable. The reasons are manifold. Perhaps most importantly, because lung cancer is the most common indication for performing lobectomy, the question of adequacy of the operation in satisfying surgical oncologic principles remains a hurdle in many surgeons' minds. The main considerations, therefore, in assessing whether to perform a minimally invasive lobectomy are adequacy as a cancer operation (as manifested by equivalent survival), safety in terms of complications and mortality, relative cost (including intraoperative and length-of-stay considerations), and benefits for the patients in terms of decreased pain and improved quality of life.

The definition of a VATS major lung resection can be problematic, or at least vague. For the purposes of this chapter, major lung resection is defined as an anatomical lung resection, segmentectomy, lobectomy, or pneumonectomy. The difficulty in the definition comes in defining the VATS component. In the literature, *VATS lobectomy* is a term used to describe a spectrum of operations from mini-thoracotomy with rib spreading and direct visualization through the wound to a completely minimally invasive approach with no rib spreading and use of only thoracoscopic techniques. In interpreting studies of VATS lobectomy, careful review of the Methods section usually sheds light as to the nature of the operation performed. This needs to be taken into account when evaluating the evidence and forming conclusions.

16.1. Summary of Evidence

The literature published to date on VATS lobectomy or major lung resections is scant and largely of a low grade on the evidence scale. A few authors from various centers around the world are responsible for the majority of studies and a large share of the data is in the form of case series (level of evidence 4).

16.1.1. Randomized, Controlled Trials

Few randomized, controlled trials (RCTs) exist in this area (Table 16.1). Of the three published trials comparing open to VATS lobectomies, two examine clinical outcomes and one investigates biochemical markers.[4,5] The first and most well-known RCT was published by Kirby and colleagues.[4] They randomized 61 patients with clinical stage I non-small cell lung cancer (NSCLC) to undergo lobectomy by VATS (31 patients) or muscle-sparing thoracotomy (30 patients). The VATS were performed without rib spreading. One patient in the open group and two patients in the VATS group had benign disease

TABLE 16.1. Randomized control trials of VATS major lung resections.

Study	Year	Level of evidence	Patients	Outcomes	Results	Comment
Kirby[4]	1995	1b	25 VATS 30 open	LOS, OR time, complications	Less complications in VATS, no other differences	Stage I tumors, 3 VATS excluded due to conversion
Sugi[5]	2000	1b	48 VATS 52 open	Survival, recurrences	No differences	All patients had MLND
Craig[6]	2001	1b	22 VATS 19 open	Acute phase reactants	Lower CRP and IL-6 in VATS	
Shigemura[7]	2004	1b	18 complete VATS 16 assisted VATS	OR time, LOS, pain, complications, markers	Longer OR, shorter LOS, lower CRP with complete	Complete VATS – no spreading

Abbreviations: VATs, video assisted thoracic surgery; LOS, length of stays; OR, operating room; CRP, C-reactive protein; IL-6, interleukin 6; MLND, mediastinal lymph node dissection.

and were excluded from analysis. In addition, three patients in the VATS group required conversion to thoracotomy and were also excluded from the analysis, leaving 30 in the open and 25 in the VATS groups. There were few differences between the groups. The incidence of postoperative complications was less in the VATS group (6 vs. 16). There were no significant differences in operating time, blood loss, duration of chest tube drainage, length of hospital stay, and incidence of disabling post-thoracotomy pain (2 in the open vs. 1 in the VATS group).

The other RCT comparing clinical outcomes between open and VATS lobectomy was published by a Japanese group.[5] Sugi and colleagues randomized 100 patients with clinical stage Ia lung cancer to open (52 patients) or VATS (48 patients) lobectomy and mediastinal lymph node dissection. The additional two patients in the open group were conversions from VATS and were analyzed in the open group. There were no significant differences in the recurrence rates or survival. The reported 3- and 5-year survivals were 93% and 85% in the open group and 90% and 90% in the VATS group, respectively. This is the only RCT examining survival differences between VATS and open lobectomies.

A study comparing acute phase responses randomized 22 patients to VATS and 19 patients to open lobectomy.[6] They used a non–rib spreading technique and all patients had mediastinoscopy preoperatively. Blood samples were taken preoperatively and at various times in the first week after surgery. Both operations increased acute phase response markers, but VATS was associated with lower rises in C-reactive protein (CRP) and interleukin (IL)-6.

A final RCT was performed comparing complete VATS (c-VATS) to assisted VATS (a-VATS).[7] Effectively, they compared a non–rib spreading approach (c-VATS, 18 patients) to a mini-thoracotomy approach with rib spreading (a-VATS, 16 patients). The authors found significantly shorter length of stay (11 vs. 15 days), longer operation times, less blood loss, and lower serum markers (CRP, white blood cells) in the c-VATS group.

16.1.2. Case Control Studies

A number of case control studies examining a variety of outcomes have been performed on VATS major lung resections (Table 16.2). Two studies investigating the effects of VATS lobectomies in high-risk patients have been performed.[8,9] A Japanese case control study done with patients 80 years of age or older, with 17 VATS cases and 15 open controls, showed no significant difference in survival or complications with trends favoring the VATS group.[8] Demmy performed a case control study comparing VATS lobectomy patients to matched controls who had open surgery.[9] Video-assisted thoracoscopic surgery was only offered to patients who were deemed high risk based on either poor pulmonary function tests (PFTs) or poor function. There were 19 patients in each group. Despite having higher risk patients, the VATS group had a shorter length of stay, a quicker return to activity, and less pain at 3 weeks postoperatively than the open group.

TABLE 16.2. Case control series of VATS major lung resections.

Study	Year	Level of evidence	Patients	Outcomes	Results	Comment
Demmy[9]	1999	3b	19 VATS 19 open	LOS, return to activity, pain	All favor VATS	High-risk pts, 3 deaths in VATS, 1 in control
Koizumi[8]	2003	3b	17 VATS 15 open	Complications, survival	Trend favors VATS	Pt age >80
Demmy[10]	2004	3b	20 VATS 38 open	Discharge independence, LOS	Shorter LOS, less pain, fewer transfers to care facilities	Groups well matched
Kawai[11]	2005	4	10 VATS 11 open	Nocturnal hypoxemia POD 3 and 14	Less hypoxemia at POD 14 with VATS	Open were >2-cm, VATS were <2-cm
Nagahiro[12]	2001	4	13 VATS 9 open	PFTs, pain, cytokines	Less pain, lower IL-6 in VATS	Open were T2, VATS were T1
Nakata[13]	2000	4	10 VATS 11 open	PFTs, early and late	PFTs better for VATS pod 7, no change at 1 year	Selection of controls ill-defined, spreading used
Yim[14]	2000	4	18 VATS 18 open	Cytokines, analgesic requirement	IL-6, IL-8, IL-10 lower and less IV narcotic in VATS	Controls were initially attempted VATS
Kaseda[15]	2000	4	44 VATS 77 open	PFTs 3 months post-op, survival	PFT changes and stage I survival better for VATS	Historical controls not well defined

Abbreviations: VATs, video assisted thoracic surgery; LOS, length of stays; OR, operating room; CRP, C-reactive protein; IL-6, interleukin 6; MLND, mediastinal lymph node dissection; POD, postoperative day; IL-8, interleukin 8; IL-10, interleukin 10; PFTs, pulmonary function tests.

A similar study by the same author evaluated patient independence after discharge.[10] Twenty VATS lobectomies were matched to 38 open controls. There were similar numbers of complications between the groups, but shorter hospital stays (4.6 vs. 6.4 days), fewer prolonged pain complaints, and fewer transfers to care facilities in the VATS group.

A number of other case control series examining pain, changes in PFTs, nocturnal hypoxemia, and various markers of inflammation have been performed and are summarized in Table 16.2.[11–15] They generally favored VATS approaches, but the selection of controls was problematic. For example, in one study of cytokines before and after surgery, the control group as made up of T2 tumors and the VATS cases were T1.[12]

16.1.3. Case Series

There are numerous case series published, many of which have been updated, reflecting the ongoing experience of the authors, follow-up of patients, and modifications in technique. The series with more than 100 patients are reviewed in Table 16.3 and discussed below.

Roviaro and colleagues from Milan have been publishing their experience with VATS for major lung resections since 1993.[1] Their most recent update looked at their 11-year experience with 344 patients (278 with NSCLC, 6 metastases, 68 benign) that went to surgery for VATS major resection. In patients with lung cancer, their indications were clinical stage I with peripheral tumors less than 3 cm in diameter.[16] Their technique does not use rib spreading and involves three to four incisions with the largest being 5cm for withdrawal of the specimen. They performed 259 procedures with a 23% conversion rate to thoracotomy. The global 5-year survival was 68.9% and for stage Ia (T1N0M0) the 5-year survival was 75%. They had 2 deaths and 20 complications.

Two recent case series have been published from different centers in Japan.[17,18] Iwasaki pub-

TABLE 16.3. Case series of VATS major lung resections (level 4 evidence).

Study	Year	Patients (ITT)	Technique	Survival	LOS days	Comment
Roviaro[16]	2004	259 (344)	No spreading	5 year 68.9	5	78 (23%) conversions, 2 deaths
Iwasaki[17]	2004	140	No spreading	5 year 77.3% I 80.9% II 70.3%	NR	100 lobes, 40 segments
Ohtsuka[18]	2004	95 (106)	Spreading	3 year 93%	7.6	Survival in only 82 patients, 1 death, 10% conversion
Walker[19]	2003	158 (178)	No spreading	5 year I 77.9% II 51.4%	6	1.8% 30-d mortality, 11% conversion
Gharagozloo[24]	2003	179	Simultaneous stapling, no spreading	5 year 83%	4.1	1 death
Solaini[20]	2001	112 (125)	No spreading	3 year 85% I 90	6.2	Survival in 86 patients with NSCLC, 10% conversion
Lewis[23]	1999	250	Simultaneous stapling, no spreading	3 year 83%	2.8	About half of patients were stage II
Yim[21]	1998	214 (266)	Spreading	2 year 93%	NR	1.8% 30-d mortality, 19% conversion
McKenna[22]	1998	298 (317)	No spreading	4 year I 70% III 65%	5.1	1 death, 6% conversion

lished their experience with 140 procedures (100 lobectomies, 40 segmentectomies).[17] Their technique did not involve rib spreading and their indications were clinical stage I disease with peripheral tumors less than 3 cm. They reported a 5-year survival of 77.3% for the VATS patients, with 80.9% for stage I and 70.3% for stage II tumors.

The other Japanese case series involved 106 patients, 95 of whom had a VATS procedure and the other 11 of whom were converted to thoracotomy (10% conversion rate).[18] Their main indication was clinical stage I, and tumor size was not a criterion. Their technique involved the use of a mini-thoracotomy and rib spreading. They reported a 3-year survival of 93%, but only included the 82 patients for whom they had follow-up data from more than 6 months.

A series published from Edinburgh, Scotland, of 178 patients with clinical stage I or II lung cancer and tumors less than 5 cm with the use of a non–rib spreading method, reported a conversion rate of 11%.[19] There were two deaths within 30 days of surgery, both after discharge. One was from pulmonary embolism and the other an adrenal infarct. No patients were lost to follow-up and the 5-year survivals were 77.9%, 51.4%, and 28.6% for stages I, II, and III, respectively.

Another series from Italy reported on 125 cases of which 112 went on to have VATS resections (10% conversion).[20] Their indications were clinical stage I for NSCLC, solitary metastasis, or carcinoid tumors. They used a non–rib spreading method and reported a complication rate of 11.6% with no deaths. In the patients who had NSCLC (86 patients), the 3-year survival was 85% and in the 72 patients with stage I it was 90%.

Yim and colleagues from Hong Kong published their series of 266 patients with tumors less than 5 cm for whom they attempted VATS resections.[21] They converted to thoracotomy 19% of the time and completed 214 VATS major lung resections. A rib spreader was used. They reported a 22% incidence of nonfatal complications, 1 postoperative death, and 93% of patients alive at 2 years.

In the largest series of completed VATS major lung resections, McKenna and colleagues reported a multi-institutional experience of 317 patients for whom they performed 298 procedures with a conversion rate of 6%.[2] Their indications were stage I or II lung cancer with tumors smaller than 6cm. They reported complications in 38 patients (12.4%) and 1 mortality due to venous mesenteric infarct (0.3%). Mean follow-up was 29 months and the reported 4-year survival was 70% for stage I patients. However, there was no comparison thoracotomy group. They also reported one recurrence at a VATS port site simultaneous with appearance of bone metastases in that patient.

Finally, two independent series using forms of simultaneous stapling have been published.[23,24] This technique involves no rib spreading, but variations on stapling the bronchus and vascular structures together without formal dissection. Lewis reported a complication rate of 11.2% and 3-year survival of 83%.[23] Of note, almost half of the patients were stage II. Gharagozloo reported 179 patients with a 5-year survival of 83%.[24] They performed 29 right upper and middle bilobectomies (16%) in the series. This high number was performed as a conscious decision after some early recurrences in the N1 nodes between upper and middle lobes.

16.2. Clinical Impact of Data

As detailed above, the bulk of the evidence is in the form of case series and case control studies with few published RCTs. By synthesizing the data we conclude the following:

- Video-assisted thorascopic surgery lobectomy can be performed safely with equivalent mortality and complication rates to open lobectomy. This is based on the results of two small RCTs and a number of case control trials and case series (recommendation grade C).[4,5,8–10,15–24]
- The survival of patients with stage I lung cancer following VATS lobectomy appears equivalent to that of patients having open surgery. This is based on one small RCT, case control studies, and the case series (recommendation grade C)[5,8,15–24]
- Based on case control studies, patients appear to experience less pain with VATS. Although one RCT did not show this, it was too small to draw a conclusion (recommendation grade C).[4,9,10,12]

- Length of hospital stay appears similar to open procedures. One RCT showed no difference and two case control studies suggested it was shorter with VATS.[4,9,10]

> VATS lobectomy can be performed safely with equivalent mortality and complication rates to open lobectomy (level of evidence 2 to 3; recommendation grade C).
>
> The survival of patients with stage I lung cancer following VATS lobectomy appears equivalent to that of patients having open surgery (level of evidence 2 to 3; recommendation grade C).
>
> Patients appear to experience less pain with VATS (level of evidence 2 to 3; recommendation grade C).

16.3. Difficult Decisions

Because the published evidence is scant, no definite recommendations can be made. The reality of the situation is that many surgeons are performing the procedure and many patients are requesting it. We feel the data supports that VATS lobectomy can be performed safely and that the survival of early-stage patients appears equivalent to thoracotomy. In terms of the postoperative course, although the data is mixed, our experience has been that VATS patients have less pain and shorter hospital stays.

The problems with the prior scientific studies are numerous. For example, proper methods of analyzing the data were not used. Patients requiring conversion from VATS lobectomy to thoracotomy were either excluded or included in the open group (ignoring a basic premise of RCTs) and the intent-to-treat principle, which must maintain patients in the group to which they were originally assigned. Deviation from this principle obscures any subsequent analysis. More importantly, the numbers designed at the outset of the trial were much too small to detect a significant difference in survival. The ideal RCT to detect a 10% difference in survival between the two arms with a power of 80% and an α of 0.05 would require a total of 385 patients to demonstrate superiority.

Differences in indications, technique, and extents of lymph node dissection make comparing across studies difficult. If one can perform the same operation in terms of anatomical dissection and lymph node removal as done through thoracotomy, then it would seem reasonable to use VATS as long as sound oncologic principles were practiced. Our practice has been to offer VATS lobectomy to patients with clinical stage I disease by computed tomography (CT) and positron emission tomography (PET) scan. Our technique uses a 4-cm utility incision with no rib spreading, two 2-cm thoracoscopic ports, and dissection performed totally under thoracoscopic visualization.[25] Dissection involves the individual ligation of hilar structures, an anatomical lobectomy, and a mediastinal node dissection or sampling. If there is any indication of oncologic compromise, a thoracotomy is performed.

Lobectomy remains the standard of care for all early lung cancers. The use of simultaneous stapling techniques is probably not warranted. In light of the increased number of bilobectomies performed by one center, due to the inadequacy of their lymph node removals, it would seem that this is not the same operation as an open lobectomy. Therefore, our recommendation is that the simultaneous stapled technique not be considered a VATS lobectomy.

16.4. Future Studies

There is certainly a need for further study. A large multicenter randomized trial comparing open lobectomy to VATS lobectomy should be performed. However, the myriad of techniques employed by different surgeons would require a standardization of the VATS lobectomy technique and probably standardization in the thoracotomy arm as well. Quality-of-life studies with validated instruments need to be performed to ascertain the impact of VATS. Another interesting avenue of investigation that has been embarked on, but requires further study, is the use of VATS in higher risk groups to see if they fare better. Also, with the recent shift in clinical practice to adjuvant chemotherapy for more and

more of our patients, there may be some additional benefit to VATS lobectomy if patients are better able to tolerate chemotherapy postoperatively.

References

1. Rovario GC, Rebuffat C, Varioli F, et al. Videoendoscopic pulmonary lobectomy for cancer. *Surg Laparosc Endosc* 1992;2:244–247.
2. Kirby TJ, Mack MJ, Landreneau RJ, et al. Initial experience with video-assisted thoracoscopic lobectomy. *Ann Thorac Surg* 1993;56;1248–1253.
3. Mack MJ, Scruggs GR, Kelly KM, et al. Video-assisted thoracic surgery: has technology found its place? *Ann Thorac Surg* 1997;64;211–215.
4. Kirby TJ, Mack MJ, Landreneau RJ, et al. Lobectomy – video-assisted thoracic surgery versus muscle-sparing thoracotomy: a randomized trial. *J Thorac Cardiovasc Surg* 1995;109:997–1002.
5. Sugi K, Kaneda Y, Esato K. Video-assisted thoracoscopic lobectomy achieves a satisfactory long-term prognosis in patients with clinical stage IA lung cancer. *World J Surg* 2000;24:27–31.
6. Craig SR, Leaver HA, Yap PL, et al. Acute phase responses following minimal access and conventional thoracic surgery. *Eur J Cardiothorac Surg* 2001;20:455–463.
7. Shigemura N, Akashi A, Nakagiri T, et al. Complete vs. assisted thoracoscopic approach: a prospective randomized trial comparing a variety of video-assisted thoracoscopic lobectomy techniques. *Surg Endosc* 2004;18:1492–1497.
8. Koizumi K, Haraguchi S, Hirata T, et al. Lobectomy by video-assisted thoracic surgery for lung cancer patients aged 80 years or more. *Ann Thorac Cardiovasc Surg* 2003;9:14–21.
9. Demmy TL, Curtis JJ. Minimally invasive lobectomy directed toward frail and high-risk patients: a case-control study. *Ann Thorac Surg* 1999;68:194–200.
10. Demmy TL, Plante AJ, Nwogu CE, et al. Discharge independence with minimally invasive lobectomy. *Am J Surg* 2004;188:698–702.
11. Kawai H, Tayasu Y Saitoh A, et al. Nocturnal hypoxemia after lobectomy for lung cancer. *Ann Thorac Surg* 2005;79:1162–1166.
12. Nagahiro I, Andou A, Aoe M, et al. Pulmonary function postoperative pain, and serum cytokine level after lobectomy: a comparison of VATS and conventional procedure. *Ann Thorac Surg* 2001;72:362–365.
13. Nakata M, Saeki H, Yokoyama N, et al. Pulmonary function after lobectomy: video-assisted thoracic

surgery versus thoracotomy. *Ann Thorac Surg* 2000;70:938–941.

14. Yim APC, Wan S, Lee TW, et al. VATS lobectomy reduces cytokine responses compared with conventional surgery. *Ann Thorac Surg* 2000;70:243–247.

15. Kaseda S, Aoki T, Hangai N, et al. Better pulmonary function and prognosis with video-assisted thoracic surgery than with thoracotomy. *Ann Thorac Surg* 2000;70:1644–1646.

16. Roviaro G, Varoli F, Vergani C, et al. Long-term survival after videothoracoscopic lobectomy for stage I lung cancer. *Chest* 2004;126:725–732.

17. Iwasaki A, Shirakusa T, Shiraishi T, et al. Results of video-assisted thoracic surgery for stage I/II non-small cell lung cancer. *Eur J Cardiothorac Surg* 2004;26:158–164.

18. Ohtsuka T, Nomori H, Horio H, et al. Is major pulmonary resection by video-assisted thoracic surgery an adequate procedure in clinical stage I lung cancer? *Chest* 2004;125:1742–1746.

19. Walker WS, Codispoti M, Soon SY, et al. Long-term outcomes following VATS lobectomy for non-small cell bronchogenic carcinoma. *Eur J Cardiothorac Surg* 2003;23:397–402.

20. Solaini L, Prusciano F, Bagioni P, et al. Video-assisted thoracic surgery major pulmonary resections. Present experience. *Eur J Cardiothorac Surg* 2001;20:437–442.

21. Yim APC, Izzat MB, Liu H, et al. Thoracoscopic major lung resection: an Asian perspective. *Semin Thorac Cardiovasc Surg* 1998;10:326–331.

22. McKenna RJ, Wolf RK, Brenner M, et al. Is lobectomy by video-assisted thoracic surgery an adequate cancer operation? *Ann Thorac Surg* 1998;66:1903–1908.

23. Lewis RJ, Caccavale RJ, Bocage JP, et al. Video-assisted thoracic surgical non-rib spreading simultaneously stapled lobectomy. *Chest* 1999;116:1119–1124.

24. Gharagozoloo F, Tempesta B, Margolis M, et al. Video-assisted thoracic surgery lobectomy for stage I lung cancer. *Ann Thorac Surg* 2003;76:1009–1015.

25. Flores RM. VATS lobectomy for early stage lung cancer. 2004. Available from: CTSNET Experts' Techniques. http://www.ctsnet.org.

17
Surgery for Non-Small Cell Lung Cancer with Solitary M1 Disease

Robert J. Downey

Almost all patients with stage IV non-small cell lung cancer (NSCLC) have diffusely metastatic disease, and therefore, the standard of care for NSCLC is chemotherapy or palliative care. A small percentage of patients with newly diagnosed and untreated stage IV disease are found to have a solitary synchronous site of extrathoracic disease, and a small number of patients who have undergone curative resections of intrathoracic disease experience metachronous solitary extrathoracic recurrences. There have been retrospective case reports or limited series that suggest that some such patients may be effectively treated by resection of both the primary tumor and the metastasis.[1-18] Most of these studies have reported patients with cerebral or adrenal metastases, although there are reports describing the surgical management of metastases to the small bowel,[1-3] spleen,[4,5] skeletal muscle, and bone.[6] Because of these reports, we conducted a prospective, single-arm study combining chemotherapy and resection of both the primary site of disease and of the M1 site. In this chapter, we will summarize the retrospective data suggesting that there may be a benefit associated with resection of M1 disease, as well as the results of our prospective trial.

17.1. Retrospective Studies of NSCLC with M1 Brain

Prior to our prospective study, there had been only retrospective reports of patients undergoing resection of a primary lung cancer NSCLC and a solitary cerebral metastasis. Magilligan[19] published the first series of patients undergoing combined resection of a primary NSCLC and a synchronous solitary cerebral metastasis in 1976, and updated his series in 1986 to include a total of 41 patients[8] with an overall survival of 55% at 1 year, 21% at 5 years, and 15% at 10 years. Similarly, Read and colleagues[9] reported in 1989 that patients with either synchronous or metachronous presentations treated with pulmonary and brain resection experienced an overall survival of 52% at 1 year, 35% at 2 years, and 21% at 5 years. Burt and colleagues in 1992[10] published a retrospective analysis of the Memorial Sloan-Kettering Cancer Center (MSKCC) experience with brain metastasectomy, which was later updated[11] to include 185 patients with NSCLC with a median survival of 27 months if the intrathoracic disease was resected, and 11 months if it was not. This report did not separate synchronous from metachronous presentations. In 1996, Mussi and coworkers[12] reported that the 5-year survival of 19 patients with surgically treated synchronous isolated cerebral metastases was 6% and of 33 patients with resected metachronous brain metastases was 19%. Finally, investigators from the Mayo Clinic[13] reported in 2001 that overall survival of 28 patients who underwent resection of synchronous solitary brain metastases was 64%, 54%, and 21% at 1, 2, and 5 years, respectively.

These studies all suffer from the deficiencies common to retrospective studies, most importantly, patient selection bias. However, taken together, these retrospective reports suggest that surgically treated metachronous disease may have a better prognosis than synchronous disease, but overall that if a complete resection of the primary site of disease and of the cerebral metastasis can be performed, that 1- and 5-year survivals of 50% and 10% to 30% may be achieved.

17.2. Retrospective Studies of NSCLC with M1 Adrenal

Similar to the reports of patients with M1 brain disease, prior to our prospective study, there had been only retrospective reports of patients undergoing resection of a primary NSCLC and a solitary adrenal metastasis. A retrospective review of our experience at MSKCC[15] suggests that the median survival of patients with isolated adrenal metastases treated with chemotherapy alone was 8.5 months, but the survival of patients treated with chemotherapy and surgical resection of the primary site and the adrenal metastases was 31 months. A subsequent review article[14] that summarized all the case reports and series to date and that included the MSKCC series reported that the adrenal metastasis was synchronous in 59%, and that the loco-regional (primary tumor) stage was stage I in 22%, stage II in 16%, stage III in 43%, and not specified in 18%. Overall, the median survival after resection of all disease was 24 months and one third of the patients survived 5 years. Finally, Porte and coauthors[20] conducted a retrospective review of 43 patients with isolated adrenal metastases treated surgically at eight institutions over 11 years. The overall survival was 29% at 2 years, 14% at 3 years, and 11% at 4 years. There was no difference in survival between patients presenting with synchronous or metachronous disease.

17.3. M1 Lung Cancer: MSKCC Prospective Trial

Because of the reports summarized above, we have considered patients seen at MSKCC with M1 disease for surgical resection. In order to assess the results attained, we conducted both a retrospective review of all patients treated in this manner,[21] as well as a prospective trial of combined modality therapy for synchronous M1 disease.[22]

The retrospective review of all patients at MSKCC treated with induction chemotherapy and surgery for NSCLC[21] during the period of 1993–1999 identified 43 patients with solitary site M1 disease treated with induction therapy and surgery. The sites of M1 disease were the brain in 16, the lung in 9, the adrenals in 7, the bone in 7, and the colon, an inguinal node, the spleen, and the subcutaneous tissues in 1 patient each. The survival of patients with M1 disease detected preoperatively was 18.8 months, which was consistent with the retrospective studies reviewed above.

However, our prospective study revealed different results. From October 1992 through December 1999, we conducted a prospective phase II study that combined chemotherapy and surgical resection for patients with NSCLC solitary synchronous M1 disease.[22] Eligibility criteria included biopsy proven, previously untreated NSCLC with potentially resectable intrathoracic disease (T1-3N0-2) and a solitary, synchronous, resectable metastatic lesion. Pretreatment evaluation included a computed tomography (CT) scan of the chest and upper abdomen, a CT or magnetic resonance (MR) scan of the brain with contrast, a bone scan, pulmonary function tests, and a bronchoscopy and mediastinoscopy. Positron emission tomography (PET) imaging was not required. All brain metastases were to be resected prior to chemotherapy, with some patients receiving postoperative whole brain irradiation. Patients with non-brain M1 sites had needle biopsies of the M1 site for histological proof of the presence of disease. Induction chemotherapy was intravenous mitomycin, vinblastine, and cisplatin. After completion of chemotherapy, if feasible, resection of all remaining sites of disease was performed. If all disease could be completely resected, patients received two cycles of vinblastine and cisplatin.

From October 1992 through February 1999, 23 patients were enrolled. Mediastinoscopy was performed in 22 patients and involved N2 nodes found in 12; the remaining patient had mediastinal adenopathy on CT thought to be highly suspicious for malignant involvement but did not undergo mediastinal nodal biopsy.

All enrolled patients received some chemotherapy, but only 12 patients completed the intended three cycles.

Resection of the primary lung tumor was performed in 14 patients. The pathological N status was N0 in six patients, N1 in one patient, and N2 in seven patients. A lung resection was not undertaken in the remaining nine patients because of a brain recurrence in five patients, and progression of disease in other sites during chemotherapy in four patients.

The surgery for the M1 site was a craniotomy in 13 patients, adrenalectomy in 1 patient, splenectomy in 1 patient, partial colectomy in 1 patient, segmental bone resection in 2 patients, and lung resection in 1 patient. One patient had a cerebral metastases treated with sterotactic irradiation without craniotomy. Three patients did not have resection of the M1 site because of progression of disease during chemotherapy.

Six of the 10 patients who had undergone complete resections of both primary and M1 sites received postoperative chemotherapy.

Overall, 20 patients had definitive treatment of the M1 site, and 13 patients had complete resections of the primary site of disease. Taken together, 10 patients had complete resections of both the primary and M1 sites of disease, 8 of whom had completed three cycles of chemotherapy.

The overall median survival for all patients entered into the study was 11 months. At last follow-up, three patients were alive: one patient was free of disease at 104 months, and two patients were alive with disease at 31 and 77 months.

We concluded first that the combination of induction therapy, surgical resection of primary and metastatic sites, and adjuvant chemotherapy was very poorly tolerated. Second, both disease-free and overall survival was poor, with only 2 out of 23 patients alive without disease at 5 years. It must be emphasized that this result is not inconsistent with the many retrospective studies previously published. If our experience had been reviewed retrospectively by a search of our databases for patients who had undergone complete resections of a solitary M1 site and intrathoracic loco-regional disease, 10 of the 23 enrolled would have been found. Of these 10 patients, 3 patients were alive at last follow-up (30%) and 2 patients were true 5-year survivors (20%). These results are similar to the retrospective report from the Mayo Clinic[13] and to the results found in our retrospective review of all patients undergoing exploration with the goal of curative resection after induction therapy[21] discussed above. For patients with synchronous primary disease, our prospective study suggests that a patient with newly diagnosed disease treated with combined modality therapy can expect a 4% to 8% chance of being alive and disease-free at 5 years, which is similar to that of patients with stage IV lung cancer treated with chemotherapy alone.

Our prospective trial does not provide information on patients with metachronous M1 disease, nor on patients with M1 disease treated only with surgical resection of all sites. Therefore, based on the retrospective reports summarized above, it is reasonable to treat patients with a solitary resectable NSCLC metastasis (either synchronous or metachronous) either with chemotherapy alone (recommendation grade A) or with surgical resection of all evident disease alone (recommendation grade C). However, given the results of our prospective study, it is difficult to support treating patients with solitary resectable M1 disease with the combination of medical therapies and surgical therapies used in our protocol (recommendation grade C). Future investigations should explore the combination of surgery with newer, less toxic chemotherapy regimens.

> It is reasonable to treat patients with a solitary resectable NSCLC metastasis (either synchronous or metachronous) either with chemotherapy alone (level of evidence 1; recommendation grade A) or with surgical resection of all evident disease alone (level of evidence 2; recommendation grade C).
>
> Treating patients with solitary resectable M1 disease with the combination of medical therapies and surgical therapies is not recommended (level of evidence 2; recommendation grade C).

References

1. Hinoshita E, Nakahashi H, Wakasugi K, Kaneko S, Hamatake M, Sugimachi K. Duondenal metastasis from large cell carcinoma of the lung: report of a case. *Surg Today (Japan)* 1999;29:799–802.
2. Berger A, Cellier C, Daniel C, et al. Small bowel metastases from primary carcinoma of the lung: clinical findings and outcome. *Am J Gastroenterol* 1999;94:1884–1887.
3. Moiser DM, Bloch RS, Cunningham PL, Dorman SA. Small bowel metastases from primary lung carcinoma: a rarity waiting to be found? *Am Surg* 1992;58:677–682.
4. Macheers SK, Mansour KA. Management of isolated splenic metastases from carcinoma of the lung: a case report and review of the literature. *Am Surg* 1992;58:683–685.
5. Edelman AS, Rotterdam H. Solitary splenic metastasis of an adenocarcinoma of the lung. *Am J Clin Path* 1990;94:326–328.
6. Luketich JD, Martini N, Ginsberg RJ, Rigberg D, Burt ME. Successful treatment of solitary extracranial metastases from non-small cell lung cancer. *Ann Thorac Surg* 1995;60:1609–1621.
7. Saitoh Y, Fujisawa T, Shiba M, et al. Prognostic factors in surgical treatment of solitary brain metastasis after resection of non-small-cell lung cancer. *Lung Cancer* 1999;24:99–106.
8. Magilligan DJ Jr, Duvernoy C, Malik G, Lewis JW Jr, Knighton R, Ausman JI. Surgical approach to lung cancer with solitary cerebral metastasis: twenty-five years' exerperience. *Ann Thorac Surg* 1986;42:360–364.
9. Read RC, Boop WC, Yoder G, Schaefer R. Management of nonsmall cell lung carcinoma with solitary brain metastasis. *J Thorac Cardiovasc Surg* 1989;98:884–890.
10. Burt ME, Wronski M, Arbit E, Galicich JH. Resection of brain metastases from non-small-cell lung carcinoma. Results of therapy. Memorial Sloan-Kettering Cancer Center Thoracic Surgical Staff. *J Thorac Cardiovasc Surg* 1992;103:399–410.
11. Wronski M, Arbit E, Burt M, Glicich JH. Survival after surgical treatment of brain metastases from lung cancer; a follow-up study of 231 patients treated between 1976 and 1991. *J Neurosurg* 1995;83:605–616.
12. Mussi A, Pistolesi M, Lucchi M, et al. Resection of single brain metastasis in non-small-cell lung cancer: prognostic factors. *J Thorac Cardiovasc Surg* 1996;112:146–153.
13. Billing PS, Miller DL, Allen MS, Deschamps C, Trastek VF, Pairolero PC. Surgical treatment of primary lung cancer with synchronous brain metastases. *J Thorac Cardiovasc Surg* 2001;122: 158–553.
14. Beitler AL, Urschel JD, Velagapudi SR, Takita H. Surgical management of adrenal metastases from lung cancer. *J Surg Oncol* 1998;69:54–57.
15. Luketich JD, Burt ME. Does resection of adrenal metastases from non-small cell lung cancer improve survival? *Ann Thorac Surg* 1996;62:1614–1616.
16. Hellman S, Weichselbaum RR. Oligometastases. *J Clin Oncol* 1995;13:8–10.
17. Urschel JD, Finley RK, Takita H. Long-term survival after bilateral adrenalectomy for metastatic lung cancer. *Chest* 1997;112:848–850.
18. Abdel-Raheem MM, Potti A, Becker WK, Saberi A, Scilley BS, Medhi SA. Late adrenal metastasis in operable non-small-cell lung carcinoma. *Am J Clin Oncol* 2002;25:81–88.
19. Magilligan DJ Jr, Rogers JS, Knighton RS, Davila JC. Pulmonary neoplasm with solitary cerebral metastasis. Results of combined excision. *J Thorac Cardiovasc Surg* 1976;72:690–698. 20. Porte H, Siat J, Guibert B, et al. Resection of adrenal metastases from non-small cell lung cancer: a multicenter study. *Ann Thorac Surg* 2001;71:981–895.
21. Martin J, Ginsberg RJ, Venkatraman ES, et al. Long-term results of combined-modality therapy in resectable non-small-cell lung cancer. *J Clin Oncol* 2002;20:1989–1995.
22. Downey RJ, Ng KK, Kris MG, et al. A phase II trial of chemotherapy and surgery for non-small cell lung cancer patients with a synchronous solitary metastasis. *Lung Cancer* 2002;38:193–197.

18
Thoracoscopy Versus the Open Approach for Resection of Solitary Pulmonary Metastases

Keith S. Naunheim

The rebirth of thoracoscopy in the 1990s led to its utilization in nearly all areas of thoracic surgery, both diagnostic and therapeutic. Because of its minimally invasive nature, thoracoscopy has been accepted as the approach of choice for many thoracic surgical procedures such as pleural biopsy and sympathectomy. There are, however, areas of great controversy in which the utility of thoracoscopy continues to be highly debated and one such area is the therapeutic resection of pulmonary metastases.

There are two scenarios in which therapeutic excision of lung metastases are undertaken. The first is resection with palliative intent in those patients with multiple metastases from sarcoma. In such patients, an open approach is accepted as standard by virtually the entire thoracic community.

However, "curative" resection most commonly involves resection of a solitary lung lesion or a limited number of pulmonary metastases (usually less than three). For such patients, a thoracoscopic approach to excision has been proposed as an acceptable minimally invasive alternative.

Opponents of the thoracoscopic approach believe that it will lead to a lower survival than can be achieved with an open procedure such as sternotomy, clamshell incision, or thoracotomy. They believe their argument to be logical and inherently obvious. Their stepwise reasoning is as follows:

1. Excision of pulmonary nodules in selective patients prolongs long-term survival.

2. The strongest predictor for success is "complete" excision of all metastases.

3. An open surgical procedure (thoracotomy, sternotomy) allows for palpation of the lung and identification and excision of radiologically occult nodules, thus allowing a more complete resection.

4. Because the open approach provides the opportunity for more complete excision, there is a greater chance for long-term survival.

5. An open surgical approach is therefore the method of choice for excision of pulmonary metastases.

Unfortunately, there exist no prospective, randomized, controlled trials which directly compare the thoracoscopic approach to the open approach for the therapeutic excision of pulmonary metastases. Neither has there been a formal systematic review of the literature regarding this issue and, thus, the above arguments can be argued only on the basis of what can be gleaned from the results from uncontrolled, prospective trials, case series, case control studies, and registry data. Each of the statements comprising this chain of logic must be evaluated individually.

18.1. Does Excision of Pulmonary Metastases Prolong Survival in Selected Patients?

No prospective, randomized trial is available to confirm or refute this assertion.

18.1.1. Pro

The argument supporting the beneficial effect of surgical resection rests on a large number of case series and individual case control studies outlining long-term results following resection of pulmonary metastases. From 1965 to the present, there have been over 400 publications in the literature addressing the results of excision of pulmonary metastases and many of these followed patients for not just for 5 years but throughout 10- and 15-year followups.[1] Perhaps the most authoritative of these is the International Registry for Lung Metastasis, the results of which were reported by Pastorino and colleagues.[2] While one might debate the relative benefits of metastasectomy on 5-year survival, the survival curves in this large registry demonstrate a survival plateau beginning at approximately 60 months and extending throughout 15 years. These results demonstrate 15-year survival in the 20% to 30% range, figures that would seem to be unachievable in patients with advanced cancer unless there was indeed some therapeutic advantage and efficacy of metastasectomy (level of evidence 2+).

18.1.2. Con

Aberg recently suggested that the beneficial effect of surgical excision of pulmonary metastasis is suspect (level of evidence 3).[3] He cited his own publication in which he compared a group of 70 surgically treated pulmonary metastasis patients with a small historical control group of 12 patients. Some of this latter group was treated with radiation therapy. Those patients treated medically had a 25% 5-year survival, not significantly different from that in the surgical group. The author went on to argue that the apparent beneficial effect of surgical resection on 5-year survival might be artifactual and due to patient selection. The exclusion of patients with multiple nodules, other distant disease, and serious medical comorbidities contraindicating surgery would lead to a select group of relatively healthy patients with limited disease that otherwise would have a reasonable chance of 5-year survival.

18.1.3. Conclusion

The assertion that pulmonary metastasectomy prolongs patient survival in selected patients would appear to be supported by the literature to date (level of evidence 2+ to 3; recommendation grade C).

> Pulmonary metastasectomy prolongs patient survival in selected patients (level of evidence 2+ to 3; recommendation grade C).

18.2. Does Open Thoracotomy Allow for More Complete Identification and Excision?

18.2.1. Pro

According to proponents for the open approach, the major drawback for thoracoscopy is that one loses the ability to digitally palpate the lungs. Thus, standard thoracoscopy is entirely dependent upon visual cues and whatever tactile feedback can be gained either with utilization of instruments for palpation or through insertion of a finger into a trochar site. With standard thoracoscopic technique, the opportunity for bimanual palpation is lost and thus it has been suggested that many small nodules will be missed.

Indeed there is fairly good evidence from case series and one prospective trial that this is the case. McCormack and colleagues performed a prospective trial to assess the efficacy of video-assisted thoracic techniques in the detection and excision of pulmonary metastases (level of evidence 2−).[4] Guidance for resection was obtained from computed tomography (CT) scans. Thoracoscopic excision was performed on patients with pulmonary metastasis and all radiologically and visually identified lesions were resected. Following this, a thoracotomy was undertaken, lung palpation performed, and any additional lesions were resected. The study was closed after only 18 of a planned 50 patients were enrolled because 56% of the patients (10 of 18) had additional malignant lesions found at thoracotomy after thoracoscopic exploration had been performed. The authors concluded that this incomplete excision would lead to an inferior survival long term.

18.2.2. Con

Thoracoscopy advocates criticize the above trial because only 2 of the 18 patients had the benefit of helical CT scanning, a technology which had just become available at that time. They believe that with the advent of rapid helical scanning requiring a single breath hold, the incidence of undetected nodules would drastically decline.

Since that trial, several papers have indeed documented that helical CT scan is superior to the old technique of high-resolution CT scanning and that more lesions are picked up. Margaritora and colleagues had a sequential series of patients, in which 78 received high-resolution CT scanning while 88 underwent helical CT scanning (level of evidence 2+).[5] The sensitivity for detection of all nodules was 82% utilizing the helical CT scanner versus 75% with a high-resolution scanner. In those nodules less than 6mm in size (those most likely to be missed with a thoracoscopic approach) the sensitivities were 61% or 48%, respectively. Similar sensitivity figures were provided by Diederich and colleagues, who found a 78% sensitivity for all nodules and a 69% sensitivity for those nodules smaller than 6mm (level of evidence 3).[6] Finally, Parsons and coworkers had confirmatory findings of noting a sensitivity of 78% for malignant nodules and 72% for all nodules (level of evidence 2–).[7]

Several adjunctive procedures have been suggested to aid in the localization of nodules when utilizing thoracoscopy.[8,9] Needle localization, methylene blue injection, and sonographic evaluation have all been used to identify nodules not easily palpable on the visceral pleural surface. However, these maneuvers would only aid in resection of radiologically detectable lesions and will not allow for detection of tiny metastases.

There is one hybrid procedure that utilizes both the thoracoscopic approach and manual palpation of the lung. This has been proposed by Mineo and colleagues, who performed an 8-cm midline subxiphoid incision, through which a hand is inserted for palpation of the lung during thoracoscopic examination.[10] In this way, one can potentially combine the advantages of both of a minimally invasive approach and the accuracy of digital palpation. In a prospective trial, these authors found that bilateral thoracoscopic exploration detected only 78% of the nodules that were detected when manual palpation was added as an adjunctive procedure (level of evidence 3).

18.2.3. Conclusion

There appears to be good evidence in case series and two prospective trials that, when compared to thoracoscopy, an open approach with manual palpation will allow the identification of additional nodules in 20% of patients and allow for more complete resection of malignant metastases in those patients (level of evidence 2+ to 3; recommendation grade C).

> Compared to thoracoscopy, an open approach with manual palpation allows the identification of additional nodules in 20% of patients and allows for more complete resection of malignant metastases (level of evidence 2+ to 3; recommendation grade C).

18.3. Is Complete Excision of the Pulmonary Metastasis a Strong Predictor of Survival?

18.3.1. Pro

Many publications have performed univariate and/or multivariate analysis to identify predictors of long-term survival following resection of pulmonary metastases. The strongest predictor of long-term success appears to be the histology of the metastatic lesions.[2] However, the second most influential predictor is the ability to completely resect all intrathoracic disease (level of evidence 2+ to 3).[2,11,12] The International Registry data demonstrated that those with complete resection had a 5-year survival three times higher than those with incomplete resections (36% vs. 13%).[2] Thus proponents of the open approach suggest that the direct digital lung palpation will allow for identification of metastases that would likely be undetected during thoracoscopy and thus are more likely to ensure "complete resection" and prolonged survival.

18.3.2. Con

Proponents for the thoracoscopy approach suggest that the above reasoning is invalid and that there is misuse of the term *complete resection*. Patients who undergo "incomplete" resection during open thoracotomy do not generally do so because of tiny resectable nodules which are not removed. It is more commonly because of large bulky disease that involves vital structures or because the disease is so extensive that major lung resections, incompatible with patient benefit, would be required to undertake resection. Most of these latter patients are currently identified at the time of CT scanning and do not even come to operation. This would appear to be the true definition of the term *unresectable* in the open situation.

In those undergoing thoracoscopic resection, the occult nodules which might be left behind (due to an inability to identify them by palpation) are not truly "unresectable"; rather they are "undetectable" utilizing thoracoscopic techniques. Proponents of thoracoscopy would suggest that these lesions that remain undetected do not necessarily portend the unfavorable prognosis that the "unresectable" definition from the open approach would imply. They would contend that it is the biological activity of the tumor rather than the anatomical considerations that truly influence long-term survival.

Small micrometastasis that go undetected at the time of thoracoscopy may certainly continue to grow and eventually present as "new" metastases subsequently. Although a subset of such patients would have concomitant distant recurrence of malignancy and would not be candidate for surgery, there would be a cohort for whom a repeat metastasectomy would be appropriate. Several case series document that a second resection of metastasis yields 5-year survivals essentially identical to those that occur following first time resection (level of evidence 2+ to 3).[2,13,14] Thus, thoracoscopy advocates suggest that even when undetected metastases are left behind, in those patients in whom they grow and present

metachronously as isolated pulmonary recurrence, a second therapeutic resection is possible and is just as likely to provide long-term survival as an upfront open approach.

18.3.3. Conclusion

Although "incomplete resection" is a predictor for therapeutic failure, the definition of incomplete resection does not equate to radiologically undetectable disease that might persist following a video-assisted thorascopic surgery (VATS) resection. No prospective trial or case series support the contention that such occult disease reliably predicts therapeutic failure (level of evidence 2+ to 3; recommendation grade C).

> Although "incomplete resection" is a predictor for therapeutic failure, the definition of incomplete resection does not equate to radiologically undetectable disease that might persist following a VATS resection. No prospective trial or case series supports the contention that such occult disease reliably predicts therapeutic failure (level of evidence 2+ to 3; recommendation grade C).

18.4. Does the Open Approach Provide a Greater Chance of Cure than the Thoracoscopic Approach?

It was hoped that this debate could be addressed and answered by a prospective, randomized trial directly comparing the treatment of pulmonary metastasis by thoracoscopic versus open techniques. There was indeed such a study proposed and instituted (Cancer and Leukemia Group B 9336), but unfortunately it was closed prematurely due to lack of accrual. Thus there are no prospective trials to address this issue.

18.4.1. Pro

Proponents for the open approach insist that the logical conclusion from the above argument is that the inability of the thoracoscopic approach to detect all malignant lesions makes it likely that metastasis will be left behind in up to one quarter of the patients. These remaining metastases will eventually take the life of the patient either due to progressive pulmonary compression/replacement by the lesions, or due to distant disease when the undetected lung metastases themselves metastasize. They believe that 5-year survival will be inferior with a VATS procedure.

18.4.2. Con

Thoracoscopy proponents do not believe this is a foregone conclusion and favor VATS resection. There are some reports with which one can gauge the efficacy of thoracoscopic resection for pulmonary metastases. Lin and colleagues gathered and published results from six institutions outlining the results of both diagnostic and therapeutic resection of pulmonary metastasis via thoracoscopy.[15] Of the 99 patients undergoing therapeutic resection, 37% were free of disease in the follow-up interval of 37 months. Just as importantly, of the 57 recurrences, 69% were distant, a number not dissimilar found by Pastorino and colleagues in the paper describing the International Registry, which encompassed over 5200 cases.[2] In Lin's paper, the incidence of extrathoracic metastasis was 46% while single or multiple intrathoracic recurrences were noted in 54% of all patients. Thus, the incidence of local recurrence following thoracoscopic resection, the supposed Achilles' heel of the technique, is lower at a mean of 37 months follow-up than that quoted by Pastorino and colleagues with the open approach. Obviously, the time of follow-up is significantly different; nonetheless, there is little in this comparison to suggest that thoracoscopic resection will provide results inferior to those of the open approach (level of evidence 3).

There have been two clinical papers comparing the thoracoscopic and open approaches to resection of pulmonary metastasis. Mutsaerts and colleagues reported on 35 patients who underwent a thoracoscopic metastasectomy for a solitary pulmonary nodule (level of evidence 2+).[16] Nineteen underwent only a minimally invasive approach while an additional 16 underwent confirmatory thoracotomy for excision of undetected nodules that could be palpated. The incidence of complications was higher in the thoracotomy cohort than the VATS cohort. The 2-year disease-free survival and overall survival rates were 50% and 60% in the thoracoscopic cohort and 42% and 70% in the thoracotomy cohort. These results suggest that at least in the early follow-up period, there appears to be little difference in the results between thoracoscopic and open approach.

A second paper from Nakajima and associates reported on a comparison of 35 patients undergoing thoracoscopic resection of pulmonary metastasis versus 55 patients undergoing an open thoracotomy approach (level of evidence 3).[17] Solitary metastases were resected more frequently with thoracoscopy than thoracotomy. The actuarial 1-, 2-, and 3-year survival rates were 83%, 70%, and 62% in the thoracoscopy group and 94%, 65% and 53% in the open group, respectively. The rates of local recurrence and actuarial survival did not differ when only patients with solitary pulmonary metastasis were analyzed. Once again, this paper provides no evidence suggesting a superior survival advantage for the open approach.

18.4.3. Conclusion

There appears to be no strong evidence supporting the assertion that an open approach to a solitary pulmonary metastasis will provide superior clinical results with regard to long-term survival. Although theoretically, the concept that the thoracoscopy will leave behind undetected metastasis and therefore lead to inferior results appears logical and conceptually attractive, there is not yet data that can definitively support this notion (level of evidence 3; recommendation grade C).

> There is no strong evidence supporting the assertion that an open approach to a solitary pulmonary metastasis will provide superior clinical results compared to a VATS approach with regard to long-term survival (level of evidence 3; recommendation grade C).

18.5. Should the Open Approach for the Resection of Pulmonary Metastasis be the Standard of Care?

18.5.1. Pro

While the concept of thoracotomy or sternotomy for curative resection of pulmonary metastasis is a time-honored and standardized technique, there is little hard evidence in the literature currently demonstrating the superiority of this approach versus minimally invasive thoracic surgical techniques. Although it may seem logical to believe that an open surgical approach that results in resection of more tissue will provide a significant survival advantage, surgical history suggests that such logical arguments do not always prove to be true. Radical mastectomy for breast cancer, pneumonectomy for lung cancer, and open thoracotomy with radical resection for esophageal cancer were, at one time, viewed as the standard of care for the treatment of their respective diseases. Currently, an open approach is likely the most commonly performed procedure for the curative treatment of pulmonary metastasis. As such, it can be considered one standard of care in the legal sense; however, it is backed by much more in the way of expert opinion than scientific fact.

18.5.2. Con

There is a minority opinion supporting a thoracoscopic approach to resection of metastases which has potential merit as well. No definitive literature exists that demonstrates inferior results from a minimally invasive approach. In fact, two clinical reports suggest that the early survival results approximate those found with an open approach.[16,17]

Lastly, it is fair to consider that the vast majority of patients undergoing resection for pulmonary metastasis will indeed not be cured by the operation. For such patients, the minimally invasive approach would appear to have significant potential benefits over thoracotomy with regard to decreased length of stay, lesser degrees of postoperative pain, and faster return to full function. This could possibly be reflected in decreased cost

of treatment and improved quality of life, although these advantages have not at present been demonstrated in this patient population.

18.5.3. Conclusion

There exist logical, theoretical arguments that an open approach for resection of lung metastases will provide a survival advantage over a minimally invasive approach. However, no literature comparing the two approaches documents inferior results with thoracoscopy. In fact, the small amount of literature available suggests equivalency. Expert opinion appears to be the primary argument supporting an open approach to resection of lung metastases (level of evidence 4; recommendation grade D). Either approach would appear appropriate for the resection of solitary lung metastases.

> That an open approach for resection of lung metastases provides a survival advantage over a minimally invasive approach is supported primarily by expert opinion (level of evidence 4; recommendation grade D).
>
> However, the small amount of literature available suggests equivalency, and either approach would appear appropriate for the resection of solitary lung metastases.

References

1. Martini N, McCormack PM. Evolution of the surgical management of pulmonary metastases. *Chest Surg Clin* 1998;8:13–27.
2. Pastorino U, Buyse M, Friedel G, et al. Long-term results of lung metastectomy: prognostic analyses based on 5206 cases. *J Thorac Cardiovasc Surg* 1997;113:37–49.
3. Aberg T, Malmberg KA, Nilsson B, et al. The effect of metastasectomy: fact or fiction? *Ann Thorac Surg* 1980;30:378–384.
4. McCormack PM, Bains MS, Begg CB, et al. Role of video-assisted thoracic surgery in the treatment of pulmonary metastases: results of a prospective trial. *Ann Thorac Surg* 1999;68:795–796.
5. Margaritora S, Porziella V, D'Andrill A, et al. Pulmonary metastases: can accurate radiologic evaluation avoid thoracotomic approach? *Eur J Cardiothorac Surg* 2002;21:1111–1114.

6. Diederich S, Semik M, Lentschig MG, et al. helical CT of pulmonary nodules in patients with extrathoracic malignancy: Ct-surgical correlation. *AJR Am J Roentgenol* 1999;172:353–360.

7. Parsons AM, Detterbeck FC, Parker LA. Accuracy of helical CT in the detection of pulmonary metastases: is intraoperative palpation still necessary? *Ann Thorac Surg* 2004;78:1910–1918.

8. Yamamoto M, Takeo M, Meguro F, et al. Sonographic evaluation for peripheral pulmonary nodules during video-assisted thoracoscopic surgery. *Surg Endosc* 2003;17:825–827.

9. Kanazawa S, Ando A, Yasui K, et al. Localization of pulmonary nodules for thoracoscopic resection: experience with a system using short hookwire and suture. *AJR Am J Roentgenol* 1998;170:332–334.

10. Mineo TC, Ambrogi V, Paci M, et al. Transxiphoid bilateral palpation in video-assisted thoracoscopic lung metastasectomy. *Arch Surg* 2001;136:783–788.

11. Jablons D, Steinberg SM, Roth J, et al. Metastasectomy for soft tissue sarcoma; further evidence for efficacy and prognostic indicators. *J Thorac Cardiovasc Surg* 1989;97:695–705.

12. Girard P, Baldeyrou P, LeChevalier T, et al. Surgery for pulmonary metastases: who are the 10-year survivors? *Cancer* 1994;74:2791–2797.

13. Jaklitsch MT, Mery CM, Lukanich JM, et al. Sequential thoracic metastasectomy prolongs survival by re-establishing local control within the chest. *J Thorac Cardiovasc Surg* 2001;121:657–667.

14. Pastorino U, Valente M, Gasparini M, et al. Median sternotomy and multiple lung resections for metastatic sarcomas. *Eur J Cardiothorac Surg* 1990;4:477–481.

15. Lin JC, Wiechmann RJ, Szwerc MF, et al. Diagnostic and therapeutic video-assisted thoracic surgery resection of pulmonary metastases. *Surgery* 1999;126:636–641.

16. Mutsaert EL, Zoetmulder FA, Meijer S, et al. Long-term survival of thoracoscopic metastasectomy versus metastasectomy by thoracotomy in patients with a solitary pulmonary lesion. *Eur J Surg Oncol* 2002;28:864–868.

17. Nakajima J, Takamoto S, Tanaka M, et al. Thoracoscopic surgery and conventional open thoracotomy in metastatic lung cancer. *Surg Endosc* 2001;15:849–853.

19
Unilateral or Bilateral Approach for Unilateral Pulmonary Metastatic Disease

Ashish Patel and Malcolm M. DeCamp, Jr.

The term *pulmonary metastasectomy* refers to surgical excision of malignant lesion(s) of the lung of extrapulmonary origin. Several retrospective studies, including the International Registry of Lung Metastases,[1] have observed increased survival following pulmonary metastasectomy when compared to historical control patient cohorts who did not undergo resection. Over the years these observations have led to widespread acceptance of pulmonary metastasectomy in appropriately selected patients. The lack of randomized, controlled trials and the continued evolution in imaging technology, chemotherapeutics, and surgical technique pose significant challenges to clinicians as they struggle with appropriate patient selection for and the optimal surgical approach to metastasectomy.

The criteria for undertaking pulmonary metastasectomy include control of the primary disease site, lack of other systemic metastatic disease, adequate physiological reserve, and the ability to resect all residual disease in the lungs. Bilateral pulmonary metastatic disease, in selected patients, is treated with bilateral resections. The obvious question, therefore, is whether to explore the contralateral lung in a patient with only unilaterally detected pulmonary metastases.

This chapter addresses the question of a unilateral or bilateral approach to unilateral pulmonary metastatic disease. Recommendations are made according to the system of evidence grading proposed by the Scottish Intercollegiate Guidelines Network (SIGN).[2] Each study cited with regard to our recommendation is assigned a level

of evidence, with 1++ being a high-quality review of randomized, controlled trials and 4 being expert opinion. Case control studies are generally assigned level 2, with 2+ given to studies with likelihood of causal relationship. Overall, recommendations are graded from A to D, with an A grade being supported by randomized, controlled trials. Grade B recommendations suggests consistency in the literature.

19.1. Unilateral or Bilateral Approach

Central to the question of a unilateral or bilateral approach to unilateral pulmonary metastatic disease is (1) the principle of achieving a complete resection of all pulmonary disease, (2) the accuracy of preoperative imaging in detecting metastatic disease, (3) the efficacy of a surgical technique in identifying and resecting all pulmonary disease, and (4) the evidence for improved outcome.

19.2. Complete Resection

The principle of resecting all pulmonary metastatic disease is based on the current understanding of cancer pathobiology coupled with decades of observations of patients undergoing pulmonary metastasectomy. Contemporary cancer biology assumes that metastases originate from cells that are shed by primary tumors and disseminated through the systemic vascular and lymphatic circulations. Hematogenous metastases are more likely to become lodged in the first capillary bed encountered following transit to the vascular system. The basis of this theory is supported by the observation that tumors of the gastrointestinal tract drained by the portal venous circulation generally metastasize first to the liver, while the tumors with venous drainage to the systemic circulation (e.g., rectum, kidney, soft-tissue sarcomas) metastasize more frequently to lungs. Histological studies support these theories as 84% of lung metastases receive their major blood supply from the pulmonary arteries while only 16% are supplied exclusively by the bronchial arteries[3] (level of evidence 3).

One of the most interesting questions in cancer pathology has been whether metastases can themselves metastasize. A retrospective review of 883 pulmonary metastasectomies performed at the Mayo Clinic identified 70 (8%) patients who had concurrent lymph node dissections at the time of metastasectomy. Fourteen (20%) of these 70 patients had positive nodes suggesting that metastases can metastasize. Three-year survival among patients with negative nodes was much higher (69%) than among patients with positive nodes (38%)[4] (level of evidence 2+). Thus, any therapy aimed at a complete and curative resection should involve evaluation of regional lymphatics around the metastasis.

Clinical experience over the last 100 years seems to support the need for complete resection. The first report of pulmonary metastasectomy is credited to Dr. Weinlechener in Germany, who, in 1882, removed an incidental metastasis of the lung during resection of a chest wall sarcoma. Unfortunately the patient only survived 24 h[5] (level of evidence 4). In 1884, Dr. Kronlein resected an incidental metastasis to the lung of a chest wall sarcoma and observed the patient survive over the next 7 years[6] (level of evidence 4). The first report of pulmonary metastasectomy in America was by Drs. Barney and Churchill in the 1930s, when they removed a metastatic focus of renal cell carcinoma. The patient survived 23 years.

Reports of improved survival among patients undergoing pulmonary metastasectomy for other cell types have led to further aggressive approaches. Osteogenic sarcoma is a highly lethal neoplasm with 5-year survival of less than 5% among patients with pulmonary metastases. When a group of patients with osteogenic sarcoma underwent pulmonary metastasectomy at Memorial Sloan-Kettering Cancer Center, the survival improved to 32% at 5 years and 18% at 20 years[7] (level of evidence 2+). All surgical efforts were focused on removal of all palpable tumors, leading to an overall impression that aggressive removal of all metastases improved survival. The most comprehensive set of retrospective data emerged with the formation of an International Registry of Lung Metastases (IRLM). The registry collected data on 5206 pulmonary metastasectomies from 18 departments of thoracic surgery around the world. The survival statistics were evaluated using Kaplan Meier estimates. The results were published in 1997 and are continually updated. Among the total of 5206 metastasectomies, 4572 were complete resections while 634 were incomplete. The survival after complete metastasectomy was 36% at 5 years, 26% at 10 years, and 22% at 15 years with a median survival of 35 months. Survival among incomplete resections was 13% at 5 years, 7% at 10 and 15 years with a median of 15 months. This observation suggests a strong correlation between survival and complete resection[1] (level of evidence 2++) and is supported by several other smaller series including a recent study by Suzuki and colleagues showing aggressive pulmonary resection of osteosarcoma metastases yielded 42% 10-year survival for complete resection and only 4.2% 6-year survival for incomplete resection[8] (level of evidence 2++).

Unfortunately, all of the above observations are affected by selection and observer bias typical of retrospective studies. Tumor-specific factors also impact survival and may dominate the salutary effect of complete resection. This hypothesis is supported by the observations that despite complete resections, overall survival is highly dependent on histology of the tumor. Among patients who had complete resection of all identifiable disease, Mountain and colleagues found 5-year survival of 54% for urinary tract and male genital tract tumors, 46% for osteogenic sarcoma, 33% for soft-tissue tumors, 24% for primary uterine cervix tumors, and only 12% for melanoma[9] (level of evidence 2+).

19.3. Imaging

The ability to detect all pulmonary metastases is central to any discussion of approach to pulmonary metastasectomy. Surgical approach has clearly been guided by the improvement in imaging, specifically single-breath-hold, helical, and/or multidetector computed tomography (CT) scans.

Early pulmonary metastasectomies, such as those by Weinlechener or Kronlein, were serendipitous. The discovery of X rays and their evolution to chest roentgenograms during the early 20th century allowed for planned metastasectomies, as those reported by Barney and Churchill. Chest roentgenograms, although helpful in the diagnosis of pulmonary lesions, were not highly sensitive. This is clearly reported by McCormack and coworkers in 1993, where 57/144 (39%) of chest roentgenograms differed in number of lesions detected from intraoperative findings. Forty-six percent of patients had more lesions than chest roentgenograms detected while 21% had fewer. The gold standard for detecting all pulmonary lesions became intraoperative palpation, which led to advocacy for operative techniques providing access to both lungs, including bilateral staged thoracotomies, median sternotomy, median sternotomy with lateral thoracotomy, and the clamshell bilateral sterno-thoracotomy[10] (level of evidence 2).

The ubiquitous availability of CT scan in the 1980s led to a re-evaluation of approaches to pulmonary metastasectomies. Some clinicians began to believe that CT could supplant palpation in terms of metastasis detection. Concerned with accuracy of CT scans, McCormack and coworkers also evaluated the sensitivity and specificity of CT scans in their review of imaging modalities in lung nodule detection. They found that CT findings differed from intraoperative findings among (30/72) 42% of patients. Twenty-five percent of patients had more malignant nodules than found on CT scan, while 17% of patients had more lesions on CT than found at operation. The authors concluded that CT was not adequate replacement for bilateral manual lung palpation. The CT images, however, were 8-mm axial images. The authors do not mention whether the lesions were unilateral or bilateral and agree that the

number of tumors found in the study failed to reach statistical significance for survival data[10] (level of evidence 2−).

The superiority of manual palpation over axial CT in detection and diagnosis of pulmonary lesions was further challenged by the advent of helical CT in the 1990s. Unlike axial CT that take axial scans over several breaths each at distance of 8mm, the helical CT takes continuous spiral scans (2.5- to 8-mm collimation) during a single breath suspended at full inspiration. Faster image acquisition results in lower distortion due to respiratory or cardiac motion and higher resolution. Several studies reported average detection of 20% more nodules by spiral CT compared to conventional CT[11] (level of evidence 3). Retrospective analyses were once again performed to resolve the sensitivity and specificity of helical CT. In a retrospective review of 34 patients who underwent both helical CT and manual lung palpation, Parsons and colleagues report only (69/88) 78% sensitivity[12] (level of evidence 2−). This is similar to sensitivity of helical CT in detecting lung lesions reported by Waters and colleagues (56%), Diederich and colleagues (77%), Ambrogi and coworkers (84%), and Margaritora and coworkers (82%)[13–16] (level of evidence 2−).

The integrated use of helical CT (2.5- to 5-mm collimation) with F-18 fluorodeoxyglucose positron tomography (FDG-PET) has become a common part of the evaluation of primary lung cancer. F-18 Fluorodeoxyglucose positron tomography scans have detected occult metastatic disease and helped patients avoid nontherapeutic resections for non-small cell lung cancer patients in up to 10% of cases. Recalling the criteria for documented control of extra thoracic disease and the increased relevance of mediastinal spread of pulmonary metastases, Pastorino and colleagues evaluated the use of FDG-PET in the workup of pulmonary metastasectomies. Eighty-six patients underwent 89 PET scans prior to surgery deemed otherwise resectable by helical CT scan. Surgery was avoided or deferred in 19 of 86 (21%) patients based on PET findings, which included 11 extra-thoracic metastases, 2 primary recurrences, 2 cases of mediastinal adenopathy, and 4 cases with confounding benign disease. FDG-PET sensitivity was 100% for detecting lung metastases and 100% for mediastinal staging compared to

95% and 71% for spiral CT scans[17] (level of evidence 2+).

Advances in imaging technology continue to provide diagnostic assistance in patient selection for pulmonary metastasectomy. The combination of improved imaging and lack of a convincing survival advantage to open palpation, along with availability of minimally invasive surgical techniques, continues to stimulate surgeons to evaluate less morbid approaches to pulmonary metastasectomy.

19.4. Surgical Approach

Once unilateral pulmonary metastases are detected radiographically, the surgeon has several therapeutic options, including bilateral thoracotomies, median sternotomy, clamshell thoracotomy, unilateral thoracotomy, or video-assisted thoracic surgery (VATS).

The decision regarding surgical approach is influenced by sensitivity and specificity of imaging, surgeon's familiarity with the technique, operative risk, and currently available literature on surgical experience. The sensitivity and specificity of imaging has been discussed above with contemporary practice favoring both an inspiratory helical CT for optimal lesion detection complimented by an integrated FDG-PET/CT study to evaluate the primary site, regional nodal basins, and to exclude other extrathoracic disease. The surgeon's familiarity with technique plays a minor role as most centers have expertise in traditional open thoracic techniques and VATS. The operative risk is minimal and acceptable regardless of the operative technique. Johnston reported no operative mortality in 53 median sternotomies in 1983[18] (level of evidence 3). Pastorino and coworkers had a similar experience with 0 early deaths in 56 consecutive sternotomies for sarcoma[19] (level of evidence 3). There are no reported, statistically relevant differences in major morbidity or mortality between thoracotomies and sternotomies for resection of lung metastases. A VATS approach has similar low morbidity and may have advantages of decreased pain, creating fewer adhesions making reintervention more feasible, and a shorter hospital stay.

The most aggressive approaches to unilateral pulmonary metastasectomy are median sternotomy, clamshell thoracotomy, or bilateral thoracotomy, each of which allow palpation of the contralateral lung. The studies supporting these approaches, however, are increasingly dated given the availability of improved imaging. Proponents of median sternotomy cite a single incision, low morbidity, and ability to palpate the contralateral lung through the same incision as advantages to the approach. Johnston, in 1983, championed median sternotomy for its low morbidity and 53% more nodules found at sternotomy than detected by chest tomography[18] (level of evidence 3). Van der Veen and colleagues report 82 sternotomies with CT discordance in 49% of cases[20] (level of evidence 2−). Reports favoring sternotomy also cite softer end points such as reduced pain and earlier recovery of pulmonary function when compared to thoracotomies[21] (level of evidence 3).

The most significant argument to challenge a bilateral approach to unilateral disease has been lack of survival advantage to the contralateral exploration. Roth and colleagues compared median sternotomy and thoracotomy for soft-tissue sarcomas in 1986. Eighty-two patients underwent complete resection of their metastases, 42 each by sternotomy and thoracotomy with a follow-up of 2 years. The groups were matched for disease-free interval, number of nodules resected, and tumor doubling time. There was no difference in survival between the two groups. The authors concluded that, although median sternotomy allows detection of unsuspected bilateral metastases, it does not offer survival advantage to unilateral thoracotomy[22] (level of evidence 2+).

Younes and colleagues evaluated the need for bilateral thoracotomy in patients with unilateral pulmonary metastases using a retrospective database from a single institution (1990–1997). Two hundred sixty-seven consecutive patients included 179 patients with unilateral lung nodules and 88 patients with bilateral nodules. Unilateral thoracotomy was performed for unilateral disease and bilateral for bilateral disease, respectively. Contralateral recurrence-free survival over 6 months, 1 year, and 5 years was 95%, 89%, and 78%, respectively. When patients with contralateral recurrence were compared with patients with bilateral metastases on admission, there was no significant difference in overall survival. Contralateral recurrence was only linked to histology and number of unilateral metastases. Given these results, the authors concluded that most patients with unilateral disease only have unilateral disease and delaying contralateral thoracotomy until lesions appear does not affect survival[23] (level of evidence 2+). These findings have been confirmed by similar observations including those by Gadd and coworkers for soft-tissue sarcoma as well as by Matthay and coworkers and Pogrebniak and colleagues[24-26] (level of evidence 2+). Additionally, there is no correlation between survival and unilateral or bilateral disease[27,28] (level of evidence 2+).

Video-assisted thoracoscopic surgery is playing an increasing role in pulmonary metastasectomy. The first reports of VATS metastasectomy were by Dowling and colleagues in 1993. Seventy-two patients with peripheral lung lesions identified by CT received wedge resections using a stapler or Nd:YAG laser. Sixty-three of 73 (86%) of resected nodules were pathologically confirmed to be metastatic lesions. Sixty-five of 72 (90%) patients underwent resection for diagnosis while only 7 underwent resection for potential survival benefit[29] (level of evidence 2). Liu and colleagues used VATS to resect lung metastases in 47 patients. Digital lung palpation was used to identify additional nodules and to locate and resect all nodules detected on preoperative imaging. Five patients were found to have additional nodules and these were resected. The authors concluded that VATS was a useful technique for metastasectomy but failed to provide follow-up survival data[30] (level of evidence 2−). In 1996, McCormack and coworkers published a prospective study comparing VATS to thoracotomy. Patients underwent VATS resection followed by immediate thoracotomy to carefully palpate the lung for missed lesions. Four (22%) patients had no additional lesions while 10 (56%) had additional malignant lesions. The remaining four (22%) had additional benign lesions. Based on these findings, VATS was not recommended for metastasectomy although the survival advantage to the resection of the "VATS-blind" nodules remains unknown[31] (level of evidence 2−).

Although the role of VATS is questioned for pulmonary metastasectomy, it is indispensable for diagnostic purposes. Pulmonary nodules in patients with a history of prior malignancy often are radiographically uncharacteristic of metastases and require diagnosis by excisional. More importantly there is a significant rate of primary lung cancer among patients with prior extrathoracic malignancy. In a study of 50 patients with a history of malignancy by Adkins and colleagues, 18% of lung lesions were benign, 18% represented a new primary lung cancer, and 64% were metastatic lesions.[32] The probability of the lesion being metastatic versus a new primary lesion is dependent on the primary histology. Ninety percent of lung lesions among patients with melanoma or sarcoma are metastatic. Fifty percent of the lung lesions are metastatic in patients with gastrointestinal, genitourinary, or gynecological malignancy. Because of the high prevalence of tobacco-related carcinogen exposure throughout the aero–digestive tract, only 33% of lung lesions in patients with head and neck cancers are metastatic.[33] With continued improvement in imaging techniques, and lack of evidence demonstrating increased survival following more radical exploratory operations, VATS will continue to play a role in pulmonary metastasectomy.

19.5. Conclusion

The field of pulmonary metastasectomy continues to evolve. Historically, it has progressed from serendipitous open resection of unexpected pulmonary metastases to planned bilateral explorations to minimally invasive resections supported by advanced imaging techniques. The justification of pulmonary metastasectomy lies in the feasibility of the procedure and the observed improvement in survival. Extensive retrospective studies point to complete resection of pulmonary metastases as a factor associated with improved survival. Traditionally this linkage has led surgeons to explore both lungs during metastasectomy. Advances in imaging technology, including helical CT and PET scans, and the integration of these anatomical and metabolic studies into a single fused image, is providing increasing diagnostic sensitivity and specificity useful in guiding selection of patients appropriate for pulmonary metastasectomy. The same images provide a useful "roadmap" for the surgeon seeking to achieve a complete resection.

19.6. Recommendation

The absence of data demonstrating improved survival after routine lung palpation without radiologically identified contralateral disease justifies a unilateral approach to unilaterally detected pulmonary nodules. A planned course of cross-sectional imaging follow-up for recurrent metastases is prudent. The precise role of VATS in pulmonary metastasectomy is poorly defined. Given continued advancement in both imaging and operative technology, this role is expected to grow. This is a grade B recommendation given the overall consistency in the literature and the presence of at least one 2++ level study.

> The absence of data demonstrating improved survival after routine lung palpation without radiographically identified contralateral disease justifies a unilateral approach to unilaterally detected pulmonary nodules (level of evidence 2++ to 3; recommendation grade B).

References

1. The International Registry of Lung Metastases. Long-term results of lung metastasectomy: prognostic analyses based on 5206 cases. *J Thorac Cardiovasc Surg* 1997;113:37–49.
2. Harbour R, Miller J, et al. A new system for grading recommendations in evidence based guidelines. *BMJ* 2001;323.
3. Downey RJ. Surgical treatment of pulmonary metastases. *Surg Oncol Clin N Am* 1999;8:341–354.
4. Ercan S, Nichols FC 3rd, Trastek VF, et al. Prognostic significance of lymph node metastasis found during pulmonary metastasectomy for extrapulmonary carcinoma. *Ann Thorac Surg* 2004;77:1786–1791.
5. Weinlechener JW. Zur Kasuistick der Tumoren ander Brustwand und deren Behandlung Wien. *Med Wchnschr* 1882;32:589–591, 624–628.
6. Kronlein RU. Ueber Lungenchirurgie. *Berl Klin Wehnschr* 1884;21:129–132.
7. Rusch VW. Pulmonary metastasectomy current indications. *Chest* 1995;107:322–331.
8. Suzuki M, Kimura H, Ando S, et al. Pulmonary metastasectomy for osteosarcomas and soft tissue sarcomas. *Gan To Kagaku Ryoho* 2004;31:1319–1323.
9. Mountain CF, McMurtrey MJ, Hermes KE. Surgery for pulmonary metastasis: a 20 year experience. *Ann Thorac Surg* 1984;38:323–330.
10. McCormack PM, Ginsberg KB, Bains M, et al. Accuracy of lung imaging in metastases with implications for the role of thoracoscopy. *Ann Thorac Surg* 1993;56:863–866.
11. Remy-Jardin J, Remy-Jardin M, Giraud F. Pulmonary nodules: detection with thick section spiral CT versus conventional CT. *Radiology* 1993;187:513–520.
12. Parsons AM, Detterbeck FC, Parker LA. Accuracy of helical CT in the detection of pulmonary metastases: is intraoperative palpation still necessary? *Ann Thorac Surg* 2004;78:1910–1918.
13. Waters DJ, Coakley FV, Cohen MD, et al. The detection of pulmonary metastases by helical CT: a clinicopathologic study in dogs. *J Comput Assist Tomogr* 1998;22:235–240.
14. Diederich S, Semik M, Lentschig MG, et al. Helical CT of pulmonary nodules in patients with extrathoracic malignancy: CT-surgical correlation. *AJR Am J Roentgenol* 1999;172:353–360.
15. Ambrogi V, Paci M, Pompeo E, Mineo TC. Transxiphoid video-assisted pulmonary metastasectomy: relevance of helical computed tomography occult lesions. *Ann Thorac Surg* 2000;70:1847–1852.
16. Margoritora S, Porziella V, D'Andrilli A, et al. Pulmonary metastases: can accurate radiological evaluation avoid thoracotomic approach? *Eur J Cardiothorac Surg* 2002;21:1111–1114.
17. Pastorino U, Veronesi G, Landoni C, et al. Flurodeoxyglucose positron emission tomography improves preoperative staging of respectable lung metastasis. *J Thorac Cardiovasc Surg* 2003;126:1906–1910.
18. Johnston MR. Median sternotomy for resection of pulmonary metastases. *J Thorac Cardiovasc Surg* 1983;85:516–522.
19. Pastorino U, Valenta M, Gasparini M, et al. Median sternotomy and multiple lung resections for metastatic sarcomas. *Eur J Cardiothorac Surg* 1990;4:477–481.
20. Van der Veen AH, van Geel AN, Hop WCJ, Wiggers T. Median sternotomy: the preferred incision for resection of lung metastases. *Eur J Surg* 1998;164:507–512.
21. Cooper JD, Nelems JM, Pearson FG. Extended indications for median sternotomy in patients requiring pulmonary resection. *Ann Thorac Surg* 1978;26:413–420.

22. Roth JA, Pass HI, Wesley MN, White D, Putnam JB, Seipp C. Comparison of median sternotomy and thoracotomy for resection of pulmonary metastases in patients with adult soft-tissue sarcomas. *Ann Thorac Surg* 1986;42:134–138.

23. Younes RN, Gross JL, Deheinzelin D. Surgical resection of unilateral lung metastases: is bilateral thoracotomy necessary? *World J Surg* 2002;26:1112–1116.

24. Gadd MA, Casper ES, Woodruff JM, McCormack PM, Brennan MF. Development and treatment of pulmonary metastases in adult patients with extremity soft tissue sarcoma. *Ann Surg* 1993;218:705–712.

25. Matthay RA, Arroglia AC. Resection of pulmonary metastases. *Am Rev Respir Dis* 1993;148:1691–1696.

26. Pogrebniak HW, Roth JA, Steinberg SM, Rosenberg SA, Pass HI. Reoperative pulmonary resectin in patients with metastatic soft tissue sarcoma. *Ann Thorac Surg* 1991;52:197–203.

27. Pogrebniak HW, Pass HI. Initial and reoperative pulmonary metastasectomy: indications, technique, and results. *Semin Surg Oncol* 1993;9:142–149.

28. Regal AM, Reese P, Antkowiak J, Hart T, Takita H. Median sternotomy for metastatic lung lesions in 131 patients. *Cancer* 1985;55:1334–1339.

29. Dowling RD, Landreneau RJ, Miller DL. Video-assisted thoracoscopic surgery for resection of lung metastases. *Chest* 1998;113:2–5.

30. Liu HP, Lin PJ, Hsieh MJ, Chang JP, Chang CH. Application of thoracoscopy for lung metastases. *Chest* 1995;107:266–268.

31. McCormack PM, Bains MS, Begg CB, et al. Role of video-assisted thoracic surgery in the treatment of pulmonary metastases: results of a prospective trial. *Ann Thorac Surg* 1996;62:213–216.

32. Adkins PC, Wessellhoeft CW Jr, Newman W, Blades B. Thoracotomy on the patient with previous malignancy: metastases or new primary? *J Thorac Cardiovasc Surg* 1968;56:351.

33. Cahan WG, Castro EB, Hajdu SI. The significance of a solitary lung shadow in patients with colon carcinoma. *Cancer* 1974;33:414–421.

20
Surgery for Bronchoalveolar Lung Cancer

Subrato J. Deb and Claude Deschamps

20.1. Definition of Bronchoalveolar Carcinoma

Bronchoalveolar carcinoma (BAC) is a distinct subtype of non-small cell lung adenocarcinoma classified by the World Health Organization (WHO) as a peripheral well-differentiated neoplasm demonstrating lepidic spread along preexisting alveolar structures.[1-4] An important histological feature is the preservation of the underlying lung architecture and the absence of invasion into stroma, pleura, or lymphatics of all pure BACs.[1-4] Lung adenocarcinomas with a BAC component are now more appropriately classified as adenocarcinomas, mixed subtype.[1] Despite the WHO designation as a subtype of adenocarcinoma, BAC has pathological, radiologic, and clinical features that are distinct from those of adenocarcinomas.

Bronchoalveolar carcinomas are rare and account for 3% to 9% of all newly diagnosed lung cancers.[1-7] Recent data suggest an increase in the occurrence of pure BAC in conjunction with lung adenocarcinoma.[3-7] Solitary peripheral BACs have an excellent prognosis, however, a consensus definition of a minimally invasive BAC with a favorable prognosis has not been achieved.[1]

20.1.1. Clinical Features of Bronchoalveolar Carcinoma

The prevalence of BAC is higher in women than other types of non-small cell lung cancer (NSCLC), comprising one third to one half of all cases reported.[6,7] Another distinct feature of BAC is the higher proportion of nonsmokers in comparison to the more common NSCLC.[6,7] Only 25% to 30% of patients with BAC have a history of heavy smoking.[6] On the basis of histological findings, BACs are divided into three subtypes: mucinous, nonmucinous, and a mixed form. Nonmucinous BAC is composed primarily of Clara cells or type 2 pneumocytes and accounts for 65% to 75% of all BAC. Mucinous BACs are differentiated toward bronchiolar goblet cells, and on gross examination these tumors have a glistening appearance. Mucin production can lead to bronchorrhea, characterized by the expectoration of water or mucoid material and is a late manifestation of advanced BAC. Three major patterns of BAC are visualized on high-resolution computerized tomography (HRCT).[5,6,8] The most common, accounting for almost half of all cases, is a solitary nodule or mass. These nodules are often ill defined and often lack a solid component, the latter being more typical of invasive adenocarcinoma. Pseudocavitation, heterogeneous attenuation, pleural tags, and spiculation may be associated findings.[6] The second most common pattern (30%) is consolidation one or more segments or lobes resembling pneumonia or air space disease. These tumors often produce mucin, which accounts for the heterogeneous attenuation on CT and has been associated with a worse outcome. Lastly, BAC can manifest radiographically as multifocal disease.[6] This multinodular form resembles that of metastatic disease or miliary tuberculosis. The nodules are often distributed in a centrilobular fashion and can range in size from 1mm to 3cm in diameter.[8] Computed tomography appearances are diverse and include well-defined or poorly defined nodules involving one or both lungs. It is uncertain whether multi-focal BAC is the result of synchronous primary lung cancers or aerogenous metastases.

Positron emission tomography (PET) has been utilized to evaluate patients with BAC. In a number of F-18 fluorodeoxyglucose positron tomography (FDG-PET) studies, BAC has been reported to have lower FDG uptake compared with other primary lung cancers.[9,10] The reason for the low uptake by BAC is unknown, but may be caused by poor cellularity or slow cell prolif-eration of the tumor. The utility of FDG-PET scan may be to identify mulitfocal BAC.[10]

20.1.1.1. Ground-Glass Opacification

Ground-glass opacity (GGO) is a finding on HRCT images that is described as a hazy, increased attenuation of the lung tissue with preservation of the bronchial and vascular margins. This non-specific finding may be noted in many types of pulmonary disease, including atypical adenoma-tous hyperplasia (AAH), defined by the WHO as a premalignant lesion.[11-13] Focal areas of ground-glass attenuation may also be an early sign of localized BAC and is considered a marker for the identification of minimally invasive BAC.[11,12] Nakajima studied 20 consecutive resected local-ized GGO for histopathological correlation.[11] These authors identified BAC in 50%, AAH in 25%, fibrosis in 15%, and invasive adenocarci-noma in 10%. Whether GGOs should be resected or followed is controversial, as the natural history of these lesions is not clearly defined. When radiographic progression of GGO on HRCT is demonstrated, as evidenced by increasing size or the appearance of a solid component or increased density, AAH or BAC is commonly identified and surgical intervention is justified.[13]

20.2. Surgical Treatment of Bronchoalveolar Carcioma

20.2.1. Available Published Data

A computerized search from the National Center for Biotechnology Information (NCBI) at the U.S. National Library of Medicine was conducted. Articles published from 1990 to the present time focusing on the surgical treatment of BAC were selected. Additional key references cited in a recent treatise were also included in the search.[14] Manuscripts focusing on radiological, pathologi-cal, or biological aspects of BAC as well as case reports were excluded from analysis. Articles cited in retrieved publications and studying a large number of patients were reviewed.

There is no meta-analysis, randomized, con-trolled trial, or systematic reviews of randomized, controlled trials in the literature encompassing the above specifications. It is not possible to provide the highest level of evidence; as such, our conclusions are based upon limited scientific foundation. For the purposes of this writing, we selected well-conducted prospective and retro-spective case control or cohort studies and case series addressing the defined criteria. Prior to the WHO classification, publications reviewing BAC applied widely varying histological criteria that has contributed to the lack of randomized data in the literature.

20.2.2. Review of Published Surgical Data for Bronchoalveolar Carcinoma

20.2.2.1. Traditional Resection of Bronchoalveolar Carcinoma

Surgery remains the cornerstone of therapy for BAC as with other forms of early-stage NSCLC. Patients with resected BAC generally have a better survival and lower recurrence rate than their NSCLC counterparts. The isolation of significant prognostic factors for BAC has been hampered by the relative rarity of pure BAC, the intermingling of BAC with adenocarcinomas in the literature, the evolution in the pathological criteria, and the variability of treatment.[3]

The Lung Cancer Study Group (LCSG) reviewed their experience with BAC between 1977 and 1988.[15] Of 1618 total patients, 235 patients with pure BAC were evaluated, representing the largest reported series of surgically resected BAC to date. Strict criteria were used to qualify patients for the study, including the demonstration of lepidic growth and the preservation of pulmonary archi-tecture. All patients underwent thoracotomy with surgical resection and lymph node staging. Of the 235 patients, 158 (67%) were T1 and 85% were N0. This study noted a higher incidence of female involvement and more nonsmokers among its cohort. The authors found that resected BAC patients were earlier stage than patients with non-BAC adenocarcinomas and squamous cell carcinoma (85% were stage I). The long-term mortality rate for stage IA BAC was reported at 7% per year, increasing to 12% per year for IB and 40% per year for stage II and III. Higher stage BAC (2 and 3) has a higher mortality rate than other types of lung cancer. The authors concluded that early resection is particularly important in patients with BAC.

Daly reviewed 134 patients with BAC who underwent surgical resection and analyzed factors that influenced survival.[16] Most of the lesions (58%) were solitary pulmonary masses, 11% were solitary pulmonary nodules, and 10% of the patients had multiple lesions. Lung carcinomas were accepted as BAC if the tumor demonstrated growth along lung architecture without evidence of invasion. Anatomical lung resections were performed in 115 patients and 19 underwent wedge excision, with 70% undergoing lobectomy. Complete mediastinal and pulmonary lymph node sampling was performed in all patients. The authors found only a 7.5% rate of lymph node metastasis, most were N2 nodal disease. Similar to the LCSG study, most patients were early stage I. The operative mortality was 1.5%. At a median follow-up of 8 years, 37.5% developed recurrent disease, primarily within the thorax. Despite early stage at resection, the authors noted 28 recurrences (62%) were among patients with stage IA and IB disease (10 T1 and 18 T2). Overall estimated 5- and 10-year survival for patients undergoing curative resection (122 patients) was 60.8% and 28.1%, respectively; 5-year survival for patients with T1N0 tumors was 90.5% compared to 55.4% for patients with T2N0 tumors. This difference was significant. Five-year survival for multicentric disease was 35.9% for unilateral and 0% for bilateral disease. It can be concluded from this study that the survival is more influenced by the extent of lung involvement (T stage) than by lymphatic metastases and that unilateral multifocal disease can be considered for resection; however, bilateral disease should not be operated upon. Additionally, these authors found that complete resection offered a significant survival advantage compared to incomplete resection and that the extent of pulmonary resection did not influence survival.

Dumont reviewed retrospectively reviewed 105 patients who underwent surgical treatment for BAC over a 19-year period.[17] Most patients presented with a solitary pulmonary nodule (85%). Surgical treatment consisted of lobectomy in 87%, bilobectomy in 3%, pneumonectomy in 7%, and 3% underwent wedge excision. All patients underwent complete mediastinal lymph node sampling. Again, the majority of patients (73%) were stage I; however, in contrast to the Daly study, there was a higher incidence of nodal disease with 28 patients (29%) having either N1 or N2 metastasis. Overall survival at 5 and 10 years was 48% and 39%, respectively, with 65% 5-year survival for stage I. Unlike Daly's study, these authors noted no statistically significant difference in survival between T1 and T2; however, there was a significant difference between N0 and N1 and between N0 and N2 metastasis. In addition, these authors found no difference between the mucinous and mucinous forms of BAC, unlike previous reports.

Another retrospective review by Regnard evaluated prognostic factors among 70 patients who underwent surgical treatment for BAC.[18] Four patients were unresectable. Of the remaining 66 remaining patients, 51 underwent lobectomy, 4 had bilobectomy, and 11 underwent pneumonectomy. There is no mention as to the extent of lymph node sampling or dissection in this paper. Similarly to previous studies, most patients were stage I (50%). This study had a large percentage of advanced cancers with 25 patients having stage III tumors. There were seven patients with diffuse disease and not staged according to TNM. The overall 5-year survival was 30%. These authors noted that tumors with nodular morphology had a better survival of 39% compared to those with pneumonic or diffuse types. In addition, those patients who were completely resected had a 5-year survival of 34% compared to 0% 5-year survival in those who were incompletely resected. Multivariate analysis confirmed the association of early TNM stage and complete resection with a favorable outcome. Of 61 patients who were completely resected, 59% developed tumor recurrence, primarily within the thorax, at a mean time period of 21 months, with most recurrence among patients with infiltrative tumors in comparison to the nodular type. Recurrence based on TNM was not determined.

Ebright reviewed 100 surgically treated patients with adenocarcinomas with various degrees of BAC features. These authors evaluated histological features that predicted surgical outcome. They classified tumors as pure BAC, BAC with focal invasion, and adenocarcinoma with BAC features.[19] This is a pathological review and the extent of surgical resection is not stated. Of the 100 patients, 47 were classified as pure BAC, 21 as BAC with focal invasion, and 32 as adenocarcinoma with BAC features. These authors confirmed the findings of Daly, that nodal metastasis was infrequent, with 2 of 47 patients with pure BAC. At a median follow-up of 86 months, the median disease free interval was 80 months without significant differences among the three groups. However, those patients exhibiting a pneumonic pattern on radiography had the shortest interval to recurrence at 19 months. Survival analysis also identified the pneumonic subtype to have the shortest survival compared to unifocal and multifocal patterns. Multivariate analysis only identified stage (I/II vs. III/IV) to have a significant impact on disease-free and overall survival. Of the 47 patients with pure BAC, 9 patients had a new cancer develop and 12 had recurrent disease. Table 20.1 summarizes some of the important findings of the above studies. From the above-mentioned studies, we can conclude that a complete resection is essential to obtaining acceptable long-term results and there appears to be a significant incidence of recurrent disease, with most recurrences occurring within the thorax, unlike other NSCLC. Lymph node sampling or dissection should be undertaken to accu-rately stage the patient, although the incidence of nodal metastasis is unclear. The pattern of radiographic appearance may be useful in determination of prognosis, as the infiltrative pneumonic form is more malignant than a solitary nodule.

20.2.3. Is Pure Bronchoalveolar Carcinoma a Candidate for Limited Resection

Several studies performed retrospective analysis of BAC, specifically examining pathological databases in a retrospective manner to compare the outcome of pure BAC and invasive adenocarcinomas of similar stage. The results uniformly reveal that pure BAC has a lower incidence of lymph node spread and better outcome in comparison to same-stage adenocarcinomas. In contrast to the historical experience noted above, it may be possible to perform lesser resection for minimally invasive pure BAC.

In the largest such study, Breathnach reviewed stage I BAC and stage I adenocarcinoma other than BAC in 138 patients.[20] There were 105 patients with adenocarcinoma and 33 patients with BAC. The pathological diagnoses of specimens were consistent with the recent WHO classification. Nineteen patients (58%) with BAC and 69% of patients with adenocarcinoma had undergone lobectomy. Additional 39% among the BAC group had limited resections and 17% in the adenocarcinoma group had wedge resections. The median follow-up for the BAC group was 6.2 years and for the adenocarcinoma group was 5.9 years. Recurrence was similar in both groups being 36% of patients with BAC and 37% among the adenocarcinoma patients. There was no significant difference in disease-free survival (DFS) in patients with BAC resected by lobectomy versus limited resection, although there was a trend toward longer DFS in patients who under-

TABLE 20.1. Comparison of published surgical series in the treatment of BAC.

Study	Year	Patients	LN Mets (%)	Recurrence rate (%)	Survival 5 year	10 years
LCSG[15]	1989	235	15	7%/year	Na	na
Daly[16]	1991	134	8	38	61	28
Dumont[17]	1998	97	29	na	48	39
Regnards[18]	1998	42	na	59	30	na
Ebright[19]	2002	100	4	45	Na	na

Abbreviations: LCSG, Lung Cancer Study Group; LN Mets, lymph node metastasis; na, not applicable.

went lobectomy (83% vs. 66%). In contrast, patients with adenocarcinoma who underwent lobectomy had a significantly longer DFS than those patients treated with limited resection (76% vs. 31%). Patients with BAC lived longer with a 5-year survival of 83% compared to adenocarcinoma with a survival of 63%. There was no significant difference in survival among BAC patients treated with lobectomy or limited resection and interestingly between patients with T1 or T2 lesions.

Two other smaller studies have examined pathological data and retrospectively compared BAC and invasive adenocarcinoma. Rena compared 28 patients with stage I peripheral nodular BAC and 80 patients with stage I peripheral adenocarcinoma.[21] Both 5-year disease-free and long-term survival were significantly higher in patients with BAC (81 vs. 51% and 86 vs. 71%, respectively). In the other study, Sakurai investigated 25 patients with BAC with 83 patients with other adenocarcinoma.[22] These authors found lymph node involvement in 36% of adenocarcinoma patients but none for any BAC lesions. At a median duration of follow-up of 5.1 years, the DFS was 100% for BAC compared to 64% for other adenocarcinomas. These studies in addition to the study by Breathnach suggest that the biological behavior of early-stage pure BAC is distinctly different than similar stage adenocarcinomas and probably NSCLC in general. The traditional approaches to NSCLC may not necessarily apply to the minimally invasive tumors.

20.2.4. Limited Resections for Bronchoalveolar Carcinoma

The LCSG published a randomized, prospective trial comparing limited resection (segmentectomy or wedge resection) with lobectomy for T1N0 NSCLC. This study clearly demonstrated the inferior results of limited resection when compared to lobectomy in survival and loco-regional recurrence.[23] More recently, Miller published the results of surgical resection for NSCLC 1 cm or less in diameter.[24] These authors identified a 7% incidence of lymph nodal spread and at 43 months median follow-up, 18% of patients developed recurrent disease. These authors note that patients who underwent lobectomy had a significantly better survival and less recurrence than patients who underwent lesser resections. Despite these results, based on the favorable behavior of pure BAC, several authors have recently published the surgical results of lesser resections for localized BAC. These results of four surgical series described below are tabulated in Table 20.2.

In a prospective review of limited resection for small peripheral BAC, the authors studied 42 patients with tumors 2 cm or less. Of these patients, 34 underwent wedge resection.[25] The authors converted to lobectomy if invasive features were identified at surgery. At 30-month follow-up, all patients who underwent lesser resection are alive and without recurrence. In another study by Watanabe, 17 patients with pure ground-glass attenuation on HRCT underwent limited pulmonary resection.[26] Fourteen underwent wedge excision and 3 underwent segmentectomy. No nodal dissection was performed. At 32-month-follow up, no death or cancer recurrence is noted. These authors recommend wedge resection with video-assisted thoracoscopic surgery (VATS) as a minimally invasive curative surgery of this type of cancer. In another prospective analysis, Nakata examined 33 patients with pure GGO lesion that were 1 cm or less.[27] Thoracoscopic wedge resection was completed in these 33 patients with the findings of BAC in 23,

TABLE 20.2. Results of limited resection.

Study	Year	Patients	Criteria for resection	Follow-up (months)	Recurrence (%)	Death (%)
Yamato[25]	2001	42	BAC <20 mm	30	0	0
Watanabe[26]	2002	17	Pure GGA	32	0	0
Nakata[27]	2003	33	Pure GGO <1 cm	18	0	0
Yamada[28]	2004	28	Pure GGO <2 cm	29	0	0

Abbreviations: BAC, bronchoalveolar carcinoma; GGA, ground-glass attenuation; GGO, ground glass opacity.

AAH in 9, and adenocarcinoma in 1. At median follow-up of 18 months, there has been no evidence of tumor recurrence or postoperative death. These authors recommend lobectomy and mediastinal dissection for mixed GGO (those revealing heterogeneous attenuation with a solid component) and pure GGO larger than 1 cm because of the higher incidence of invasive adenocarcinoma among these lesions. Yamada evaluated 39 patients who demonstrated pure GGO less than or equal to 2 cm on HRCT.[28] Twenty-eight patients underwent wedge excision and 11 underwent segmentectomy or lobectomy, 9 patients had multiple lesions. The authors divided the final pathology based on the extend of fibroblastic proliferation and utilized Naguchi's classification for small adenocarcinomas to stratify their results. Of the 39 patients, 29 patients had localized BAC without active proliferation (Noguchi A or B). At a mean follow-up of 29 months, no death or recurrence was noted among the localized BAC patients. The above studies support the notion that limited resections can be performed pure BAC, however, direct comparison with formal anatomical resection has not been made in a prospective manner.

20.2.5. Limited Resection Versus Traditional Resection

Three retrospective studies have compared limited resection by wedge excision to anatomical resection by lobectomy or segmentectomy. The major limitation of all three studies are the small number of patients undergoing limited resections and the last study described below failed to reach a statistical difference.

In the evaluation by Okubo, the authors studied 119 patients with BAC. Among this group, 58 patients had lesions larger than 3 cm and 14 patients had multiple lesions.[29] The median follow-up was 7 years; these authors noted an overall survival of 69% at 5 years and 57% at 10 years among the 107 patients who underwent resection. The authors identified wedge resection and nodal involvement as having a negative impact on survival. Although this is a large study of patients, it should be noted that the study group included only 17 patients with pure BAC, with the remainder of patients having adenocar-

cinoma and various percentages of BAC. In another retrospective analysis, Liu reviewed 153 patients with BAC, of which 93 underwent surgical resection.[30] Most patients presented with a solitary pulmonary nodule (85%). Eighty patients underwent either lobectomy or bilobectomy and 7 were treated with pneumonectomy. Only 7 patients underwent wedge excision, for reasons not clearly defined. Most patients (66%) were stage I. Patients who underwent lobectomy or bilobectomy noted a higher survival although the wedge group was very small. Nodal involvement was noted to have a significant negative impact on survival. Lastly, Furak analyzed 67 patients with BAC in a retrospective analysis.[31] Among the 55 patients without multifocal disease, surgical procedures included anatomical resection in 49 patients and only 6 patients underwent wedge excision. Histological analysis conformed to current WHO guidelines. Almost 30% of patients had lymph node metastasis and the overall 5-year survival was 62%. When comparison between wedge resection was made against lobectomy and pneumonectomy, the 5-year survival favored anatomical resection (60% vs. 37%) but did not reach statistical significance.

20.2.6. Defining Criteria for Limited Resection

As evident in the previous reviewed studies, the criteria applied to select patients for limited resection are unclear, with some parameters influenced by subjective bias. To better define objective criteria, several authors have focused on HRCT findings that may better predict those patients who should undergo limited resection.[32-37] The specific criteria found in these studies are summarized in Table 20.3.

20.2.7. Multifocal and Advanced Bronchoalveolar Carcinoma

Mulitfocal disease has been shown to have favorable outcomes in several published series evaluating BAC.[16,17,19] In addition, investigators have reported the efficacy of resecting multiple synchronous or metachronous NSCLC.[38-40] Daly found a survival around 36% at 5-year survival for unilateral multicentric disease but no survi-

TABLE 20.3. Preoperative predictors of favorable outcome to limited resection.

Study	Year	Total patients analyzed	Predictor for favorable outcome
Nakamura	2004	100	Pure GGO <2 cm
Nakata[37]	2005	146	GGO opacity ration >90%
Higashiyama[36]	1999	206	BAC component of peropheral Ad Ca >50%
Suzuki[35]	2002	1540	Pure GGO component
Namori[34]	2003	100	Single peak at low CT number on histogram
Kodama[33]	2001	104	BAC with GGO area >50%
Matsuguma[32]	2004	90	GGO area >50%

Abbreviations: Ad Ca, adenocarcinoma; BAC, bronchoalveolar carcinoma; CT, computed tomography; GGO, ground glass opacity.

vors with bilateral multicentric disease.[16] Donker evaluated the impact of surgery and chemotherapy in patients with advanced BAC.[41] These authors' evaluated 126 patients, and 51 patients (41%) had advanced disease (stages IIIb and IV). Surgery was associated with prolonged survival in patients with mulitfocal disease in comparison to supportive care. The median survival reported was better among patients with multifocal lesions confined to a single lobe than multiple lobes. Interestingly, those patients who underwent surgery plus chemotherapy did not demonstrate a survival advantage to those who underwent surgery alone. One significant limitation to this retrospective analysis is that the pathology specimens were not re-reviewed to confirm the diagnosis of BAC. In another analysis, Roberts evaluated 73 patients with BAC, of whom 14 patients had multifocal disease without evidence of lymph node metastasis.[42] These authors note an overall 5-year survival after resection of multifocal BAC at 64%; in contrast to the previous study, these authors found no difference is survival between unilateral and bilateral distribution.

With more diffuse and bilateral disease, the survival is dismal and often less than 1 year. The tendency of BAC to metastasize locally within the thorax has prompted evaluation of radical local therapy. Patients with the mucinous variety of BAC can experience severe disabling bronchorrhea or refractory hypoxia, decreasing the quality of life. Zorn and others have reported successful single- and double-lung transplant for patients with advanced BAC.[43,44] Although symptom relief was impressive, the recurrence rate of the original tumor is high. The indication for lung transplantation in this situation remains controversial. Others have reported successful palliative pneumonectomy in select patients with unequal distribution of disease.[45] The efficacy of this procedure remains to be proven.

20.2.8. Molecular Targeting Therapy for Advanced Bronchoalveolar Carcinoma

The epidermal growth factor receptor (EGRF) has recently emerged as a leading target for the treatment of NSCLC. The EGRF tyrosine kinase inhibitors, gefitinib and erlotinib, have been found to be effective in some patients with in advanced BAC.[46–48] Interestingly, the greatest response rates have been reported in women and never smokers.

20.3. Summary of Surgical Data

Prior to 1999, the WHO classification of BAC surgical series included pure BAC as well as adenocarcinoma with various degrees of BAC. This conglomeration may have contributed to the discrepancies in outcome and the overall poor outcome of resected BAC. There is no randomized level 1 data to draw definite conclusions. The following is a synopsis of the major findings and conclusions.

1. Bronchoalveolar carcinoma is curable with appropriate surgical therapy; incomplete resection results in dismal prognosis.
2. The incidence and value of lymph node dissection is not clearly defined.
3. The prognosis of BAC is dependent on its presenting CT appearance.
4. Stage I pure BAC biologically behaves in a more favorable manner than similar stage invasive adenocarcinomas and may be a candidate for lesser resections. Level of evidence is 2+ and recommendation grade is B.
5. Patients with pure BAC, presenting as GGO less than 1cm, may be candidates for limited resection with excellent early results. These patients will have to be identified prior to surgery based on specific HRCT characteristics. Level of evidence is 2++ and recommendation grade is B.

> Stage I pure BAC biologically behaves in a more favorable manner than similar stage invasive adenocarcinomas and may be a candidate for lesser resections (level of evidence 2+; recommendation grade B).
>
> Patients with pure BAC presenting as GGO less than 1 cm may be candidates for limited resection (level of evidence 2++; recommendation grade B).
>
> All other patients with BAC should undergo standard anatomical lung resection based on pulmonary function capacity (level of evidence 1+; recommendation grade A).

6. All other patients with BAC should undergo standard anatomical lung resection based on pulmonary function capacity. This is supported by randomized data. Level of evidence is 1+ and recommendation grade is A.

7. Patients with ipsilateral or bilateral multifocal disease may be candidates for aggressive surgical resection if complete resection can be accomplished.

8. There may be a role for palliative surgical intervention with pneumonectomy or lung transplantation in select patients for symptom control. This is controversial.

9. Patients with unresectable advanced disease should be enrolled into appropriate clinical trials. EGFR tyrosine kinase inhibitors hold future promise.

20.4. Opinion of the Authors

It is our opinion that until longer follow-up and randomized, prospective data is available, the standard therapy for patients presenting with early-stage BAC should be complete anatomical resection and complete mediastinal lymph node dissection. Patients with GGO that are observed to change after a period of 3 to 6 months should undergo resection. If adenocarcinoma is identified on intraoperative frozen section analysis, complete surgical resection should be performed. As we have shown previously,[24] even cancers less than 1 cm can result in recurrence and systemic metastasis. We reserve limited resection only for

those patients with compromised lung function who would not tolerate a formal lung resection. Thorascopic techniques can be applied successfully in the management of early-stage lung cancer without compromising the oncologic principles and should be tailored to each individual surgeon's comfort level.

Patients with multifocal disease, either unilateral or bilateral, are candidates for parenchymal-sparing lung resection. The benefit of lobectomy in these patients is not supported and in our practice, multiple wedge resections and mediastinal lymph node dissection is performed. Palliative pneumonectomy should be performed for patients with severe incapacitating bronchorrhea or refractory hypoxia.

Future studies will need to evaluate in a randomized prospective analysis, if patients with pure BAC presenting as GGO should undergo limited resection or traditional surgery. With the survival benefit demonstrated for early-stage lung cancer treated with postoperative adjuvant therapy, further studies need to be done using EGFR inhibitors in this application specifically in patients with BAC.

References

1. Travis WD, Garg K, Franklin WA, et al. Evolving concepts I the pathology and computed tomography imaging of lung adenocarcinoma and bronchioalveolar carcinoma. *J Clin Oncol* 2005;23: 3279–3287.
2. Jackman DM, Chirieac LR, Janne PA. Bronchioalveolar carcinoma: a review of the epidemiology, pathology and treatment. *Semin Respir Crit Care Med* 2005;26:342–352.
3. Laskin JJ. Bronchoalveolar carcinoma: current treatment and future trends. *Clin Lung Cancer* 2004;S75–S79.
4. Read WL, Page NC, Tierney RM, et al. The epidemiology of bronchioalveolar carcinoma over the past two decades: analysis of the SEER database. *Lung Cancer* 2004;45:137–142.
5. Sabloff BS, Truong MT, Wistuba II, et al. Bronchioalveolar cell carcinoma: radiologic appearance and dilemmas in the assessment of response. *Clin Lung Cancer* 2004;6:108–112.
6. Lee KS, Kim Y, Han J, et al. Bronchioloalveolar carcinoma: clinical, histopathologic, and radiologic findings. *Radiographics* 1997;17:1345–1357.

7. Patel JD. Role of epidermal growth factor receptor tyrosine kinase inhibitors in the treatment of bronchoalveolar carcinoma. *Clin Lung Cancer* 2004;6:S43–S47.

8. Akira M, Atagi S, Kawahara M, et al. High-resolution CT findings of diffuse bronchoalveolar carcinoma in 38 patients. *AJR Am J Roentgenol* 1999;173:1623–1629.

9. Yap CS, Schiepers C, Fishbeln MC, et al. FDG-PET imaging in lung cancer: how sensitive is it for bronchoalveolar carcinoma? *Eur J Nucl Med* 2002;29:1166–1173.

10. Heyneman LE, Patz EF. PET imaging in patients with bronchioalveolar cell carcinoma. *Lung Cancer* 2002;38:261–266.

11. Nakajima R, Yokose T, Kakinuma R, et al. Localized pure ground-glass opacity on high-resolution CT: histologic characteristics. *J Comput Assisted Tomogr* 2002;26:323–329.

12. Jang HJ, Lee KS, Kwon OJ, et al. Bronchioalveolar carcinoma: focal area of ground glass attenuation at thin-section CT as an early sign. *Radiology* 1996;199:485–488.

13. Kakinuma R, Oshmatsu H, Kaneko M, et al. Progression of focal pure ground-glass opacity detected by low dose helical computed tomography screening for lung cancer. *J Comput Assist Tomogr* 2004;28:17–23.

14. Altorki NK. Bronchioalveolar carcinoma and ground glass opacities. *Ann Thorac Surg* 2005;80:1560–1561.

15. Grover FL, Piantadosi S, and The Lung Cancer Study Group. Recurrence and survival following resection of bronchioalveolar carcinoma of the lung. The Lung Cancer Study Group experience. *Ann Surg* 1989;206:779–790.

16. Daly RC, Trastek VF, Pairolero PC, et al. Bronchoalveolar carcinoma: factors affecting survival. *Ann Thorac Surg* 1991;51:368–377.

17. Dumont P, Gasser B, Roughe C, et al. Bronchoalveolar carcinoma. Histopathologic study of evolution in a series of 105 surgically treated patients. *Chest* 1998;113:391–395.

18. Regnards JF, Santelmo N, Romdhani N, et al. Bronchioalveolar lung carcinoma. Results of lsurgical treatment and prognostic factors. *Chest* 1998;114:45–50.

19. Ebright MI, Zakowski MF, Martin J, et al. Clinical pattern and pathologic stage but not histologic features predict outcome for bronchoalveolar carcinoma. *Ann Thorac Surg* 2002;74:1640–1647.

20. Breathnach OS, Kwiatkowski DJ, Finkelstein DM, et al. Bronchioloalveolar carcinoma of the lung: recurrences and survival in patients with stage I disease. *J Thorac Cardiovasc Surg* 2001;121:42–47.

21. Rena O, Papilia E, Ruffini E, et al. Stage I pure bronchioloalveolar carcinoma: recurrences, survival and comparison with adenocarcinoma of the lung. *Eur J Cardiothorac Surg* 2003;23:409–414.

22. Sakurai H, Dobashi Y, Mizutani E, et al. Bronchioloalveolar carcinoma of the lung 3 centimeters or less in diameter: a prognostic assessment. *Ann Thorac Surg* 2004;78:1728–1733.

23. Ginsberg R, Rubinstein L. Randomized trial of lobectomy versus limited resection for T1 N0 non-small cell lung cancer. Lung Cancer Study Group. *Ann Thorac Surg* 1995;60:615–622.

24. Miller DL, Rowland CM, Deschamps C, et al. Surgical treatment of non-small cell lung cancer 1 cm or less in diameter. *Ann Thorac Surg* 2002;73:1545–1550.

25. Yamato Y, Tsuchida M, Watanabe T, et al. Early results of a prospective study of limited resection for bronchoalveolar adenocarcinoma of the lung. *Ann Thorac Surg* 2001;71:971–974.

26. Watanabe S, Watanabe T, Arai K, et al. Results of wedge resection for focal bronchioloalveolar carcinoma showing pure ground-glass attenuation on computed tomography. *Ann Thorac Surg* 2002;73:1071–1075.

27. Nakata M, Sawada S, Saeki H, et al. Prospective study of thorascopic limited resection for ground-glass opacity selected by computed tomography. *Ann Thorac Surg* 2003;75:1601–1606.

28. Yamada S, Kohno T. Video-assisted thoracic surgery for pure ground-glass opacities 2 cm or less in diameter. *Ann Thorac Surg* 2004;77:1911–1915.

29. Okubo K, Mark EJ, Flieder D, et al. Bronchoalveolar carcinoma: clinical, radiologic, and pathologic factors and survival. *J Thorac Cardiovasc Surg* 1999;118:702–709.

30. Liu YY, Chen YM, Huang MH, et al. Prognosis and recurrent patterns in bronchioloalveolar carcinoma. *Chest* 2000;118:940–947.

31. Furak J, Trojan I, Szoke T, et al. Bronchioloalveolar lung cancer: occurrence, surgical treatment and survival. *Eur J Cardiothorac Surg* 2003;23:818–823.

32. Matsuguma H, Nakahara R, Anraku M, et al. Objective definition and measurement method of ground-glass opacity for planning limited resection in patients with clinical stage IA adenocarcinoma of the lung. *Eur J Cardiothorac Surg* 2004;25:1102–1106.

33. Kodama K, Higashiyama M, Yokouchi H, et al. Prognostic valve of ground-glass opacity found in

small lung adenocarcinoma on high-resolution CT scanning. *Lung Cancer* 2001;33:17–25.

34. Namori H, Ohtsuka T, Naruke T, et al. Histogram analysis of computed tomography numbers of clinical T1 N0 M0 lung adenocarcinoma with special reference to lymph node metastasis and tumor invasiveness. *J Thorac Cardiovasc Surg* 2003;126:1584–1589.

35. Suzuki K, Asamua H, Kusumoto M, et al. Early peripheral lung cancer: prognostic significance of ground glass opacity on thin-section computed tomographic scan. *Ann Thorac Surg* 2002;74:1635–1639.

36. Higashiyama M, Kodama K, Yokouchi H, et al. Prognostic value of bronchiolo-alveolar carcinoma component of small lung adenocarcinoma. *Ann Thorac Surg* 1999;68:2069–2073.

37. Nakata M, Sawada S, Yamashita M, et al. Objective radiologic analysis of ground-glass opacity aimed at curative limited resection for small peripheral non-small cell lung cancer. *J Thorac Cardiovasc Surg* 2005;129:1226–1231.

38. Nakata M, Sawada S, Yamashita M, et al. Surgical treatments for multiple primary adenocarcinoma of the lung. *Ann Thorac Surg* 2004;78:1194–1199.

39. Okada M, Tsubota N, Yoshimura M, et al. Operative approach for multiple primary lung carcinomas. *J Thorac Cardiovasc Surg* 1998;115:836–840.

40. Battafarano RJ, Meyers BF, Guthrie TJ, et al. Surgical resection of multifocal non-small cell lung cancer is associated with prolonged survival. *Ann Thorac Surg* 2002;74:988–994.

41. Donker R, Stewart DJ, Dharouge S, et al. Clinical characteristics and the impact of surgery and chemotherapy on survival of patients with advanced and metastatic bronchioloalveolar carcinoma: a retrospective study. *Clin Lung Cancer* 2000;1:211–215.

42. Roberts PF, Straznicka M, Lara PN, et al. Resection of multifocal non-small cell lung cancer when the bronchioloalveolar subtype is involved. *J Thorac Cardiovasc Surg* 2003;126:1597–1602.

43. Zorn GL, McGiffin DC, Young RK, et al. Pulmonary transplantation for advanced bronchioloalveolar carcinoma. *J Thorac Cardiovasc Surg* 2003;125:45–48.

44. Paloyan EB, Swinnen LJ, Montoya A, et al. Lung transplantation for advanced bronchioloalveolar carcinoma confined to the lungs. *Transplantation* 2000;69:2446–2448.

45. Barlesi F, Doddoli C, Thomas P, et al. Bilateral bronchioloalveolar lung carcinoma: is there a place for palliative pneumonectomy? *Eur J Cardiothorac Surg* 2001;20:1113–1116.

46. DeGrendele H, Belani CP, Perry MC. Epidermal growth factor inhibitors, gefitinib and erlotinib (Tarceva, OS1-774), in the treatment of bronchioloalveolar carcinoma. *Clin Lung Cancer* 2003; 83–85.

47. Miller VA, Kris MG, Shah N, et al. Bronchioloalveolar pathologic subtype and smoking history predict sensitivity to gefitinib in advanced non-small cell lung cancer. *J Clin Oncol* 2004;22:1103–1109.

48. Gandara DR, West H, Chansky K, et al. Bronchioloalveolar carcinoma: a model for investigating the biology of epidermal growth factor receptor inhibition. *Clin Cancer Res* 2004;10:4205–4209.

21
Lung Volume Reduction Surgery in the Candidate for Lung Transplantation

Christine L. Lau and Bryan F. Meyers

Emphysema is a progressive, unrelenting disease that results in a continued decline in pulmonary function. When pulmonary function testing documents a forced expiratory volume in 1s (FEV_1) of less than 30% predicted values, the 3-year mortality risk has been estimated at 40% to 50%.[1-4] Because of the increased mortality and the decreased quality of life seen with severe emphysema, multiple surgical treatments have been devised for patients with emphysema. The majority of these surgical interventions have been subsequently abandoned because of the lack of reproducible benefits and the false physiological principles upon which they were based. An excellent published review on the history of emphysema surgery has been provided by Deslauriers.[5] As surgeons and physicians gained a better understanding of the pathophysiology of emphysema, most of these procedures would be considered of historical interest with no current practical value. Today, two surgical options exist for patients with severe emphysema: lung volume reduction surgery (LVRS) and lung transplantation. In the properly identified recipient, both procedures provide an improvement in quality of life, exercise tolerance, and, possibly, survival. Combinations of LVRS and lung transplantation, either simultaneously or sequentially, may be considered under rare circumstances. This chapter will review the results achieved with lung transplantation and LVRS and then attempt to address the specific question: which of the two surgical strategies is best supported by the evidence as the initial approach for the candidate with dual eligibility? It is beyond the scope of this

chapter to review the specific evidence supporting lung transplantation or LVRS as a therapy for emphysema. While this work will presuppose eligibility for either procedure and address the evidence guiding selection of an initial operation, the tables supporting the text will reiterate commonly accepted exclusion criteria for either procedure.

21.1. Patient Selection for Lung Volume Reduction Surgery Versus Lung Transplantation

Lung transplantation and LVRS are invasive procedures with a risk of both morbidity and mortality to patients receiving such operations, thus both procedures are directed only at patients who remain symptomatic despite optimal medical treatment. Pulmonary rehabilitation programs have been shown to relieve subjective dyspnea, increase functional capabilities, and improve subjective quality of life. All patients considered for surgical treatment of emphysema should be enrolled in a supervised pulmonary rehabilitation program and their subsequent consideration for surgery should be based on their compliance and progress with rehabilitation. Because lung transplantation and LVRS carry an increased perioperative risk of morbidity and mortality, and because increased life expectancy has only been shown in a subset of patients undergoing LVRS, patients considering an operation must be willing to accept the possibility of a shortened life in exchange for an anticipated relief from dyspnea and an improvement in quality of life. Specific indications for lung transplantation or LVRS are mentioned with regard to each operation.

21.1.1. Transplantation for End-stage Emphysema

Pulmonary emphysema was once thought to be a contraindication for lung transplantation. During the era preceding bilateral transplantation, the perceived difficulties of ventilation and perfusion mismatching with the native and newly transplanted lung were thought to be too great an obstacle. After the initial success with single-lung transplantation for emphysema was reported[6] and after the development of techniques to allow safer bilateral lung transplantation,[7,8] the use of lung transplantation for patients with emphysema quickly increased. Emphysema quickly became the leading diagnosis cited as an indication for transplant, partly due to the prevalence of emphysema and partly due to the survival advantage that emphysema patients demonstrate while awaiting lungs after being listed for transplantation.

Emphysema and α1-antitrypsin deficiency have become the most common indications for pulmonary transplantation. These two indications together account for 61.2% of the adult single-lung transplants and 32.1% of the bilateral lung transplants reported in the 2005 Registry of the International Society for Heart and Lung Transplantation (ISHLT), as reported by Trulock and colleagues.[9] General criteria for transplantation in these patients have been reported by Trulock.[10] Most patients considered for transplant have deteriorated to a point at which oxygen supplementation is required. In experience described by Trulock, the mean supplemental oxygen requirement at the time of transplantation was slightly in excess of 4L/min. The obstructive physiology in these patients resulted in a FEV_1 of well under 1L, or approximately 16% of predicted normal values for the average patient. This particular patient group usually has a stable course with excellent survival on the waiting list while awaiting pulmonary transplantation. Progressive elevation in PCO_2 has been observed in some patients, however, with several of these individuals undergoing transplantation with the

PCO_2 in excess of 100mmHg. The current criteria used at Washington University for evaluating potential lung transplant candidates are recorded in Table 21.1.

The advantages of lung transplantation are obvious: complete replacement of the diseased and nonfunctional lung with a new and healthy donor lung. Initial and long-term function of patients with single- or bilateral lung transplants for emphysema show a dramatic improvement in pulmonary function and exercise tolerance with elimination of the need for supplementary oxygen. The experience at Washington University is recorded in Table 21.2, showing survival of 88% at 1 year and 59% at 5 years after transplant for emphysema. Together, patients with emphysema and α1-antitrypsin deficiency emphysema comprise 55% of those undergoing transplantation over the past 16 years and the results in this subset are superior to those observed in the overall cohort of transplant recipients.

The disadvantages of lung transplant are well known but worth reviewing. First, the lack of

TABLE 21.1. Indications and contraindications for lung volume reduction surgery and lung transplantation.

Indications common to both procedures
  Emphysema with destruction and hyperinflation
  Marked impairment (FEV_1 <35% predicted)
  Marked restriction in activities of daily living
  Failure of maximal medical treatment to correct symptoms
Contraindications to both procedures
  Abnormal body weight (<70% or >130% of ideal)
  Co-existing major medical problems increasing surgical risk
  Inability or unwillingness to participate in pulmonary rehabilitation
  Unwillingness to accept the risk of morbidity and mortality of surgery
  Tobacco use within the last 6 months
  Recent or current diagnosis of malignancy
  Increasing age (>65 years for transplant, >70 years for volume reduction)
  Psychological instability, such as depression or anxiety disorder
Discriminating conditions favoring lung volume reduction surgery
  Marked thoracic distension
  Heterogeneous disease with obvious apical target areas
  FEV_1 >20% predicted
  Age between 60 and 70 years
Discriminating conditions favoring lung transplantation
  Diffuse disease without target areas
  FEV_1 <20% predicted
  Hypercarbia with $Paco_2$ >55 mm Hg
  Pulmonary hypertension
  Age less than 60 years
  α1-Antitrypsin deficiency

TABLE 21.2. Patient actuarial survival: Washington University Lung Transplant Program, 1988–2004.

Diagnosis	Number	Kaplan–Meier Survival		
		1 year	3 years	5 years
COPD	316	88%	76%	59%
ATDef	108	83%	73%	59%
All transplants	764	85%	73%	58%

Abbreviations: ATDef, α1-antitrypsin deficiency; COPD, chronic obstructive pulmonary disease.

available donor lungs has created a situation in which the waiting time for a transplant recipient in our program routinely exceeds 2 years. The changes in the lung allocation rules in May 2005 may make this waiting time even longer for emphysema patients as it has been devised to prioritize patients based on severity of disease rather than time on the list. There have not been reports on the disease-specific impact of the new allocation algorithm, but most suspect that patients with emphysema will suffer decreased donor lung availability. Once lungs become available, the initial morbidity and mortality of lung transplant is higher than that reported for lung volume reduction, with mortality variously described as 5% to 15% for the first 30 days and somewhat higher for the first year. For the survivors, the presence of allograft lungs creates the need for lifelong immunosuppression, which carries with it high medical costs to the individual and society and an increased risk of hypertension, renal dysfunction, hyperlipidemia, neoplasm, and infection when compared with nonimmunosuppressed patients. Finally, the risk of developing chronic allograft dysfunction, or bronchiolitis obliterans syndrome (BOS), increases with time since transplant and reaches 50% to 60% by 5 years after transplant. The cumulative 5-year survival of our lung transplant experience for emphysema is 58%, a fact that clearly demonstrates the imperfect solution that transplant offers to emphysema patients.

Early reports on the efficacy of lung transplant for pulmonary emphysema compared the merits and risks of bilateral (BLT) versus single (SLT) lung transplantation and demonstrated a higher perioperative risk for the bilateral operation without a demonstrable functional benefit to the

recipients.[11,12] For that reason and for the reason of better utilization of graft lungs, SLT quickly became the preferred operation for obstructive lung disease. More recent reports, however, have made BLT appear a better option for obstructive lung disease, although the comparisons are not randomized. The 2005 ISHLT registry data reports significantly improved survival of bilateral rather than single-lung procedures over 10 years after transplantation for chronic obstructive pulmonary disease (COPD; $p < 0.001$) and for α1-antitrypsin deficiency emphysema ($p = 0.007$).[9] Single center data from Washington University shows a 5-year survival of 65% for patients undergoing bilateral lung transplantation for emphysema compared to only 45% for those undergoing single-lung transplantation ($p <0.001$). The in-hospital mortality is not different between SLT (7.0%) and BLT (5.9%; $p = 0.79$). The freedom from BOS for patients transplanted for emphysema was 30.6% at 5 years for SLT compared to 53.0% of BLT ($p = 0.006$).[13] The Duke Lung Transplant group has also shown an increased rate of BOS in recipients undergoing SLT compared to those receiving BLT.[14] Table 21.2 shows the survival data for all patients with lung transplants performed by Washington University. As demonstrated, COPD and α1-antitrypsin deficiency emphysema affect more than half of the total recipients and have outcomes that meet or exceed the group of transplant recipients as a whole. The functional status of transplant recipients in our program was reviewed by Gaissert and colleagues.[15] Figure 21.1 shows the effect of BLT and SLT on the FEV_1, with both groups starting below 20% of predicted values and both enjoying a sustained benefit over the first 12 months of observation. Figure 21.2 shows the results of the measured 6-min walk for the same patients.

21.1.2. Lung Volume Reduction Surgery

The advantages of lung volume reduction for suitable candidates are numerous, including the relief of dyspnea and improvement of functional capabilities without the cost and adverse side effects of organ transplantation. There is no built-in waiting time as seen with transplantation; as soon as candidates can reach the

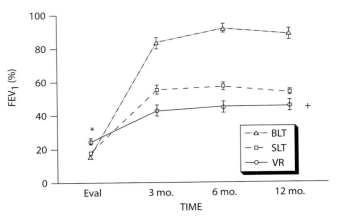

Figure 21.1. Percentage of predicted forced expiratory volume in 1s (FEV_1) before and after volume reduction (VR), single-lung transplantation (SLT), and bilateral lung transplantation (BLT). At evaluation (Eval): VR vs. SLT, $p < 0.05$; VR vs. BLT, $p < 0.001$. At 6 months: VR vs. SLT, $p < 0.001$; VR vs. BLT, $p < 0.001$. (From Gaissert et al.[15])

pulmonary rehabilitation exercise goals they are ready for the procedure. The early and late mortality for lung volume reduction are lower than those reported for transplantation. Without the concern for distribution of a scarce commodity such as donor lungs, lung volume reduction can be offered with slightly less rigid adherence to selection criteria. For example, a 72-year-old who is otherwise an acceptable volume reduction candidate would be considered for the procedure, whereas such a patient would likely not be added to a transplant waiting list. The drawback of volume reduction is that it is dependent on stringent anatomical and pathological characteristics in the patient's lungs. Early work has shown that the lack of specific target areas and, to a lesser extent, the absence of apical target areas in particular decrease the likelihood of a good result. Specific indications and contraindications for

lung volume reduction surgery are listed in Table 21.1. The refinements of the selection criteria that resulted from the National Emphysema Treatment Trial (NETT)[16] have made the overlap in indications for LVRS and transplant even smaller. Patients deemed at high risk for death after LVRS include those with an FEV_1 less than 20% predicted and either homogeneous emphysema or a diffusing capacity of carbon monoxide (DLCO) less than 20% predicted. The specific subgroup of FEV1 less than 20% and DLCO less than 20% with ideal heterogeneity of emphysematous obstruction was not specifically addressed by the NETT high-risk paper, but it is likely the risk in not greatly elevated over baseline risk faced by most patients.[17]

Multiple prospective observational studies as well as several randomized, controlled trials have shown the benefits of LVRS, including

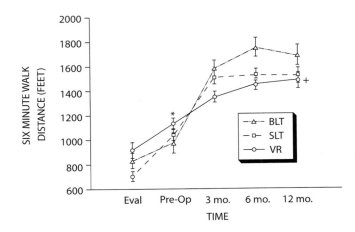

Figure 21.2. Comparison of 6-min walk distance before and after volume reduction (VR), single-lung transplantation (SLT), and bilateral lung transplantation (BLT). At evaluation: VR vs. SLT, not significant; VR vs. BLT, $p < 0.05$. At 6 months: VR vs. SLT, not significant; VR vs. BLT, $p < 0.001$. (From Gaissert et al.[15])

improvement in functional status and quality of life.[18-20] Most studies in the literature report a postoperative mortality of 3% to 8% for LVRS.[21] The remarkable finding is that these fairly uniform results have been obtained despite the use of a wide array of surgical strategies including bilateral and unilateral approaches, open and thoracoscopic operations, and buttressed or unbuttressed staple lines. The consistent theme among reports of successful lung volume reduction programs has been meticulous patient selection, methodical patient preparation with reduction of risk factors, and attentive postoperative care.

Even prior to the recent release of the NETT results, at least five randomized and controlled trials compared medical treatment to LVRS and showed improvements in physiological and functional parameters in the surgically treated arm. These studies were all designed to evaluate the short-term benefits.[22-26] The results of the NETT, a multi-institutional randomized trial comparing medical treatment to LVRS for select patients with emphysema, were released in 2003.[16] Although the trialists had originally planned to enroll 4700 patients, poor recruitment resulted in substantially fewer enrollees (1218 patients).[27]

Following an interim analysis of results,[28] 140 patients with high risk of death following surgery were excluded. After excluding this group, the 538 non–high-risk patients that were randomly assigned to surgery were more likely to have improvements in exercise capacity and quality of life compared to the 540 non–high-risk patients randomly assigned to medical therapy. For the entire group there was no reduction in mortality in the surgical group during an average 29 months of follow-up (risk ratio, 0.89; $p = 0.31$).[16] Exercise capacity was improved in the surgically treated group, with an improvement after 24 months in the surgical group of more than 10W in 16% of patients, as compared to 3% of patients in the medically treated group ($p < 0.001$).

Subgroup analysis of results revealed some interesting findings among distinct cohorts within the trial participants.[29] Four subgroups were defined according to the presence or absence of upper lobe predominant emphysema and the exercise capacity (low or high) at the time of baseline evaluation. The effect of LVRS surgery

on mortality varied among these four subgroups. An improvement in survival was seen for LVRS recipients in the subgroup of patients with predominantly upper-lobe emphysema and low baseline exercise tolerance. In this group the risk ratio of death in the LVRS-treated group compared to the medically treated group was 0.47 ($p = 0.005$), showing a significant survival benefit of surgery. In the subgroup with non–upper-lobe predominance emphysema and high exercise capacity, the risk of death was significantly higher in the surgical group compared to the medical group (risk ratio 2.06; $p = 0.02$). In the two remaining subgroups, surgery appeared to have little effect on the risk of death [risk ratio of LVRS to medical care in the subgroup with upper-lobe emphysema and high baseline exercise tolerance was 0.98 ($p = 0.70$), while in the subgroup with non–upper-lobe predominance emphysema and low exercise capacity the risk ratio was 0.81 ($p = 0.49$)]. All four subgroups experienced improvement in exercise capability and self-reported quality of life.

The NETT trial added additional weight to the preponderance of evidence in support of LVRS for properly selected patients. The specific inclusion and exclusion criteria for the NETT have been adopted in the national coverage decision for LVRS by the Center for Medicare Services. Therefore, pending any adjustments, the criteria for LVRS are well mapped out and the question remains: what does one offer a patient who appears to be a suitable candidate for both procedures?

21.2. Optimal Surgical Management of End-Stage Emphysema

There are several permutations in which lung transplantation and lung volume reduction can be combined to optimize treatment for patients with emphysema. These combinations have all been tried and have been anecdotally reported for clusters of patients. The combined approaches can be summarized as follows: volume reduction as a bridge to transplant, simultaneous single-lung transplant and unilateral volume reduction to prevent native lung hyperexpansion, early post-transplant unilateral volume reduction to treat acute native lung hyperexpansion, and late unilateral volume reduction to treat chronic native lung hyperexpansion. Todd and colleagues reported the Toronto experience[30] with simultaneous unilateral volume reduction to improve overall lung function prospectively after a single-lung transplant. They experienced no postoperative problems, and the pulmonary function at 3 months was better than expected based on historical controls receiving a single lung for emphysema. Yonan and colleagues retrospectively analyzed 27 patients who received 31 single-lung transplants for emphysema.[31] They identified 12 patients who experienced early or late native lung hyperexpansion, and they performed two early lung volume reduction operations to combat this problem. Their analysis included an assessment of risk factors, and they concluded that low pretransplant FEV$_1$, high residual volume, and relative pulmonary hypertension were all associated with a higher risk for native lung hyperexpansion. They did not perform or advocate volume reduction simultaneous with a single-lung transplant for emphysema. The use of LVRS for late native lung hyperexpansion after single-lung transplantation can be described as rare and anecdotal. Kroshus and colleagues reported three patients who were treated with unilateral LVRS for native lung hyperinflation and post-transplant dyspnea that was not attributable to infection or rejection. The patients represented a small fraction of the 66 single-lung transplants performed at that center for emphysema. The volume reduction operations were performed 12, 17, and 42 months after the initial lung transplantation; and all patients experienced substantial relief of their dyspnea with an improvement in exercise tolerance and in the appearance of the chest radiograph.[32] A similar report by Le Pimpec-Barthes and coworkers described successful treatment of symptomatic native lung hyperexpansion by volume reduction of the native side in the form of a right upper lobectomy.[33]

The use of volume reduction as a bridge to transplant is the form of combined procedures that has been most frequently attempted. The concept was introduced to the medical literature by Zenati and colleagues in 1995 when they reported two patients who received single-lung transplants 17 months and 4 months, respectively, after laser ablation of emphysematous bullae.[34] One group has prospectively performed volume reduction in patients thought to be also eligible for transplantation.[35] This center found 31 patients eligible for both procedures; at the same time, they identified 20 patients who were suitable for LVRS alone and 139 who were thought to be transplant candidates only. Twenty-four patients had successful LVRS, and 7 (including 1 death) were considered LVRS failures. Follow-up was too short at the time of the report to know how frequently late transplants would be performed and the series has not been followed-up with the long-term results.

Our own results with LVRS in transplant-eligible patients have been reported.[36] We retrospectively identified 99 of 200 patients who underwent bilateral LVRS and who were thought to have been transplant eligible. With a median follow-up of 5.1 years, 32 of the 99 had been listed for transplant, and 15 had undergone transplantation without a peri-operative mortality. The only preoperative or operative factor that was predictive for the subsequent need for transplantation was a lower-lobe, rather than an upper-lobe, LVRS procedure. The actuarial survival results from the Washington University Lung Volume Reduction Program are shown in Figure 21.3.[37] Pulmonary function and the 6-min walk test results before and after lung volume reduction are shown in Table 21.3.[37]

Others have shown prior LVRS does not preclude subsequent successful lung transplantation.[38,39] Bilateral LVRS appears to be a more effective bridge.[39] Initial LVRS in candidates for LVRS or transplantation should have the goal of providing relief from dyspnea, improved functional status, and allow the patients to get into improved physical condition for transplantation. Lung volume reduction surgery is used to palliate these patients during their long waiting period. Senbaklavaci and colleagues[38] reported their results of 27 patients who underwent LVRS followed by lung transplantation at their institution. In the group that had a FEV$_1$ increase greater than 20% after LVRS, they found these patients were brought into a better pretransplant condition that resulted in a decreased mortality at the

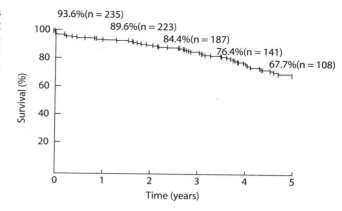

FIGURE 21.3. Kaplan–Meier survival of 250 patients after bilateral lung volume reduction surgery at Washington University School of Medicine. Data were censored for missing data (1 patient), lung transplantation (18 patients), or end of follow-up. (From Ciccone et al[37]).

time of lung transplantation. Patients who failed LVRS, however, were poor candidates for lung transplantation as their pretransplant condition was not improved. In a multi-institutional experience of 35 lung transplant patients who had previously undergone LVRS, the median time from LVRS to transplant was 4.1 years (range, 1.1–8.2).[40]

Many patients have had LVRS as a functional bridge to transplant, but it has occurred not so much as part of an a priori plan to bridge them

as it was additional treatment for crippling dyspnea that was not improved sufficiently by lung volume reduction. The concept is attractive on the surface: patients obtain volume reduction initially and relieve part of the crunch for available lungs to transplant. The benefit for the patient successfully volume reduced initially is the possibility that transplant might be avoided altogether by an excellent response to the reduction. A second possibility is that transplant is delayed by several years and the patient is

TABLE 21.3. Pulmonary function and exercise test results before and after surgery.

	Evaluation baseline (n = 249)	After rehabilitation (n = 249)	6-month PO (n = 231)	1-year PO (n = 225)	3-year PO (n = 178)	5-year PO (n = 106)
Time from surgery (days, mean ± SD)	−124 ± 79	−6 ± 5	193 ± 36	401 ± 60	1076 ± 133	1799 ± 217
FEV1 Mean ± SD (L)	0.7 ± 0.2	0.7 ± 0.3	1.1 ± 0.5	1.0 ± 0.5	0.9 ± 0.5	0.8 ± 0.5
% predicted	25%*	26%	39%**	38%**	34%**	30%***
RV Mean ± SD (L)	5.9 ± 1.4	5.8 ± 1.3	4.0 ± 1.2	4.1 ± 1.3	4.2 ± 1.3	4.8 ± 1.8
% predicted	282%*	277%	189%**	193%**	198%**	222%**
RV/total lung capacity (%, mean ± SD)	72 ± 7*	70 ± 7	−57 ± 9**	−58 ± 10**	−61 ± 11**	−66 ± 11**
DLCO Mean ± SD (mL/[min · mm Hg])	9.1 ± 3.7	8.9 ± 3.9	10.4 ± 4.6	10.3 ± 4.3	9.2 ± 4.1	8.6 ± 4.2
% predicted	34%*	33%	39%*	39%**	36%*	34%*
6-min walk (mean ± SD, ft)	−919 ± 335**	1142 ± 291	1345 ± 316*	−1341 ± 310**	1271 ± 305**	348*

Abbreviation: DLCO, diffusive capacity of carbon monoxide; PO, postoperative.

*$p \geq 0.05$ for paired analyses with scores after rehabilitation.

**$p \leq 0.001$ for paired analyses with scores after rehabilitation.

***p 0.02 for paired analyses with scores after rehabilitation.

Source: Ciccone et al.[37]

given a transplant with a later cohort, with the possibility of improved techniques, better immunosuppression, and overall better survival. Finally, because the falloff in the survival curve is steeper for lung transplant recipients that it is for LVRS recipients, anything that can safely delay entry onto the steeper survival curve is worth pursuing.

The logic of the potential benefits of LVRS as a bridge to transplant falls apart when faced with some aspects of reality. First, the anatomical and physiological criteria for volume reduction are much more restrictive than those for transplantation, so it is unlikely that a large fraction of transplant candidates could be safely and successfully treated with volume reduction. Also, the dilemma remains as to how to treat a patient at the upper limit of acceptability with regard to age. It is possible that a patient who is acceptable for both procedures at age 62 might face ineligibility for future lung transplantation years later when lung function declines. Results have confirmed this: of the 15 patients in one center who have undergone transplantation after bilateral LVRS, only one was older than 60 years of age at the time of LVRS evaluation. The next oldest was 58, and the mean age for the group was 54 years.[36]

It is worth noting that some factors in this decision-making process are in flux. The system of allocation of graft lungs to potential recipients was formally changed in the United States in May 2005. As a result, priority for donor lungs is based on a score determined by an algorithm that favors patients with high risk of pretransplant death and high likelihood of pretransplant survival. It is unclear how this will affect emphysema patients, but it is likely to lower the priority of most emphysema patients when compared to patients with other diagnoses leading to transplantation. The system is too new to allow meaningful conclusions, but it certainly has the potential to change strategies for the patients who are the subjects of this review.

21.3. Conclusions

There are currently two surgical therapies aimed at crippling, end-stage emphysema: lung trans-

plantation and LVRS. We favor a meticulous selection process in which both options are considered and the best option is selected for each patient. Patients with ideal circumstances for LVRS have hyperinflation, heterogeneous distribution of disease, FEV_1 20% or greater, and a normal PCO_2; they are offered LVRS (level of evidence 4; recommendation grade D). In contrast, patients with diffuse disease, low FEV_1, hypercapnia, and associated pulmonary hypertension are directed toward a transplant (level of evidence 4; recommendation grade D). Lung volume reduction surgery has not been a satisfactory option for patients with α1-antitrypsin deficiency, and transplantation must be considered in these cases (level of evidence 4; recommendation grade D). With these considerations, we find that few patients are serious candidates for both procedures. The literature supporting decision making in this field is mostly the case-series level of evidence (Table 21.4) Lessons from prospective randomized trials are available, but applying them to decision making in treatment allocation requires creativity because they are usually side issues or subset analyses that apply to the patients in question here. Finally, the recent changes in the allocation system for lung transplantation may have an impact on decision making for the patients who are currently viewed as viable candidates for the two procedures.

> Patients with ideal circumstances for LVRS have hyperinflation, heterogeneous distribution of disease, FEV_1 20% or greater, and a normal PCO_2; they should be offered LVRS (level of evidence 4; recommendation grade D).
>
> Patients with diffuse disease, low FEV_1, hypercapnia, and associated pulmonary hypertension are directed towards lung transplantation (level of evidence 4; recommendation grade D).
>
> Lung reduction volume surgery has not been a satisfactory option for patients with α1-antitrypsin deficiency, and transplantation should be considered in these cases (level of evidence 4; recommendation grade D).

TABLE 21.4. Evidence table for the decision of lung volume reduction surgery versus lung transplantation for severe emphysema.

Patient subset	LVRS considered?	Lung transplant considered?	Evidence level
FEV_1 greater than 40%	No, disease not severe enough	No, disease not severe enough	Opinion favors no surgical therapy Evidence level: 4 Recommendation grade: D
FEV_1 25%–40% predicted	Yes, depending on symptoms	No, disease not severe enough	Opinion favors LVRS as initial approach Evidence level: 3 Recommendation grade: D
FEV_1 20%–25%	Yes, depending on anatomy and symptoms. Increasing age, additional comorbidities, heterogeneous target areas all favor LVRS	Yes, depending on anatomy and symptoms. Youth, fewer comorbidities, homogeneous emphysema and history of pleural space surgery would favor transplant	Opinion favors LVRS as initial approach Evidence level: 3 Recommendation grade: D
FEV_1 less than 20%, upper lobe predominant, DLCO greater than 20% predicted	Yes. Increasing age, additional comorbidities, heterogeneous target areas all favor LVRS	Yes. Youth, fewer comorbidities, homogeneous emphysema and history of pleural space surgery would favor transplant	Opinion favors LVRS as initial approach Evidence level: 4 Recommendation grade: D
FEV_1 less than 20%, and either DLCO less than 20% or homogeneous emphysema	No, considered too high risk	Yes, if free from contraindications	RCT suggests high risk for LVRS in this subset Evidence level: 2+ Recommendation grade: C
FEV_1 20%–25%, α1-antitrypsin deficiency, hypercapnea, or pulmonary hypertension	Yes, but these factors increase risk and decrease long-term benefit	Yes	Opinion favors lung transplant as initial approach when pulmonary comorbidities are high Evidence level: 4 Recommendation grade: D
FEV_1 20%–40%, High exercise capacity, non-upper-lobe predominant emphysema	No, increased risk of death versus medical therapy alone	No, exercise capacity suggests insufficient impairment to justify transplant	RCT suggests no LVRS in this group; opinion suggest no transplant Evidence level: 2+ Recommendation grade: C

Abbreviations: DLCO, diffusine capacity of carbon monoxide; FEV_1, forced expiratory volume in 1 s; LVRS, lung volume reducing surgery; RCT, randomized, controlled trial.

References

1. Diener CF, Burrows B. Further observations on the course and prognosis of chronic obstructive pulmonary disease. *Am Rev Respir Dis* 1975;111:719–724.

2. Traver GA, Cline MG, Burrows B. Predictors of mortality in chronic obstructive pulmonary disease. *Am Rev Respir Dis* 1979;119:895–902.

3. Burrows B, Earle RH. Course and prognosis of chronic obstructive lung disease: a prospective study of 200 patients. *N Engl J Med* 1969;280:397–404.

4. Nocturnal-Oxygen-Therapy-Trial-Group. Continuous or nocturnal oxygen therapy in hypoxemic chronic obstructive lung disease. *Ann Intern Med* 1980;93:391–398.

5. Deslauriers J. History of surgery for emphysema. *Semin Thorac Cardiovasc Surg* 1996;8:43–51.

6. Mal H, Andreasian B, Pamela F. Unilateral lung transplantation in end stage pulmonary emphysema. *Am Rev Respir Dis* 1989;140:797–802.

7. Patterson GA, Cooper JD, Goldman B, et al. Technique of successful clinical double-lung transplantation. *Ann Thorac Surg* 1988;45:626–633.

8. Pasque MK, Cooper JD, Kaiser LR, Haydock DA, Triantafillou A, Trulock EP. An improved technique for bilateral lung transplantation: rationale and initial clinical experience. *Ann Thorac Surg* 1990;49:785–791.

9. Trulock EP, Edwards LB, Taylor DO, Boucek MM, Keck BM, Hertz MI. The Registry of the International Society for Heart and Lung Transplantation: twenty-second official adult lung and

heart-lung transplant report – 2005. *J Heart Lung Transplant* 2005;24:956–967.

10. Trulock EP. Lung transplantation. *Am J Respir Crit Care Med* 1997;155:789–818.

11. Low DE, Trulock EP, Kaiser LR, et al. Morbidity, mortality, and early results of single versus bilateral lung transplantation for emphysema. *J Thorac Cardiovasc Surg* 1992;103:1119–1126.

12. Patterson GA, Maurer JA, Williams TJ, et al. Comparison of outcomes of double and single lung transplantation for obstructive lung disease. *J Thorac Cardiovasc Surg* 1991;101:623–632.

13. Cassivi SD, Meyers BF, Battafarano RJ, et al. Thriteen-year experience in lung transplantation for emphysema. *Ann Thorac Surg* 2002;74:1663–1670.

14. Hadjiliadis D, Davis RD, Palmer SM. Is transplant operation important in determining posttransplant risk of bronchiolitis obliterans syndrome in lung transplant recipients?[see comment]. *Chest* 2002;122:1168–1175.

15. Gaissert HA, Trulock EP, Cooper JD, Sundaresan RS, Patterson GA. Comparison of early functional results after volume reduction or lung transplantation for chronic obstructive pulmonary disease. *J Thorac Cardiovasc Surg* 1996;111:296–307.

16. Fishman A, Martinez F, Naunheim K, et al. A randomized trial comparing lung-volume-reduction surgery with medical therapy for severe emphysema [comment]. *N Engl J Med* 2003;348:2059–2073.

17. Meyers BF, Yusen RD, Guthrie TJ, et al. Results of lung volume reduction surgery in patients meeting a national emphysema treatment trial high-risk criterion [see comment]. *J Thorac Cardiovasc Surg* 2004;127:829–835.

18. Cooper JD, Trulock EP, Triantafillou AN, et al. Bilateral pneumectomy (volume reduction) for chronic obstructive pulmonary disease. *J Thorac Cardiovasc Surg* 1995;109:106–116; discussion16–19.

19. Cooper JD. Clinical trials and future prospects for lung volume reduction surgery. *Semin Thorac Cardiovasc Surg* 2002;14:365–370.

20. Sciurba FC, Rogers RM, Keenan RJ, et al. Improvement in pulmonary function and elastic recoil after lung-reduction surgery for diffuse emphysema [comment]. *N Engl J Med* 1996;334:1095–1099.

21. Meyers BF. Complications of lung volume reduction surgery. *Semin Thorac Cardiovasc Surg* 2002;14:399–402.

22. Geddes D, Davies M, Koyama H, et al. Effect of lung-volume-reduction surgery in patients with severe emphysema. *N Engl J Med* 2000;343:239–245.

23. Criner GJ, Cordova FC, Furukawa S, et al. Prospective randomized trial comparing bilateral lung volume reduction surgery to pulmonary rehabilitation in severe chronic obstructive pulmonary disease. *Am J Respir Crit Care Med* 1999;160:2018–2027.

24. Pompeo E, Marino M, Nofroni I, Matteucci G, Mineo TC. Reduction pneumoplasty versus respiratory rehabilitation in severe emphysema: a randomized study. Pulmonary Emphysema Research Group. *Ann Thorac Surg* 2000;70:948–953; discussion 954.

25. Goodnight-White S, Jones WJ, Baaklini J, et al. Prospective randomized controlled trial comparing bilateral lung volume reduction surgery (LVRS) to medical therapy alone in patients with severe emphysema. *Chest* 2000;118(suppl 4):102S.

26. Lofdahl CG, Hillerdal G, Strom K. Randomized controlled trial of volume reduction surgery-preliminary results up to12 months. *Am J Respir Crit Care Med* 2000;161:A585.

27. Anonymous. Rationale and design of the National Emphysema Treatment Trial (NETT): a prospective randomized trial of lung volume reduction surgery. *J Thorac Cardiovasc Surg* 1999;118:518–528.

28. National Emphysema Treatment Trial Research Group. Patients at high risk of death after lung-volume-reduction surgery [comment]. *N Engl J Med* 2001;345:1075–1083.

29. Ware JH. The National Emphysema Treatment Trial – how strong is the evidence? [comment]. *N Engl J Med* 2003;348:2055–2056.

30. Todd TRJ, Perron J, Winton TL, Keshavjee SH. Simultaneous single-lung transplantation and lung volume reduction. *Ann Thorac Surg* 1997;63:1468–1470.

31. Yonan NA, El-Gamel A, Egan J, Kakadellis J, Rahman A, Deiraniya AK. Single lung transplantation for emphysema: predictors for native-lung hyperinflation. *J Heart Lung Transplant* 1998;17:192–201.

32. Kroshus TJ, Bolman RM, Kshettry VR. Unilateral volume reduction after single-lung transplantation for emphysema. *Ann Thorac Surg* 1996;62:363–368.

33. Le Pimpec-Barthes F, Debrosse D, Cuenod C-A, Gandjbakhch I, Riquet M. Late contralateral lobectomy after single-lung transplantation for emphysema. *Ann Thorac Surg* 1996;61:231–234.

34. Zenati M, Keenan RJ, Landreneau RJ, Paradis IL, Ferson PF, Griffith BP. Lung reduction as a bridge to lung transplantation in pulmonary emphysema. *Ann Thorac Surg* 1995;59:1581–1583.

35. Bavaria JE, Pochettino A, Kotloff RM, et al. Effect of volume reduction on lung transplant timing and selection for chronic obstructive pulmonary disease. *J Thorac Cardiovasc Surg* 1998;115:9–18.

36. Meyers BF, Yusen RD, Guthrie TJ, et al. Outcome of bilateral lung volume reduction in patients with emphysema potentially eligible for lung transplantation. *J Thorac Cardiovasc Surg* 2001;122:10–17.

37. Ciccone AM, Meyers BF, Guthrie TJ, et al. Long-term outcome of bilateral lung volume reduction in 250 consecutive patients with emphysema [comment]. *J Thorac Cardiovasc Surg* 2003;125:513–525.

38. Senbaklavaci O, Wisser W, Ozpeker C, et al. Successful lung volume reduction surgery brings patients into better condition for later lung transplantation. *Eur J Cardiothorac Surg* 2002;22:363–367.

39. Burns KE, Keenan RJ, Grgurich WF, Manzetti JD, Zenati MA. Outcomes of lung volume reduction surgery followed by lung transplantation: a matched cohort study. *Ann Thorac Surg* 2002;73:1587–1593.

40. Lau CL, Guthrie TJ, Chaparro C, et al. Lung transplantation in recipients with previous lung volume reduction surgery. *J Heart Lung Transplant* 2003;22(suppl 1):S183.

22
Pleural Sclerosis for the Management of Initial Pneumothorax

Richard W. Light

A pneumothorax occurs when there is air in the pleural space. Pneumothoraces are classified as spontaneous, which occur without preceding trauma or other obvious cause, or traumatic, which occur as a result of trauma to the chest. Spontaneous pneumothoraces are subclassified as primary or secondary. A primary spontaneous pneumothorax occurs in an otherwise healthy person without underlying lung disease. A secondary spontaneous pneumothorax complicates an underlying lung disease, most commonly chronic obstructive pulmonary disease.

Because there is a high rate of recurrence after an initial primary spontaneous pneumothorax, consideration should be given to preventing a recurrence when the patient is initially seen. Sadikot and associates[1] followed 153 patients with primary spontaneous pneumothorax for a mean of 54 months and reported that the ipsilateral recurrence rate was 39% and most recurred within the first year. In this same study, 15% of the 153 patients developed a pneumothorax on the contralateral side.[1] Patients who are tall and those who continue to smoke are more likely to have a recurrence.[1] However, there is no relationship between the number of blebs or the size of the blebs on computed tomography (CT)[2] or the appearance of the lung at thoracotomy[3] and the risk of recurrence. Once a patient has had one recurrence, the risk of another recurrence increases to more than 50%.[4]

The recurrence rates after secondary spontaneous pneumothorax are higher than those after primary spontaneous pneumothorax. Guo and coworkers[5] used the Cox proportional hazard model to assess the factors associated with recurrence of pneumothorax in 138 patients and found that recurrence was significantly more frequent in patients with secondary spontaneous pneumothorax, in taller patients, and in patients with lower weight. Other authors have also reported that the recurrence rates with secondary spontaneous pneumothorax without treatment are slightly higher than those for primary spontaneous pneumothorax without treatment.[6,7]

The main difference in the treatment of primary and secondary spontaneous pneumothoraces is that it is more important to prevent recurrences with secondary pneumothoraces because a recurrence of a secondary pneumothorax may be life threatening. In contrast, the recurrence of a primary pneumothorax is usually not life threatening.

22.1. Summary of Published Data

There are several ways by which one can try to prevent recurrence of a pneumothorax. These include the injection of various sclerosing agents such as a tetracycline derivative or talc suspended in saline (talc slurry) through a chest tube, medical thoracoscopy with the insufflation of talc, and video-assisted thoracic surgery (VATS) with the treatment of subpleural blebs and a concomitant procedure to produce a pleurodesis. The pleurodesis can be produced by pleural abrasion, partial parietal pleurectomy, talc insufflation, or the intrapleural instillation of another sclerosing agent such as tetracycline, silver nitrate, or iodopovidone.

Unfortunately, there are a very limited number of randomized, controlled studies, as outlined in Table 22.1, comparing the various methods for preventing a recurrent pneumothorax. In the discussion that follows, the results from three randomized studies, eight uncontrolled studies, and two statements from thoracic societies are summarized. There are many other studies on the prevention of recurrent pneumothorax that are uncontrolled, but the selected ones are most pertinent.

A large Veterans Administration (VA) cooperative study in the 1980s[6] demonstrated that the intrapleural administration of 1500mg tetracycline when a patient had a chest tube for treatment of a pneumothorax decreased the overall

TABLE 22.1. Summary of published data on management of spontaneous pneumothorax.

First citation	Summary	No. of patients	Conclusion	Level of evidence	Reference no.
Light RW. *JAMA* 1990;264:2224–2230.	Patients with CT randomized to tetracycline or only CT; multicenter	229	25% reccurrence in tetracycline group, <41% recurence in controls	1++	6
Almind M. *Thorax* 1989;44:627–630.	Patients randomized to tetracycline, talc slurry, or CT	96	13%, 8%, and 36% recurrence after talc, tetracycline, and CT, respectively	1+	8
Alfageme I. *Chest* 1994;106:347–350.	Nonrandomized with 66 with tetracycline and 51 with CT	117	9% recurrence after tetracycline and 35% recurrence after CT	2–	9
Guo Y. *Respirology* 2005;10:378–384.	Nonrandomized with 45 tetracycline, 23 gentamicin, and 70 CT	138	33%, 26%, and 50% recurrence after tetracycline, gentamicin, and CT	2+	5
Tschopp JM. *Thorax* 1997;52:329–332.	Uncontrolled talc pleurodesis via medical thoracoscopy	89	7.4% recurrence in patients that had follow-up	3	10
Tschopp JM. *Eur Respir J* 2002;20:1003–1009.	Randomized talc pleurodesis via medical thoracoscopy vs. CT; multicenter	108	5% recurrence after talc and 34% recurrence after CT	1+	11
Yim AP. *Surg L Endosc* 1997;7:236–240.	Uncontrolled VATS with pleural abrasion ± treatment of blebs	483	1.7% recurrence, all received mechanical pleurodesis	3	12
Cardillo G. *Ann Thorac Surg* 2000;69:357–361.	Uncontrolled VATS with talc poudrage or parietal pleurectomy	432	4.4% recurrence 1.79% with talc 9.15% with parietal pleurectomy	2+	13
Waller DA. *Ann R Coll Surg Engl* 1999;81:387–392.	Uncontrolled VATS with stapling of blebs and parietal pleurecdtomy	173	6.9% recurrence, but decreased with increasing experience	3	14
Margolis M. *Ann Thorac Surg* 2003;76:1661–1663.	Uncontrolled VATS with stapling of blebs and pleural abrasion	156	No recurrences All primary spontaneous pneumothoraces	3	15
Lee P. *Chest* 2004;125:1315–1320.	Uncontrolled talc via medical thoracoscopy, mean age >70 years	41	3.4% recurrence 30-day morality 10%	3	16
Henry M. *Thorax* 2003;58(suppl 2): II39–II52.	BTS guidelines for management of spontantous pneumothorax	NA	Chemical pleurodesis with tetracycline if patient is not a surgical candidate	4	18
Baumann MH. *Chest* 2001;119:590–602.	ACCP statement on management of spontaneous pneumothorax	NA	Thoracoscopy with bleb stapling and pleural abrasion for preventing recurrence.	4	17

Abbreviations: ACCP, American College of Chest aphysicians; BTS, British Thoracic Society; CT, chest tube; VATS, video-assisted thoracoscopic surgery.

recurrence rate for the pneumothorax from 41% to 25% when the patients were followed for 30 months. The intrapleural administration of tetracycline effected a reduction in the recurrence rates in patients with primary spontaneous pneumothorax from 32% to 10%, in patients with secondary spontaneous pneumothorax from 43% to 28%, and in patients with recurrent pneumothorax from 50% to 21%.[6]

The randomized, controlled study by Almind and associates[8] also demonstrated that the injection of either talc slurry or tetracycline through a chest tube resulted in a significant reduction in the recurrence rate after a first spontaneous pneumothorax. In their study, 34 patients received simple drainage, 33 patients received in addition tetracycline 550mg in 20mL, and 29 patients received in addition 5g of talc suspended in 250mL saline. The recurrence rates during the follow-up period were as follows: simple drainage 36%, tetracycline 13%, and 8% in the talc group. The patients in the talc group tended to have more pain and more temperature elevation than the patients in the tetracycline group.

A nonrandomized study by Alfageme and coworkers[9] also suggested that the intrapleural injection of tetracycline reduced the recurrence rate in patients with spontaneous pneumothorax. These authors injected tetracycline (either 20mg/kg or a total dose of 2g) in 150mL saline. For one control group, they used 66 patients who had active pleural or pulmonary infections or refused surgery. A second control group consisted of 32 patients who were treated by observation because the pneumothorax size was less than 20%. The recurrence rate in the tetracycline group (9%) was significantly less than that in the chest tube group (35%) or the observation group (36%).

Guo and associates[5] performed multiple risk factor analysis on factors related to the recurrence of pneumothorax in 138 patients who had a spontaneous pneumothorax. They reported that the most important characteristic associated with recurrence was increased height ($p < 0.0045$) followed by decreased weight ($p < 0.0051$), the presence of pre-existing lung disease ($p < 0.0073$), and the absence of a pleurodesis procedure ($p < 0.017$). The recurrence rate after 3 years in

the 68 patients who had pleurodesis was 27% while the recurrence rate in the 70 patients who had only chest tubes was 50%. The recurrence rates were similar for the 23 patients who received gentamicin 16mg as a sclerosing agent and the 45 patients who received tetracycline 1000mg.[5]

The efficacy of pleurodesis induced by the insufflation of talc at the time of medical thoracoscopy was demonstrated by Tschopp and coworkers.[10] In an uncontrolled study of 93 procedures in 89 patients, 3 to 5g of pure talc were insufflated into the pleural space at the time of medical thoracoscopy under local anesthesia. In the immediate postoperative period, two patients required an additional surgical procedure because the lung did not expand, three patients had tetracycline instilled because of persistent bubbling, two patients had a third drain inserted, and two patients had a second medical thoracoscopy because of relapse or persistent bubbling. During the follow-up period for a mean of 5.1 years, 6 of 81 patients (7.4%) available for follow-up had a recurrence.[10]

The effectiveness of talc insufflation at medical thoracoscopy was compared to chest tube drainage in a prospective, randomized multicenter study of 108 patients with primary spontaneous pneumothorax, the majority of which were recurrent.[11] Patients with bullae more than 5cm in diameter were excluded. In this study, the recurrence rate was 5% in the group that received talc and 34% in the group that received chest tubes. However, it should be noted that 10 of the 16 recurrences in the chest-tube group occurred during the initial hospitalization while only 1 recurrence occurred in the talc group during hospitalization. The recurrence rates after the initial hospitalization were 5% in the talc group and 13% in the chest-tube group, although 10 of the 47 patients in the chest-tube group also got talc during their initial hospitalization. This study also concluded that medical thoracoscopy with the insufflation of talc was cost effective in comparison to chest tube alone in patients with primary spontaneous pneumothorax requiring a chest tube.[11]

Although there have been no randomized, controlled studies evaluating the effectiveness of

VATS in the prevention of recurrent pneumothorax, there have been many case series and some of the largest are summarized. Yim and Liu[12] reported their experience with 518 VATS procedures in 483 patients with primary spontaneous pneumothorax. They treated the blebs in various ways including stapled bullectomy (196), endoloop ligation (261), argon beam coagulation (6), and endoscopic suturing (35). All patients received mechanical abrasion of their pleura. The overall recurrence rate with a mean follow-up of 20 months was 1.74%. Twenty of their patients received only mechanical pleurodesis and the recurrence rate was 25% in this subgroup.[12]

Cardillo and associates[13] reviewed their experience with VATS in 432 patients for primary spontaneous pneumothorax. They treated the blebs with stapling or ligation, and they attempted to induce pleurodesis via partial parietal pleurectomy or talc insufflation (2g). They reported that the overall recurrence rate with a mean follow-up of 38 months was 4.16%. The recurrence rates in patients who received ligation was 11 of 104 (10.6%), while the recurrence rates in patients who received stapling was 3 of 235, or 1.27%. The recurrence rates in patients who received subtotal pleurectomy was 14 of 153 (9.15%), while the recurrence rates in patients who received t alc insufflation was 5 of 279 (1.79%). However, most of the difference in the recurrence rates between talc and subtotal pleurectomy was due to the fact that many more ligations were performed in the group that received the subtotal pleurectomy.[13]

In another uncontrolled study, Waller[14] reported his experience with VATS in 173 patients for spontaneous pneumothorax, including 55 patients with secondary spontaneous pneumothoraces. He performed stapling of the bullae and an apical parietal pleurectomy on all patients. Overall, the recurrence rate with a mean follow-up of 2 years was 6.6%. Most of the recurrences occurred in patients who were operated upon early in the experience. The late recurrence rate was lower for the secondary spontaneous pneumothorax than it was for the primary spontaneous pneumothorax.[14]

The best results with VATS were reported by Margolis and associates,[15] who treated 156 young adults with primary spontaneous pneumothorax via VATS with stapling of blebs and pleural abrasion. In this uncontrolled study there were no postoperative air leaks and the mean hospital stay was only 2.4 days. During the median follow-up 62 months, there were no recurrences.

In an uncontrolled study, Lee and coworkers[16] evaluated the effectiveness of medical thoracoscopy with the insufflation of talc in the treatment of secondary spontaneous pneumothorax in patients with advanced chronic obstructive pulmonary disease (COPD). They insufflated 3g of talc in 41 patients with a mean age of 70.7 years and a mean forced expiratory volume in 1s (FEV_1) of 0.88L. The 30-day mortality in this group of patients was 10% and all the patients that died had an FEV_1 between 0.5L and 0.7L. The recurrence rate in the survivors was 2 of 37 (5.4%).

The American College of Chest Physicians (ACCP) and the British Thoracic Society (BTS) have both published guidelines for the management of spontaneous pneumothorax in the past few years. The ACCP guidelines were generated by pulmonologists, thoracic surgeons, emergency room physicians, and interventional radiologists and used the Delphi process.[17] The consensus of these physicians was that procedures to prevent the recurrence of primary spontaneous pneumothorax should be reserved for the second pneumothorax occurrence. This guideline felt that thoracoscopy was the preferred intervention for primary spontaneous pneumothorax and that patients with apical bullae should undergo intraoperative bullectomy. They also recommended that parietal pleural abrasion should be performed in most patients to induce a pleurodesis. They felt that instillation of sclerosing agents through a chest tube was an acceptable approach for pneumothorax prevention in patients who decline surgery or who have an increased surgical risk. The ACCP guidelines for patients with secondary spontaneous pneumothorax recommended an intervention to prevent pneumothorax recurrence after the first occurrence because of the potential lethality of secondary pneumothoraces.[17] Otherwise, the recommendations for primary and secondary pneumothorax were very similar.

The British Thoracic Society concluded that chemical pleurodesis is best achieved with the insufflation of 5g sterile talc.[18] They also concluded that chemical pleurodesis can prevent recurrent pneumothorax, but that is should be performed only if the patient is unwilling or unable to undergo surgery. The BTS gave the following indications for operative intervention: (1) second ipsilateral pneumothorax, (2) first contralateral pneumothorax, (3) bilateral spontaneous pneumothorax, (4) persistent air leak (>5–7 days of tube drainage; (5) air leak or failure to completely re-expand), (6) professions at risk (e.g., pilots, divers).

22.2. How Should Published Data Impact on Clinical Practice

The data summarized in the above section and in the table demonstrate the paucity of randomized studies comparing the different methods for pleurodesis. Nevertheless, several conclusions can be made. First, the instillation of a tetracycline derivative or talc suspended in saline through a chest tube will decrease the risk of recurrent pneumothorax from ~50% to ~20% (recommendation grade A). Second, no agent has been shown to have clear-cut superiority in inducing a pleurodesis when injected through a chest tube (recommendation grade A). Third, medical thoracoscopy with the insufflation of talc will decrease the risk of recurrence of primary spontaneous pneumothorax to less than 10% (recommendation grade B) and this procedure was also effective in preventing recurrences in one small study of patients with secondary spontaneous pneumothorax (recommendation grade C). Fourth, VATS with the stapling of blebs and the application of some procedure to create a pleurodesis will decrease the risk of recurrence to less than 5% (recommendation grade A). There are no randomized, controlled studies comparing the effectiveness of medical thoracoscopy with VATS for the prevention of recurrent pneumothorax. Likewise there are no randomized studies comparing medical thoracoscopy with VATS in the management of patients with pneumothorax.

The instillation of a tetracycline derivative or talc suspended in saline through a chest tube will decrease the risk of recurrent pneumothorax from ~50% to ~20% (level of evidence 1; recommendation grade A).

No agent has been shown to have clear-cut superiority in inducing a pleurodesis when injected through a chest tube (level of evidence 1; recommendation grade A).

Thoracoscopy with insufflation of talc decreases the risk of recurrence of primary spontaneous pneumothorax to less than 10% (level of evidence 2 to 3; recommendation grade B).

Thoracoscopy with insufflation of talc decreases the risk of recurrence of secondary spontaneous pneumothorax (level of evidence 3; recommendation grade C).

Video-assisted thorascopic surgery with the stapling of blebs and pleurodesis will decrease the risk of recurrence to less than 5% (level of evidence 1; recommendation grade A).

22.3. My View of the Data

My personal view of the clinical data presented above and my recommendations based on this data are as follows: When one is dealing with a patient with a pneumothorax who has a chest tube in place, consideration should be given to doing something to prevent a recurrence because a recurrence can be expected in approximately 50% of patients. The simplest and least expensive procedure is to inject a sclerosant through the chest tube that will reduce the recurrence rate to less than 25%. The two agents that have been used most commonly are talc slurry and doxycycline. I prefer doxycycline because the intrapleural administration of talc has been associated with the development of the acute respiratory distress syndrome (ARDS).[19,20] If parenteral doxycycline is not available, then the contents of doxycycline tablets or capsules can be injected after they are dissolved in saline and passed through a filter.[21] I recommend this procedure for patients with their first primary spontaneous pneumothorax and for patients who refuse or are thought not to be candidates for medical thoracoscopy or VATS. If a tetracycline derivative is used as a pleurodesing agent, conscious sedation should be administered as the intrapleural injection of a tetracycline derivative can be very painful.[6]

Patients with a recurrent primary spontaneous pneumothorax or a secondary spontaneous pneumothorax should be considered for a more aggressive procedure, which could be medical thoracoscopy with the insufflation of talc or a VATS procedure. In general, if everything else is equal, I prefer a VATS procedure. The two main reasons that I prefer the VATS procedure are the following: (1) I worry about the possibility of ARDS after the insufflation of talc intrapleurally, and (2) from a purely theoretical viewpoint, it makes more sense to me to treat the blebs that are responsible for the pneumothorax as well as to try to create a pleurodesis. At the time of VATS, the blebs should be stapled and a procedure done to crea te a pleurodesis, such as mechanical pleural abrasion or partial parietal pleurectomy. There are other factors that can affect whether to perform medical thoracoscopy or a VATS procedure. Certainly, medical thoracoscopy with the insufflation of talc is less expensive than a VATS procedure. Stapling of the blebs is very expensive.[22] The availability of individuals capable of performing medical thoracoscopy or VATS at a given institution also affects the choice of procedure.

22.4. Future Studies

There are several clinical studies that could be performed that would be important aids in decision making in the future. The effectiveness of transforming growth factor β, the agent that is most effective in producing pleurodesis in animals,[23] should be compared to doxycycline or talc slurry injected through chest tubes for reducing recurrence rates. The effectiveness (and the cost) of medical thoracoscopy should be compared with VATS in patients with both primary and secondary spontaneous pneumothoraces. The effectiveness of mechanical pleural abrasion should be compared to that of partial parietal pleurectomy and other procedures advocated by some to produce a pleurodesis at the time of VATS. Lastly, the cost effectiveness of medical thoracos-

copy compared with tube thoracostomy with the instillation of a sclerosing agent at the time that a patient has an initial primary or secondary spontaneous pneumothorax should be compared.

References

1. Sadikot RT, Greene T, Meadows K, et al. Recurrence of primary spontaneous pneumothorax. *Thorax* 1997;52:805–809.
2. Smit HJ, Wienk MA, Schreurs AJ, et al. Do bullae indicate a predisposition to recurrent pneumothorax? *Br J Radiol* 2000;73:356–359.
3. Janssen JP, Schramel FM, Sutedja TG, et al. Videothoracoscopic appearance of first and recurrent pneumothorax. *Chest* 1995;108:330–334.
4. Gobbel WGJ, Rhea WGJ, Nelson IA, et al. Spontaneous pneumothorax. *J Thorac Cardiovasc Surg* 1963;46:331–345.
5. Guo Y, Xie C, Rodriguez RM, et al. Factors related to recurrence of spontaneous pneumothorax. *Respirology* 2005;10:379–384.
6. Light RW, O'Hara VS, Moritz TE, et al. Intrapleural tetracycline for the prevention of recurrent spontaneous pneumothorax. Results of a Department of Veterans Affairs cooperative study. *JAMA* 1990;264:2224–2230.
7. Lippert HL, Lund O, Blegvad S, et al. Independent risk factors for cumulative recurrence rate after first spontaneous pneumothorax. *Eur Respir J* 1991;4:324–331.
8. Almind M, Lange P, Viskum K. Spontaneous pneumothorax: comparison of simple drainage, talc pleurodesis, and tetracycline pleurodesis. *Thorax* 1989;44:627–630.
9. Alfageme I, Moreno L, Huetas C, et al. Spontaneous pneumothorax. Long-term results with tetracycline pleurodesis. *Chest* 1994;106:347–350.
10. Tschopp JM, Brutsche M, Frey JG. Treatment of complicated spontaneous pneumothorax by simple talc pleurodesis under thoracoscopy and local anaesthesia. *Thorax* 1997;52:329–332.
11. Tschopp JM, Boutin C, Astoul P, et al. Talcage by medical thoracoscopy for primary spontaneous pneumothorax is more cost-effective than drainage: a randomised study. *Eur Respir J* 2002;20:1003–1009.
12. Yim AP, Liu HP. Video assisted thoracoscopic management of primary spontaneous pneumothorax. *Surg Laparosc Endosc* 1997;7:236–240.
13. Cardillo G, Facciolo F, Giunti R, et al. Videothoracoscopic treatment of primary spontaneous pneumothorax: a 6-year experience. *Ann Thorac Surg* 2000;69:357–361.

14. Waller DA. Video-assisted thoracoscopic surgery for spontaneous pneumothorax – a 7-year learning experience. *Ann R Coll Surg Engl* 1999;81:387–392.

15. Margolis M, Gharagozloo F, Tempesta B, et al. Video-assisted thoracic surgical treatment of initial spontaneous pneumothorax in young patients. *Ann Thorac Surg* 2003;76:1661–1663.

16. Lee P, Yap WS, Pek WY, et al. An audit of medical thoracoscopy and talc poudrage for pneumothorax prevention in advanced COPD. *Chest* 2004;125:1315–1320.

17. Baumann MH, Strange C, Heffner JE, et al. Management of spontaneous pneumothorax: An American College of Chest Physicians Delphi Consensus Statement. *Chest* 2001;119:590–602.

18. Henry M, Arnold T, Harvey J. BTS guidelines for the management of spontaneous pneumothorax. *Thorax* 2003;58(suppl 2):II39–II52.

19. Light RW. Talc should not be used for pleurodesis. *Am J Respir Crit Care Med* 2000;162:2023–2026.

20. Dresler CM, Olak J, Herndon JE 2nd, et al. Phase III intergroup study of talc poudrage vs talc slurry sclerosis for malignant pleural effusion. *Chest* 2005;127:909–915.

21. Bilaceroglu S, Guo Y, Hawthorne ML, et al. Oral forms of tetracycline and doxycycline are effective in producing pleurodesis. *Chest* 2005;128:3750–3756.

22. Yim AP. Video-assisted thoracoscopic suturing of apical bullae. An alternative to staple resection in the management of primary spontaneous pneumothorax. *Surg Endosc* 1995;9:1013–1016.

23. Lee YCG, Teixeira LR, Devin CJ, et al. Transforming growth factor-beta(2) induces pleurodesis significantly faster than talc. *Am J Respir Crit Care Med* 2001;163:640–644.

Part 3
Esophagus

23
Staging for Esophageal Cancer: Positron Emission Tomography, Endoscopic Ultrasonography

Jarmo A. Salo

Survival rates in esophageal cancer are closely related to the stage of the disease at the beginning of treatment and the completeness of surgical R0 resection. Preoperative staging is reasonable only if it allows selection between different treatment options. Accurate pretreatment staging is critical for optimal choice of treatment. Today's stage-adjusted treatment of advanced esophageal cancers requires a meticulous diagnostic workup. Multimodal therapy may improve the outcome even in more advanced cases.[1–3] Hence, the exact role of positron emission tomography (PET) and endoscopic ultrasonography (EUS) in restaging after neoadjuvant treatment needs to be determined. In esophageal cancer, EUS represents the gold standard for T staging, crucial when less radical approaches, such as endoscopic mucosa resection or limited resection for early carcinoma, are considered.[4,5] Positron emission tomography is a promising new method based on changes in the glucose metabolism of cancer tissue. However, any advantage offered by PET in the staging of esophageal cancer is unclear, and its supplemental value in the routine clinical preoperative workup of esophageal cancer patients is unknown.

23.1. Positron Emission Tomography

Positron emission tomography is based on accumulation of fluorinated glucose analog (F-18 fluorodeoxyglucose) in malignant cells.[6] The method provides a means of detecting altered tissue metabolism in malignant tumors using a positron camera.[6] The sensitivity of PET in detecting primary esophageal carcinoma is high (level of evidence 2−).[7] Secondary primary neoplasms can sometimes also be diagnosed with PET.

PET does, however, have a low sensitivity in the diagnosis of small-volume tumors and metastases. Cancer T status, small metastatic lesions in locoregional lymph nodes, and intra-abdominal carcinomatosis are difficult to diagnose (level of evidence 2+ to 2−).[8–11] These diagnostic limitations are partially due to the spatial resolution of PET, which is only 6 mm. However, spatial resolution is not the sole limitation of PET because tumors of up to 30 mm (mean diameter, 13.5 mm) can occasionally go undetected.[8,9] Thus, the primary indication for PET is not diagnosis of esophageal cancers, especially small-volume carcinomas.

The sensitivity of PET in diagnosing loco-regional metastases is only 51% and the specificity is 84% (level of evidence 1−).[12] Therefore, PET is unsuitable for detecting loco-regional lymph node metastases (level of evidence 2−).[11] In fact, PET is inferior to EUS in this regard (level of evidence 2+).[8] PET's sensitivity and specificity in diagnosing distant lymph node metastases and hematogenous metastases are 67% and 97%, respectively.[11,12] Metastatic sites missed by PET are usually less than 1 cm in diameter.[11] In addition, peritoneal carcinomatosis is difficult to diagnose with this technique.[8] The accuracy of PET may be improved by the use of combined PET and computed tomography (CT; level of evidence 2–).[13] Only a few studies have investigated the ability of PET to diagnose cancer recurrence. In one report, PET gave additional information in 27% of cases (level of evidence 2+).[14]

The limitations of PET in detecting small carcinomas can, however, offer benefits in clinical practice. Patients with PET-detectable primary tumors are mostly unsuitable candidates for modern, less radical surgical approaches such as endoscopic mucosa resection or limited resection. Adding PET to standard staging improves detection of stage IV esophageal cancer, which is associated with poor survival (level of evidence 2–).[9–11,15,16] However, the modest sensitivity for distant lymph node metastases and the false-positive judgment of cervical and supraclavicular nodes must be taken into consideration. Positive PET findings in distant lymph nodes should be verified by histology or cytology before making a diagnosis of inoperability.[8,9]

23.2. PET in Restaging after Neoadjuvant Therapy

Positon emission tomography is a promising noninvasive tool for the assessment and prediction of pathological response in locally advanced esophageal cancer after neoadjuvant treatment.[17] The pathological response of an initially highly metabolic tumor correlates with the metabolic response in PET and provides additional information about the effect of treatment (level of evidence 2–).[18,19] In addition, the standardized uptake value of F-18 fluorodeoxyglucose may be used to predict tumor resectability (level of evidence 2+).[20] In a systematic review of the literature, PET and EUS offered an equally high accuracy after neoadjuvant treatment, but EUS was not always feasible (level of evidence 2+).[21] In restaging patients after neoadjuvant therapy, PET/CT may be more accurate than EUS-assisted fine needle aspiration (level of evidence 2–).[22]

23.3. Endoscopic Ultrasonography

Endoscropic ultrasonography provides a 360° view of all five to nine layers (depending on the feature of the probe) of the esophageal wall and paraesophageal tissues. Endoscopic ultrasonography is an effective method for detecting invasion depth of esophageal cancer and represents the gold standard for T staging (level of evidence 2–).[23–27] The accuracy of EUS in T staging ranges from 63% to 90%,[11,21,25,26,28] therefore being better than that of CT scans.[26] The EUS probes used and the depth of the tumor infiltration influence the accuracy, which is best in T4 tumors and worst in T1 and T2 tumors (level of evidence 2– to 1–).[25,26,29] The low accuracy achieved by standard lower-frequency ultrasound endoscopes in differentiating T1 (mucosal and submucosal cancer) and T2 may be increased to more than 90% with high-frequency ultrasound probes (level of evidence 2–).[30–32] This is very important when endoscopic mucosal resections or limited surgery are being considered. Although high-frequency miniprobes allow better superficial visualization, their drawback is limited depth of penetration. Evaluation of N stage should therefore be performed with conventional EUS (level of evidence 2–).[33] Overstaging is usually more common than understaging in EUS.[25] The most important weakness of EUS in investigating a malignant stenosis is that the large probe (dip diameter, 12–13mm) often cannot pass the tumor. In cases such as this, the accuracy is only half of that of traversable tumors (level of evidence 2–).[34] In addition, the evaluation of tracheal or bronchial infiltration is problematic due to air causing reflection of the ultrasonic waves.

The EUS procedure is based on the diameter, form, and echoic pattern being different in malignant and benign lymph nodes. Metastatic lymph nodes are typically larger than 10mm in diameter and have a round shape, sharp borders, and a uniform hypoechogenicity.[35] When all four of these characteristics are present, the accuracy of nodal involvement is supposed to be nearly 100% (level of evidence 2–).[36] However, the diagnostic accuracy of these findings is usually less than 80% (level of evidence 2– to 2+).[37,38] The reported higher accuracies of lymph node staging originate from studies including greatly advanced carcinomas with lymph node metastasis.

The loco-regional N staging can be improved (accuracy, sensitivity, and specificity >90%) by transmural EUS-assisted fine needle puncture cytology (level of evidence 2+).[39] In the diagnosis of distant metastases especially, the ability to confirm malignant involvement of celiac axis lymph nodes (M1 disease) is important (level of evidence 2−).[40] In distant metastasis outside the celiac axis, the role of EUS is rather limited.

23.4. EUS in Restaging after Neoadjuvant Treatment

Restaging of esophageal cancer with EUS after neoadjuvant treatment is often difficult because scars and inflammation cannot be distinguished from the primary tumor. Volume reduction of the tumor may be present but is not distinguishable with EUS. This leads to overstaging as well as to understaging because microscopic foci of residual tumor within the esophageal wall are common. After neoadjuvant treatment, the T-stage accuracy with EUS has been found to vary from 27% to 73% and the N-stage accuracy from 38% to 71% (level of evidence 2− to 2+).[41–43] Recently, the proportion of reduction of maximal tumor thickness exceeding 30% with EUS was reported to correctly predict 94% of responders (level of evidence 2−).[44] The postoperative detection of local tumor recurrence by EUS is also difficult because of anatomical changes and scars.

23.5. Summary

The sensitivity of PET in detecting primary esophageal carcinoma is high. Positron emission tomography has, however, a low sensitivity in the diagnosis of small-volume (less than 5mm in diameter) tumors, metastases, and intra-abdominal carcinomatosis. Therefore, PET is unsuitable for detecting loco-regional lymph node metastases and is inferior to EUS for this purpose (level of evidence 2− to 1−; recommendation grade B). PET's sensitivity and specificity in diagnosing distant lymph node metastases and hematogenous metastases are 67% and 97%, respectively. Adding PET to standard staging improves detection of stage IV esophageal cancer, which is associated with poor survival (level of evidence 2−; recommendation grade C).

> Positron emission tompgraphy is unsuitable for detecting loco-regional lymph node metastases and is inferior to EUS for this purpose (level of evidence 1− to 2−; recommendation grade B).
>
> Adding PET to standard staging improves detection of stage IV esophageal cancer, which is associated with poor survival (level of evidence 2−; recommendation grade C).

Endoscopic ultrasonography is an effective method for detecting invasion depth of esophageal cancer and represents the gold standard for T staging. The accuracy of EUS in T staging ranges from 63% to 90%, therefore being better than that of CT scans (level of evidence 2−; recommendation grade C). The most important weakness of EUS in investigating a malignant stenosis is that the large probe (tip diameter, 12–13mm) often cannot pass the tumor. In restaging patients after neoadjuvant therapy the T-stage accuracy with EUS has been found to vary from 27% to 73% and the N-stage accuracy from 38% to 71%. In restaging patients after neoadjuvant therapy, PET/CT may be more accurate than EUS-assisted fine needle aspiration (level of evidence 2−; recommendation grade C).

> Endoscopic ultrasonography is an effective method for detecting invasion depth of esophageal cancer and represents the gold standard for T staging (level of evidence 2−; recommendation grade C).
>
> In restaging patients after neoadjuvant therapy, PET/CT is more accurate than EUS-assisted fine needle aspiration (level of evidence 2−; recommendation grade C).

23.6. Personal View

In routine clinical practice, EUS is an essential tool in planning treatment strategy for most patients with esophageal cancer. Ascertaining the exact T stage of the tumor with mucosal or submucosal infiltration is important before deciding the extent of resection (mucosal or limited resection, or radical surgery with lymphadenectomy). Endoscopic ultrasonography is more suitable than PET in diagnosing metastatic loco-regional lymph nodes, findings of which indicate consideration of neoadjuvant treatment. Use of EUS is not advisable in the diagnosis of distant metastasis, in restaging after neoadjuvant therapy, or in postoperative situations.

Today, we use PET in preoperative staging of most patients with esophageal cancer despite not knowing its actual value in preventing unnecessary resections or its cost effectiveness. Positron emission tompgraphy does help to diagnose inoperative stage IV cancer and should thus be performed at least in patients with operative risk factors. On the other hand, positive findings in PET suggesting distant metastases in operable patients should be confirmed by cytology or histology, particularly in cases where CT and EUS have negative findings. In restaging after neoadjuvant treatment, in spite of a few sound studies, PET is not yet used to discriminate between responders and nonresponders because of the lack of standardization in cutoff values.

References

1. Ajani JA, Komaki R, Putnam JB, et al. A three-step strategy of induction chemotherapy then chemoradiation followed by surgery in patients with potentially resectable carcinoma of the esophagus or gastroesophageal junction. *Cancer* 2001;92:279–286.
2. Walsh TN, Noonan N, Hollywood D, et al. A comparison of multimodal therapy and surgery for esophageal adenocarcinoma. *N Engl J Med* 1996;335:462–467.
3. Lew JI, Gooding WE, Ribeiro U Jr, et al. Long-term survival following induction chemoradiotherapy and esophagectomy for esophageal carcinoma. *Arch Surg* 2001;136:737–742; discussion 743.
4. Stein HJ, Feith M, Mueller J, et al. Limited resection for early adenocarcinoma in Barrett's esophagus. *Ann Surg* 2000;232:733–742.
5. Ell C, May A, Gossner L, et al. Endoscopic mucosal resection of early cancer and high-grade dysplasia in Barrett's esophagus. *Gastroenterology* 2000;118:670–677.
6. Pauwels EK, McCready VR, Stoot JH, et al. The mechanism of accumulation of tumour-localising radiopharmaceuticals. *Eur J Nucl Med* 1998;25:277–305.
7. Kim K, Park SJ, Kim BT, et al. Evaluation of lymph node metastases in squamous cell carcinoma of the esophagus with positron emission tomography. *Ann Thorac Surg* 2001;71:290–294.
8. Rasanen JV, Sihvo EIT, Knuuti MJ, et al. Prospective analysis of accuracy of positron emission tomography, computed tomography, and endoscopic ultrasonography in staging of adenocarcinoma of the esophagus and the esophagogastric junction. *Ann Surg Oncol* 2003;10:954–960.
9. Sihvo EIT, Rasanen JV, Knuuti MJ, et al. Adenocarcinoma of the esophagus and the esophagogastric junction: positron emission tomography improves staging and prediction of survival in distant but not in locoregional disease. *J Gastrointest Surg* 2004;8:988–996.
10. Flanagan FL, Dehdashti F, Siegel BA, et al. Staging of esophageal cancer with 18F-fluorodeoxyglucose positron emission tomography. *AJR Am J Roentgenol* 1997;168:417–424.
11. Flamen P, Lerut A, Van Cutsem E, et al. Utility of positron emission tomography for the staging of patients with potentially operable esophageal carcinoma. *J Clin Oncol* 2000;18:3202–3210.
12. van Westreenen HL, Westerterp M, Bossuyt PMM, et al. Systematic review of the staging performance of 18F-fluorodeoxyglucose positron emission tomography in esophageal cancer. *J Clin Oncol* 2004;22:3805–3812.
13. Bar-Shalom R, Guralnik L, Tsalic M, et al. The additional value of PET/CT over PET in FDG imaging of oesophageal cancer. *Eur J Nucl Med Mol Imaging* 2005;32:918–924.
14. Flamen P, Lerut A, Van Cutsem E, et al. The utility of positron emission tomography for the diagnosis and staging of recurrent esophageal cancer. *J Thorac Cardiovasc Surg* 2000;120:1085–1092.
15. Kole AC, Plukker JT, Nieweg OE, et al. Positron emission tomography for staging of oesophageal and gastroesophageal malignancy. *Br J Cancer* 1998;78:521–527.
16. Rankin SC, Taylor H, Cook GJ, et al. Computed tomography and positron emission tomography in the pre-operative staging of oesophageal carcinoma. *Clin Radiol* 1998;53:659–665.
17. Kato H, Kuwano H, Nakajima M, et al. Usefulness of positron emission tomography for assessing the response of neoadjuvant chemoradiotherapy in patients with esophageal cancer. *Am J Surg* 2002;184:279–283.
18. Brucher BL, Weber W, Bauer M, et al. Neoadjuvant therapy of esophageal squamous cell carcinoma: response evaluation by positron emission tomography. *Ann Surg* 2001;233:300–309.
19. Song SY, Kim JH, Ryu JS, et al. FDG-PET in the prediction of pathologic response after neoadju-

vant chemoradiotherapy in locally advanced, resectable esophageal cancer. *Int J Radiat Oncol Biol Phys* 2005;63:1053–1059.

20. van Westgreenen HL, Plukker JT, Cobben DC, et al. Prognostic value of the standardized uptake value in esophageal cancer. *AJR Am J Roentgenol* 2005;185:436–440.

21. Westerterp M, van Westreenen HL, Reitsma JB, et al. Esophageal cancer: CT, endoscopic US, and FDG PET for assessment of response to neoadjuvant therapy – systematic review. *Radiology* 2005;236:841–851.

22. Cerfolio RJ, Bryant AS, Ohja B, et al. The accuracy of endoscopic ultrasonography with fine-needle aspiration, integrated positron emission tomography with computed tomography, and computed tomography in restaging patients with esophageal cancer after neoadjuvant chemoradiotherapy. *J Thorac Cardiovasc Surg* 2005;129:1232–1241.

23. Richards DG, Brown TH, Manson JM. Endoscopic ultrasound in the staging of tumours of the oesophagus and gastro-oesophageal junction. *Ann R Coll Surg Engl* 2000;82:311–317.

24. Botet JF, Lightdale CJ, Zauber AG, et al. Preoperative staging of gastric cancer: comparison of endoscopic US and dynamic CT. *Radiology* 1991;181:426–432.

25. Salminen JT, Farkkila MA, Ramo OJ, et al. Endoscopic ultrasonography in the preoperative staging of adenocarcinoma of the distal oesophagus and oesophagogastric junction. *Scand J Gastroenterol* 1999;34:1178–1182.

26. Rosch T. Endosonographic staging of esophageal cancer: a review of literature results. *Gastrointest Endosc Clin N Am* 1995;5:549–557.

27. Vickers J, Alderson D. Influence of luminal obstruction on oesophageal cancer staging using endoscopic ultrasonography. *Br J Surg* 1998;85:999–1001.

28. Luketich JD, Schauer P, Landreneau R, et al. Minimally invasive surgical staging is superior to endoscopic ultrasound in detecting lymph node metastases in esophageal cancer. *J Thorac Cardiovasc Surg* 1997;114:817–821; discussion 821–823.

29. Saunders HS, Wolfman NT. Esophageal cancer [review]. *Radiologic Staging* 1997;35:281–294.

30. Hasegawa N, Niwa Y, Arisawa T, et al. Preoperative staging of superficial esophageal carcinoma: comparison of an ultrasound probe and standard endoscopic ultrasonosgraphy. *Gastrointest Endosc* 1996;44:388–393.

31. Inoue H, Kawano T, Takeshita K, et al. Modified soft-balloon methods during ultrasonic probe examination for superficial esophageal cancer. *Endoscopy* 1998;30(suppl 1):A41–A43.

32. Murata Y, Suzuki S, Ohta M, et al. Small ultrasonic probes for determination of the depth of superficial esophageal cancer. *Gastrointest Endosc* 1996;44:23–28.

33. Menzel J, Domschke W. Gastrointestinal miniprobe sonography: the current status. *Am J Gastroenterol* 2000;95:605–616.

34. Hordijk ML, Zander H, van Blankenstin M, et al. Influence of tumor stenosis on the accuracy of endosonography in preoperative T staging of esophageal cancer. *Endoscopy* 1993;25:171–175.

35. Tio TL, Coene PP, den Hartog Jager FC, et al. Preoperative TNM classification of esophageal carcinoma by endosonography. *Hepatogastroenterology* 1990;37:376–381.

36. Catalano MF, Sivak MV Jr, Rice T, et al. Endosonographic features predictive of lymph node metastasis. *Gastrointest Endosc* 1994;40:442–446.

37. Kelly S, Harris KM, Berry E, et al. A systematic review of the staging performance of endoscopic ultrasound in gastro-oesophageal carcinoma. *Gut* 2001;49:534–539.

38. Monig SP, Schroder W, Baldus SE, et al. Preoperative lymph-node staging in gastrointestinal cancer—correlation between size and tumor stage. *Onkologie* 2002;25:342–344.

39. Wiersema MJ, Vilmann P, Giovanni M, et al. Endosonography-guided fine-needle aspiration biopsy: diagnostic accuracy and complication assessment. *Gastroenterology* 1997;112:1087–1095.

40. Eloubeidi MA, Wallace MB, Reed CE, et al. The utility of EUS and EUS-guided fine needle aspiration in detecting celiac lymph node metastasis in patients with esophageal cancer: a single center experience. *Gastrointest Endosc* 2001;54:714–719.

41. Lightdale CJ, Kulkarni KG. Role of endoscopic ultrasonography in the staging and follow-up of esophageal cancer. *J Clin Oncol* 2005;23:4483–4489.

42. Hirata N, Kawamoto K, Ueyama T, et al. Using endosonography to assess the effects of neoadjuvant therapy in patients with advanced esophageal cancer. *AJR Am J Roentgenol* 1997;169:485–491.

43. Isenberg G, Chak A, Canto MI, et al. Endosonographic ultrasound in restaging of esophageal cancer after neoadjuvant chemoradiation. *Gastrointest Endosc* 1998;48:158–163.

44. Ota M, Murata Y, Ide H, et al. Useful endoscopic ultrasonography to assess the efficacy of neoadjuvant therapy for advanced esophageal carcinoma: based on the response evaluation criteria in solid tumors. *Dig Endosc* 2005;17:59–63.

24
Induction Therapy for Resectable Esophageal Cancer

Sarah E. Greer, Philip P. Goodney, and John E. Sutton

Despite advances in treatment regimens, overall 5-year survival rates for esophageal cancer remain low, averaging less than 30%.[1-5] Although surgery remains the standard treatment and the only hope for cure, there is growing support for multimodality therapy.

While there has been little significant progress in improving overall survival in esophageal cancer despite new chemotherapeutics and surgical techniques, induction chemotherapy and/or radiotherapy followed by surgery offers several potential advantages over surgery with or without adjuvant treatment.

First, up-front chemotherapy and radiation may be better tolerated than therapy following extensive surgery. Second, a preoperative strategy allows those with occult distant disease to declare themselves, avoiding delay in systemic treatment for micrometastases as well as avoiding major surgical procedures which may not be curative. Third, preoperative therapy allows delivery of chemotherapy or radiation to a relatively well-perfused tumor bed, thus improving its efficacy. It may also cause sufficient tumor destruction, particularly at the periphery, to improve resectability. By increasing the likelihood of a margin-negative resection, induction therapy may improve local control.

However, there are disadvantages to induction therapy. Preoperative treatment is associated with significant morbidity and mortality. In attempts to minimize this toxicity, especially in preoperative combination therapy with chemotherapy and radiation, dose reductions may be necessary, potentially compromising the efficacy of the treatment. Definitive local control is also delayed, which may be an important clinical consideration in patients who are symptomatic with dysphagia and poor preoperative nutritional status.

24.1. Published Evidence

24.1.1. Preoperative Radiotherapy

While preoperative radiation (without chemotherapy) has been studied in the past, it failed to show a benefit for overall survival, and in many cases[6-8] proved to increase the morbidity and mortality associated with treatment. For these reasons, more recent trials have evaluated preoperative radiation only in combination with chemotherapy.

24.1.1.1. Randomized, Controlled Trials

At least six randomized trials comparing preoperative radiotherapy and surgery with surgery alone for esophageal carcinoma have been performed.[6-11] Radiotherapy regimens varied, with low-to-moderate doses ranging from 20Gy to 53Gy over a period of 1 to 4 weeks prior to surgery. Accrual of patients in randomized, controlled trials of preoperative radiotherapy took place prior to 1989 (Table 24.1).

No statistically significant survival benefit for groups receiving preoperative radiotherapy was seen. In fact, some studies found a small reduction in overall survival following preoperative radiotherapy, which may have been due in part to

TABLE 24.1. Single modality induction therapy – randomized, controlled trials of preoperative chemotherapy or radiation versus surgery alone.

Author and year	Study type	Type of cancer	Accrual	Level of evidence	Treatment groups	Patients enrolled	Median survival (months)	OS 1 year	OS 2 year	OS 3 year	OS 4 year	OS 5 year	Statistical significance
Launois et al.[6] 1981	RCT	Squamous	1973–1976	1+	40-Gy / Surgery	67	4.5	46	20	15	14	10	p=ns
Gignoux et al.[7] 1987	RCT	Squamous	1976–1982	1+	Surgery alone	57	8.2 (mean)	50	35	25	20	12	p=0.94
					33-Gy / Surgery	115	12.3	55	24	20	17	10	
Wang et al.[9] 1989	RCT	Squamous	1977–1985	1+	40-Gy / Surgery	114	12 (mean)	57	30	14	11	9	p=ns
					Surgery	104						35	
Nygaard et al.[11] 1992	RCT	Squamous	1983–1988	1−	Surgery alone	102							p=0.08
					35-Gy / Surgery	58	10	44	25	21		30	
Arnott et al.[12] 1992	RCT	Squamous / Adenocarcinoma	1979–1983	1+	Surgery alone	50	7	34	13	9	9	9	p=0.4
					20-Gy / Surgery	90	8	40	22	13			
Fok et al.[8] 1994	RCT	Squamous	1968–1981	1+*	Surgery alone	86	8	40	28	23	21	17	p=ns
					24–53-Gy / Surgery	40	11	42	34	24	10	10	
Nygaard et al.[11] 1992	RCT	Squamous	1983–1988	1−	Surgery alone	39	22	58	36	24	16	16	p=ns
					Cisplatin, bleomycin / Surgery	56	7	31	6	3			
Schlag et al.[17] 1992	RCT	Squamous		1+	Surgery alone	50	7	34	13	9			p=ns
					Cisplatin, 5-FU / Surgery	22	7.5	20					
Maipang et al.[18] 1994	RCT	Squamous	1988–1990	1+	Surgery alone	24	5	32	31				p=ns
					Cisplatin, vinblastin, bleomycin / Surgery	24	17	58		31			
Law et al.[22] 1997	RCT	Squamous	1989–1995	1+	Surgery alone	22	17	85	40	36	28	28	p=ns
					Cisplatin, 5-FU / Surgery	74	16.8	60	44	38			
Ancona et al.[19] 2001	RCT	Squamous	1992–1997	1+	Surgery alone	73	13	50	31	14	14		p=0.55
					Cisplatin, 5-FU / Surgery	47	25	75	55	44	42	34	
MRC 2002	RCT	Squamous / Adenocarcinoma	1992–1998	1++	Surgery alone	400	16.8	75	55	41	38	22	p=0.004; HR=0.79 (95% CI, 0.67–0.93)
					Cisplatin, 5-FU / Surgery	402	13.3	59	43	35	28	26	
					Surgery			54	34	27	20	15	

Abbreviations: 5-FU, 5 fluoro uracil; ns, not significant; RCT, randomized controlled trial; MRC = Medical Research Council.

treatment related mortality that exceeded 20% in some trials.[6-8]

24.1.1.2. Meta-analyses

Because the number of patients treated in clinical trials was small, a Cochrane Review meta-analysis was performed using individual patient data to determine conclusively whether there is any effect for preoperative radiotherapy.[12] This study included 1147 patients with updated survival data and a median follow-up of 9 years. The overall hazard ratio was 0.89 [$\chi^2(1) = 3.48$, $p = 0.06$], suggesting a trend towards a modest benefit for preoperative radiotherapy, but with a small absolute improvement in survival of 4% at 5 years.

A second meta-analysis was performed by Malthaner and colleagues.[13] Again, no statistically significant difference in the risk of mortality with preoperative radiotherapy compared with surgery alone was detected [relative risk (RR) = 1.01; 95% confidence interval (95% CI), 0.88–1.16; $p = 0.87$], but overall survival was evaluated only at 1 year.

24.1.1.3. Systematic Reviews

A number of systematic reviews also address the clinical question of the efficacy of preoperative radiotherapy in resectable esophageal cancer.[13-16] These reviews uniformly conclude that there is no benefit from preoperative radiotherapy with respect to resectability, treatment-related mortality, or overall survival as demonstrated by randomized, clinical trials.

24.1.1.4. Recommendation

It appears unlikely that single-modality preoperative therapy with radiation will be resurrected as a meaningful therapeutic option with curative intent. Given the body of work available, as a guideline for clinical practice, we recommend against the use of preoperative radiotherapy as standard of care, with a grade A for the level of recommendation.

> There is no benefit to preoperative radiotherapy as standard of care in the management of resectable esophageal cancer (level of evidence 1; recommendation grade A).

24.1.2. Preoperative Chemotherapy

Preoperative chemotherapy initially appeared more promising than preoperative radiotherapy. However, following multiple randomized trials and meta-analyses, no overall survival benefit has been shown for preoperative chemotherapy, with one exception. A wide variety of chemotherapeutic agents have been studied, including cisplatin, fluorouracil, leucovorin, paclitaxel, vinblastin, etoposide, epirubicin, mitomycin, and bleomycin. While most trials enrolled patients with squamous cell carcinoma,[17-19] the largest studies included both squamous cell and adenocarcinoma.[20,21] Accrual of patients occurred between 1983 and 1998 (Table 24.1).

24.1.2.1. Randomized, Controlled Trials

At least six randomized trials of preoperative chemotherapy and surgery versus surgery alone have been performed.[11,17-20,22] Five of the six showed no significant survival benefit.[11,17-19,22] However, a large multicenter study including both squamous cell and adenocarcinoma showed improved results using a regimen of fluorouracil and cisplatin in the arm receiving induction therapy.[20] The investigators reported a median survival of 16.8 months versus 13.3 months (difference, 107 days; 95% CI, 30–196), and 2-year survival of 43% and 34% (difference, 9%; 95% CI, 3–14) in the group receiving chemotherapy. Estimated 5-year survival based on Kaplan–Meier curves was also significantly improved (hazard ratio 0.79; 95% CI, 0.67–0.93); estimated reduction in risk of death was 21%.

Two additional randomized clinical trials examined preoperative chemotherapy and found no statistically significant difference in overall survival. However, in these two trials patients in the induction therapy arm also received postoperative chemotherapy.[21,23] One of these trials[21] included the same chemotherapeutics, at higher doses, that showed a survival benefit in the trial described above.[20] It is difficult to reconcile these results, but a more intense chemotherapy regimen could have adversely affected the outcome in the induction therapy arm in the latter trial.

24.1.2.2. Meta-analyses

Four meta-analyses have been performed examining preoperative chemotherapy versus surgery alone,[13,24-26] with only one showing a significant improvement in survival.

The meta-analysis by Urschel and colleagues[25] included 1976 patients from 11 randomized, controlled trials and found no statistically significant difference between preoperative chemotherapy with surgery over surgery alone for survival at 1, 2, or 3 years. A Cochrane Review meta-analysis[26] included 2051 patients from 11 trials and calculated the relative risk for survival at 1, 2, 3, 4, and 5 years. A statistically significant difference in survival for patients who received preoperative chemotherapy was detected only at 5 years (RR = 1.44; 95% CI, 1.05–1.97; $p = 0.02$). However, both of these analyses included trials that used postoperative chemotherapy in addition to preoperative treatment.

Bhansali and colleagues[24] analyzed eight randomized controlled trials and found an odds ratio for risk of death of 0.96 (95% CI, 0.75–1.22). The systematic review and meta-analysis performed by Malthaner and coworkers[13] included a total of 1241 patients from six trials that studied only preoperative chemotherapy versus surgery alone, and showed no survival benefit at 1 year (RR = 1.00; 95% CI, 0.83–1.19; $p = 0.98$).

24.1.2.3. Systematic Reviews

A number of systematic reviews address the efficacy of preoperative chemotherapy in resectable esophageal cancer.[13-16] The majority of these reviews conclude that despite the benefit seen in the most recent large randomized trial,[20] there is not yet sufficient evidence to institute preoperative chemotherapy as standard of care.

24.1.2.4. Recommendation

For patients with resectable esophageal cancer for whom surgery is considered appropriate, we recommend surgery alone (without preoperative chemotherapy) as standard practice, with a grade of A for level of recommendation.

> For patients with resectable esophageal cancer for whom surgery is considered appropriate, surgery alone (without preoperative chemotherapy) is standard practice (level of evidence 1; recommendation grade A).

24.1.3. Preoperative Chemoradiotherapy

The preoperative therapy that has shown the most promise and has generated much interest is combination chemotherapy and radiation. In fact, despite a lack of definitive evidence, it has become the de facto standard of care at many institutions.

Six randomized trials compared preoperative chemoradiotherapy to surgery alone.[11,27-31] These trials have been small, thus limiting the power of each study to detect differences in overall survival. Furthermore, the design, therapeutic regimens, surgical approaches, and histologies varied widely across studies, making comparison of the trials difficult. Accrual of patients occurred between 1983 and 1995 (Table 24.2).

24.1.3.1. Randomized, Controlled Trials

Five of the six trials failed to show a statistically significant benefit in overall survival for the groups receiving preoperative chemoradiotherapy.

Initial results reported high treatment-related mortality of more than three times that of surgery alone in one trial,[28] and exceeding 24% in another.[11] Lack of stratification by stage and unequal distribution of patients makes results difficult to interpret.[11] Inadequate power to detect small differences also plagued many studies. Patient accrual based on promising large differences between phase II studies and historical controls that ultimately failed to show a statistically significant survival benefit may simply be due to type II error.

The one trial that has shown a significant survival benefit included both squamous cell and adenocarcinoma, and used various techniques for surgical resection.[31] The authors found a 3-year survival of 32% in the group who received preoperative chemoradiotherapy versus 6% in the surgery alone arm ($p = 0.01$), with a median

TABLE 24.2. Multimodality induction therapy – randomized, controlled trials of preoperative chemoradiation versus surgery alone.

Author and year	Study type	Type of cancer	Accrual	Level of evidence	Treatment groups	Patients enrolled	Median survival (months)	Overall survival (percentage)					Statistical significance
								1 year	2 year	3 year	4 year	5 year	
Nygaard et al. 1992	RCT	Squamous	1983–1988	1–	Cisplatin, bleomycin, 35-Gy Surgery	53	7	39	23	17			p = 0.3
					Surgery alone	50	7	34	13	9			
Apinop et al. 1994	RCT	Squamous	1986–1992	1+	Cisplatin, 5-FU 40-Gy Surgery	35	9.7	49	30	26	24	24	p = 0.4
					Surgery alone	34	7.4	39	23	20	19	10	
LePrise et al. 1994	RCT	Squamous	1988–1991	1+	Cisplatin, 5-FU 20-Gy Surgery	41	11	47	27	19			p = 0.56
					Surgery alone	45	11	47	33	14			
Walsh et al. 1996	RCT	Adenocarcinoma	1990–1995	1–	Cisplatin, 5-FU 40-Gy Surgery	58	16	52	37	32			p = 0.01
					Surgery alone	55	11	44	26	6			
Bossert et al. 1997	RCT	Squamous	1989–1995	1+	Cisplatin 37-Gy Surgery	143	18.6	69	48	39	35	33	p = 0.78
					Surgery alone	139	18.6	67	43	37	34	32	
Urba et al. 2001	RCT	Squamous Adenocarcinoma	1989–1994	1++	Cisplatin, 5-FU 45-Gy Surgery	50	17.6	72	42	30	25	20	p = 0.15
					Surgery alone	50	16.9	58	38	16	14	10	

5-FU, 5 fluoro uracil; RCT, randomized, controlled trial.

follow-up of 11 months. However, the 6% 3-year survival in the control arm was lower than other published survival rates for surgery alone, with most centers reporting between 20% and 30% 3-year survival. Only after patients had received preoperative chemoradiotherapy and were re-evaluated was stage reported. This may have resulted in an overall downstaging of patients in the NCRT group and a false impression that patients in the surgery alone arm had more advanced disease. Uncertainty regarding the true baseline characteristics of patients limits our ability to interpret the effect of preoperative stage on outcome. However, despite these problems, the cited benefit in this trial carried a significant impact and widely influenced clinical practice. A 5-year follow-up study was also published with the finding of a significantly improved median survival from 12 months for surgery alone to 17 months for multimodal therapy ($p = 0.002$).[32]

24.1.3.2. Meta-analyses

A meta-analysis by Urschel and colleagues[33] included 1116 patients from nine randomized clinical trials, though three had been published only in abstract form. There was no statistically significant difference in 1-year or 2-year survival. However, a statistically significant improvement in 3-year survival was found for the group receiving preoperative chemoradiation [odds ratio (OR) = 0.66; 95% CI, 0.47–0.92; $p = 0.016$].

A meta-analysis by Malthaner and coworkers[13] included 753 patients in six trials. No significant difference in the 1-year survival for preoperative chemoradiation and surgery compared to surgery alone was detected. However, at 3 years a statistically significant difference in the risk of mortality was found favoring neoadjuvant chemoradiation (RR = 0.87; 95% CI, 0.80–0.96, $p = 0.004$).

In the meta-analysis by Fiorica and coworkers,[34] 3-year survival was improved in the group receiving preoperative chemoradiotherapy (OR 0.53; 95% CI, 0.31–0.93, $p = 0.03$), but the magnitude of the benefit was small. Two other meta-analyses showed a trend towards improved survival with preoperative chemoradiotherapy, but which failed to reach statistically significant benefit.[35,36]

24.1.3.3. Systematic Reviews

Based on the body of evidence available and lack of consistently demonstrated survival benefit, systematic reviews have recommended against using preoperative chemoradiotherapy as standard of care.[13–15]

24.1.3.4. Recommendation

For patients with resectable esophageal cancer for whom surgery is considered appropriate, surgery alone (without preoperative chemoradiotherapy) is recommended as standard practice, with a grade of A for level of recommendation.

> For patients with resectable esophageal cancer for whom surgery is considered appropriate, surgery alone (without preoperative chemoradiotherapy) is standard practice (level of evidence 1; recommendation grade A).

24.1.4. Other Treatments

24.1.4.1. Combinations of Neoadjuvant and Adjuvant Therapy

Because the design of clinical trials has varied substantially with respect to comparisons of neoadjuvant or adjuvant therapy versus surgery alone or one regimen versus another, Malthaner and colleagues performed a systematic review and meta-analysis of 12 such combinations.[13] None were found to be superior, and the authors concluded that surgery alone should remain the standard of care for treatment of resectable esophageal cancer.

24.1.4.2. Hyperthermia

A novel modality in esophageal carcinoma that has been shown to have a role in the treatment of other cancers, such as peritoneal malignancies and melanoma, is hyperthermia.[37–39] When studied in combination with preoperative chemoradiotherapy versus preoperative chemoradiotherapy alone, the 3-year survival was doubled in one trial.[40] While these results bear further investigation, this modality may provide renewed enthusiasm for induction therapy.

24.2. Impact on Clinical Practice

Every patient deserves an optimistic surgeon. However, this optimism must be tempered by first principles, namely, to do no harm.

While it is difficult to dismiss the theoretical advantages of induction therapy, there is currently not sufficient evidence to recommend its use as standard practice. Furthermore, the increased cost as well as quality of life associated with chemotherapy and radiation must be considered in judging the clinical significance of the small survival benefits that have been shown in a few cases.

However, as new chemotherapeutic agents become available, and as improvements in molecular diagnostics allow for more careful patient selection, there may be a role for further study of induction therapy. Thus it is crucial to maintain clinical equipoise.

The question that lies at the heart of proper utilization of evidenced-based medicine, is "how much evidence is enough?" In the face of multiple negative studies, is one well-designed positive trial sufficient to be paradigm shifting? Although improved methodologies have been developed for categorizing data, evaluating trials, and creating guidelines, there is no clear answer to these questions. In the context of continuing to strive for advances in scientific knowledge, we must remember that medicine is a profoundly human profession – at the end of the day, it is the competent and compassionate clinician who must understand the intersection between scientific evidence and individual values in order to lead a patient to an informed decision.

References

1. *SEER Cancer Statistics Review, 1973–1999*. Bethesda, MD: National Cancer Institute, 2002. Available from: http://seer.cancer.gov/csr/1973_1999.
2. Parker SL, Tong T, Bolden S, Wingo PA. Cancer statistics, 1997. *CA Cancer J Clin* 1997;47:5–27.
3. Wingo PA, Ries LA, Parker SL, Heath CW Jr. Long-term cancer patient survival in the United States. *Cancer Epidemiol Biomarkers Prev* 1998;7:271–282.
4. Farrow DC, Vaughan TL. Determinants of survival following the diagnosis of esophageal adeno-
carcinoma (United States). *Cancer Causes Control* 1996;7:322–327.
5. Thomas RM, Sobin LH. Gastrointestinal cancer. *Cancer* 1995;75(suppl 1):154–170.
6. Launois B, Delarue D, Campion JP, Kerbaol M. Preoperative radiotherapy for carcinoma of the esophagus. *Surg Gynecol Obstet* 1981;153:690–692.
7. Gignoux M, Roussel A, Paillot B, et al. The value of preoperative radiotherapy in esophageal cancer: results of a study of the E.O.R.T.C. *World J Surg* 1987;11:426–432.
8. Fok M, McShane J, Law S, Wong J. Prospective randomised study in the treatment of oesophageal carcinoma. *Aust N Z J Surg* 1994;17:223–229.
9. Wang M, Gu XZ, Yin WB, Huang GJ, Wang LJ, Zhang DW. Randomized clinical trial on the combination of preoperative irradiation and surgery in the treatment of esophageal carcinoma: report on 206 patients. *Int J Radiat Oncol Biol Phys* 1989;16:325–327.
10. Arnott SJ, Duncan W, Kerr GR, et al. Low dose preoperative radiotherapy for carcinoma of the oesophagus: results of a randomized clinical trial. *Radiother Oncol* 1992;24:108–113.
11. Nygaard K, Hagen S, Hansen HS, et al. Pre-operative radiotherapy prolongs survival in operable esophageal carcinoma: a randomized, multicenter study of pre-operative radiotherapy and chemotherapy. The second Scandinavian trial in esophageal cancer. *World J Surg* 1992;16:1104–1109.
12. Arnott SJ, Duncan W, Gignoux M, et al. Preoperative radiotherapy in esophageal carcinoma: a meta-analysis using individual patient data (Oesophageal Cancer Collaborative Group). *Int J Radiat Oncol Biol Phys* 1998;41:579–583.
13. Malthaner RA, Wong RK, Rumble RB, Zuraw L. Neoadjuvant or adjuvant therapy for resectable esophageal cancer: a systematic review and meta-analysis. *BMC Med* 2004;2:35.
14. Law S, Wong J. Current management of esophageal cancer. *J Gastrointest Surg* 2005;9:291–310.
15. Visser BC, Venook AP, Patti MG. Adjuvant and neoadjuvant therapy for esophageal cancer: a critical reappraisal. *Surg Oncol* 2003;12:1–7.
16. Lehnert T. Multimodal therapy for squamous carcinoma of the oesophagus. *Br J Surg* 1999;86:727–739.
17. Schlag P. [Randomized study of preoperative chemotherapy in squamous cell cancer of the esophagus. CAO Esophageal Cancer Study Group]. *Chirurg* 1992;63:709–714.
18. Maipang T, Vasinanukorn P, Petpichetchian C, et al. Induction chemotherapy in the treatment of

patients with carcinoma of the esophagus. *J Surg Oncol* 1994;56:191–197.

19. Ancona E, Ruol A, Santi S, et al. Only pathologic complete response to neoadjuvant chemotherapy improves significantly the long term survival of patients with resectable esophageal squamous cell carcinoma: final report of a randomized, controlled trial of preoperative chemotherapy versus surgery alone. *Cancer* 2001;91:2165–2174.

20. A comparison of chemotherapy and radiotherapy as adjuvant treatment to surgery for esophageal carcinoma. Japanese Esophageal Oncology Group. *Chest* 1993;104:203–207.

21. Kelsen DP, Ginsberg R, Pajak TF, et al. Chemotherapy followed by surgery compared with surgery alone for localized esophageal cancer. *N Engl J Med* 1998;339:1979–1984.

22. Law S, Fok M, Chow S, Chu KM, Wong J. Preoperative chemotherapy versus surgical therapy alone for squamous cell carcinoma of the esophagus: a prospective randomized trial. *J Thorac Cardiovasc Surg* 1997;114:210–217.

23. Roth JA, Pass HI, Flanagan MM, Graeber GM, Rosenberg JC, Steinberg S. Randomized clinical trial of preoperative and postoperative adjuvant chemotherapy with cisplatin, vindesine, and bleomycin for carcinoma of the esophagus. *J Thorac Cardiovasc Surg* 1988;96:242–248.

24. Bhansali MS, Vaidya JS, Bhatt RG, Patil PK, Badwe RA, Desai PB. Chemotherapy for carcinoma of the esophagus: a comparison of evidence from meta-analyses of randomized trials and of historical control studies. *Ann Oncol* 1996;7:355–359.

25. Urschel JD, Vasan H, Blewett CJ. A meta-analysis of randomized controlled trials that compared neoadjuvant chemotherapy and surgery to surgery alone for resectable esophageal cancer. *Am J Surg* 2002;183:274–279.

26. Malthaner R, Fenlon D. Preoperative chemotherapy for resectable thoracic esophageal cancer. *Cochrane Database Syst Rev* 2001;1:CD001556.

27. Apinop C, Puttisak P, Preecha N. A prospective study of combined therapy in esophageal cancer. *Hepatogastroenterology* 1994;41:391–393.

28. Bosset JF, Gignoux M, Triboulet JP, et al. Chemoradiotherapy followed by surgery compared with surgery alone in squamous-cell cancer of the esophagus. *N Engl J Med* 1997;337:161–167.

29. Le Prise E, Etienne PL, Meunier B, et al. A randomized study of chemotherapy, radiation therapy, and surgery versus surgery for localized squamous cell carcinoma of the esophagus. *Cancer* 1994;73:1779–1784.

30. Urba SG, Orringer MB, Turrisi A, Iannettoni M, Forastiere A, Strawderman M. Randomized trial of preoperative chemoradiation versus surgery alone in patients with locoregional esophageal carcinoma. *J Clin Oncol* 2001;19:305–313.

31. Walsh TN, Noonan N, Hollywood D, Kelly A, Keeling N, Hennessy TP. A comparison of multimodal therapy and surgery for esophageal adenocarcinoma. *N Engl J Med* 1996;335:462–467.

32. Walsh TN, Grennell M, Mansoor S, Kelly A. Neoadjuvant treatment of advanced stage esophageal adenocarcinoma increases survival. *Dis Esophagus* 2002;15:121–124.

33. Urschel JD, Vasan H. A meta-analysis of randomized controlled trials that compared neoadjuvant chemoradiation and surgery to surgery alone for resectable esophageal cancer. *Am J Surg* 2003;185:538–543.

34. Fiorica F, Di Bona D, Schepis F, et al. Preoperative chemoradiotherapy for oesophageal cancer: a systematic review and meta-analysis. *Gut* 2004;53:925–930.

35. Kaklamanos IG, Walker GR, Ferry K, Franceschi D, Livingstone AS. Neoadjuvant treatment for resectable cancer of the esophagus and the gastroesophageal junction: a meta-analysis of randomized clinical trials. *Ann Surg Oncol* 2003;10:754–761.

36. Greer SE, Goodney PP, Sutton JE, Birkmeyer JD. Neoadjuvant chemoradiotherapy for esophageal carcinoma: a meta-analysis. *Surgery* 2005;137:172–177.

37. Alexander HR Jr, Fraker DL, Bartlett DL. Isolated limb perfusion for malignant melanoma. *Semin Surg Oncol* 1996;12:416–428.

38. Bartlett DL, Ma G, Alexander HR, Libutti SK, Fraker DL. Isolated limb reperfusion with tumor necrosis factor and melphalan in patients with extremity melanoma after failure of isolated limb perfusion with chemotherapeutics. *Cancer* 1997;80:2084–2090.

39. Park BJ, Alexander HR, Libutti SK, et al. Treatment of primary peritoneal mesothelioma by continuous hyperthermic peritoneal perfusion (CHPP). *Ann Surg Oncol* 1999;6:582–590.

40. Kitamura K, Kuwano H, Watanabe M, et al. Prospective randomized study of hyperthermia combined with chemoradiotherapy for esophageal carcinoma. *J Surg Oncol* 1995;60:55–58.

25
Transthoracic Versus Transhiatal Resection for Carcinoma of the Esophagus

Jan B.F. Hulscher and J. Jan B. van Lanschot

Esophageal carcinoma is still a dreadful disease with a dismal prognosis. Surgery remains the mainstay of curative treatment. Optimizing the surgical treatment of esophageal cancer patients consists of different strategies such as early diagnosis, optimal patient selection, optimal peri-operative care, and possibly the application of (neo)adjuvant chemoradiation therapy. The treatment of esophageal carcinoma therefore warrants a multidisciplinary approach to optimize care for these patients.

Whereas surgery is generally considered as offering the best chance for cure in the absence of local unresectablility and/or distant metastasis, opinions on how to improve survival rates with surgery are conflicting. For years the procedure of choice for esophageal resection has been the Lewis–Tanner operation, in which the tumor and peri-esophageal tissue with its adjacent lymph nodes are resected through a right-sided thoracotomy in combination with a laparotomy. In the last decades, two major surgical strategies to improve survival rates have emerged.

The first strategy aims to minimize surgical trauma and thus to decrease early morbidity and mortality. This might be achieved by performing a transhiatal esophagectomy. During this procedure the esophagus is resected via a laparotomy combined with a cervical incision, thus avoiding a formal thoracotomy with its alleged (mainly pulmonary) complications. The second strategy aims to improve the long-term cure rate by performing a more radical (transthoracic) resection, with a wide excision of the tumor and its adjacent tissues in combination with a lymph node dissec-

tion in the upper abdomen and chest, thereby accepting a potential increase in early morbidity and mortality. This rests on the belief that in some patients with lymphatic dissemination cure can be obtained by an aggressive surgical resection of peri-tumoral tissue combined with a dissection of all possibly involved nodes. Also, staging may be improved by performing a more radical resection, offering a better insight into prognosis, and possibly a more tailored allocation of adjuvant therapy in the near future.

The purpose of this chapter is to assess the present literature and offer suggestions for the surgical treatment of esophageal carcinoma, based on the differences between transthoracic and transhiatal resections with respect to staging of the tumor, peri-operative morbidity, early mortality, and long-term survival.

25.1. Methods

We published a meta-analysis of the English literature between 1990 and 1999 comparing transthoracic esophagectomy with transhiatal esophagectomy for carcinoma of the thoracic esophagus and/or the gastro-esophageal junction.[1] In that paper, randomized clinical trials, comparative studies, and case series describing 50 or more patients were included.[2–51] The different transthoracic procedures were considered as one entity, without paying attention to differences between the transthoracic approaches. We did not review adeno- and squamous cell carcinoma separately because tumor behavior, surgical approach, and long-term prognosis are generally considered to be comparable.[52-54]

Studies were divided into three groups: randomized trials, comparative trials (including the randomized trials), and all studies (including the randomized, nonrandomized comparative, and noncomparative studies). Overall event rates were calculated as weighted averages of the trial-specific rates with weights proportional to the total sample sizes of the studies.[55] After calculating values for the noncomparative studies concerning transthoracic and transhiatal resections, these results were considered together as one comparative study in the overall group. Evidence from this meta-analysis is considered level 1.

Since the publication of this meta-analysis, one large randomized clinical trial comparing transhiatal and transthoracic resection for adenocarcinoma of the mid/distal esophagus has been published.[56] Evidence from this trial is level 1+. For the purpose of this chapter, data from this trial, more than doubling the total number of randomized patients in the literature, have been added to the data of the meta-analysis.

25.2. Effect of Transthoracic Resection on Staging

In multivariate analyses lymph node status and radicality of the resection (R0, microscopically radical resection; R1, macroscopically radical but microscopically irradical resection; R2, macroscopic tumor remaining) are often the predominant prognostic factors.[53,57-59] A transthoracic resection with extended lymph node dissection might offer better insight in the lymphatic dissemination of the tumor. This might influence staging of the tumor. A thoracotomy also offers an improved access to the tumor and surrounding tissues, which might increase the number of macro- and microscopically radical (R0) resections.

Patients with four or less involved lymph nodes appear to have a survival advantage over patients with more than four metastatic nodes, which is correlated with the finding that patients with more than four involved nodes have a higher risk of distant lymphatic dissemination.[60,61] The extent of lymphatic dissemination is also correlated

with survival: patients with involvement of only the abdominal lymph nodes have a survival advantage over patients with metastatic lymph nodes in both abdomen and chest.[57] Other authors argue that it is not (or not only) the absolute number of positive lymph nodes, but the ratio of positive to removed nodes. This might better reflect the state of disease than the absolute number of positive nodes, especially when one takes into account that the number of lymph nodes removed per patient or per surgeon may vary substantially.[58,62]

This issue also underlies the phenomenon of stage migration. Dissecting more lymph nodes increases the chance of finding a tumor positive node. The finding of a tumor positive node when performing an extended dissection might influence the pTNM stage significantly, especially as tumor-positive lymph nodes near the celiac axis are considered distant metastases for esophageal carcinoma, and these nodes are only resected during an extended resection.

During a transhiatal resection the subcarinal nodes may sometimes be reached via the widened hiatus of the diaphragm, but they often form the cranial boundary of the lymph node dissection. Unresected tumor-positive lymph nodes may therefore remain in the chest, which might lead to understaging. The specimens obtained after transhiatal resections might therefore not reflect the true state of disease. When in the same patient a formal lymph node dissection would have been performed, a positive lymph node might have been found, leading to a different pTNM stage, the so-called stage migration (see Table 25.1).

When the results of the different resection forms are compared, this is frequently done on a stage-by-stage basis. Stage migration might seriously hamper this comparison, because patients with the same stage might be staged differently based on the extent of the lymph node dissection and the increased possibility of finding a positive node in more extended resections.

In a recent analysis of patients undergoing a transthoracic resection with two-field lymph node dissection, 37% of patients showed tumor-positive nodes in extended fields: 20% in the abdomen, 20% in the mediastinum.[63] Subcarinal nodes were most affected (19%). Extended resection led to tumor upstaging in 23% of the patients;

TABLE 25.1. Age (in years) and clinicopathological staging of patients undergoing either transthoracic (TTE) or transhiatal esophagectomy (THE) for malignancy.

	TTE	THE
Age (mean)	*64*	*69*
	60	62
Stage 0/I	*16%*	*13%*
	22%	19%
Stage II	*15%*	*30%*
	27%	36%
Stage III	*54%*	*50%*
	41%	37%
'Stage IV	*15%*	*7%*
	10%	8%

Data from the Amsterdam trial are in **bold italic**; data from the earlier meta-analysis are in roman type.
Staging according to the 1997 UICC TNM classification.

mainly due to positive nodes near celiac axis, hepatic- or splenic artery. These nodes can also be resected during a transhiatal resection. Tumor positivity in paratracheal – or aorta – pulmonary nodes occurred in 8% of patients, rarely influencing staging.[63]

Another theoretical advantage of a transthoracic resection is the improved exposure, possibly leading to an increase in microscopically radical (R0) resections. However, in the Amsterdam trial there was no increase in R0 resections after transthoracic resection when compared with transhiatal resection (72% vs. 71%), despite the allegedly improved access to the esophagus

and surrounding tissues.[56] It should be noted, however, that in the Amsterdam trial only tumors distal to the carina were included.

Based on the evidence reviewed, we would recommend a formal lymph node dissection in the abdomen including the lymph nodes near the celiac axis when performing a transhiatal resection (recommendation grade C).

25.3. Clinical Effect of Transthoracic Resection

25.3.1. Perioperative Complications

The avoidance of a thoracotomy during a transhiatal resection might decrease the peri-operative surgical morbidity and mortality. However, due to the partially blunt dissection during the removal of the thoracic esophagus, the risk of perioperative complications such as injury to the trachea might be increased. Both the earlier meta-analysis and the recent Amsterdam trial did not show a difference in perioperative complications. However, blood loss and operative time were significantly increased after transthoracic resection (Table 25.2).

25.3.2. Postoperative Complications

The most important postoperative complications are depicted in Table 25.3. Over the last decade

TABLE 25.2. Mean peri-operative blood loss and operative time in patients undergoing either transthoracic esophagectomy (TTE) or transhiatal esophagectomy (THE).

	Number of patients		TTE outcome	THE outcome	p value
	TTE	THE			
Blood loss (mL)					
Recent Amsterdam	*114*	*106*	*1918 ± 1011*	*1223 ± 976*	*<0.001*
Earlier randomized	35	36	1402	847	
Earlier comparative	577	440	1105	859	
Comparative and noncomparative	949	1922	1001 ± 575	728 ± 438	
Overall including Amsterdam	**1063**	**2020**	**1099 ± 621**	**754 ± 468**	**<0.001**
Operative time (h)					
Recent Amsterdam	*114*	*106*	*6.0 ± 1.4*	*3.5 ± 1.2*	*<0.001*
Earlier randomized	70	68	5.2	3.5	
Earlier comparative	674	568	5.6	4.0	
Comparative and noncomparative	1291	808	5.0 ± 1.6	4.2 ± 1.5	
Overall including Amsterdam	**1405**	**914**	**5.1 ± 1.6**	**4.1 ± 1.5**	**<0.001**

Data from the Amsterdam trial are in **bold italics**; data from the earlier meta-analysis are in roman type.
The results of the Amsterdam study are included in the overall group.

TABLE 25.3. Hospital mortality, postoperative complications, stay in the Intensive Care Unit (ICU)/Medium Care Unit (MCU) and hospital stay in patients undergoing either transthoracic esophagectomy (TTE) or transhiatal esophagectomy (THE).

Qualitative outcomes	Number of patients		Percentage of patients with complications		Relative risk (RR)	Statistics (95% CI)	p value
	TTE	THE	TTE	THE			
In-hospital mortality							
Amsterdam	*114*	*106*	*4%*	*2%*	*2.32*	*0.46–11.73*	
Earlier randomized	70	68	1.4%	8.8%	0.12	0.04–1.12	
Earlier comparative	1375	1164	9.8%	7.2%	–	–	
Comparative and noncomparative	3942	3301	9.2%	5.7%	1.60	1.42–1.89	
Overall including Amsterdam	**4056**	**3407**	**9.0%**	**5.6%**	**1.61**	**1.36–1.90**	
Cardiac complications							
Amsterdam	*114*	*106*	*26%*	*16%*	*1.64*	*0.96–2.80*	
Earlier randomized	35	36	17.1%	22.2%	0.77	0.30–1.90	
Earlier comparative	563	458	10.3%	9.0%	–	–	
Comparative and noncomparative	1638	1084	6.6%	19.5%	0.34	0.27–0.41	
Overall including Amsterdam	**1740**	**1190**	**7.8%**	**19.9%**	**0.39**	**0.32–0.48**	
Pulmonary complications							
Amsterdam	*114*	*106*	*57%*	*27%*	*2.08*	*1.47–2.95*	
Earlier randomized	51	48	37.3%	43.8%	0.85	0.53–1.38	
Earlier comparative	765	698	22.9%	26.1%	–	–	
Comparative and noncomparative	2070	2397	18.7%	12.7%	1.47	1.29–1.68	
Overall including Amsterdam	**2184**	**2503**	**20.6%**	**11.3%**	**1.82**	**1.59–2.09**	
Anastomotic leakage							
Amsterdam	*114*	*106*	*16%*	*14%*	*1.09*	*0.58–2.06*	
Earlier randomized	70	68	7.3%	6.0%	1.20	0.34–4.25	
Earlier comparative	907	891	8.6%	14.8%	–	–	
Comparative and noncomparative	2594	3068	7.2%	13.6%	0.53	0.45–0.63	
Overall including Amsterdam	**2708**	**3174**	**7.9%**	**13.6%**	**0.58**	**0.50–0.68**	
Vocal cord paralysis							
Amsterdam	*114*	*106*	*21%*	*13%*	*1.59*	*0.8–2.92*	
Earlier randomized	54	52	3.7%	3.9%	0.98	0.14–6.59	
Earlier comparative	712	736	5.1%	11.9%	–	–	
Comparative and noncomparative	1743	2753	3.5%	9.5%	0.36	0.27–0.47	
Overall including Amsterdam	**1857**	**2859**	**4.5%**	**9.6%**	**0.47**	**0.37–0.60**	
Chylous leakage							
Amsterdam	*114*	*106*	*10%*	*2%*	*5.11*	*1.16–22.54*	
Earlier randomized	–	–	–	–	–	–	
Earlier comparative	595	465	2.8%	1.5%	–	–	
Comparative and noncomparative	1626	2260	2.4%	1.4%	1.70	1.07–2.69	
Overall including Amsterdam	**1740**	**2366**	**2.8%**	**2.0%**	**1.42**	**0.96–2.11**	
Wound infection							
Amsterdam	*114*	*106*	*10%*	*8%*	*1.27*	*0.53–3.06*	
Earlier randomized	–	–	–	–	–	–	
Earlier comparative	688	634	7.7%	4.1%	–	–	
Comparative and noncomparative	1744	2327	7.7%	4.3%	1.76	1.37–2.27	
Overall including Amsterdam	**1858**	**2433**	**7.8%**	**4.9%**	**1.60**	**1.26–2.02**	
ICU-stay [days]							
Amsterdam	*114*	*106*	*8.9±11.7*	*3.9±5.5*	–	–	*<0.001*
Earlier randomized	35	32	8.6	9.2	–	–	0.67
Earlier comparative	371	287	5.8	6.2	–	–	
Comparative and noncomparative	1033	618	11.2±6.2	9.1±5.3	–	–	<0.001
Overall including Amsterdam	**1147**	**724**	**10.7±6.8**	**8.1±5.3**	–	–	**<0.001**
Hospital stay [days]							
Amsterdam	*114*	*106*	*22.6±23.0*	*17.3±9.4*	–	–	*<0.001*
Earlier randomized	54	52	21.2	19.5	–	–	0.52
Earlier comparative	679	654	20.6	19.3	–	–	
Comparative and noncomparative	1198	1397	21.0±16.2	17.8±10.3	–	–	<0.001
Overall including Amsterdam	**1312**	**1503**	**22.2±16.8**	**17.7±10.2**	–	–	**<0.001**

Data from the Amsterdam trial are in ***bold italics***; data from the earlier meta-analysis are in roman type.
The results of the Amsterdam study are included in the overall group.

perioperative care has improved significantly. As more experience is gained, mortality rates for complex surgery tend to decrease. Twenty years ago the average hospital mortality rate following resection of esophageal carcinoma was 29%.[62] Ten years later the resection mortality rate was more than halved to 13%.[1] Today the average hospital mortality rate is almost halved again: when all data are combined a hospital mortality rate of 7.5% is achieved. Mortality rates vary widely (0%–27.8%), and decrease with growing experience and a higher hospital volume.[66–68] In experienced centers hospital mortality should be below 5%.

Although most individual reports do not find significant differences in in-hospital mortality between transthoracic and transhiatal approaches, overall in-hospital mortality is significantly higher after transthoracic resections, despite the fact that many surgeons perform transhiatal resections preferably on older patients with more comorbidity.[4,5,15,21] In the Amsterdam trial, there was no difference in preoperative characteristics such as age or American Society of Anesthesiologists' classification. There was also no difference in mortality after transthoracic resection (4%) versus transhiatal resection (2%, $p = 0.45$).[56]

Theoretically, transthoracic resections carry the disadvantages of a formal thoracotomy, which might result in a higher number of pulmonary complications. This is confirmed by the present data. Transthoracic resections may be associated with a transient deterioration of pulmonary function during one-lung ventilation in the left-lateral position, although this might be (partly) compensated for during the intervention when two-lung ventilation is resumed.[4] With modern anesthesiologic techniques (early extubation, epidural analgesia) and improved perioperative respiratory care, the incidence of cardiopulmonary complications might further decrease.

The incidence of anastomotic leakage varies widely in the literature, which is partly due to a discrepancy in definitions: some authors mention only the clinically significant leaks, while others include both subclinical and clinical leaks. Overall there is a significant difference favoring transthoracic approaches. This is at least partly due to the location of the anastomosis. In transthoracic resections, the anastomosis can be made cervically, but often it is made in the chest. During transhiatal procedures, the anastomosis is always made in the neck. A cervical anastomosis carries a higher risk of leakage than an intrathoracic anastomosis, but diminishes the risk of mediastinitis when leakage occurs.[6,8,11,16,17,32] In the Amsterdam trial, all anastomoses were made in the neck, and there was no difference in incidence of (sub)clinical anastomotic leaks (16% and 14%).[56] Most cervical leakages are minor, that is, subclinical (only seen radiologically) and do not require surgical exploration as they often resolve spontaneously 10 to 35 days after operation.[7,14,26,17,32,56] When surgical drainage is required, opening of the cervical incision almost always suffices. Unfortunately, approximately one third of the patients who develop anastomotic leakage in the neck will develop a subsequent stricture that jeopardizes the long-term functional result.[41]

Vocal cord paralysis due to injury of the recurrent laryngeal nerve is another frequent complication of esophagectomy, but most of the time the paralysis disappears within a few months.[6,69] A high incidence of vocal cord paralysis is mentioned after a cervical anastomosis, both after transthoracic and after transhiatal procedures, indicating that the recurrent nerve is mainly at risk during the cervical dissection and the construction of the anastomosis.[69–71] In the Amsterdam trial, the incidence of vocal fold paralysis was slightly but not significantly higher after transthoracic resection, reflecting the combination of a cervical anastomosis with a lymph node dissection in the aorta-pulmonary window (during which the left recurrent nerve is at risk).[56]

In the published literature of the last decade, patients stay slightly but significantly longer on the ventilator and in the intensive care unit/medium care unit (ICU/MCU) after transthoracic resection. In the Amsterdam trial there was also a clear difference in ICU/MCU stay favoring the transhiatal approach.[56] This also reflects on the total hospital stay, which is prolonged after transthoracic resection, while the stay on the surgical ward after patient had left the ICU/MCU was not prolonged.

In conclusion, pulmonary complications occur more frequently after transthoracic resection, leading to an increased intensive care and hospital stay (level of evidence 1+). Overall mortality may also be increased after transthoracic resection, although individual randomized trials do not demonstrate this increased mortality.

25.3.3. Long-term Survival

When all data of the last decade are combined for all tumor stages, there is no difference in 3-year survival rates between transthoracic and transhiatal resections [27.6% vs. 26.1%; relative risk (RR) 1.06; 95% confidence interval (95% CI), 0.94–1.19; see Table 25.4). When only the comparative trials are considered, there is a statistically significant difference in 5-year survival favoring transthoracic resection, but when all studies are included the 5-year survival rate is not significantly higher: 23.6% versus 23.3%; RR 1.01; 95% CI, 0.92–1.12. These results are comparable with the results of an early meta-analysis by Müller and coworkers in 1990, covering the decade 1980 to 1989.[65]

In the Amsterdam trial, 142/220 patients had died at the end of follow-up: 74 (69%) after transhiatal resection and 68 (60%) after transthoracic resection ($p = 0.12$). Although the difference in survival was not statistically significant, there

was a trend towards a survival benefit of the extended approach at 5 years: disease-free survival was 27% versus 39%, while overall survival was 29% versus 39%.[56]

The long-term benefit of transthoracic resection in the Amsterdam trial could be fully attributed to patients with a mid/distal esophageal carcinoma (Siewert type I), in whom the estimated 5-year survival benefit for transthoracic resection was 17% (95% CI of the difference, 3%–37%; see Figure 25.1).[72] The survival benefit of a transthoracic resection for patients with a carcinoma of the cardia/gastro-esophageal junction (Siewert type II) was only 1%.

A recent paper discusses the outcomes of transhiatal resection for early (T1) adenocarcinoma of the esophagus or gastro-esophageal junction.[73] In this paper, it is shown that only 1% of the tumors confined to the mucosa or superficial submucosa (T1M1–M3/SM1) have lymph node metastases, versus 44% of tumors confined to the deeper layers of the submucosa (T1SM2-SM tumors). This was also reflected in the 5-year survival rates of these tumors: 97% and 57%, respectively. These data suggest that T1M1-M3/SM1 tumors may be eligible for local endoscopic therapy such as endoscopic mucosal resection (EMR).[74] Currently we perform a diagnostic EMR for small tumors. When a T1M1-M3/SM1 tumor is found, we consider this a curative resection.

TABLE 25.4. Long-term survival after transthoracic esophagectomy (TTE) or transhiatal esophagectomy (THE) for all tumor stages combined.

	Number of patients		Percentage of surviving patients		Statistics	
	TTE	THE	TTE	THE	Relative risk	95% CI
3-year survival						
Amsterdam	*114*	*106*	*42.8%*	*38.5%*	*1.11*	*0.8–1.53*
Earlier randomized	35	32	28.6%	25.6%	1.83	0.70–4.78
Earlier comparative	375	250	29.1%	22.0%	–	–
Comparative and noncomparative	1914	1119	26.7%	25.0%	1.07	0.94–1.21
Overall including Amsterdam	**2028**	**1225**	**27.6%**	**26.1%**	**1.06**	**0.94–1.19**
5-year survival						
Amsterdam	*114*	*106*	*39%*	*29%*	*1.32*	*0.9–1.92*
Earlier randomized	–	–	–	–	–	–
Earlier comparative	807	499	35.2%	24.9%	1.41	1.68–1.89
Comparative and noncomparative	2677	2264	23.0%	21.7%	1.06	0.96–1.18
Overall including Amsterdam	**2791**	**2370**	**23.6%**	**23.3%**	**1.01**	**0.92–1.12**

Results of the Amsterdam trial are in ***bold italics***; results from the earlier meta-analysis are in roman type.
The results of the Amsterdam study are included in the overall group.

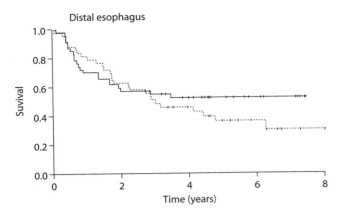

FIGURE 25.1. Survival curves after transthoracic and transhiatal resection for adenocarcinoma of the mid-/distal esophagus of the Amsterdam trial ($p = 0.14$). (Reprinted from Hulscher JB, Van Lanschot JJ. Individualised surgical treatment of patients with an adenocarcinoma of the distal oesophagus or gastro-oesophageal junction. *Dig Surg* 2005;22:130–134, with permission from S. Karger AG, Basel.)

When a tumor larger than T1-SM1 is found, the patient is scheduled for esophagectomy. In almost half of the patients with T1SM2-SM3 tumors, recurrent disease develops within 5 years after transhiatal resection. This substantial recurrence rate after transhiatal resection, including both locoregional and distant dissemination, might be an argument in favor of more extensive surgery, and/or neoadjuvant chemoradiation therapy in this patient group.

25.4. Conclusion

With only four randomized trials, amounting to 358 patients, there is a clear lack of properly conducted large randomized studies comparing transhiatal and transthoracic resection. All other comparative studies except three are retrospective, often extending over many years with relatively small numbers of selected patients. Definitions of peri-operative events are rarely given, making exact comparison difficult. Comparison of different series is further hampered because results are not presented in a standardized format, often including different histological subtypes and stages. Based on the present state of evidence, the following conclusions can be drawn.

Esophageal carcinoma remains a disease with a grim prognosis. Surgery remains the mainstay of potentially curative treatment, but postoperative morbidity is still high. Based on the similar in-hospital mortality and the clinically relevant

(albeit not statistically significant) 17% higher survival rates as demonstrated in the Amsterdam trial, we now prefer the transthoracic approach combined with a two-field lymph node dissection for patients with a tumor of the mid/distal esophagus who are fit for major surgery (level of evidence 1– to 2++; recommendation grade C). We reserve the transhiatal route for patients with a cardia/junction carcinoma, unless tumor-positive lymph nodes have been identified at or proximal to the carina during preoperative workup. In those cases we perform a transthoracic resection with two-field lymphadenectomy, just as we do for patients with a tumor of the mid/distal esophagus. Both transthoracic and transhiatal resections have their firm protagonists, but until further randomized trials have been performed to confirm these results, the choice for a certain surgical approach to esophageal cancer still rests on the individual preference of the surgeon, not on solid evidence.

Based on the similar in-hospital mortality and the clinically relevant (albeit not statistically significant) higher survival rates, we prefer the transthoracic approach combined with a two-field lymph node dissection for patients with a tumor of the mid/distal esophagus, and reserve the transhiatal route for patients with a cardia/junction carcinoma, unless positive lymph nodes have been identified at or proximal to the carina (level of evidence 1– to 2++; recommendation grade C).

References

1. Hulscher JBF, Tijssen JG, Obertop H, Van Lanschot JJ. Transthoracic versus transhiatal resection for carcinoma of the esophagus: a meta-analysis. *Ann Thorac Surg* 2001;72:306–313.
2. Goldminc M, Maddern G, LePrise E, Meunier B, Campion JP, Launois B. Oesophagectomy by transhiatal approach or thoracotomy: a prospective randomized trial. *Br J Surg* 1993;80:367–370.
3. Chu KM, Law SY, Fok M, Wong J. A prospective randomized comparison of transhiatal and transthoracic resection for lower-third esophageal carcinoma. *Am J Surg* 1997;174:320–324.
4. Jacobi CA, Zieren HU, Müller M, Pichlmaier H. Surgical therapy of oesophageal carcinoma: the influence of surgical approach and oesophageal resection on cardiopulmonary function. *Eur J Cardiothoracic Surg* 1997;11:32–37.
5. Junginger T, Dutkowski P. Selective approach to the treatment of oesophageal cancer. *Br J Surg* 1996;83:1473–1477.
6. Horstmann O, Verreet PR, Becker H, Ohmann C, Röher HD. Transhiatal oesophagectomy compared with transthoracic resection and systematic lymphadenectomy for the treatment of oesophageal cancer. *Eur J Surg* 1995;161:557–567.
7. Svanes K, Stangeland L, Viste A, Varhaug JE, Gronbech JE, Soreide O. Morbidity, ability to swallow, and survival, after oesophagectomy for cancer of the oesophagus and cardia. *Eur J Surg* 1995;161:669–675.
8. Tilanus HW, Hop WCJ, Langenhorst BLAM, Van Lanschot JJB. Esophagectomy with or without thoracotomy. *J Thorac Cardiovasc Surg* 1993;105:898–903.
9. Bonavina L. Early oesophageal cancer: results of a European multicentre survey. *Br J Surg* 1995;82:98–101.
10. Paç M, Basoglu A, Koçak H, et al. Transhiatal versus transthoracic esophagectomy for oesophageal cancer. *J Thorac Cardiovasc Surg* 1993;106:205–209.
11. Putnam JB, Suell DM, McMurtey MJ, et al. Comparison of three techniques of esophagectomy within a residency training program. *Ann Thorac Surg* 1994;57:319–325.
12. Thomas P, Doddoli C, Lienne P, et al. Changing patterns and surgical results in adenocarcinoma of the oesophagus. *Br J Surg* 1997;84:119–125.
13. Millikan KW, Silverstein J, Hart V, et al. A 15-year review of esophagectomy for carcinoma of the oesophagus and cardia. *Arch Surg* 1995;30:617–624.
14. Daniel TM, Fleisher KJ, Flanagan TL, Tribble CG, Kron IL. Transhiatal esophagectomy: a safe alternative for selected patients. *Ann Thorac Surg* 1992;54:686–690.
15. Gluch L, Smith RC, Bambach CP, Brown AR. Comparison of outcomes following transhiatal or Ivor Lewis esophageactomy for oesophageal carcinoma. *World J Surg* 1999;23:271–276.
16. Moon MR, Schulte WJ, Haasler GB, Condon RE. Transhiatal and transthoracic esophagectomy for adenocarcinoma of the oesophagus. *Arch Surg* 1992;127:951–955.
17. Jauch KW, Bacha EA, Denecke H, Anthuber M, Schildberg FW. Oesophageal carcinoma: prognostic features and comparison between blunt transhiatal dissection and transthoracic resection. *Eur J Surg Oncol* 1992;18:553–562.
18. Bolton JS, Ochsner JL, Abdoh A. Surgical management of esophageal cancer: a decade of change. *Ann Surg* 1994;219:475–480.
19. Pommier RF, Vetto JT, Ferris BL, Wilmarth TJ. Relationships between operative approaches and outcomes in esophageal cancer. *Am J Surg* 1998;175:422–425.
20. Hagen JA, Peters JH, DeMeester TR. Superiority of extended en bloc esophagectomy for carcinoma of the lower esophagus and cardia. *J Thorac Cardiovasc Surg* 1993;106:850–859.
21. Torres AJ, Sanchez-Pernaute A, Hernande F, et al. Two-field radical lymphadenectomy in the treatment of esophageal carcinoma. *Dis Esophagus* 1999;12:137–143.
22. Hansson LE, Gustavsson S, Haglund U. Postoperative morbidity and mortality after surgical treatment of advanced carcinoma of the oesophagus and the gastro-oesophageal junction. *Dig Surg* 1997;14:506–511.
23. Stark SP, Romberg MS, Pierce GE, et al. Transhiatal versus transthoracic oesophagectomy for adenocarcinoma of the distal esophagus and cardia. *Am J Surg* 1996;172:478–482.
24. Berdejo L. Transhiatal versus transthoracic oesophagectomy for clinical stage I oesophageal carcinoma. *Hepatogastroenterology* 1995;42:789–791.
25. Naunheim KS, Hanosh J, Zwishenberger J, et al. Esophagectomy in the septuagenarian. *Ann Thorac Surg* 1993;56:880–884.
26. Collard JM, Otte JB, Reynaert M, Fiasse R, Kestens PJ. Feasibility and effectiveness of en bloc resection of the oesophagus for oesophageal cancer. Results of a prospective study. *Int Surg* 1991;76:209–213.
27. Liedman BL, Bennegard K, Olbe LC, Lundell LR. Predictors of postoperative morbidity and

mortality after surgery for gastro-oesophageal carcinomas. *Eur J Surg* 1995;161:173–180.

28. Griffin SM, Woods SDS, Chan A, Chung SCS, Li AKC. Early and late surgical complications of subtotal oesophagectomy for squamous cell carcinoma of the oesophagus. *J R Coll Surg Edinb* 1991;36:170–173.

29. Sharpe DAC, Moghissi K. Resectional surgery in carcinoma of the oesophagus and cardia: what influences long-term survival? *Eur J Cardiothorac Surg* 1996;10:359–364.

30. Wang LS, Huang MH, Huang BS, Chien KY. Gastric substitution for respectable carcinoma of the esophagus: an analysis of 368 cases. *Ann Thorac Surg* 1992;53:289–294.

31. Rahamin J, Cham CW. Oesophagogastrectomy for carcinoma of the oesophagus and cardia. *Br J Surg* 1993;80:1305–1309.

32. Lerut T, DeLeyn P, Coosemans W, Raemdonck D van, Scheys I, LeSaffre E. Surgical strategies in esophageal carcinoma with emphasis on radical lymphadenectomy. *Ann Surg* 1992;216:583–590.

33. Sutton DN, Wayman J, Griffin SM. Learning curve for oesophageal cancer surgery. *Br J Surg* 1998;85: 1399–1402.

34. Tsutsui S, Moriguchi S, Morita M, et al. Multivariate analysis of postoperative complications after esophageal resection. *Ann Thorac Surg* 1992;53: 1052–1056.

35. Mannell A, Becker PJ. Evaluation of the results of oesophagectomy for oesophageal cancer. *Br J Surg* 1991;78:36–40.

36. Page RD, Khalil JF, Whyte RI, Kaplan DK, Donnelly RJ. Esophagogastrectomy via left thoracophrenotomy. *Ann Thorac Surg* 1990;49:763–766.

37. Altorki NK, Skinner DB. En bloc esophagectomy: the first 100 patients. *Hepatogastroenterology* 1990;37:360–363.

38. Ahmed ME. The surgical management and outcome of oesophageal cancer in Khartoum. *J R Coll Surg Edinb* 1993;38:16–18.

39. Lozac'h P, Topart P, Etienne J, Charles JF. Ivor Lewis operation for epidermoid carcinoma of the esophagus. *Ann Thorac Surg* 1991;52:1154–1157.

40. Paricio PP, Marcilla JAG, Haro LM de, Escandell MAO, Escrig GC. Results of surgical treatment of epidermoid carcinoma of the thoracic esophagus. *Surg Gynecol Obstet* 1993;177:398–404.

41. Orringer MB, Marshall B, Iannettoni MD. Transhiatal esophagectomy: clinical experience and refinements. *Ann Surg* 1999;230:392–403.

42. Gupta NM. Oesophagectomy without thoracotomy: first 250 patients. *Eur J Surg* 1996;162:455–461.

43. Moreno GE, Garcia GI, Pinto GAI, et al. Results of transhiatal oesophagectomy in cancer of the esophagus and other diseases. *Hepatogastroenterology* 1992;39:439–442.

44. Gelfland GAJ, Finley RJ, Nelems B, Inculet R, Evans KG, Fradet G. Transhiatal esophagectomy for carcinoma of the oesophagus and cardia. *Arch Surg* 1992;127:1164–1168.

45. Gürkan N, Terzioglu T, Tezelman S, Sasman O. Transhiatal oesophagectomy for esophageal cancer. *Br J Surg* 1991;78:1348–1351.

46. Vigneswaran WT, Trastek VF, Pairolero PC, Deschamps C, Daly RC, Allen MS. Transhiatal esophagectomy for carcinoma of the oesophagus. *Ann Thorac Surg* 1993;56:838–846.

47. Gillinov AM, Heitmiller RF. Strategies to reduce pulmonary complications after transhiatal esophagectomy. *Dis Esophagus* 1998;11:43–47.

48. Gertsch P, Vauthey JN, Lustenberger AA, Friedlander-Klar. Long-term results of transhiatal esophagectomy for esophageal carcinoma. *Cancer* 1993;72:2312–2319.

49. Dudhat SB, Shinde SR. Transhiatal esophagectomy for squamous cell carcinoma of the oesophagus. *Dis Esophagus* 1998;11:226–230.

50. Beik AI, Jaffray B, Anderson JR. Transhiatal oesophagectomy: a comparison of alternative techniques in 68 patients. *J R Coll Surg Edinb* 1996;25:25–29.

51. Gottley DC, Beard J, Cooper MJ, Britton DC, Williamson RCN. Abdominocervical (transhiatal) oesophagectomy in the management of oesophageal carcinoma. *Br J Surg* 1990;77:815–819.

52. Law SY, Fok M, Cheng SW, Wong J. A comparison of outcome after resection for squamous carcinomas and adenocarcinomas of the esophagus and cardia. *Surg Gynecol Obstet* 1992;175:107–112.

53. Hulscher JBF, Van Sandick JW, Tijssen TP, Obertop H, Van Lanschot JJ. The recurrence pattern after transhiatal resection. *J Am Coll Surg* 2000;191:143–148.

54. Ellis FH, Heatley GJ, Krasna MJ, Williamson WA, Balogh K. Esophagogastrctomy for carcinoma of the esophagus and cardia: a comparison of findings and results after standard resection in three consecutive eight-year intervals with improved staging criteria. *J Thorac Cardiovasc Surg* 1997;113: 836–848.

55. Kleinbaum DG, Kupper LL, Morgenstern H. *Epidemiologic research: Principles and Quantitative Methods*. New York: Van Nostrand Reinhold, 1982.

56. Hulscher JBF, Van Sandick JW, de Boer AG, et al. Extended transthoracic resection compared with

limited transhiatal resection for adenocarcinoma of the esophagus. *N Engl J Med* 2002;347:1662–1669.

57. Steup WH, De Leyn P, Deneffe G, Van Raemdonck D, Coosemans W, Lerut T. Tumours of the esophagogastric junction. Long-term survival in relation to the pattern of lymph node metastasis and a critical analysis of the accuracy of pTNM classification. *J Thorac Cardiovasc Surg* 1996;111:85–95.

58. Van Sandick JW, Van Lanschot JJB, Ten Kate FJW, Tijssen JGW, Obertop H. Indicators of prognosis after transhiatal esophageal resection without thoracotomy for cancer. *J Am Coll Surg* 2002;114:28–36.

59. Abe S, Tachibana M, Shiraishi M, Nakamura T. Lymph node metastasis in resectable esophageal cancer. *J Thorac Cardiovasc Surg* 1990;100:287–291.

60. Matsubara T, Ueda M, Nagao N, Takahashi T, Nakajima T, Nishi M. Cervicothoracic approach for total meso-esophageal dissection in cancer of the thoracic esophagus. *J Am Coll Surg* 1998;187:238–245.

61. Nishimaki T, Tanaka O, Suzuki T, Aizawa K, Hatakeyama K, Muto T. Patterns of lymphatic spread in thoracic esophageal cancer. *Cancer* 1994;74:4–11.

62. Roder JD, Busch R, Stein HJ, Fink U, Siewert JR. Ratio of invaded to removed lymph nodes as a predictor of survival in squamous cell carcinoma of the oesophagus. *Br J Surg* 1994;81:410–413.

63. Hulscher JB, Van Sandick JW, Offerhaus GJ, Tilanus HW, Obertop H, Van Lanschot JJ. Prospective analysis of the diagnostic yield of extended en bloc resection for adenocarcinoma of the oesophagus or gastric cardia. *Br J Surg* 2001;88:715–719.

64. Earlam R, Cunha-Melo JR. Oesophageal squamous cell carcinoma: I. a critical review of surgery. *Br J Surg* 1980;67:381–390.

65. Müller JM, Erasmi H, Stelzner M, Zieren U, Pichlmaier H. Surgical therapy of oesophageal carcinoma. *Br J Surg* 1990;77:845–857.

66. Van Lanschot JJ, Hulscher JB, Buskens CJ, Tilanus HW, Ten Kate FJ, Obertop H. Hospital volume and hospital mortality for esophagectomy. *Cancer* 2001;91:1574–1578.

67. Patti MG, Corvera CU, Glasgow RE, Way LW. A hospital's annual rate of esophagectomy influences the operative mortality rate. *J Gastrointest Surg* 1998;2:186–192.

68. Miller JD, Jain MK, De Gara CJ, Morgan D, Urschel JD. Effect of surgical experience on results of esophagectomy for esophageal carcinoma. *J Surg Oncol* 1997;65:20–21.

69. Hulscher JBF, Van Sandick JW, DeVriese PP, Van Lanschot JJB, Obertop H. Vocal cord paralysis after subtotal oesophagectomy. *Br J Surg* 1999;86:1583–1586.

70. Vigneswaran WT, Trastek VF, Pairolero PC, Deschamps C, Daly RC, Allen MS. Extended esophagectomy in the management of carcinoma of the upper thoracic esophagus. *J Thorac Cardiovasc Surg* 1994;107:901–907.

71. McLarty AJ, Deschamps C, Trastek VF, Allen MS, Pairolero PC, Harmsen WS. Esophageal resection for cancer of the esophagus: long-term function and quality of life. *Ann Thorac Surg* 1997;63:1568–1572.

72. Hulscher JB, Van Lanschot JJ. Individualised surgical treatment of patients with an adenocarcinoma of the distal oesophagus or gastro-oesophageal junction. *Dig Surg* 2005;22:130–134.

73. Westerterp M, Koppert LB, Buskens CJ, et al. Outcome of surgical treatment for early adenocaricnoma of the esophagus or gastro-esophageal junction. *Virchows Arch* 2005;446:497–504.

74. Van Lanschot JJ, Bergman JJ. Tailored therapy for early Barrett's lesions. *Br J Surg* 2005;92:791–792.

26
Minimally Invasive Versus Open Esophagectomy for Cancer

Ara Ketchedjian and Hiran Fernando

Despite advances in medical and radiation oncology, esophagectomy continues to remain the cornerstone of therapy for esophageal cancer when cure is the goal. The surgical approaches to esophagectomy, however, vary by institution. In many cases patients with esophageal cancer are older with significant comorbid diseases. Open approaches to esophagectomy can often carry significant morbidity and mortality for these compromised patients. Minimally invasive strategies, bolstered by improving techniques and technology, have made minimally invasive esophagectomy (MIE) a feasible operative strategy for esophageal cancer surgery. Minimally invasive surgery offers the potential for faster postoperative recovery and fewer pulmonary complications. Much like open surgery, MIE approaches and techniques differ based on institution and surgeon. The goal, however, regardless of the approach, is complete resection of all cancer. Whether MIE can provide added benefit to morbidity, mortality, or postoperative recovery without compromising oncologic resection continues to be a topic of debate.

Minimally invasive esophagectomy remains a relatively new approach for the treatment of esophageal cancer with a paucity of level 1 evidence comparing it to standard open esophageal surgery. A majority of the literature on MIE reflects institutional-based observations and experience. This chapter will review the literature on both open and minimally invasive esophagectomy, comparing the relevant factors that may influence a surgeon's approach to esophageal cancer surgery.

26.1. Operative Procedure and Feasibility

Minimally invasive esophagectomy techniques require advanced laparoscopic and thoracoscopic skills for optimal outcomes. Due to the inherent limitations in visualization and instrumentation, operative times are often longer and vary widely (3.7–7.5h; Table 26.1). The earliest descriptions of MIE involved a combination of open surgery with either thoracoscopy or laparoscopy. In 1993, Collard demonstrated that esophageal dissection could be carried out thoracoscopically when combined with laparotomy for gastric mobilization.[1] The disadvantage of a hybrid approach such as this is that the patient is still subjected to the morbidity of the open approach in the abdomen. The first report of a completely minimally invasive approach was by Depaula, who described a laparoscopic transhiatal esophagectomy.[2] Swanstrom and colleagues later described the first North American experience using the same approach as Depaula.[3] Luketich and coworkers further modified the approach utilizing both laparoscopy and thoracoscopy to achieve esophagectomy.[4] This modification was added to help with visualization and dissection of the thoracic esophagus, as well as to achieve a more complete lymph node dissection. As with most new technologies and procedures, there is a continuous evolution of technique in an attempt to improve operative outcome and ease of surgery. Other techniques such as robotic esophagectomy have been reported, but currently the experience with this approach is relatively small.[5]

TABLE 26.1. Minimally invasive esophagectomy – surgical outcome.

Surgeon	n	Evidence	Operative approach (h)	Operation time	LOS (days)	Mortality (%)
Total						
MIE						
DePaula[2]	12	Retrospective	Lap THE	4.3	7.6	0
Swanstrom[3]	9	Retrospective	Lap THE	6.5	6.4	0
Watson[29]	7	Retrospective	MIE	4.4	12	0
Luketich[15]	222	Retrospective	MIE	–	7	1.4
Nguyen[30]	46	Retrospective	MIE	5.8	8	4.3
Avital[23]	22	Retrospective	Lap THE	6.3	8	4.5
Hybrid						
Liu[31]	20	Retrospective	VATS/laparotomy	4.6[a]	19	0
Peracchia[32]	18	Retrospective	VATS/laparotomy	5.6	–	5.5
Law[33]	18	Retrospective	VATS/laparotomy	4	–	0
Kawahara[34]	23	Retrospective	VATS/laparotomy	1.8[a]	26	0
Smithers[35]	153	Retrospective	VATS/laparotomy	5.0	12	3.3
Osugi[12]	80	Retrospective	VATS/laparotomy	3.7	–	0
Open						
Mathisen[36]	104	Retrospective	TA (64)/IL (40)	–	–	2.9
Lerut[37]	198	Retrospective	Open (varied)	–	18	9.6
Orringer[17]	1085	Retrospective	THE	–	10	4
Swanson[38]	250	Retrospective	Three-hole	–	13	3.6
Bailey[16]	1777	Retrospective	Open (varied)	–	–	9.8
Rizk[19]	510	Retrospective	Open (varied)	–	23[b]	6.1
					11[c]	

IL, Ivor Lewis; Lap, laparoscopic; MIE, minimally invasive esophagectomy; TA, left thoraco-abdominal; THE, transhiatal esophagectomy; VATS, video-assisted thorascopic surgery.
[a]VATS portion only.
[b]Patients with complications.
[c]Patients without complications.

Even for open esophagectomy there is some controversy as to which operative approach is best. Prospective, randomized trials comparing transhiatal and transthoracic procedures have demonstrated no significant difference in survival.[6–8] Additionally, there are differences in outcome when comparing low-volume to high-volume esophageal centers. Birkmeyer and colleagues, in reviewing a national database, reported mortality rates ranging from 8% in high-volume centers to as high as 23% in low-volume centers.[9] In the absence of a randomized trial, the differences in outcome between centers is an additional source of bias when trying to compare surgical approaches.

With regards to techniques for open esophagectomy, surgeons tend to prefer one approach over another. Advocates of transhiatal esophagectomy favor this approach because it avoids thoracotomy and all its associated morbidities. In comparison, achieving an R0 resection has been stressed by others as the most important factor for attaining cure, suggesting that a more exten-

sive dissection accomplished by an open thoracotomy approach is superior.[10] Extended (three-field) lymph node dissection and en bloc resection are being used to optimize the number of harvested lymph nodes in an attempt to accomplish R0 resection. Some groups have also reported en bloc resections using minimally invasive techniques, although they failed to demonstrate any improvement in morbidity.[11,12] Although en bloc resections have been demonstrated to be safe at high-volume centers, they are associated with higher morbidity.

26.2. Studies Comparing Open and Minimally Invasive Esophagectomy

There have been no randomized studies that compare MIE to open esophagectomy (OE). There are two retrospective studies that have compared MIE to OE.[13,14] In the first study, 18 MIE were compared to 16 OE. The authors found that the mean operative time (364min), blood loss (297mL), and length of intensive care unit stay (6.1 days) were decreased compared with open transthoracic esophagectomy (437min, 1046mL, 9.9 days) and blunt transhiatal esophagectomy (391min, 1142mL, 11.1 days).[14] The incidence of respiratory complications (pneumonia, pulmonary embolism, respiratory failure) was similar among the groups. It should be emphasized, however, that there were significant differences between the groups in this retrospective comparison. The open patients had more advanced cancers whereas the MIE group had more patients with high-grade dysplasia or a benign disorder requiring esophagectomy. Additionally, the open operations were performed by a group of four surgeons with variable experience with esophageal surgery, whereas the MIE procedures were performed by a single surgeon with specific expertise in minimally invasive esophageal surgery. The open operations were performed several years before the MIE procedures, so there may also have been differences in practice patterns accounting for the longer lengths of stay. The second comparative study included 25 laparoscopic transhiatal (with the use of a handport) and 20 open transhiatal esophagectomies. It should be noted that there was a relatively high incidence (36%) of conversions to laparotomy in the MIE group. Not unexpectedly, the authors demonstrated a significantly longer operative

time in the MIE group (300 vs. 257min). In favor of MIE, however, there was a significantly shorter intensive care unit stay (1 vs. 2 days) and blood loss (600 vs. 900mL) in these patients compared to the open procedures. Otherwise there was no difference in perioperative outcome.

In the MIE series by Luketich, the median ICU stay was 1 day, time to oral intake was 4 days, and hospital stay was 7 days. This minimally invasive approach which utilizes thoracoscopy compares favorably with outcomes after laparoscopic transhiatal and is better than most series of open esophagectomy (Table 26.1).[15]

26.3. Morbidity and Mortality

As discussed above, there are no randomized or published prospective trials involving MIE. In the absence of such data the best option is to compare the best published results with those reported after open operation. Although mortality is usually reported in esophagectomy series, total morbidity is not. Reports of morbidity typically target specific outcomes such as anastomotic leak and pneumonia rates, making comparisons of morbidity challenging. For this reason, rather than comparing overall morbidity, we have compared the reported rates of specific complications after MIE, hybrid, and OE from different series in Tables 26.2 and 26.3.

TABLE 26.2. Minimally invasive esophagectomy – recurrence and survival.

	Year	n	Evidence	Approach	Follow-up (months)	Survival (%) Median (mos)	1 year	3 years	5 years	Loco-regional recurrence
I MIE										
Swanstrom[3]	1997	9	Retrospective	Lap THE	13	–	–	–	–	22.2
Nguyen[30]	2003	46	Retrospective	MIE (41 IL)	26	–	87	57	–	26.1
Luketich[15]	2003	222	Retrospective	MIE	19	26	69%	45%	36	–
Hybrid										
Peracchia[32]	1997	18	Retrospective	VATS/laparotomy	17	–	–	–	–	16.6
Law[33]	1997	18	Retrospective	VATS/laparotomy	13.7	–	81	–	–	44.4
Kawahara[34]	1999	23	Retrospective	VATS/laparotomy	–	–	–	–	–	30.4
Smithers[35]	2001	153	Retrospective	VATS/laparotomy	21	29	70	–	40	–
Open										
Mathisen[36]	1988	104	Retrospective	TA (64)/IL (40)	–	–	–	–	15	5.8
Lerut[37]	1992	198	Retrospective	Open (varied)	>24	–	63	–	30	–
Orringer[17]	1999	1085	Retrospective	THE	27	–	67	34	23	–
Swanson[38]	2001	250	Retrospective	Three-hole	24	25	44	–	–	5.6
Rizk[19]	2004	510	Retrospective	Open (varied)	–	–	44	–	–	–

IL, Ivor Lewis; Lap, laparoscopic; MIE, minimally invasive esophagectomy; TA, left thoraco-abdominal; THE, transhiatal esophagectomy; VATS, video-assisted thoracoscopic surgery.

TABLE 26.3. Postoperative complications after esophagectomy.

Author	Number of patients	Type of procedure	Pneumonia	Myocardial infarction	Anastomotic leak	Chylothorax	Atrial fibrillation
Whooley[39]	710	Open	17	8	3.5	1.7	23
Atkins[20]	NA	Open	15.8	1.1	14	3	13.7
Ferguson[40]	269	Open	27	2	16	4	36
Luketich[15]	222	MIE	7.7	1.8	11.7	3.2	12
Nguyen[30]	46	MIE	2.1	2.1	8.7	na	na

Abbreviation: na, not applicable.

26.3.1. Mortality

Mortality was 1.5% in the Pittsburgh series and 4.5% from the University of California, Davis series, the two largest MIE reported experiences to date. This compares favorably with other open series, where typically mortality is 5% or less when reported from large-volume esophageal centers. Bailey recently reported on a prospective multicenter series of 1777 patients all from the Veterans Administration (VA) system.[16] This is one of the largest studies of its kind. Mortality in this study was higher at 9.8%. Similarly, the report analyzing outcomes from the Leapfrog database indicated that mortality even in high-volume esophageal centers was around 8%.[9] A prospective, nonrandomized phase II study of MIE currently is being conducted by the Eastern Cooperative Oncology Group and the Cancer and Leukemia Group B (E2202). The goal of E2202 is look at the feasibility of MIE in a multicenter setting, with perioperative mortality being the primary end point.

26.3.2. Complications

In the largest series of MIE, major complications occurred in 32% of patients.[15] The most common major complication was anastomotic leak, which occurred in 11% of patients overall. The leak rate in this series was influenced by technique. Mid-series a narrow gastric tube (4cm or less) was utilized and resulted in a very high leak rate of 25.9%. Because of these results the authors subsequently reverted back to a wider gastric tube (6cm or more) and reported a lower leak rate of 6.1%. In the University of Michigan series of 1085 transhiatal esophagectomies, the overall leak rate was 13%.[17] More recently, the same group has reported a significant reduction in the

leak rate to 2.7% using a side-to-side stapled anastomosis.[18] Risk and colleagues recently reported the results from Memorial Sloan-Kettering in 510 open esophagectomies.[19] Anastomotic leak rates were higher (21%) in this group of patients.

Pneumonia has been shown to be a significant predictor of mortality and morbidity after esophagectomy.[20] Pneumonia was the second most common major complication in the Pittsburgh series of MIE, occurring in 7.7% of patients.[15] This pneumonia rate is lower than the reported rates after open approaches that include a significant number of thoracotomies (15%–30%) but is higher than the 2% pneumonia rate reported after the largest series of transhiatal esophagectomies.[17] In the University of California Davis series of MIE, the most frequent complications were anastomotic leaks (11%) and respiratory failure (11%), which are similar to those in other series. The most frequent minor complication in the Pittsburgh MIE series was atrial fibrillation occurring in 12%.[15] Atrial fibrillation has been reported to occur in between 20% to 25% of patients after OE.[21]

26.4. Recurrence and Survival

There is scant data on long-term survival and recurrence patterns following minimally invasive approaches to esophagectomy. In the single institution MIE series by Luketich and associates, Kaplan–Meier estimates of survival based on stage were similar to those in the open literature.[15] Although not presented in that original publication, re-analysis of the original dataset of 222 patients with esophageal cancer demonstrated 1-, 3-, and 5-year survivals of 69%, 45%, and 36%, respectively, which are similar if not better than for some open series (Table 26.3). In the University of California at Davis MIE series, there were 87% 1-year and 57% 3-year survival rates in 46 patients.[22] Avital and colleagues in the most recently published MIE series reported a 61% survival at 30-month follow-up.[23] It should be emphasized, however, that this study included a relatively large number of early-stage cancers, with 84% of the patients having either stage I or II tumors. Loco-regional recurrence rates of between 16% and 44% have been documented in minimally invasive series, which is on par with the known natural history of resected esophageal cancer using open techniques. Prospective, controlled studies will be required to more accurately delineate the survival and recurrence patterns afforded by MIE compared to open techniques (Table 26.2).

26.5. Pain and Quality of Life

There are no specific analyses of postoperative pain in the MIE literature. Studies comparing video-assisted thorascopic surgery (VATS) or thoracotomy for lung resection have demonstrated less pain, better preservation of lung function, and improved shoulder function with VATS.[24,25] Whether this holds true after MIE needs to be determined.

Quality of life (QOL) is a critical factor in the management of patients with esophageal cancer. Headrick and associates have found that on long-term follow-up, esophagectomy can be performed with little to no impairment in QOL compared with normal patients based on SF36 scoring.[26] Similarly, Blazeby and co-authors found that QOL initially was diminished in patients undergoing resection for esophageal carcinoma, but improved back to baseline in those patients surviving for 2 years following esophagectomy.[27] In the Pittsburgh series of 222 MIE patients, the mean postoperative dysphagia score was 1.4 on a scale from 1 (no dysphagia) to 5 (severe dysphagia).[15] The presence of dysphagia after esophagectomy, particularly if performed in a relatively asymptomatic patient such as those with high-grade dysplasia, can have a significant effect on QOL. Overall QOL using the SF36 were also measured and were not significantly different com-

pared to age-matched normal values during follow-up after MIE.

26.6. Summary

Currently, experience with MIE is relatively small, and published results are mostly single institution reports. It should be emphasized that there is no level 1 data comparing OE and MIE. The only trials that have compared MIE to OE were level 3b (single-institution case control) studies.[13,14] The first study was biased in terms of case mix and surgeon experience favoring the MIE cases, whereas the second study included a relatively large number of conversions in the MIE group, suggesting that this was early in the surgeons learning curve. Otherwise, the data supporting MIE is primarily level 4 (single institution case series). However, this is also the case for OE where the best reported results in terms of morbidity and mortality are from single institution high-volume esophageal centers. Comparison of such MIE and OE reports indicates that MIE is associated with at least equivalent results in terms of mortality, morbidity, and survival after esophagectomy (recommendation grade C). Although pain control and pulmonary function have not been compared after different esophagectomy approaches, there is level 3B evidence suggesting that both of these outcomes are better with VATS compared to thoracotomy (recommendation grade C).[24,25] Similarly, QOL has rarely been addressed in esophagectomy studies. The data that exists is primarily level 4 for both OE and MIE and indicate that with longer follow-up that QOL is similar to normal value patients (recommendation grade C).[15,26,27]

Minimally invasive esophagectomy is associated with at least equivalent results in terms of mortality, morbidity, and survival as open esophagectomy (level of evidence 3b to 4; recommendation grade C).

Pain control and pulmonary function may be better after VATS compared to thoracotomy for esophagectomy (level of evidence 3b; recommendation grade C).

The differences in case mix, experiences of the surgeon and centers involved, as well as a number of alternative open approaches make it difficult to draw definitive conclusions about whether MIE has real advantages over OE. The prospective E2202 trial will answer some questions about the utility of MIE. It should be emphasized that esophagectomy, whether performed by an open or minimally invasive approach, is a complex procedure and outcomes are better in high-volume centers. Another issue with MIE is the steep learning curve required to master these minimally invasive techniques, so it is likely that only a few centers with expertise in both minimally invasive techniques and open esophageal surgery will adopt this approach. Nevertheless, the results are encouraging and may broaden the applicability of this technique to higher-risk patient groups such as the elderly.[28] Prospective studies will be required to determine whether postoperative pain, recovery time, and cost are improved. As with VATS lobectomy, there will likely be a cadre of surgeons performing MIE and another group performing OE, all with excellent results. A randomized study may not be feasible because of institutional preferences, and so a prospective registry oriented series may be the best option to help elucidate whether the perceived advantages of MIE hold true.

References

1. Collard JM, Lengele B, Otte JB, Kestens PJ. En bloc and standard esophagectomies by thoracoscopy. *Ann Thorac Surg* 1993;56:675–679.
2. DePaula AL, Hashiba K, Ferreira EA, de Paula RA, Grecco E. Laparoscopic transhiatal esophagectomy with esophagogastroplasty. *Surg Laparosc Endosc* 1995;5:1–5.
3. Swanstrom LL, Hansen P. Laparoscopic total esophagectomy. *Arch Surg* 1997;132:943–947; discussion 7–9.
4. Luketich JD, Nguyen NT, Schauer PR. Laparoscopic transhiatal esophagectomy for Barrett's esophagus with high grade dysplasia. *JSLS* 1998;2:75–77.
5. Elli E, Espat NJ, Berger R, Jacobsen G, Knoblock L, Horgan S. Robotic-assisted thoracoscopic resection of esophageal leiomyoma. *Surg Endosc* 2004;18:713–716.
6. Goldminc M, Maddern G, Le Prise E, Meunier B, Campion JP, Launois B. Oesophagectomy by a

transhiatal approach or thoracotomy: a prospective randomized trial. *Br J Surg* 1993;80:367–370.
7. Chu KM, Law SY, Fok M, Wong J. A prospective randomized comparison of transhiatal and transthoracic resection for lower-third esophageal carcinoma. *Am J Surg* 1997;174:320–324.
8. Hulscher JB, van Sandick JW, de Boer AG, et al. Extended transthoracic resection compared with limited transhiatal resection for adenocarcinoma of the esophagus. *N Engl J Med* 2002;347:1662–1669.
9. Birkmeyer JD, Siewers AE, Finlayson EV, et al. Hospital volume and surgical mortality in the United States. *N Engl J Med* 2002;346:1128–1137.
10. Hermanek P. pTNM and residual tumor classifications: problems of assessment and prognostic significance. *World J Surg* 1995;19:184–190.
11. Akaishi T, Kaneda I, Higuchi N, et al. Thoracoscopic en bloc total esophagectomy with radical mediastinal lymphadenectomy. *J Thorac Cardiovasc Surg* 1996;112:1533–1540; discussion 40–41.
12. Osugi H, Takemura M, Higashino M, Takada N, Lee S, Kinoshita H. A comparison of video-assisted thoracoscopic oesophagectomy and radical lymph node dissection for squamous cell cancer of the oesophagus with open operation. *Br J Surg* 2003;90:108–113.
13. Nguyen NT, Follette DM, Wolfe BM, Schneider PD, Roberts P, Goodnight JE Jr. Comparison of minimally invasive esophagectomy with transthoracic and transhiatal esophagectomy. *Arch Surg* 2000;135:920–925.
14. Van den Broek WT, Makay O, Berends FJ, et al. Laparoscopically assisted transhiatal resection for malignancies of the distal esophagus. *Surg Endosc* 2004;18:812–817.
15. Luketich JD, Alvelo-Rivera M, Buenaventura PO, et al. Minimally invasive esophagectomy: outcomes in 222 patients. *Ann Surg* 2003;238:486–494; discussion 94–95.
16. Bailey SH, Bull DA, Harpole DH, et al. Outcomes after esophagectomy: a ten-year prospective cohort. *Ann Thorac Surg* 2003;75:217–222; discussion 222.
17. Orringer MB, Marshall B, Iannettoni MD. Transhiatal esophagectomy: clinical experience and refinements. *Ann Surg* 1999;230:392–400; discussion 403.
18. Orringer MB, Marshall B, Iannettoni MD. Eliminating the cervical esophagogastric anastomotic leak with a side-to-side stapled anastomosis. *J Thorac Cardiovasc Surg* 2000;119:277–288.
19. Rizk NP, Bach PB, Schrag D, et al. The impact of complications on outcomes after resection for

esophageal and gastroesophageal junction carcinoma. *J Am Coll Surg* 2004;198:42–50.

20. Atkins BZ, Shah AS, Hutcheson KA, et al. Reducing hospital morbidity and mortality following esophagectomy. *Ann Thorac Surg* 2004;78:1170–1176; discussion 1176.

21. Murthy SC, Law S, Whooley BP, Alexandrou A, Chu KM, Wong J. Atrial fibrillation after esophagectomy is a marker for postoperative morbidity and mortality. *J Thorac Cardiovasc Surg* 2003;126:1162–1167.

22. Nguyen NT, Roberts P, Follette DM, Rivers R, Wolfe BM. Thoracoscopic and laparoscopic esophagectomy for benign and malignant disease: lessons learned from 46 consecutive procedures. *J Am Coll Surg* 2003;197:902–913.

23. Avital S, Zundel N, Szomstein S, Rosenthal R. Laparoscopic transhiatal esophagectomy for esophageal cancer. *Am J Surg* 2005;190:69–74.

24. Ninomiya M, Nakajima J, Tanaka M, et al. Effects of lung metastasectomy on respiratory function. *Jpn J Thorac Cardiovasc Surg* 2001;49:17–20.

25. Landreneau RJ, Mack MJ, Hazelrigg SR, et al. Prevalence of chronic pain after pulmonary resection by thoracotomy or video-assisted thoracic surgery. *J Thorac Cardiovasc Surg* 1994;107:1079–1085; discussion 85–86.

26. Headrick JR, Nichols FC 3rd, Miller DL, et al. High-grade esophageal dysplasia: long-term survival and quality of life after esophagectomy. *Ann Thorac Surg* 2002;73:1697–1702; discussion 1702–1703.

27. Blazeby JM, Farndon JR, Donovan J, Alderson D. A prospective longitudinal study examining the quality of life of patients with esophageal carcinoma. *Cancer* 2000;88:1781–1787.

28. Perry Y, Fernando HC, Buenaventura PO, Christie NA, Luketich JD. Minimally invasive esophagectomy in the elderly. *Jsls* 2002;6:299–304.

29. Watson DI, Jamieson GG, Devitt PG. Endoscopic cervico-thoraco-abdominal esophagectomy. *J Am Coll Surg* 2000;190:372–378.

30. Nguyen NT, Roberts PF, Follette DM, et al. Evaluation of minimally invasive surgical staging for esophageal cancer. *Am J Surg* 2001;182:702–706.

31. Liu HP, Chang CH, Lin PJ, Chang JP. Video-assisted endoscopic esophagectomy with stapled intrathoracic esophagogastric anastomosis. *World J Surg* 1995;19:745–747.

32. Peracchia A, Rosati R, Fumagalli U, Bona S, Chella B. Thoracoscopic esophagectomy: are there benefits? *Semin Surg Oncol* 1997;13:259–262.

33. Law S, Fok M, Chu KM, Wong J. Thoracoscopic esophagectomy for esophageal cancer. *Surgery* 1997;122:8–14.

34. Kawahara K, Maekawa T, Okabayashi K, et al. Video-assisted thoracoscopic esophagectomy for esophageal cancer. *Surg Endosc* 1999;13:218–223.

35. Smithers BM, Gotley DC, McEwan D, Martin I, Bessell J, Doyle L. Thoracoscopic mobilization of the esophagus. A 6 year experience. *Surg Endosc* 2001;15:176–182.

36. Mathisen DJ, Grillo HC, Wilkins EW Jr, Moncure AC, Hilgenberg AD. Transthoracic esophagectomy: a safe approach to carcinoma of the esophagus. *Ann Thorac Surg* 1988;45:137–143.

37. Lerut T, De Leyn P, Coosemans W, Van Raemdonck D, Scheys I, LeSaffre E. Surgical strategies in esophageal carcinoma with emphasis on radical lymphadenectomy. *Ann Surg* 1992;216:583–590.

38. Swanson SJ, Batirel HF, Bueno R, et al. Transthoracic esophagectomy with radical mediastinal and abdominal lymph node dissection and cervical esophagogastrostomy for esophageal carcinoma. *Ann Thorac Surg* 2001;72:1918–1924; discussion 1924–1925.

39. Whooley BP, Law S, Murthy SC, Alexandrou A, Wong J. Analysis of reduced death and complication rates after esophageal resection. *Ann Surg* 2001;233:338–344.

40. Ferguson MK, Martin TR, Reeder LB, Olak J. Mortality after esophagectomy: risk factor analysis. *World J Surg* 1997;21:599–603; discussion 604.

27
Lymph Node Dissection for Carcinoma of the Esophagus

Nasser K. Altorki

The controversy surrounding the surgical treatment of esophageal cancer focuses, almost exclusively, on the extent of lymph node dissection required during esophagectomy. The majority view holds that an extended or a radical lymph node dissection will not improve overall or disease-free survival because the disease is systemic at the time of diagnosis and that long-term outcomes are largely determined by the biological behavior of the tumor; an issue that cannot be influenced by the extent of surgical dissection. Advocates of this view embrace the conventional techniques of esophageal resection where the esophagus is extracted from its mediastinal bed along with the adjacent periesophageal and lesser curvature nodes.[1-18] This extent of lymph node excision is easily achieved by either a transhiatal or a transthoracic approach and thus, the terms *transhiatal* or *transthoracic* are descriptive only of the means of surgical access rather than the extent of lymph node dissection which is, for all intents and purposes, similar in extent. In contrast, the opposing view held by a minority of surgeons in the West, states that a radical lymphadenectomy may improve local disease control and survival in a small, but significant, proportion of patients. The extent of lymph node dissection, as generally proposed by Japanese and some Western surgeons includes at least two nodal basins (two-field dissection) and occasionally three nodal basins (three-field dissection). These nodal regions or fields include:

1. The abdominal field, which encompasses the paracardial, lesser curvatures, left gastric, celiac, common hepatic, and splenic artery nodes.

In addition, all retroperitoneal tissues between the superior border of the pancreas and the crus of the diaphragm are included within the dissection.

2. The mediastinal field, which includes the middle and lower periesophageal nodes, the subcarinal nodes, and the thoracic duct with its associated lymph nodes as it courses through the middle and lower mediastinum. Resection of the trunk of the azygous vein, as previously proposed, is no longer considered a necessary component of the operation.[19]

3. The third field, which includes the chain of lymph nodes along both recurrent nerves throughout their mediastinal and cervical course, as well as the deep cervical nodes posterior and lateral to the jugular vein and the supraclavicular nodes. Thus, the third field encompasses a group of nodal stations that span the superior posterior mediastinum and the lower neck.

The purpose of this chapter is to review the published evidence supporting either of these two surgical strategies. For purposes of clarity, the data from transhiatal and transthoracic resections are presented separately, despite the earlier contention that the two procedures differ only slightly in the extent of the associated lymph node dissection.

27.1. Transhiatal Esophagectomy

This procedure is one of the more common techniques for esophagectomy in North America and Europe. In a study of the National Cancer

Database of the American College of Surgeons, transhiatal esophagectomies were performed in 25% to 30% of patients with carcinoma of the esophagus.[20] The procedure entails extirpation of the intrathoracic esophagus without a thoracotomy and advancement of the esophageal substitute, usually a greater curvature gastric tube, to the neck for reconstruction. The extent of nodal dissection with this operation is essentially limited to the periesophageal nodes and those perigastric nodes along the cardia, the lesser gastric curve, and the left gastric artery.

The largest single experience with transhiatal esophagectomy is that of Orringer, who reported on 800 patients with cancer of the intrathoracic esophagus and cardia.[1] Adenocarcinoma was present in 69% of the patients, while 28% had epidermoid cancer. Hospital mortality was 4.5% and morbidity was 27%. Overall survival at the 2-, 3-, and 5-year mark was 47%, 34%, and 23%, respectively. Five-year survival was 59% for stage I patients and 22% for stage IIA patients. Patients with stage III disease had a 2- and 5-year survival rate of 32% and 10%, respectively. There was an overall statistically significant survival advantage for patients with adenocarcinoma (24% vs. 17%).

This study by the University of Michigan group is considered the benchmark for transhiatal esophagectomy and represents the best expected outcome following transhiatal resections for carcinoma. However, it is clear from reviewing the literature that these survival rates are quite consistent with the experience of most surgeons who practice a similar approach[2-7] (Table 27.1). Gelfand reported on 160 patients who underwent transhiatal esophagectomy for carcinoma of the lower esophagus and cardia.[2] Most tumors were adenocarcinoma and most were in earlier stages. Survival rates at 2 years and 5 years were 40% and 21%, respectively. Gertsch reported on 100 patients with esophageal carcinoma who were uniformly treated with transhiatal esophagectomy without adjuvant therapy over a 10-year period.[3] Hospital mortality was 3% and morbidity 68%. The median survival was 18 months and the overall 5-year survival was 23%. There was no difference in survival between patients with adenocarcinoma compared to those with squamous histology. Survival was better for T1 and T2 tumors (63% 5-year survival). Vigneswaran reported on the results after transhiatal esophagectomy in 131 patients, the majority of whom had adenocarcinoma.[4] Operative mortality was 2%. Overall 5-year survival was 21%. Patients with stage I disease had a 47.5% 5-year survival compared to patients with stage III disease, whose 5-year survival was 5.8%. Patients with adenocarcinoma had a 5-year survival of 27%, while not a single patient with squamous cell cancer was alive at the 5-year mark.

A few studies reported the local recurrence rates following transhiatal resection.[21-23] Urba and colleagues reported the results of a randomized trial comparing transhiatal esophagectomy alone to transhiatal esophagectomy following induction chemoradiotherapy.[21] More than 75% of patients in both study arms had adenocarcinoma. There was no statistically significant difference in either overall survival or disease-free

TABLE 27.1. Transhiatal esophagectomy for esophageal cancer.

Author	Year	Patients	Cell type	Hospital mortality (%)	5-year survival (%)	Median survival
Orringer[1]	1999	800	A/S	4.5	23	ns
Chu[5,a]	1997	20	S	15	ns	16 months
Horstmann[6]	1995	46	A/S	15	20	12 months
Putnam[10]	1994	42	A/S	4.8	18	14 months
Gertsch[3]	1993	100	A/S	3	23	ns
Vigneswaran[4]	1993	131	A/S	2.3	21	ns
Goldminc[7,a]	1993	32	S	6.25	30 (3 years)	ns
Gelfand[2]	1992	160	A	0.9	21	ns

Abbreviations: A/S, adenocarcinoma/squamous cell carcinoma; ns, not significant; S, squamous cell carcinoma.
[a]Randomized trials comparing transhiatal and transthoracic esophagectomy.

survival between the two arms of the study. Overall survival and disease-free survival were both 16% after transhiatal esophagectomy alone. Local recurrence as a component of treatment failure occurred in 42% of patients in the surgery alone arm. This figure is almost identical to the local failure rate reported by Barbier, who prospectively evaluated the recurrence rate in 50 patients that underwent transhiatal resection for cancer by serial CT scans.[22] Local recurrence was detected in 39% of patients. More recently, Hulscher reported a loco-regional recurrence rate of 37% among 137 esophageal cancer patients treated by transhiatal esophagectomy without preoperative therapy.[23]

In summary, it appears that for patients with esophageal adenocarcinoma, transhiatal esophagectomy can usually be performed with an operative mortality of 5% or less in the hands of experienced esophageal surgeons (Table 27.1). Five-year survival rates are generally in the 20% to 25% range. Survival for patients with stage I tumors is in the 60% to 70% range, while patients with stage III disease have a 5% to 10% 5-year survival. Finally, the procedure is associated with failure to control or eradicate local disease in nearly 40% of patients.

27.2. Standard Transthoracic Esophagectomy

Transthoracic esophagectomy is probably the most widely performed operation for cancer of the esophagus worldwide. In the United States, 50% to 60% of all surgically treated tumors of the esophagus are performed using a transthoracic approach.[20] The procedure can be carried out either through a right or left thoracotomy incision, depending on the preference of the surgeon and the location of the tumor within the esophagus. Generally, a right thoracotomy is required for adequate exposure of tumors in the middle or upper thirds that are anatomically intimately related to the membranous trachea or the arch of the aorta. Tumors located at the gastroesophageal junction or in the lower third of the esophagus can also be approached through a left thoracotomy incision combined with a left phrenotomy, or, alternatively, with a left thoracoab-

dominal incision. Regardless of the side of the thoracotomy, the extent of lymph node dissection is usually limited to the immediate periesophageal, cardial, and perigastric nodes.

One of the largest experiences in North America with this approach is that of Ellis and coworkers.[8] The authors reported their experiences with nearly 500 patients who received a transthoracic esophagectomy employing standard surgical techniques. One third had squamous cell carcinoma, while the majority had adenocarcinoma of the esophagus or gastroesophageal junction. Hospital mortality was 3.3%. Complications occurred in 34% of patients. Overall 5-year survival including operative mortality and non–cancer-related deaths was 24.7%. Patients who had a complete (R0) resection had a 5-year survival of 29%, while no patients with either residual microscopic (R1) or macroscopic disease (R2) survived 5 years. Median and 5-year survival for patients with adenocarcinoma was 18 months and 25%, respectively. The corresponding figures for squamous cell cancers were 18 months and 20%, respectively, and were not statistically different from those for adenocarcinoma. Five-year survival was 79% for patients with stage I disease, 38% for those with stage IIA, and 27% for those with stage IIB. Patients with stage III disease had a 3- and 5-year survival of 20% and 13.7%, respectively.

This series by Ellis is generally representative of the results achievable using this surgical technique in many esophageal centers across the United States. For example, a recent study from the Mayo Clinic reported on the results after transthoracic esophagectomy in 220 patients, of whom 188 had adenocarcinoma.[9] Notwithstanding an impressively low hospital mortality and morbidity (1.4% and 37%, respectively), the survival rates remained essentially similar to those reported by Ellis nearly a decade previously. Overall 5-year survival was 25% and survival at 5 years for stages I, IIa, IIb, and III was 94%, 36%, 14%, and 10%, respectively. A review of some of the surgical series reported within the past decade from North America and Europe is shown in Table 27.2. Resectability rates ranged from 60% to 90% and hospital mortality ranged from 3.2% to 23%. Five-year survival rates varied between 8% and 24%. The variability in rates of

TABLE 27.2. Transthoracic esophagectomy for esophageal cancer.

Author	Year	Patients	Cell type	Hospital mortality %	5-year survival %	Median survival
Hofstetter[15]	2002	994	A/S	7%	34% (3 years)	20 months
Visbal[9]	2001	220	A/S	1.4%	25.2%	1.9 years
Karl[11]	2000	143	A/S	2.1%	29.6 (3 years)	1.6 years
						18 months (A)
Ellis[8]	1999	455	A/S	3.3%	24.7%	18 months (S)
Kelsen[17]	1998	227	A/S	6%	26% (3 years)	16.1 months
Adam[16]	1996	597	A/S	6.9%	16.3%	ns
Sharpe[14]	1996	562	A/S	9%	18%	ns
Walsh[18]	1996	113	A	2%	6% (3 years)	11 months
Lieberman[12]	1995	258	A/S	5%	27%	27 months
Putnam[10]	1994	134	A/S	8.2%	19%	22 months
Wright[13]	1994	91	A	2%	8%	ns

Abbreviations: A, adenocarcinoma; A/S, adenocarcinoma/squamous cell carcinoma; ns, not significant; S, squamous cell carcinoma.

resectability, hospital mortality, and 5-year survival likely represents inherent differences in patient selection, surgical expertise, and the retrospective nature of nearly all of these studies.

More instructive to review are the survival results achieved by the surgical arms of randomized trials comparing various preoperative regimens to surgical resection alone. The most recent of these trials was the North American Intergroup trial that compared chemotherapy followed by surgery with surgery alone.[17] There were 467 eligible patients of which 227 underwent primary surgical resection. The majority of resections were through a transthoracic approach. One hundred six patients had squamous cell cancer (47%) and 121 had adenocarcinoma (53%). Hospital mortality was 6%. Major complications occurred in 26% of patients. Overall survival at 1-, 2-, and 3-years was 60%, 37%, and 26%, respectively. Actuarial 5-year survival was 20%. There was no difference in outcome between patients with adenocarcinoma and those with epidermal cancer. In the trial by Walsh et al, 113 patients, all of whom had adenocarcinoma, were randomized to receive either surgery alone or chemoradiation followed by transthoracic esophagectomy.[18] Hospital mortality in the control arm was 2% and 3-year survival was 6%. In 2002, the Medical Research Council Esophageal Cancer Working Group reported the results of a large multicenter controlled, randomized trial of preoperative chemotherapy followed by esophagec-

tomy versus esophagectomy alone.[24] Although the details of the operative procedures were not described, the assumption may be made that the majority of cases had been done using a transthoracic approach, a common surgical strategy in most European centers. Survival in the surgery alone arm was 34% at 2 years and 15% at 5 years, with no difference in survival between adenocarcinoma and squamous cell cancer.

Local recurrences following standard transthoracic resections have been reported in 30% to 60% of patients. Most of the data regarding local recurrences are obtained from the surgical control arms of the various randomized trials. In the previously mentioned Intergroup trial comparing esophagectomy alone with chemotherapy followed by esophagectomy, the local recurrence rate in the control arm was 31% among 135 patients who received a complete (R0) resection. An additional 68 patients had an R1 or R2 resection. The overall local failure rate (persistent or recurrent disease) in all 227 patients in the control arm was 61%.[17]

27.3. Comparison of Transhiatal and Transthoracic Esophagectomy

Several retrospective studies have shown little difference in the peri-operative and survival outcomes between transhiatal and transthoracic esophagectomy. Rindani reviewed the results from 44 series published between 1986 and 1996.[25]

Thirty-three articles reported results on 2675 patients who underwent transhiatal resection while 29 articles reported results of transthoracic resections done in 2808 patients. Thirty-day mortality was 6.3% after transhiatal and 9.5% after transthoracic esophagectomy. Overall 5-year survival was 24% after transhiatal esophagectomy and 26% following transthoracic resection. More recently, Hulscher and colleagues reported a meta-analysis of the results of all comparative studies of transhiatal and transthoracic esophagectomy.[26] Their analysis included data abstracted from 50 articles published in the English literature between 1990 and 1999, with a total of 7500 patients. There was no statistically significant difference in overall 3-year and 5-year survival between the two procedures. There are two small, randomized trials that compared transhiatal and transthoracic resections with survival as an end point. The study by Chu and colleagues[5] comprised 39 patients, while the one by Goldminc had a total of 67 patients.[7] Neither study described the statistical details by which these small sample sizes were calculated. In the study by Goldminc and coworkers,[7] 67 patients were randomly assigned to receive either a transhiatal or transthoracic (non–en bloc) esophagectomy. Although the median operating time for transthoracic esophagectomy (TTE) was significantly longer than that for transhiatal resection (THE; 4h vs. 6h) there was no difference in other intra- and postoperative outcome measures including the need for blood transfusions, intensive care unit stay, and postoperative complications. Pulmonary complications occurred with similar frequency in both groups (THE, 19%; TTE, 20%), as did anastomotic leaks (THE, 6%; TTE, 9%) and recurrent nerve injuries (3% each). The 2-year overall survival was identical in both groups (40%). No information was given regarding disease-free survival or adequacy of local control. The study by Chu and colleagues[5] randomized an even smaller group of patients to either a THE ($n = 20$) or a TTE ($n = 19$). There was no difference in intraoperative or postoperative complications including transfusion requirements, cardiopulmonary complications, or anastomotic leaks between the two groups. There was no difference between both arms of the study in either local recurrence rates (25% for THE and

21% for TTE) or median survival times (THE, 16 months; TTE, 13.5 months).

In summary, it is clear that there are no important differences in survival between transhiatal and transthoracic esophagectomy. Given the similarity in the extent of nodal dissection between the two procedures these results may have been predictable.

27.4. En Bloc Esophagectomy

Logan introduced the en bloc concept in 1963 and it was re-introduced by Skinner in 1979.[19,27] The basic premise of the en-bloc operation is to maximize local tumor control by resection of the tumor-bearing esophagus within a wide envelope of adjoining tissues that includes both pleural surfaces laterally and the pericardium anteriorly where these structures are intimately related to the esophagus. Posteriorly, the lymphatics wedged dorsally between the esophagus and the aorta, including the thoracic duct throughout its mediastinal course, are resected en bloc with the specimen. This posterior mediastinectomy necessarily results in a complete mediastinal node dissection from the tracheal bifurcation to the esophageal hiatus. Additionally, an upper abdominal lymphadenectomy is performed including the common hepatic, celiac, left gastric, lesser curvature, parahiatal, and the retroperitoneal nodes. Local recurrence rates reported by proponents of this approach have been in the 2% to 10% range.[28,29] This is a strikingly low local failure rate when compared to local recurrences reported following either transhiatal esophagectomy or standard transthoracic resections, or those reported following chemoradiation delivered with curative intent.[30]

Critics have argued that the procedure is associated with a high operative mortality and morbidity, without an apparent survival advantage. In fact, in the earliest report by Skinner, the operative mortality for 80 patients with cancer of the cardia treated by an en bloc resection was 11% and the 5-year survival only 18%.[19] However, the past decade has witnessed a significant reduction in hospital mortality to the 5% range.[30–32] Several investigators have also reported survival rates exceeding those achievable by conventional techniques of esophageal resection. Lerut reported his experience with 195 patients who had an R0 (curative) resection for adenocarcinoma of the distal esophagus and gastroesophageal junction.[31] All patients had transmural disease (T3) and none received preoperative therapy. Five-year survival was 57% for node-negative patients and 26% for patients with nodal metastases. A prospective or cohort study by Altorki and Skinner reported on 111 patients who had an en bloc resection, the majority of which had adenocarcinoma and stage III disease.[32] Hospital mortality was 3.6%. Overall 5-year survival was 40%. Stage-specific survival was 78%, 72%, and 39%, respectively, for stages I, IIa, and III disease. Hagen reported similar results in a smaller group of patients with adenocarcinoma of the distal esophagus and gastroesophageal junction.[33] En bloc resection was performed in 30 patients and transhiatal resection was done in 16 patients. Overall survival was significantly better after en bloc resection (41% vs. 14%, $p = 0.001$). A survival advantage was observed in patients with early lesions (T1 and T2) where 5-year survival was 75% versus 21%, in favor of en bloc resection. Similarly patients with transmural tumors (T3) associated with 5 or less positive nodes had a significantly better survival after en bloc resection (27% vs. 9%).

An important criticism of most of these studies is the failure to clearly define the criteria for patient selection for one procedure versus another. For example, in the study by Hagen and colleagues, the patients receiving a transhiatal resection were either significantly older than the en bloc group or had a worse performance status with respect to cardiopulmonary function.[33] Additionally, a selection bias towards inclusion of patients with early-stage disease in the en bloc groups may have favorably biased survival outcome. The only randomized trial reported to date comparing transthoracic en bloc resection with transhiatal esophagectomy was reported by Hulscher and coworkers in 2002.[34] The authors randomly assigned 220 patients with adenocarcinoma of the mid to distal esophagus, or adenocarcinoma of the cardia, to either a transhiatal resection or a transthoracic esophagectomy with extended en bloc lymphadenectomy. The mean number of resected lymph nodes was 31 nodes after en bloc resection and 16 after transhiatal resection. There was no difference between the two arms in hospital mortality but morbidity was significantly higher after the extended en bloc procedure. The study was powered to detect a 50% relative improvement in survival in favor of the en bloc procedure. Although there was an important trend favoring the transthoracic (en bloc) group in both overall (39% vs. 29%) and disease-free survival (39% vs. 27%) at 5 years, the resultant 25% relative improvement in survival did not achieve statistical significance. A subsequent report by the same group suggested that with continued follow-up the difference in overall and disease-free survival achieved statistical significance for adenocarcinoma of the esophagus, but not that of the cardia.[35] Interestingly in this randomized trial there was no difference in either the rate of loco-regional recurrence or the time to recurrence between the two arms of the study.

27.5. Three-Field Lymphadenectomy

The concept of three-field lymph node dissection for esophageal cancer was developed by Japanese surgeons in the 1980s in response to the observation that as many as 40% of patients with resected squamous cell esophageal cancer developed isolated cervical lymph node metastases.[36] A nationwide retrospective study was subsequently reported describing the findings and potential benefits of esophagectomy with three-field dissection.[37] The additional third field of dissection included excision of the nodes along both recurrent nerves as they course through the mediastinum and neck, as well as a modified cervical node dissection. Previously, unsuspected cervical nodal metastases, primarily in the recurrent nodes, were seen in approximately one third of patients. Furthermore, the authors reported a significantly higher overall 5-year survival after three-field dissection in comparison to two-field dissection. The largest Japanese study from a single institution was reported by Akiyama in 1994.[38] The authors reported their experience with 717 patients in whom a complete (R0) resection was performed using either a two-field ($n = 393$) or a three-field technique ($n = 324$). Five-year survival in node-negative patients was 84% after the three-field procedure compared to 55% after two-field lymphadenectomy ($p = 0.004$). Patients with node-positive disease also fared better after three-field dissection with a 5-year survival rate of 43% compared to a 28% 5-year survival rate after two-field dissection ($p = 0.0008$). Two prospective studies have been reported.[39,40] The study by Nishihira was a prospective, randomized trial that showed a survival advantage for three-field over two-field lymph node dissection (65% vs. 48%); however the difference was not statistically significant.[39] The study from the National Cancer Hospital in Tokyo was a prospective, nonrandomized, case-matched study that showed that 5-year survival was significantly better after three-field dissection (48% vs. 33%; $p = 0.03$).[40] Five-year survival in the group of patients with cervical nodal disease was an impressive 30%. The relevance of these findings to a Western population afflicted primarily by esophageal adenocarcinoma remains unknown.

The only experience in North America with this technique was reported by Altorki and colleagues in 2002.[41] A prospective database was established in 1994 to examine survival and recurrence after esophagectomy with three-field dissection. The procedure was performed in 80 patients, 60% of which had adenocarcinoma of the esophagus. Hospital mortality was 5% and morbidity 47%. Recurrent nerve injury occurred in 6% of patients. An average of 60 nodes were resected per patient. The prevalence of cervical nodal metastases was 37% in patients regardless of cell type or location of the tumor within the esophagus. Overall and disease-free survival was 50% and 46%, respectively, and was not influenced by cell types. Patients with adenocarcinoma who had metastases to the recurrent laryngeal lymph nodes had a 3- and 5-year survival of 30% and 15%, respectively. In contrast patients with squamous cell carcinoma and positive recurrent laryngeal nodes had a 5-year survival of 40%. Lerut reported the only European experience with esophagectomy and three-field lymph node dissection.[42] One hundred and seventy-four patients had an R0 three-field esophagectomy with a hospital mortality of 1.4% and morbidity of 57%. Fifty-five percent of patients had adenocarcinoma of the esophagus or cardia. Overall and disease-free survival at 5

years was 42% and 46%, respectively. There was no difference in survival between patients with adenocarcinoma compared to those with squamous carcinoma (35% vs. 44%, $p = 0.5$). The incidence of positive cervical nodes in patients with adenocarcinoma was 23% and was slightly higher for those with esophageal versus cardial tumors (26% vs. 18%). Four- and five-year survival for patients with adenocarcinoma and positive cervical nodes were 35% and 11%, respectively.

27.6. Perspective

The above discussion of the results of the various surgical approaches suggests that there is no substantive difference in mortality, morbidity, recurrence, or survival between limited lymph node dissection performed through a transhiatal or a conventional transthoracic approach. The data supporting this conclusion are derived from the two small, randomized trials by Chu and Goldminc[5,7] that compared transhiatal and transthoracic resections with survival as an endpoint (level of evidence 1). Despite the small sample sizes in both studies, the consistency of their results with those reported by a large number of retrospective studies (level of evidence 3) suggests that there is most likely no important differences between these two surgical approaches in the extent and results of lymph node dissection and that survival is likely to be in the 25% to 30% range. It is also apparent that with the exception of two cohort studies by Altorki and colleagues[32,41] (level of evidence 2) and the single randomized trial by Hulscher and coworkers[34] (level of evidence 1), the evidence supporting an extended lymph node dissection is derived from case series (level of evidence 3) with a variable number of patients and undefined selection criteria. However, the survival of results in the two cohort studies reported by Altorki and colleagues (5-year survival of 40%) are consistent with similar results reported by other Japanese and European centers practicing a similar surgical strategy. Interestingly, these survival figures are also identical to the 39% survival reported by Hulscher and colleagues[34] in the en bloc arm of their randomized trial.[34] This constitutes a 25% to 30% *relative* improvement in survival for the en bloc procedure in patients with adenocarcinoma of the middle and distal esophageal thirds.[35]

Based on these data, patients with esophageal carcinoma (stages I–III), with good performance status (ECOG performance status 0–1) and no prohibitive comorbidities, should undergo an esophagectomy with at least a two-field en bloc dissection (recommendation grade B). The evidence suggests that the procedure provides the most complete staging information (level of evidence 1) and improves survival (level of evidence 2), but does so at the expense of an increase in perioperative morbidity (level of evidence 1). The role of a three-field dissection remains to be more clearly defined.

> Patients with esophageal carcinoma should undergo an esophagectomy with at least a two-field en bloc dissection (level of evidence 1 to 2; recommendation grade B). There is insufficient evidence to make recommendations regarding the role of a three-field dissection.

References

1. Orringer, MB, Marshall B, Iannettoni MD. Transhiatal esophagectomy: clinical experience and refinements. *Ann Surg* 1999;230:392–403.
2. Gelfand GA, Finley RJ, Nelems B, Inculet R, Evans KG, Fradet G. Transhiatal esophagectomy for carcinoma of the esophagus and cardia. Experience with 160 cases. *Arch Surg* 1992;127:164–167.
3. Gertsch P, Vauthey JN, Lustenberger AA, Friedlander-Klar H. Long-term results of transhiatal esophagectomy for esophageal carcinoma. A multivariate analysis of prognostic factors. *Cancer* 1993;72:2312–2319.
4. Vigneswaran WT, Trastek VF, Pairolero PC, Deschamps C, Daly RC, Allen MS. Transhiatal esophagectomy for carcinoma of the esophagus. *Ann Thorac Surg* 1993;56:838–844.
5. Chu KM, Law SY, Fok M, Wong J. A prospective randomized comparison of transhiatal and transthoracic resection for lower-third esophageal carcinoma. *Am J Surg* 1997;174:320–324.
6. Horstmann O, Verreet PR, Becker H, Ohmann C, Roher HD. Transhiatal oesophagectomy compared with transthoracic resection and systematic lymphadenectomy for the treatment of oesophageal cancer. *Eur J Surg* 1995;161:557–567.
7. Goldminc M, Maddern G, Le Prise E, Meunier B, Campion JP, Launois B. Oesophagectomy by a transhiatal approach or thoracotomy: a prospective randomized trial. *Br J Surg* 1993;80:367–370.
8. Ellis FH Jr. Standard resection for cancer of the esophagus and cardia. *Surg Oncol Clin N Am* 1999;8:279–294.
9. Visbal AL, Allen MS, Miller DL, Deschamps C, Trastek VF, Pairolero PC. Ivor Lewis esophagogastrectomy for esophageal cancer. *Ann Thorac Surg* 2001;71:1803–1808.
10. Putnam JB Jr, Suell DM, McMurtrey MJ, et al. Comparison of three techniques of esophagectomy within a residency training program. *Ann Thorac Surg* 1994;57:319–325.
11. Karl RC, Schreiber R, Boulware D, Baker S, Coppola D. Factors affecting morbidity, mortality, and survival in patients undergoing Ivor Lewis esophagogastrectomy. *Ann Surg* 2000;231:635–643.
12. Lieberman MD, Shriver CD, Bleckner S, Burt M. Carcinoma of the esophagus. Prognostic significance of histologic type. *J Thorac Cardiovasc Surg* 1995;109:130–138.
13. Wright CD, Mathisen DJ, Wain JC, et al. Evolution of treatment strategies for adenocarcinoma of the esophagus and gastroesophageal junction. *Ann Thorac Surg* 1994;58:1574–1578.
14. Sharpe DA, Moghissi K. Resectional surgery in carcinoma of the esophagus and cardia: What influences long-term survival? *Eur J Cardiothorac Surg* 1996;10:359.
15. Hofstetter W, Swisher SG, Correa AM, et al. Treatment outcomes of resected esophageal cancer. *Ann Surg* 2002;236:376–384.
16. Adam DJ, Craig SR, Sang CT, Walker WS, Cameron EW. Esophagogastrectomy for carcinoma in patients under 50 years of age. *J R Coll Surg Obstet* 1996;41:371–373.
17. Kelsen DP, Ginsberg R, Pajak TF, et al. Chemotherapy followed by surgery compared with surgery alone for localized esophageal cancer. *N Engl J Med* 1998;339:1979–1984.
18. Walsh TN, Noonan N, Hollywood D, Kelly A, Keeling N, Hennessy TP. A comparison of multimodal therapy and surgery for esophageal adenocarcinoma. *N Engl J Med* 1996;335:462–467.
19. Skinner DB. *En-bloc resection for neoplasms of the esophagus and cardia.* J Thorac Cardiovasc Surg 1983;85:59–69.
20. Daly JM, Fry WA, Little AG, et al. Esophageal cancer: results of an American College of Surgeons

Patient Care Evaluation Study. *J Am Coll Surg* 2000;190:562–572; discussion 572–573.

21. Urba SG, Orringer MB, Turrisi A, et al. Randomized trial of preoperative chemoradiation versus surgery alone in patients with locoregional esophageal carcinoma. *J Clin Oncol* 2001;19:305–313.

22. Barbier PA, Luder PJ, Schupfer G, Becker CD, Wagner HE. Quality of life and patterns of recurrence following transhiatal esophagectomy for cancer: results of a prospective follow-up in 50 patients. *World J Surg* 1988;12:270–276.

23. Hulscher JB, van Sandick JW, Tijssen JG, Obertop H, van Lanschot JJ. The recurrence pattern of esophageal carcinoma after transhiatal resection. *J Am Coll Surg* 2000;191:143–148.

24. Medical Research Council Oesophageal Cancer Working Party. Surgical resection with or without preoperative chemotherapy in oesophageal cancer: a randomized controlled trial. *Lancet* 2002;359: 1727–1733.

25. Rindani R, Martin, CJ, Cox MR. Transhiatal versus Ivor-Lewis esophagectomy: is there a difference? *Aust N Z J Surg* 1999;69:187–194.

26. Hulscher JB, Tijssen JG, Obertop H, van Lanschot JJ. Transthoracic versus transhiatal resection for carcinoma of the esophagus: a meta-analysis. *Ann Thorac Surg* 2001;72:306–313.

27. Logan A. The surgical treatment of carcinoma of the esophagus and cardia. *J Thorac Cardiovasc Surg* 1963;46:150–161.

28. Nigro JJ, De Meester SR, Hagen JA, et al. Node status in transmural esophageal adenocarcinoma and outcome after en-bloc esophagectomy. *J Thorac Cardiovasc Surg* 1999;117:960–968.

29. Altorki NK, Girardi L, Skinner DB. En-bloc esophagectomy improves survival for stage III esophageal cancer. *J Thorac Cardiovasc Surg* 1997;114:948–955.

30. Herskovic A, Martz K, Al-Sarraf M, et al. Combined chemotherapy and radiotherapy compared with radiotherapy alone in patients with cancer of the esophagus. *N Engl J Med* 1992;326:1593–1598.

31. Lerut T, Moons J, Fieuws S. Extracapsular lymph node involvement in esophageal cancer and number of involved nodes. *J Thorac Cardiovasc Surg* 2004;127:1855–1856.

32. Altorki N, Skinner D. Should en bloc esophagectomy be the standard of care for esophageal carcinoma? *Ann Surg* 2001;234:581–587.

33. Hagen JA, Peters JH, De Meester TR. Superiority of extended en bloc esophagogastrectomy for carcinoma of the lower esophagus and cardia. *J Thorac Cardiovasc Surg* 1993;106:850–858.

34. Hulscher JB, van Sandick JW, de Boer AG, et al. Extended transthoracic resection compared with limited transhiatal resection for adenocarcinoma of the esophagus. *N Engl J Med* 2002;347:1662–1669.

35. Hulscher JB, van Lanschot JJ. Individualised surgical treatment of patients with an adenocarcinoma of the distal oesophagus or gastro-oesophageal junction. *Dig Surg* 2005;22:130–134.

36. Isono K, Onada S, Okuyama K, et al. Recurrence of intrathoracic esophageal cancer. *Jpn J Clin Oncol* 1985;15:49–60.

37. Isono K, Sato H, Nakayama K. Results of nationwide study of the three-field lymph node dissection of esophageal cancer. *Oncology* 1991;48:411–420.

38. Akiyama H, Tsurumaru M, Udagawa H, Kajiyama Y. Radical lymph node dissection for cancer of the thoracic esophagus. *Ann Surg* 1994;220:364–372.

39. Nishihira T, Hirayama K, Mori S. A prospective randomized trial of extended cervical and superior mediastinal lymphadenectomy for carcinoma of the thoracic esophagus. *Am J Surg* 1998;175:47–51.

40. Kato H, Watanabe H, Tachimori Y, Iizuka T. Evaluation of the neck lymph node dissection for thoracic esophageal carcinoma. *Ann Thorac Surg* 1991;51:931–935.

41. Altorki N, Kent M, Ferrara C, Port J. Three-field lymph node dissection for squamous cell and adenocarcinoma of the esophagus. *Ann Surg* 2002;236:177–183.

42. Lerut T, Nafteux P, Moons J, et al. Three-field lymphadenectomy for carcinoma of the esophagus and gastroesophageal junction in 174 R0 resections: impact on staging, disease-free survival, and outcome: a plea for adaptation of TNM classification in upper-half esophageal carcinoma. *Ann Surg* 2004;240:962–972.

28
Intrathoracic Versus Cervical Anastomosis in Esophageal Replacement

Christian A. Gutschow and Jean-Marie Collard

Subtotal esophagectomy may consist of either resection of the lower 90% of the thoracic segment of the esophagus with subsequent esophagogastrostomy at the apex of the chest, or resection of the whole thoracic segment plus the lower segment of the cervical part of the esophagus with subsequent cervical esophagogastrostomy.

This chapter aims at establishing scientific evidence in pros and cons of cervical and high intrathoracic esophagogastrostomy, addressing three different aspects: the initial perioperative course, long-term postoperative function, and oncologic outcome.

28.1. Current Beliefs

28.1.1. Belief Number 1

Individual surgical experience and data from noncomparative studies[1] suggest that both anastomotic fistula and stricture are more common after construction of the anastomosis in the neck, whereas postoperative mortality is higher after leakage of an intrathoracic esophagogastrostomy.

Arguments supporting this belief are:

- The need for preservation of the poorly vascularized upper part of the fundus to reach the cervical esophageal stump.[2]
- The relative shortness of the gastric transplant is liable to put the cervical suture line under undue tension with subsequent collapse of intramural microvessels.[3,4]
- External compression of the gastric conduit at the thoracic inlet may compromise blood flow to the cervical anastomosis.[5]

Indeed, Liebermann-Meffert[2] showed that the uppermost 20% of the gastric transplant is vascularized only through microvascular venous and arterial networks within both the mucosa and submucosa of the gastric wall, so that the author recommends resection of the fundus prior to constructing the cervical anastomosis. This is supported by the observation of Pierie[3,4] that tailoring of the stomach into an esophageal substitute reduces parietal blood flow to the fundus as assessed by laser–Doppler velocimetry by 48% on average. Likewise, Nabeya[6] showed that fundic blood flow at the time of completion of the gastric transplant, in reference to predissection values, drops by 29% on average when the stomach is maintained in its entirety, and by 33% when it is shaped into a greater curvature tube. Moreover, Pierie[3,4] showed that the risk for the development of an anastomotic stricture is far higher in patients having a blood perfusion lower than 70% of preconstruction values. This observation is in line with the one of Kudo[7] that fundic blood flow is lower in patients who develop a cervical fistula compared to those who do not develop a cervical fistula. This is confirmed by Mori,[8] who reported that the risk for the development of a cervical fistula correlated well with the distance between the anastomotic site in the fundus and the uppermost pulsatile branch of the vascular arcade along the greater curvature.

The most common explanation for the higher mortality attributed to intrathoracic leakage is the development of mediastinitis.[1,9] In contrast, leaks from a cervical esophagogastrostomy usually consist of external salivary weeping only.[9]

28.1.2. Belief Number 2

It is generally believed that the ability of gastric contents to reflux into the esophagus is linked to the level (intrathoracic vs. cervical) of the esophagogastrostomy. Those surgeons who think that esophageal exposure to gastric contents is higher after intrathoracic anastomosis refer to the concept that the pressure gradient between the chest and the neck opposes reflux into the cervical esophageal remnant.[10] Conversely, those who believe that exposure of the esophagus to gastric contents is greater after neck esophagogastrostomy point to motility studies showing that the longer the residual esophageal segment, the better the propulsive activity, esophageal clearance, and resistance to gastroesophageal reflux.[11]

28.1.3. Belief Number 3

It is commonly accepted that the difference in length of the esophageal remnant after intrathoracic esophagogastrostomy and that after cervical anastomosis is so great that it substantially influences functional outcome. In contrast, other surgeons believe that it does not make any substantial difference because of the spontaneous tendency of cervical esophagogastrostomy to move downwards during the postoperative course.[12]

28.1.4. Belief Number 4

Upper resection margin above the tumor on the resected specimen is much longer after neck transsection of the esophagus than after its division at the apex of the chest. As a consequence, it is believed that neoplastic recurrence at the level of the anastomosis is substantially lower after cervical esophagogastrostomy.[13]

28.2. Evidence-Based Knowledge

28.2.1. Perioperative Course

This section addresses both intra- and postoperative outcomes of patients after subtotal esophagectomy and cervical or intrathoracic anastomosis. The parameters analyzed were operating time, blood loss, number of transfused blood units, anastomotic time, anastomotic leakage rate, rates of pulmonary and cardiac complications, overall complication rate, incidences of vocal cord palsy, chylothorax, and reoperations, duration of hospital stay, mortality, and mortality due to leakage. A detailed analysis can be found in Table 28.1.

Fourteen comparative studies, out of which three prospective, randomized, controlled trials (level of evidence 2b), three prospective, nonrandomized trials (level of evidence 3b), and eight other studies (level of evidence 3b) were analyzed. In studies showing a statistically significant difference between the thoracic and the cervical approach, this significance was unequivocal in favor of intrathoracic anastomosis for anastomotic time,[14] rate of anastomotic leakage,[12,15,16] and frequency of pulmonary complications.[17] In contrast, unambiguous significance in favor of cervical esophagogastrostomy was found for the parameter "mortality due to anastomotic leakage."[15] Other comparative studies did not show any significant difference between both types of anastomosis for all the parameters listed in Table 28.1 (first column), especially for operative time, blood loss, need for transfusion, cardiac complications, vocal cord palsy, incidence of chylothorax, need for operative reintervention, duration of hospital stay, postoperative mortality, and overall morbidity.

Our main conclusions are that an intrathoracic anastomosis is quicker to perform with lower risk for the development of anastomotic leakage and pulmonary complications (recommendation grade B). On the other hand, mortality due to a cervical anastomotic insufficiency appears to be less lethal (recommendation grade C). Analysis of the other intra- and postoperative parameters does not allow for further valid conclusions.

An intrathoracic anastomosis is quicker to perform with lower risk for the development of anastomotic leakage and pulmonary complications (level of evidence 2b to 3b; recommendation grade B).

Mortality due to a cervical anastomotic insufficiency is less lethal (level of evidence 3b; recommendation grade C).

TABLE 28.1. Perioperative parameters.

Evidence level	2b	2b	2b	3b	3b	3b	3b	3b	3b	3b	3b	3b	3b	3b
Study design	1	1	1	2	2	2	3	3	3	3	3	3	3	3
Reference	12	17	14	25	26	27	15	16	28	22	20	32	34	33
n (CA/TA)	43/49	30/30	41/42	99/289	62/33	50/57	108/444	44/1921	19/55	56/153	62/46	248/58	273/22	122/301
Operating time	Ns		ns											
Blood loss			ns		ns									
Transfusions	Ns		ns		ns									
Anastomotic time	TA better, $p < 0.02$		TA better, $p < 0.0001$											
Anastomotic leak	ns	ns	ns	ns	ns	ns	TA better	TA better, $p < 0.001$	ns	ns	ns	ns	ns	ns
Pulmonary complications	ns	TA better, $p = 0.01$	ns	ns									ns	
Cardiac complications			ns		ns									
Vocal cord palsy		ns	ns		ns									
Chylothorax	ns		ns		ns									
Reoperation			ns		ns									
Hospital stay	ns		ns		ns									
Mortality	ns	ns	ns	ns	ns		ns		ns			ns	ns	
Mortality due to leakage	ns	ns	ns	ns	ns	CA better	ns		ns			CA better, $p < 0.001$	ns	ns
Overall complications	ns	ns	ns		ns	ns	ns				ns			

Abbreviations: 1, prospective, randomized study; 2, prospective, nonrandomized study; 3, other study design; CA, cervical anastomosis; ns, not significant; TA, thoracic anastomosis.

28.2.2. Functional Aspects

This section aims at covering the functional outcome of patients after subtotal esophagectomy and cervical or intrathoracic anastomosis. Parameters analyzed were rates of esophagitis, stricture, and dilations; incidence of heartburn, regurgitation, and dysphagia; results of esophageal pH-metry and scintigraphic tests; anastomotic diameter; weight loss; and quality of life. A detailed analysis can be found in Table 28.2.

Fifteen comparative studies, out of which 2 randomized, controlled trials (level of evidence 2b), 1 prospective, nonrandomized trial (level of evidence 3b), and 12 other studies (level of evidence 3b) were analyzed. In all studies showing statistically significant differences between the thoracic and the cervical approach, patients with cervical esophagogastrostomy had lower incidences of esophagitis,[18,19] heartburn,[15,19,20] regurgitation,[19,20] and dysphagia.[15] Likewise, all significant results were in favor of cervical esophagogastrostomy for results of esophageal pH-metry[21] and quality of life.[20] Discrepant, though significant results were found for the incidence of stricture formation in favor of cervical anastomosis in one study[19] and in favor of intrathoracic anastomosis in another study.[22] Other comparative studies did not show any significant difference between the types of anastomosis for all the parameters listed in Table 28.2, especially for need for dilations, esophageal diameter, weight loss, and parameters assessed via scintigraphic methods (esophageal swallowing function, gastric emptying, gastroesophageal reflux).

Our main conclusions from this section are that cervical anastomosis provides functional advantages concerning the incidence of heartburn and regurgitation combined with a lower rate of esophagitis (recommendation grade C). Analysis of the other functional parameters does not allow for further valid recommendations.

A cervical anastomosis provides functional advantages concerning the incidence of heartburn and regurgitation, combined with a lower rate of esophagitis (evidence level 3b; recommendation grade C).

28.2.3. Oncologic Outcome

This section aims at covering the oncologic outcome of patients after subtotal esophagectomy and cervical or intrathoracic anastomosis. Parameters analyzed were mean, median, and 5-year-survival; survival with positive abdominal lymph nodes; rates of local recurrence; length of the esophageal remnant and the upper resection margin; and rate of complete resection. A detailed analysis can be found in Table 28.3.

The issue of whether three-field lymph node dissection would provide patients with better long-term survival compared to two-field dissection is beyond the scope of the chapter.

Ten comparative studies, out of which three prospective, randomized, controlled trials (level of evidence 2b), two prospective, nonrandomized trials (level of evidence 3b), and five other studies (level of evidence 3b) were analyzed. The esophageal remnant was shorter and the healthy upper resection margin of the surgical specimen was found to be significantly longer after subtotal esophagectomy, including resection of the lower segment of the cervical esophagus.[12,14,17,23] Unequivocal significant differences were found in favor of the intrathoracic anastomosis for survival of patients with positive abdominal lymph nodes,[12] and in favor of cervical esophagogastrostomy for the incidence of local tumor recurrence.[23] However, no significant difference between both types of anastomosis was found for all the parameters listed in Table 28.3, especially for mean and median survival, 5-year survival, and prevalence of completely resected tumors (R0 resection).

Our conclusion is that a cervical anastomosis allows for a longer esophageal margin from the proximal extent of tumor (recommendation grade B). However, this did not translate into a lower local recurrence rate in most studies. Therefore, in daily clinical practice, this information appears of little value to the operating surgeon. Analysis of the other oncologic parameters does not allow for further valid recommendations.

A cervical anastomosis allows for a longer esophageal margin from the proximal extent of tumor. However, this does not translate into a lower local recurrence rate (level of evidence 2b to 3b; recommendation grade B).

TABLE 28.2. Functional parameters.

Evidence level	2b	2b	3b	3b	3b	3b	3b	3b	3b	3b	3b	3b	3b	3b	3b
Study design	1	1	2	3	3	3	3	3	3	3	3	3	3	3	3
Reference	12	14	27	15	22	20	24	31	30	18	31	21	19	34	33
n (neck/thorax)	43/49	41/42	50/57	108/444	56/153	62/46	20/27	5/5	78/13	39/35	15/19	51/19	50/30	273/22	122/301
Esophagitis							ns		ns	CA better $p=0.0039$		ns	CA better $p=0.0001$ at 12 m		
Stricture	ns	ns			TA better $p=0.03$		ns						CA better $p=0.0458$ at 3 m		ns
Dilations	ns	ns	ns				ns								
Heartburn				CA better		CA better $p<0.03$						ns	CA better $p=0.001$ at 12 m	ns	
Regurgitation						CA better $p<0.02$	ns						CA better $p=0.001$ at 12 m		
Dysphagia		ns					ns						CA better $p=0.0256$ at 3 m		
Esophageal pH-metry							ns					CA better			
Swallow fx (scinti)								ns	ns		ns				
GER (scinti)								ns							
Gastric emptying (scinti)								ns	ns		ns				
Anastomotic diameter		ns	ns												
Weight loss	ns	ns													
Quality of life				CA better											

Abbreviations: 1, prospective, randomized study; 2, prospective, nonrandomized study; 3, other study design; CA, cervical anastomosis; ns, not significant; TA, thoracic anastomosis.

TABLE 28.3. Oncologic parameters.

Evidence level	2b	2b	2b	3b	3b	3b	3b	3b	3b	3b
Study design	1	1	1	2	2	3	3	3	3	3
Reference	12	17	14	25	27	15	23	20	24	32
n (neck/thorax)	43/49	30/30	41/42	99/289	50/57	108/444	19/55	62/46	20/27	248/58
Mean survival			ns							
Median survival	ns	ns					ns	ns		
5-year survival			ns			ns		ns		
Survival with positive abdominal lymphnodes	TA > CA $p < 0.05$									
Local recurrence			ns	ns	ns		CA > TA $p = 0.04$			ns
Length esophageal remnant			TA > CA $p < 0.0001$						TA > CA $p < 0.001$	
Length upper resection margin	CA > TA $p < 0.05$	CA > TA		ns						
Complete resection	ns	ns	ns				ns	ns		

Abbreviations: 1, prospective, randomized study; 2, prospective, nonrandomized study; 3, other study design; CA, cervical anastomosis; ns, not significant; TA, thoracic anastomosis.

28.3. Summary

The aim of this chapter was to analyze the available evidence as to whether cervical or intrathoracic anastomosis after subtotal esophageal resection provide patients with a better outcome in terms of perioperative, functional, and oncologic parameters.

For this purpose, a Medline literature search was performed for comparative studies in this field. Twenty-one references were found, out of which 3 prospective, randomized studies,[12,14,17] 3 prospective, nonrandomized studies,[25–27] and 16 trials using another study design.[15,16,18–24,28–34]

For certain parameters, unequivocal evidence could be found among those studies showing significant results. Accordingly, several existing beliefs were substantiated: cervical esophagogastrostomy is quicker to perform, carries a higher risk for anastomotic fistula, and has a lower mortality due to anastomotic leakage than intrathoracic esophagogastrostomy. Furthermore, unequivocal significant evidence was found for several functional parameters: cervical anastomosis carries a lower incidence of esophagitis, heartburn, positive esophageal pH-metry, and dysphagia. Likewise, general quality-of-life status was found to be better after cervical esophagogastrostomy. Evidence available shows that upper esophageal resection margin is significantly longer and the remaining cervical esophageal stump is shorter after cervical esophagogastrostomy. However, this translated in a significantly lower local recurrence rate in only one retrospective study,[23] whereas this rate was not different in several other trials.[14,25,27,32] Moreover, there was no trial that showed a higher R0 resection rate after cervical anastomosis.

In conclusion, although our results indicate that some of the widely held beliefs cited above might be true, currently available data provided by the evidence-based literature are not sufficient to give clear advice to the surgeon which principle to follow. In addition to discrepant data, most studies fail to show any statistically significant difference for most perioperative, functional, and oncologic parameters.

References

1. Borst HG, Dragojevic D, Stegmann T, et al. Anastomotic leakage, stenosis, and reflux after esophageal replacement. *World J Surg* 1978;2:861–866.
2. Liebermann-Meffert D, Siewert JR. Vascular anatomy of the gastric tube used for esophageal reconstruction. *Ann Thorac Surg* 1992;54:1110–1115.
3. Pierie JPEN, de Graaf PW, Poen A, et al. Gastric blood flow perfusion predicts healing of oesophagogastrostomies [abstract]. *Fourth International Congress of the O.E.S.O.* Paris: O.E.S.O.; 1993:119.

4. Pierie JPEN, de Graaf PW, Poen H, et al. Incidence and management of benign anastomotic stricture after cervical oesophagogastrostomy. *Br J Surg* 1993;80:471–474.

5. Siewert JR, Stein HJ, Liebermann-Meffert D, et al. Esophageal reconstruction: the gastric tube as an esophageal substitute. *Dis Esophagus* 1995;8:11–19.

6. Nabeya K, Hanaoka T, Onozawa K, et al. Two-stage esophagogastrostomy for esophageal reconstruction. In: Ferguson MK, Little AG, Skinner DB, eds. *Diseases of the Esophagus, Malignant Diseases.* Vol. 1. New York: Futura;1990:247–252.

7. Kudo T, Abo S, Itabashi T. Prognosis of esophageal substitute in tissue variability and anastomotic leakage. In: Siewert JR, Hölscher AH, eds. *Diseases of the Esophagus. Pathophysiology, Diagnosis, Conservative and Surgical Treatment.* Berlin: Springer Verlag; 1988:522–525.

8. Mori T. An experimental study of the hemodynamics of the gastric tube for esophageal reconstruction. *Nippon Geka Hokan* 1991;60:250–263.

9. Urschel JD. Esophagogastrostomy anastomotic leaks complicating esophagectomy: a review. *Am J Surg* 1995;169:634–640.

10. Hölscher AH, Voit H, Buttermann G, et al. Function of the intrathoracic stomach as esophageal replacement. *World J Surg* 1988;12:835–844.

11. Maier G, Jehle C, Becker HD. Functional outcome following oesophagectomy for oesophageal cancer: a prospective manometric study. *Dis Esophagus* 1995;8:64–69.

12. Chasseray VM, Kiroff GK, Buard JL, et al. Cervical or thoracic anastomosis for esophagectomy for carcinoma. *Surg Gynecol Obstet* 1989;169:55–62.

13. Tam PC, Siu KF, Cheung HC, et al. Local recurrences after subtotal esophagectomy for squamous cell carcinoma. *Ann Surg* 1987;205:189–194.

14. Walther B, Johansson J, Johnsson F, et al. Cervical or thoracic anastomosis after esophageal resection and gastric tube reconstruction. *Ann Surg* 2003;238:803–814.

15. Chen J, Wei G Shao L. A comparative study of cervical and thoracic anastomoses after esophagectomy for esophageal carcinoma. *Zhonghua Zhong Liu Za Zhi* 1996;18:131–133.

16. Sun Y, Ding B, Zhou N. Stapled anastomosis in esophageal resections with Chinese staplers: a retrospective study of 1965 consecutive cases. *Chin Med J* 1998;111:867–869.

17. Ribet M, Debrueres B, Lecomte-Houcke M. Resection for advanced cancer of the thoracic esophagus: cervical or thoracic anastomosis? *J Thorac Cardiovasc Surg* 1992;103:784–788.

18. Shibuya S, Fukudo S, Shineha R, et al. High incidence of reflux esophagitis observed by routine endoscopic examination after gastric pull-up esophagectomy. *World J Surg* 2003;27:580–583.

19. De Leyn P, Coosemans W, Lerut T. Early and late functional results in patients with intrathoracic gastric replacement after oesophagectomy for carcinoma. *Eur J Cardiothorac Surg* 1992;6:79–85.

20. Schmidt CE, Bestmann B, Küchler T, et al. Quality of life associated with surgery for esophageal cancer: differences between collar and intrathoracic anastomoses. *World J Surg* 2004;28:355–360.

21. Gutschow CA, Romagnoli R, Schröder W, Hoelcher A, Collard J-M. Gastroesophageal reflux after esophageal replacement by gastric pull-up: cervical vs high intrathoracic anastomosis. In press.

22. Law S, Suen D, Wong KH, et al. A single-layer, continuous, hand-sewn method for esophageal anastomosis. *Arch Surg* 2005;140:33–39.

23. Blewett CJ, Miller JD, Ramlawi B, et al. Local recurrence after total and subtotal esophagectomy for esophageal cancer. *J Exp Clin Cancer Res* 2001;20:17–19.

24. Johansson J, Johnsson F, Groshen S, et al. Pharyngeal reflux after gastric pull-up esophagectomy with neck and chest anastomoses. *J Thorac Cardiovasc Surg* 1999;118:1078–1083.

25. Lam TCF, Fok M, Cheng S, et al. Anastomotic complications after esophagectomy for cancer. *J Thorac Cardiovasc Surg* 1992;104:395–400.

26. Schilling MK, Eichenberger M, Wagener V, et al. Impact of fundus rotation gastroplasty on anastomotic complications after cervical and thoracic oesophagogastrostomies: a prospective non-randomized study. *Eur J Surg* 2001;167:110–114.

27. Johansson J, Zilling T, Staël von Holstein C, et al. Anastomotic diameters and strictures following esophagectomy and total gastrectomy in 256 patients. *World J Surg* 2000;24:78–85.

28. Blewett CJ, Miller JD, Young JEM, et al. Anastomotic leaks after esophagectomy for esophageal cancer: a comparison of thoracic and cervical anastomoses. *Ann Thorac Cardiovasc Surg* 2001;7:75–78.

29. Foltýnová V, Brousil J, Velátová A, et al. Swallowing function and gastric emptying in patients undergoing replacement of the esophagus. *Hepatogastroenterology* 1993;40:48–51.

30. Gutschow CA, Collard JM, Romagnoli R, et al. Denervated stomach as an esophageal substitute recovers intraluminal acidity with time. *Ann Surg* 2001;233:509–514.

31. Johansson J, Sloth M, Bajc M, et al. Radioisotope evaluation of the esophageal remnant and the gastric conduit after gastric pull-up esophagectomy. *Surgery* 1999;125:297–303.
32. Wang LS, Huang MH, Huang BS, et al. Gastric substitution for resectable carcinoma of the esophagus: an analysis of 368 cases. *Ann Thorac Surg* 1992;53:289–294.
33. Fok M, Ah-Chong AK, Cheng SWK, et al. Comparison of a single-layer, continuous handsewn method and circular stapling in 580 oesophageal anastomoses. *Br J Surg* 1991;78:342–345.
34. Finley RJ, Lamy A, Clifton J, et al. Gastrointestinal function following esophagectomy for malignancy. *Am J Surg* 1995;169:471–475.

29
Jejunostomy after Esophagectomy

Lindsey A. Clemson, Christine Fisher, Terrell A. Singleton, and Joseph B. Zwischenberger

Esophageal resection is indicated most often for treatment of localized esophageal cancer and Barrett's esophagus with high grade dysplasia.[1,2] Despite the improved techniques utilized for resection, Karl and colleagues[3] report esophagectomy continues to be associated with a 30-day mortality of 2.1% and a 3-year survival of 29.6%. Overall, 29% of patients experience complications such as anastomotic leaks (3.5%) and pulmonary complications (19%). Approximately 58% of patients with esophageal cancer present with significant weight loss.[4] These patients often have nutritional deficiencies due to the obstructive nature of the tumor and the catabolic effects of the malignancy.[5] Poor preoperative nutritional status may increase the risk of postoperative complications and therefore nutritional support is a treatment modality that may directly impact outcomes.

Historically, gastrointestinal surgery in which an anastomosis was performed involved a period of postoperative starvation with feeding initiated after evidence of gastric motility. This practice was presumed to decrease postoperative nausea and vomiting and to allow up to a week after surgery for the anastomosis to sufficiently heal.[6–8] Perioperative nutrition in surgical patients over the past few decades has evolved into three basic approaches (or combinations thereof): (1) short-term starvation; (2) intravenous (parenteral)-based nutrition; or (3) gastrointestinal (enteral) based feedings.

The natural gastrointestinal (enteral) route is currently the preferred method for supplying nutritional supplementation. Infusion of even suboptimal nutritional supplements into the intestinal tract helps to maintain mucosal integrity,[9] prevents loss of the mucosal barrier associated with catabolic stress, attenuates inflammatory responses postoperatively by reducing bacterial exotoxin translocation from the gut,[10] and reduces the incidence of acalculous cholecystitis by maintaining gut motility.[11] There are instances, however, in which oral intake may be precluded, including depressed mentation, incompetence of swallowing with aspiration, upper gastrointestinal (GI) tract obstruction, and gastric paresis. These circumstances require higher levels of nutritional support, usually via an enteral route.

Enteral nutrition can be delivered by a variety of tubes, generally classified as either nasoenteric or tube enterostomy. Nasoenteric tubes are indicated for short-term feeding in patients who are unable to maintain adequate oral intake, but who retain normal gut motility. The nasogastric approach is associated with a greater risk of aspiration than nasointestinal feeding. Nasoduodenal and nasojejunal tubes are preferred for patients with a high risk of aspiration, delayed gastric emptying, or gastroparesis. These tubes may require endoscopy, image guidance, laparoscopy, or laparotomy for placement.

Total parenteral nutrition (TPN) utilizes intravenous central catheters to deliver nutrients to the patient, bypassing the GI tract.[12] Absolute indications for TPN include severe short bowel syndrome, radiation enteritis, high-output gastrointestinal fistulas, persistent postoperative ileus, intestinal pseudoobstruction unresponsive to enteral feeding (i.e., scleroderma), and nonop-

TABLE 29.1. Options of methods of nutritional support for esophagectomy patients.

Method	Placement	Risks	Benefit	Level of evidence	Recommendation
Short-term starvation	None	Progressive starvation; missed opportunity	Low initial risk; delayed enteral feeds	Heslin[16] 1b Page[5] 1b Carr[18] 1b Lewis[17] 1a	Grade A Outcomes equal to nutritional supplementation in most patients
Total parenteral nutrition	Central venous access	Increased hospital stay; hyperglycemia; access complications; sepsis; expense	Immediate supplemental nutrition	Salvino[23] 1a Bozzetti[19] 1b Veterans Cooperative Study[20] 1b Bozzetti[21] 1b Braunschweig[22] 1a	Grade A TPN is beneficial for the perioperative nutrition of severely malnourished patients and better tolerated by this population.
Enteral Nasojejunal tubes	Intraoperative or image-guided placement	Aspiration; blockage	Immediate enteral feeds	Sand[25] 1b Gabor[26] 2b Carr[18] 2b	Grade A NJ tubes are relatively safe and inexpensive forms of nutrition for the postesophagectomy patient. Enteral feeding improves gut function and decreases complications
Feeding jejunostomy	Intraoperative bowel procedure	Small bowel torsion/ obstruction/adhesions	Immediate long-term enteral access	Baigrie[6] 1b Watters[27] 1b Finley[28] 2b McCarter[32] 2b Brock[33] 4	Grade A Jejunostomy is an effective form of feeding for postesophagectomy patients with infrequent but serious complications relative to TPN or short-term starvation.

erative mechanical intestinal obstruction.[13] Risks of infectious complications, sepsis, and mortality were found to be higher in patients supplemented on TPN versus enteral feeding.[14] The parenteral route is considered acceptable when enteral access cannot be safely obtained or when enteric feeding cannot be tolerated.

A jejunostomy is indicated when enteral access to the upper GI tract is unobtainable or contraindicated due to impaired gastric motility or aspiration risk. There are unique complications associated with an open or laparoscopic jejunostomy because an abdominal stoma is required that may leak or create a fulcrum for a potential volvulus.[15] Despite the risks associated with this additional procedure intraoperatively or postoperatively, open jejunostomy tubes are frequently placed in patients who have undergone esophagectomy for esophageal cancer to provide early nutritional support and potentially long-term enteral access if recurrent obstruction or anastomotic complications occur.

Given this background, our chapter will investigate the controversy surrounding the use of a feeding jejunostomy in a postesophagectomy patient utilizing an evidence-based evaluation of the literature. Table 29.1 summarizes our findings and we will discuss each section in detail.

29.1. Postoperative Starvation

Temporary postoperative starvation plus intravenous fluids and glucose (3–5 days) is a simple form of nutritional support (NS) in the postoperative period. Heslin and colleagues[16] performed a randomized, controlled trial (RCT), rated 1b, comparing intravenous crystalloid versus immediate enteral feeds via either jejunostomy or feeding tube on 195 patients who underwent laparotomy for upper gastrointestinal malignancies (esophageal, gastric, peripancreatic, and bile duct) at Memorial Sloan-Kettering Cancer Center. There was no significant difference between minor or major complications, infection rates, or length of hospital stay between control and experimental groups. However, there was one bowel necrosis associated with enteral feeding by jejunostomy requiring reoperation.

Page and colleagues[5] likewise performed a RCT, rated 1b, with 40 patients undergoing transthoracic esophagectomy by one surgeon over 1 year randomized to an enterally fed group (double lumen nasojejunal tube was placed intra-operatively) or an intravenous crystalloid group. No significant difference existed between groups, but 7 out of 20 were removed from the study prematurely because of nasojejunal tube dislodgement.

Lewis and coworkers[17] investigated whether or not postoperative starvation is beneficial after gastrointestinal surgery with a review and meta-analysis of RCTs involving 837 patients in 11 studies. No major benefit was identified to enteral feeds over nil by mouth.

Carr and coworkers[18] assessed 30 patients undergoing elective laparotomies in a RCT, rated 1b, comparing postoperative enteral feeding via a nasojejunal tube versus postoperative fluids by one surgeon. Significantly fewer postoperative complications were seen in the enterally fed group ($p < 0.005$); however, the study failed to define these complications.

29.1.1. Comments

In these prospective, randomized, but unblinded outcomes studies there is no proven benefit of enteral feeding or TPN over short-term postoperative starvation, following gastrointestinal surgery (level of evidence 1a to 1b; recommendation grade A). The randomized, controlled trials that were reviewed were limited by their use of small populations. Most of the trials listed, except Page and associated,[5] included GI resections of all types. Therefore, future trials are needed to focus on identified malnourished patients undergoing esophagectomy.

> There is no proven benefit of enteral feeding or TPN over short-term postoperative starvation following gastrointestinal surgery (level of evidence 1A to 1B; recommendation grade A).

29.2. Total Parenteral Nutrition

Certain populations cannot tolerate enteral feeding or are so malnourished that preoperative nutrition may improve their prognosis. The proper method and utilization of nutritional support in a malnourished esophagectomy patient has yet to be determined. Many investigators have studied the role of TPN in malnourished populations.

In a randomized, controlled trial, Bozzetti and colleagues,[19] level 1b, investigated the potential benefits of perioperative TPN for reducing the risk after surgery in malnourished cancer patients. Ninety elective surgical patients with gastrointestinal cancer were randomly assigned to 10 days of preoperative and 9 days of postoperative nutrition versus a simple control group, which received only postoperative hypocaloric intraveneous (IV) fluids with adequate nitrogen support until able to take postoperative feeds. Malnourished gastrointestinal cancer patients (mean weight loss of 15%–16%) showed a one third decrease in overall complication rate with preoperative TPN that was continued postoperatively (37%) compared to controls (57%). Despite these promising results, the need for hospitalization 10 days preoperatively is often unavailable and always expensive.

The Veterans Affairs Total Parenteral Nutrition Cooperative Study Group[20] published a RCT in the *New England Journal of Medicine*, graded 1b. Malnourished patients (on the basis of objective nutritional assessment, $n = 395$) were selected who required either a laparotomy or noncardiac thoracotomy. The TPN group was treated 7 to 15 days before surgery and 3 days afterwards and the control group received no perioperative TPN. Patients who received optimal courses of TPN had fewer major complications after 30 days than those with suboptimal courses of TPN (19.2% vs. 38.7%; $p < 0.05$). In a retrospective analysis, 33 patients defined as severely malnourished (in accordance with the Nutritional Risk Index <83.5) showed that preoperative TPN decreased postoperative noninfectious complications from 42.9% to 5.3% ($p = 0.3$) and there was no increase in the frequency of infectious complications. Although TPN does appear favorable in severely malnourished patients, this study does not consider length of hospital stay or cost in its analysis.

In a more recent randomized, multicenter study by Bozzetti and coworkers,[21] graded 1b, TPN and total enteral nutrition (TEN) were compared in 317 malnourished patients who had surgery for gastrointestinal cancer. Isocaloric and isonitrogenous formulas of TEN (by jejunostomy tube or nasogastric tube) and TPN were both started the morning after surgery and continued until the patient could tolerate adequate postoperative intake. Postoperative complications [relaparotomy, transfer to intensive care unit (ICU), and percutaneous drainage of fluid collections by interventional radiology] occurred in 34% of TEN compared with 49% of TPN ($p < 0.05$). Total enteral nutrition, however, was associated with a higher frequency of gastrointestinal adverse effects (abdominal distension, abdominal cramps, diarrhea, and vomiting) requiring a switch-over to TPN in 9% of cases. The length of stay was a mean of 1.6 days shorter in the TEN-fed group. This study supports the benefit of early TEN over TPN in reducing complications in postoperative malnourished gastrointestinal cancer patients provided that there are no contraindications for TEN, even though TPN has better GI tolerance. Unfortunately, this study was not stratified by levels of malnourished patients.

Braunschweig and colleagues[22] published a meta-analysis on 27 prospective RCTs in 1,828 patients regarding the effects of parenteral nutrition compared with tube feeding or standard care IV dextrose, followed by conventional diets when tolerated. The overall assessment showed that tube feeding and standard care is associated with a lower risk of infection than is parenteral nutrition. In populations with high percentages of protein energy malnutrition (PEM), TPN was associated with a lower risk of mortality and a trend toward lower risk of infection than standard care. The authors stated two rather general points: "(1) failure to provide adequate nutrition to a population with PEM is associated with untoward consequences, and (2) TPN should not be initiated in normally nourished populations, unless there is a good reason to do so". The limitations of this analysis are different outcome variable definitions, small sample sizes, small numbers of prospective randomized controlled trials (PRCTs) with populations of PEM, few comparisons of standard care with TPN, and the variability of reported complications. Cost analysis was not included in this review.

Salvino and colleagues[23] reviewed several studies on perioperative TPN and postoperative TPN. To receive preoperative TPN, a severely malnourished patient must require elective surgery (safe to delay 7–10 days) shown to have an improved clinical outcome with nutritional support. Postoperative nutritional support should be started when a mild to moderately malnourished patient cannot tolerate an oral diet 7 to 10 days after surgery (5–7 days after surgery for a severely malnourished patient). Their review supported the use of TEN over TPN whenever possible due to its association with safer and better outcomes and increased cost effectiveness.

29.2.1. Comments

Due to the lack of studies in malnourished esophagectomy patients, our recommendation must be extrapolated from studies in similar populations. Perioperative TPN may reduce postoperative complication rates in severely malnourished patients with gastrointestinal cancer (level of evidence 1a to 1b; recommendation grade A). The literature soundly supports the use of TPN to decrease preoperative surgical morbidity in severely malnourished patients, even though TEN is generally preferred over TPN due to a decrease in complications and cost effectiveness. We acknowledge the practice guidelines on nutritional support (NS) summarized by the American Society of Parenteral and Enteral Nutrition[24] that only moderately to severely malnourished patients who are scheduled for major GI surgery should receive 7 to 14 days of preoperative NS if surgery can be safely postponed, taking the modality of nutritional support into consideration. Because many esophageal cancer patients can still tolerate liquids, oral supplements would be the first choice for preoperative nutritional supplementation. For patients with inadequate oral intake, a cost/benefit analysis must be done if it is necessary to extend the length of hospitalization by 7 to 10 days for preoperative nutrition. Total parenteral nutrition, on average, costs five times more than enteral feeds, not including the added cost of extended hospital stay. The use of preoperative enteral feeding may be a more cost-effective method in treating severely malnourished esophagectomy candidates if enteral access is possible. However, TPN is certainly appropriate when indicated.

> Perioperative TPN may reduce postoperative complication rates in severely malnourished patients with gastrointestinal cancer (level of evidence 1a to 1b; recommendation grade A).

29.3. Enteral Feeding

The per oral (PO) route is delayed in a postoperative esophagectomy patient for a short time period in order to allow the initiation of anastomotic healing. These patients, however, may be malnourished and need NS or may be unable to begin PO intake in a timely manner. Hence, a decision must be made between which method of enteral feeding, nasojejunal tube or jejunostomy tube, is best for a postesophagectomy patient.

Baigrie and colleagues[6] conducted a prospective, randomized trial (PRT), graded 1b, comparing enteral (jejunostomy) to parenteral nutrition after esophagectomy or gastrectomy in 97 patients. The TPN group demonstrated a 45% incidence of major morbidity which included catheter-related complications and sepsis as well as life threatening non–catheter-related complications such as respiratory failure, renal failure, and myocardial infarction. Complications attributable to enteral nutrition were relatively minor, such as cramping, abdominal pain, and diarrhea. Benefits of enteral nutrition include the simplicity of intra-operative jejunostomy placement and the low cost of jejunostomy feeding relative to parenteral nutrition.

Sand and colleagues[25] conducted a PRT, graded 1b, comparing parenteral and nasojejunal feeding in 29 patients after total gastrectomy for gastric cancer. One died in the parenteral group of infection after an esophagojejunal leak. The incidence of diarrhea was similar in both groups. Enteral nutrition by nasojejunal catheter was shown to be safe and well tolerated with fewer infectious complications ($p = 0.7$), and was four times less expensive than TPN.

Gabor and coworkers[26] performed a prospective study, graded 2b, of 44 consecutive patients with esophagectomy for esophageal carcinoma who began early enteral nasojejunal feeding compared to 44 historical patients as a control parenteral feeding group. Patients in the enteral group received 10mL/h by nasojejunal tube starting 6 hours after surgery, increasing in a stepwise fashion until total nutrition was reached at day 6. The control group was given total parenteral nutrition until postoperative day 7, when patients were then switched to enteral nutrition. Both the average postoperative ICU stay and total hospital stay were high in this study, however, patients who began early enteral feeding had a shorter stay than those on total parenteral nutrition (19 to 10 days and 43 to 26 days, respectively). There was no difference in 30-day mortality between groups.

In a randomized trial of the safety and efficacy of immediate postoperative enteral feeding in 14 patients undergoing elective laparotomies and GI resection by one surgeon, graded 2b, Carr and associates[18] compared postoperative enteral feeding via a nasojejunal tube versus postoperative intravenous fluids. There was no difference in length of stay (9.3 days vs. 9.8 days) and there was not a significant difference in clinical outcomes.

Watters and colleagues[27] conducted a RCT, graded 1b, comparing the value of nutrition by jejunostomy to replacement intravenous fluids only as measured by strength of grip, respiratory strength, mobility, and urine biochemistry. Patients fed by jejunostomy had the same fatigue level, measured by grip strength and maximal inspiratory pressure, as the control group. Immediate postoperative jejunal feeding was associated with impaired respiratory mechanics and reduced postoperative mobility, perhaps due to slight abdominal distension. Intensive care unit and postoperative hospital stay did not differ between groups.

In a retrospective review, evidence level 2b, Finley and associates[28] assessed the frequency and causes of GI complications in 228 patients fed by open jejunostomy following esophagectomy. J tubes were not associated with delayed emptying, leaks, early satiety, or pneumonia. At 3-month follow-up, the patients denied symptoms of dysphagia, reflux, dumping, diarrhea, or hoarseness. Two of the 228 (1%) required laparotomies for bowel torsion and obstruction at the site of the J tube. They support sewing a broad base of the jejunum to the abdominal wall at the site of the J tube to prevent torsion at the site of the jejunostomy, as recommended by others.[29–31]

McCarter and colleagues[32] evaluated the feasibility and tolerance of early jejunal feeding in an analysis, graded 2b, of prospectively collected data from 167 patients following major upper gastrointestinal surgery. On postoperative day 1, patients were started on full-strength enteral feeds at 25mL/h by jejunostomy. Diets were advanced to a calculated target rate (25kcal/kg/day) by postoperative day 4. Patients experienced cramping, distension, nausea, and diarrhea; however, most of the symptoms were described by patients as mild.

In a 350 patient case series, graded 4, Brock and colleagues[33] report excellent safety profile and ease of placement of the percutaneous J tube in patients following esophagectomy. Only 4.9% required J tube replacement.

29.3.1. Comments

In comparison to parenteral nutrition, enteral devices are simple to place and are associated with fewer complications and lower cost, both in terms of nutritional expense and length of hospital stay. Enteral nutrition is also associated with more rapid return of bowel function and decreased major morbidity. However, there are specific complications associated with various enteral feeding modalities.

Historically, jejunostomy feeding has been commonly associated with mild gastrointestinal symptoms and occasional serious complications such as obstruction or torsion. Jejunostomy, however, carries a substantial risk of mortality, estimated to be as high as 10%.[29,34–36] Adams and coworkers[34] reported 7 of 73 patients died as a direct result of complications from jejunostomy for GI tract obstruction or dysfunction. Serious complications of jejunostomy feeding are greatly reduced by sewing a broad base of the jejunum to the abdominal wall when the tube is placed. The risks of jejunostomy feeding often do not outweigh the benefits. In comparison to IV fluids

alone, the benefit of nasojejunal feeding provides decreased postoperative complications in select patients, but similar clinical outcomes. There is level 2a evidence supporting the use of both a nasojejunal tube and a jejunostomy tube in post-esophagectomy patients.

Which form of enteral feeding is best for a patient following esophagectomy? Because there is no study directly comparing nasogastric and jejunostomy feeding methods in esophagectomy patients, we must extrapolate a decision based on the relative safety, tolerability, and efficacy of enteral feeding options. We recommended that if enteral feeding is indicated, NJ tubes should be used postoperatively to feed patients following esophagectomy (level of evidence 1b to 2b; recommendation grade B). This recommendation primarily stems from the serious nature of complications associated with jejunostomy feeding in comparison to the relatively mild gastrointestinal symptoms of nasojejunal feeding. An uncomplicated patient can be advanced on oral feeds 5 to 7 days following surgery, allowing time for appropriate healing of the esophageal anastomosis.

> If enteral feeding is indicated, nasojejunal tubes should be used postoperatively to feed patients following esophagectomy (level of evidence 1b to 2b; recommendation grade B).

29.4. Authors' Recommendation

When treating a patient who is a candidate for an esophagectomy, his/her total health should be taken into consideration. Their nutritional status is of supreme importance due to the fact that many patients are malnourished from the combination of esophageal obstruction and the ravages of cancer. The algorithm in Figure 29.1 lays out the various nutritional treatment plans for an esophagectomy patient. A patient who can tolerate PO intake should be given oral supplements during workup and treated expectantly after surgery. Per oral intake can be initiated 3 to 5 days to resume full feeling 5 to 7 days postoperatively, giving time for the anastomosis to heal.

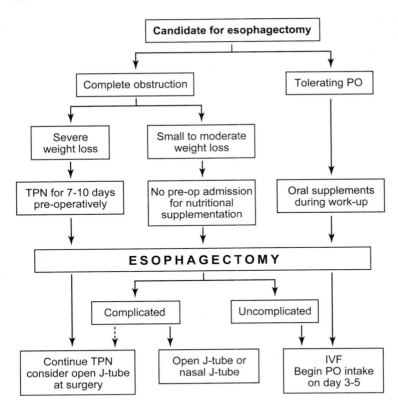

FIGURE 29.1. Algorithm for management of nutritional support for esophagectomy patients.

The treatment of a patient with esophageal obstruction and concomitant malnutrition is much more complex. The patient's level of malnutrition stratification based on the Nutritional Risk Index or other anthropometric indices determines the treatment. Only patients with severe malnutrition need preoperative hospital admission 7 to 10 days before surgery for TPN supplementation. During surgery it is wise to consider placing a jejunostomy tube or nasojejunal tube if there is a thought that the patient may struggle with postoperative malnutrition or will be unable to tolerate appropriate PO intake after the operation. Postoperative esophagectomy complications may warrant the placement of a nasojejunal or jejunostomy tube in order to resume nutritional support.

As the literature describes (Table 29.1), the decision to feed a patient with a jejunostomy after esophagectomy should be on a patient by patient basis, taking into account nutritional status, ease of insertion, and postoperative complications.

References

1. Bueno JT, Schattner MA, Barrera R, et al. Endoscopic placement of direct percutaneous jejunostomy tubes in patients with complications after esophagectomy. *Gastrointest Endosc* 2003;57:536–540.
2. DeCamp MM Jr, Swanson SJ, Jaklitsch MT. Esophagectomy after induction chemoradiation. *Chest* 1999;116(suppl 6):466S–469S.
3. Karl RC, Schreiber R, Boulware D, et al. Factors affecting morbidity, mortality, and survival in patients undergoing Ivor Lewis esophagogastrectomy. *Ann Surg* 2000;231:635–643.
4. Gurski RR, Schirmer CC, Rosa AR, et al. Nutritional assessment in patients with squamous cell carcinoma of the esophagus. *Hepatogastroenterology* 2003;50:1943–1947.
5. Page RD, Oo AY, Russell GN, et al. Intravenous hydration versus naso-jejunal enteral feeding after esophagectomy: a randomised study. *Eur J Cardiothorac Surg* 2002;22:666–672.
6. Baigrie RJ, Devitt PG, Watkin DS. Enteral versus parenteral nutrition after oesophagogastric

surgery: a prospective randomized comparison. *Aust N Z J Surg* 1996;66:668–670.

7. Gerndt SJ, Orringer MB. Tube jejunostomy as an adjunct to esophagectomy. *Surgery* 1994;115:164–169.

8. Wakefield SE, Mansell NJ, Baigrie RJ, et al. Use of a feeding jejunostomy after oesophagogastric surgery. *Br J Surg* 1995;82:811–813.

9. Lacey JM, Wilmore DW. Is glutamine a conditionally essential amino acid? *Nutr Rev* 1990;48:297–309.

10. Takagi K, Yamamori H, Toyoda Y, et al. Modulating effects of the feeding route on stress response and endotoxin translocation in severely stressed patients receiving thoracic esophagectomy. *Nutrition* 2000;16:355–360.

11. Ephgrave KS, Brasel KJ, Cullen JJ, et al. Gastric mucosal protection from enteral nutrients: role of motility. *J Am Coll Surg* 1998;186:434–440.

12. Dudrick SJ, Wilmore DW, Vars HM, et al. Long-term total parenteral nutrition with growth, development, and positive nitrogen balance. *Surgery* 1968;64:134–142.

13. Scolapio JS. A review of the trends in the use of enteral and parenteral nutrition support. *J Clin Gastroenterol* 2004;38:403–407.

14. Finck C. Enteral versus parenteral nutrition in the critically ill. *Nutrition* 2000;16:393–394.

15. Trahan K, Gore DC. Nutritional support. *Chest Surg Clin N Am* 2002;12:227–249, v.

16. Heslin MJ, Latkany L, Leung D, et al. A prospective, randomized trial of early enteral feeding after resection of upper gastrointestinal malignancy. *Ann Surg* 1997;226:567–580.

17. Lewis SJ, Egger M, Sylvester PA, et al. Early enteral feeding versus "nil by mouth" after gastrointestinal surgery: systematic review and meta-analysis of controlled trials. *BMJ* 2001;323:773–776.

18. Carr CS, Ling KD, Boulos P, et al. Randomised trial of safety and efficacy of immediate postoperative enteral feeding in patients undergoing gastrointestinal resection. *Br Med J* 1996;312:869–871.

19. Bozzetti F, Gavazzi C, Miceli R, et al. Perioperative total parenteral nutrition in malnourished, gastrointestinal cancer patients: a randomized, clinical trial. *JPEN J Parenter Enteral Nutr* 2000;24:7–14.

20. Perioperative total parenteral nutrition in surgical patients. The Veterans Affairs Total Parenteral Nutrition Cooperative Study Group. *N Engl J Med* 1991;325:525–532.

21. Bozzetti F, Braga M, Gianotti L, et al. Postoperative enteral versus parenteral nutrition in mal-nourished patients with gastrointestinal cancer: a randomised multicentre trial. *Lancet* 2001;358:1487–1492.

22. Braunschweig CL, Levy P, Sheean PM, et al. Enteral compared with parenteral nutrition: a meta-analysis. *Am J Clin Nutr* 2001;74:534–542.

23. Salvino RM, Dechicco RS, Seidner DL. Perioperative nutrition support: who and how. *Cleve Clin J Med* 2004;71:345–351.

24. Guidelines for the use of parenteral and enteral nutrition in adult and pediatric patients. *JPEN J Parenter Enteral Nutr* 2002;26(suppl 1):1SA–138SA.

25. Sand J, Luostarinen M, Matikainen M. Enteral or parenteral feeding after total gastrectomy: prospective randomised pilot study. *Eur J Surg* 1997;163:761–766.

26. Gabor S, Renner H, Matzi V, et al. Early enteral feeding compared with parenteral nutrition after oesophageal or oesophagogastric resection and reconstruction. *Br J Nutr* 2005;93:509–513.

27. Watters JM, Kirkpatrick SM, Norris SB, et al. Immediate postoperative enteral feeding results in impaired respiratory mechanics and decreased mobility. *Ann Surg* 1997;226:369–380.

28. Finley FJ, Lamy A, Clifton J, et al. Gastrointestinal function following esophagectomy for malignancy. *Am J Surg* 1995;169:471–475.

29. Smith RC, Hartemink RJ, Hollinshead JW, et al. Fine bore jejunostomy feeding following major abdominal surgery: a controlled randomized clinical trial. *Br J Surg* 1985;72:458–461.

30. Yagi M, Hashimoto T, Nezuka H, et al. Complications associated with enteral nutrition using catheter jejunostomy after esophagectomy. *Surg Today* 1999;29:214–218.

31. Zapas JL, Karakozis S, Kirkpatrick JR. Prophylactic jejunostomy: a reappraisal. *Surgery* 1998;124:715–720.

32. McCarter MD, Gomez ME, Daly JM. Early postoperative enteral feeding following major upper gastrointestinal surgery. *J Gastrointest Surg* 1997;1:278–285.

33. Brock MV, Venbrux AC, Heitmiller RF. Percutaneous replacement jejunostomy after esophagogastrectomy. *J Gastrointest Surg* 2000;4:407–410.

34. Adams MB, Seabrook GR, Quebbeman EA, et al. Jejunostomy. A rarely indicated procedure. *Arch Surg* 1986;121:236–238.

35. Cogen R, Weinryb J, Pomerantz C, et al. Complications of jejunostomy tube feeding in nursing facility patients. *Am J Gastroenterol* 1991;86:1610–1613.

36. Smith-Choban P, Max MH. Feeding jejunostomy: a small bowel stress test? *Am J Surg* 1988;155:112–117.

30
Gastric Emptying Procedures after Esophagectomy

Jeffrey A. Hagen and Christian G. Peyre

In the 1940s, Dragstedt reported a 20% to 25% frequency of delayed gastric emptying after truncal vagotomy alone for peptic ulcer disease.[1,2] A similarly high frequency of delayed gastric emptying was reported by Bergin in 1959 in a series of 32 patients.[3] Based on this experience, it seemed reasonable, as many authorities have, to expect prolonged gastric emptying after esophagectomy and reconstruction by gastric pullup – an operation in which bilateral truncal vagotomy is inevitable – unless a pyloroplasty or pyloromyotomy is performed.[4,5]

More recently, a number of arguments have been made against routine gastric drainage. It has been argued that the stomach loses its reservoir function when placed in the chest, acting as a passive conduit that drains by gravity. The risk of peri-operative complications (leak, graft shortening, damage to the vascular pedicle) and the long-term consequences of bile reflux and dumping have also been proposed as justification for omitting a drainage procedure.[6-8] Opponents argue further that when symptoms of delayed gastric emptying do occur, they often improve with time,[9] and if not, they commonly respond to medical therapy[10-12] or endoscopic balloon dilatation.[13]

Proponents of routine gastric drainage argue that a pyloroplasty or pyloromyotomy results in fewer symptoms of gastric stasis such as regurgitation, fullness, or distention, and patients return to a normal diet faster. They also argue that gastric drainage prevents potentially serious long-term complications due to pulmonary aspiration events.[14,15] They contend that the proce-

dure is safe in experienced hands and that the higher complication rate associated with a delayed pyloroplasty can be avoided.[16]

30.1. Published Clinical Data

The purpose of this chapter is to review the evidence regarding the need to perform a pyloroplasty or pyloromyotomy after esophagectomy and gastric reconstruction. The review is based on a Medline search from 1950 to 2005 for English language articles that address the subject of gastric drainage following esophagectomy and reconstruction (three foreign language articles were not reviewed). The review includes five case series, four cohort studies, eight randomized controlled trials, and one meta-analysis (Table 30.1).[6,11,14-29]

30.2. Symptoms of Gastric Stasis

Proponents of routine gastric drainage argue that symptoms of gastric stasis are more common if a pyloroplasty is not performed. The results of published case series do suggest that symptoms such as early satiety, nausea, fullness, and regurgitation do occur in patients without drainage. Velanovich and colleagues[17] reported outcomes in a case series that included 58 patients who had esophagectomy and reconstruction without gastric drainage, with 19% experiencing symptoms due to gastric stasis. Three other case series have reported a frequency of these stasis symp-

TABLE 30.1. Clinical studies examining role of pyloroplasty after esophagectomy.

| Author (year) | Type of study | Number Patients Studied | | Level of evidence |
		No drainage	Drainage	
Urschel[15] (2002)	Meta-analysis of RCTs	553 total		1a−
Fok[16] (1991)	RCT	100	100	1b
Cheung[22] (1987)	RCT	37	35	1b
Mannell[14] (1990)	RCT	20	20	1b
Kao[25] (1994)	RCT	19	19	1b−
Gupta[29] (1989)	RCT	12	12	2b−
Chattopadhyay[21] (1991)	RCT	12	12	2b−
Chattopadhyay[28] (1993)	RCT	12	12	2b−
Huang[23] (1985)	RCT	15	20	2b−
Gutschow[27] (2001)	Cohort	40	18	2b−
Finley[24] (1995)	Cohort	46	249	2b−
Bemelman[13] (1995)	Cohort	111	23	2b−
Wang[20] (1992)	Cohort	58	18	2b−
Mannell[19] (1984)	Case series	15		4
Golematis[18] (1982)	Case series	14		4
Velanovich[17] (2003)	Case series	58		4
Angorn[6] (1975)	Case series	10		4
Hinder[26] (1976)	Case series		10	4

Abbreviation: RCT, randomized, controlled trial.

toms of 21% to 53%.[6,18,19] A similar frequency of gastric stasis symptoms was reported in a cohort study by Wang and colleagues.[20] Outcome was reported for 18 patients with and 58 patients without a drainage procedure. When a gastric emptying procedure was not performed 38% experienced abdominal fullness and 41% experienced regurgitation. However, in this cohort study, these symptoms were no more common than in patients who had a pyloroplasty performed.

Five of the eight randomized, controlled trials report the frequency of obstructive foregut symptoms in patients with and without a gastric drainage procedure. While three of these trials showed no significant difference,[21–23] the randomized, controlled trials by Mannell and colleagues[14] and Fok and colleagues[16] showed a significantly higher frequency of symptoms of gastric stasis if gastric drainage was omitted. In the latter series, the largest randomized, controlled trial reported a total of 200 patients. Those who had a gastric drainage procedure were significantly more likely to be free of abdominal pain, distention, or regurgitation compared to patients without a pyloroplasty (86% vs. 53%). As a consequence of these two trials, the meta-analysis by Urschel and colleagues[15] showed that early complications related to pyloric outlet obstruction were significantly

less common if a pyloroplasty was routinely performed [relative risk (RR) = 0.018; 95% confidence interval (95% CI), 0.03–0.97; $p = 0.046$). In addition, long-term outcome assessment indicated a nonsignificant trend toward fewer obstructive symptoms in patients who had a gastric drainage procedure (RR = 0.97).

30.3. Respiratory Complications

Poor drainage of the gastric pullup can also result in regurgitation of gastric contents into the tracheobronchial tree, resulting in respiratory complications including chronic cough, pneumonia, and aspiration. These respiratory complications were first reported in 1984 in the case series by Mannell and colleagues,[19] in which 15 patients were assessed between 6 and 30 months after esophagectomy without a drainage procedure. Seven patients experienced a cough following meals or when supine, with clinical evidence of pneumonitis in four. Two additional patients had documented episodes of pneumonia, resulting in a frequency of respiratory complications of 60%. The remainder of the case series do not report the frequency of respiratory complications, but in the case series by Velanovich and coworkers,[17] one patient (2%) was reported to die postoperatively from pulmonary aspiration.

In spite of the concerns raised regarding the risk of aspiration in the case series, the cohort studies and randomized, controlled trials do not indicate a significantly higher risk of potentially fatal respiratory events when a gastric drainage procedure is not performed. Interestingly, the two cohort studies that specifically addressed this issue both reported a slightly higher rate of aspiration when gastric drainage was performed. The difference was not statistically significant. Wang and coworkers[20] reported signs or symptoms of aspiration in 17% of patients who had a gastric drainage procedure compared to only 3% when drainage was not performed. Finley and colleagues[24] reported an identical 17% frequency of aspiration in 249 patients who had a pyloroplasty compared to an 11% frequency of aspiration in the 46 patients who did not have a gastric drainage procedure.

The frequency of respiratory complications has been reported in two randomized, controlled trials. In the first, Mannell and colleagues[14] randomized 40 patients to reconstruction with and without a pyloroplasty. Clinical outcome was assessed 8 months after surgery. Three patients in the no pyloroplasty group died of postoperative aspiration, with an additional death during late follow-up due to aspiration. There were no major pulmonary complications early or late when a pyloroplasty was performed. This difference in frequency of aspiration (20% without pyloroplasty vs. 0% with pyloroplasty) did not reach statistical significance ($p = 0.11$), most likely due to the small number of patients randomized. In the second randomized, controlled trial, Fok and associates[16] randomized 200 patients each to pyloroplasty or gastric reconstruction without a drainage procedure. Once again, pulmonary aspiration was more common in the no pyloroplasty group (including two deaths), but the difference did not reach statistical significance (23% vs. 16%; $\chi^2 = 1.56$; $p = 0.21$). As a consequence, the meta-analysis by Urschell and coworkers[15] found a nonsignificant reduction in pulmonary complications overall (RR = 0.69; 95% CI, 0.42–1.14; $p = 0.15$) and in fatal pulmonary aspiration (RR = 0.25; 95% CI, 0.4–1.6; $p = 0.14$) when a pyloroplasty was performed.

30.4. Impact on Diet

Proponents of adding a gastric drainage procedure also express concern regarding the adverse effects of delayed gastric emptying on dietary function. Early dietary function was assessed in the cohort study by Bemelman and colleagues[30] that reported outcome in 140 patients following esophagectomy and reconstruction using the whole stomach in 40 patients (9 with and 31 without pyloroplasty), the distal stomach in 65 (20 with and 45 without pyloroplasty), and a narrow gastric tube without pyloroplasty in 35 patients. When the time to resumption of a normal diet was assessed, they found no significant difference between patients with and without a gastric drainage procedure (6/29 vs. 18/76; $p = 0.80$).

Long-term dietary function was assessed in two of the randomized, controlled trials. Cheung and colleagues[22] randomized 35 patients to a pyloroplasty and 37 to reconstruction without gastric drainage. At 6 months, more patients in the pyloroplasty group were tolerating a regular diet (18/22 vs. 17/25; $p = 0.33$) but this difference disappeared by 2 years when all patients in both groups were tolerating a solid food diet. A similar trend was seen when meal capacity was assessed, with a minor (nonsignificant) difference noted at 6 months but with all patients in both groups tolerating a normal meal capacity by 2 years. Fok and coworkers[16] have also compared the time to resumption of a normal diet in patients with and without gastric drainage. At 2 weeks, more patients in the gastric drainage group were taking a regular diet (65% vs. 41%; $p < 0.01$), and the meal capacity was more likely to be normal (73% vs. 52%; $p < 0.01$). While these authors also found that these differences decreased over time, there was still a significantly higher percentage of patients who complained of foregut symptoms during meals when a pyloroplasty was not performed (47% vs. 14% at 6 months; $p < 0.01$).

30.5. Impact of a Gastric Drainage Procedure on Gastric Emptying

Formal assessment of gastric emptying after esophagectomy without gastric drainage was first reported by Angorn and colleagues.[6] In this case

TABLE 30.2. Evaluation of gastric emptying by radionuclide scintigraphy.

Author (year)	Type of radionuclide-labeled meal	Drainage (n)	No drainage (n)	Drainage (mean ± SD in min)	No drainage (mean ± SD in min)	p value
Cheung[22] (1987)	Semi-solid	16	21	11.6 ± 9.6	40.8 ± 38.0	<0.01
Fok[16] (1991)	Semi-solid	42	44	6.5 ± 7.5	24.3 ± 31.5	<0.001
Gupta (1989)	Liquid	12	12	161.21 ± 3.10	378.89 ± 26.16	Not reported
Kao (1994)	Solid	19	19	175.9 ± 284	250.6 ± 336	Not reported
Mannell[14] (1990)	Solid	14	10	54	63	>0.05

Abbreviation: SD, standard deviation.

series, 10 patients had liquid barium transit studies. Using this relatively crude test, the authors concluded that emptying of the stomach was faster after gastric pullup without gastric drainage than that measured in asymptomatic volunteers. Two additional case series specifically assessed gastric emptying and arrived at similar conclusions.[18,19] However, all three of these series compared emptying from the gastric conduit to that measured in an intact innervated stomach in normal subjects. It should not be surprising that emptying is more rapid from a stomach that has been at least partially tubularized and positioned more vertically in the chest cavity.

The two cohort studies that have assessed emptying of the gastric conduit show no difference in emptying in patients with and without a drainage procedure. Wang and colleagues[20] compared gastric emptying by nuclear medicine scanning in 10 patients with and 23 without gastric drainage, finding no difference in emptying in the upright position (15 vs. 18s, respectively). Using the time to clearance of liquid barium, Finley and coworkers[24] reported similar clearance rates in the supine position in patients who had undergone pyloroplasty compared to those who had not.

When gastric emptying is compared in the randomized, controlled trials, a different picture emerges. In all but one of these trials, emptying was more rapid after a gastric drainage procedure than when a drainage procedure was omitted (Table 30.2). In the largest of these trials, Fok and associates[16] compared gastric emptying at 6 months in 42 patients with and 44 without gastric drainage. Using a labeled solid meal in the upright position, the emptying halftime was significantly shorter in patients who had a gastric drainage procedure (6.6 vs. 24.3 min; $p < 0.001$).

30.6. Perioperative Complications Related to the Pyloroplasty

One of the main arguments against routine gastric drainage is the concern that performing a pyloroplasty may increase the risk of postoperative complications including leakage from the pyloroplasty site or injury to the vascular pedicle and that it may shorten the stomach graft. While complications related to a pyloroplasty can certainly occur, the available literature does not support the conclusion that pyloroplasty should be avoided on this basis. None of the case series or cohort studies report any complications related to the pyloroplasty, nor do the three randomized, controlled trials that specifically detail perioperative complications rates.[14,16,22] In the meta-analysis by Urschell and associates,[15] a nonsignificant trend was identified toward an increased risk of complications related to pyloric drainage (RR = 2.55; 95% CI, 0.34–18.98; $p = 0.36$). This was based on 3 patients who experienced pyloroplasty complications reported in a non-English language publication of a randomized trial not included in our review.

30.7. Dumping Symptoms and Diarrhea

Troublesome symptoms of dumping and a tendency toward diarrhea have also been proposed as reasons not to perform gastric drainage. It is interesting to note, however, that the case series reporting outcome in patients without pyloroplasty suggest that dumping and diarrhea can occur even when a gastric drainage procedure is not performed. Mannell and colleagues[19] reported dumping in 2/15 (13%) of patients without gastric drainage and Angorn and coworkers[6] reported diarrhea in 20%. Clearly, not all dumping and diarrhea experienced after gastric pullup can be attributed to the pyloric drainage procedure.

The evidence from cohort studies is mixed with regard to the relative frequency of dumping and diarrhea. Wang and colleagues[20] reported a significant increase in the frequency of dumping when a pyloroplasty was added [6/18 (33%) vs. 4/58 (6.9%); $p = 0.0094$]. However, the larger cohort study by Finley and colleagues[24] reported no difference in the frequency of either dumping [13/238 (5%) vs. 2/45 (4%)] or diarrhea [44/238 (18%) vs. 7/45 (16%)].

Data from the randomized trials, although limited, indicate that the addition of a pyloroplasty does not increase the frequency of dumping symptoms or diarrhea. Mannell and associates[14] reported dumping in only 1/20 patients after a pyloroplasty, with a similarly low frequency of dumping symptoms in the trial reported by Chattopadhyay and colleagues.[21] Dumping symptoms were experienced by 2/12 patients who had a pyloroplasty compared to 1/12 without, with an equal frequency of diarrhea whether or not a pyloroplasty was performed (2/12 in each group).

30.8. Bile Reflux

It has also been suggested that adding a pyloroplasty will result in increased gastric exposure to bile, leading to symptoms of bilious regurgitation and the development of gastritis. It is clear that reconstruction with the addition of gastric drainage will increase gastric exposure to bile when compared to normal subjects, based on the case series of 10 patients reported by Hinder and coworkers.[26] In this series, 5 patients had overnight aspiration studies for bile, with increased bile exposure documented in 3 patients. However, there are two case series that show that bile reflux and gastritis also occur in patients without a drainage procedure. Mannell and colleagues[19] reported results of overnight gastric aspiration studies for bile in 15 patients who had reconstruction without gastric drainage, demonstrating an increased mean bile exposure. There was endoscopic evidence of gastritis in 8/15 with an additional 3 patients manifesting gastritis on biopsy.

Further, of the 4 patients without gastritis at the initial endoscopy, 3 had a follow-up endoscopy a year later, with an ulcer in one and gastritis in another. Golematis and colleagues[18] also reported a high frequency of gastritis (7/11 patients at 1 year) in patients who did not have pyloric drainage.

The results of the cohort studies are mixed with respect to the frequency of abnormal bile reflux in patients with and without gastric drainage. Wang and coworkers[20] reported a higher frequency of symptomatic bile reflux in patients who had a pyloroplasty (56% vs. 9%), with Tc 99m HIDA scanning performed in a subgroup of these patients to assess bile reflux. The frequency of abnormal enterogastric reflux was higher in the pyloroplasty group (60% vs. 9%). In contrast, Gutschow and coworkers[27] performed a detailed assessment of bile exposure after gastric pullup, using Bilitec 2000® monitoring in 79 patients. They found abnormal bile exposure in 54% overall, with no difference in bile exposure whether or not a pyloroplasty was performed. Interestingly, they did demonstrate improvement in bile exposure with the administration of erythromycin in patients who had a pyloroplasty, with return of bile exposure to levels comparable to normal healthy control subjects. Such an effect was not seen with erythromycin in patients who did not have a gastric drainage procedure. The authors concluded that from the perspective of bile reflux, a gastric drainage procedure is advantageous when combined with prokinetic therapy.

Only one randomized, controlled trial specifically addressed bile reflux in a relatively limited number of patients.[28] Overnight bile aspiration studies were performed 6 months after gastric pullup in 12 patients with and 12 without a pyloroplasty. Bile exposure was increased in all 24 patients, and although the mean bile acid concentration was slightly higher in the pyloroplasty group, the difference was not statistically significant.

30.9. Summary of the Published Data

Of the concerns cited by proponents of routine pyloroplasty or pyloromyotomy, the published data indicate that symptoms of gastric stasis are more common when gastric drainage is omitted (level of evidence 1b). Complications related to pyloric outlet obstruction are also more common (level of evidence 1a). The development of respiratory complications including fatal aspiration does not appear to be more common based on either cohort studies or randomized, controlled trials, although the number of patients studied is small. There is, however, level 1b evidence to suggest patients that have a pyloroplasty return to a normal diet faster with fewer foregut symptoms during meals.

Opponents to routine gastric drainage argue that adding a pyloroplasty increases the risk of postoperative complications, damage to the vascular pedicle, and may shorten the gastric graft. This concern is not supported by any evidence other than expert opinion (level of evidence 5). It has also been argued that the dumping symptoms and diarrhea are more common with gastric drainage, an assertion supported by a single case control study (level of evidence 3b). The limited information available from the randomized, controlled trials, reporting a total of only 54 patients, would suggest there is no difference in the frequency of dumping symptoms or diarrhea whether a pyloroplasty is performed or not (level of evidence 1b–).

Objective assessment of gastric emptying has been reported in five randomized, controlled trials and in each, emptying was slower in patients who did not have a gastric drainage procedure (level of evidence 1b). However, the heterogeneity in methods used to measure gastric emptying in the published trials makes it difficult to collectively analyze the disparate types of gastric emptying data, limiting the ability of meta-analysis to detect a significant difference.

Finally, it has been suggested that the performance of a pyloroplasty or pyloromyotomy will result in increased gastric exposure to bile. This assertion is supported by a single case series and a small cohort study (level of evidence 4). A larger case control study and a single randomized, controlled trial showed no difference in gastric bile exposure whether or not a gastric drainage procedure was performed.

30.10. Impact on Clinical Practice

In our opinion, the sum of the evidence appears to favor the routine addition of a pyloroplasty or pyloromyotomy when performing a reconstruc-

tion following esophagectomy. It does not appear to increase the rate of early complications and may prevent the occasional mortality related to early gastric outlet obstruction and aspiration that are reported in 2% of patients without pyloroplasty in the largest randomized, controlled trial. While this difference did not achieve statistical significance even with 100 patients randomized to each arm, this study was under powered to detect a clinically meaningful reduction in mortality given the low frequency of this complication. The data also suggest that symptomatic outcome and dietary function are improved when gastric drainage is performed.

> The sum of the evidence favors the routine addition of a pyloroplasty or pyloromyotomy when performing a reconstruction following esophagectomy (level of evidence 1a to 1b; recommendation grade B).

The major objections to a gastric drainage procedure do not appear to be well supported by the available literature. Dumping symptoms and diarrhea do occur but are no more common than in patients without drainage. The major unanswered question relates to the development of bile reflux and complications of gastritis or gastric ulcer. While the evidence in the literature is unclear, with small numbers of patients studied in cohort studies or randomized, controlled trials, a few important observations do emerge. First, there is clear evidence to suggest that reflux of bile into the stomach is increased when a pyloroplasty is performed. However, because of the effects of a drainage procedure on gastric emptying, these reflux episodes are likely to be short lived. Contrast this to the situation when a drainage procedure is not performed, where there is clear evidence to suggest that abnormal bile reflux can still occur. In these patients, it is likely that transposition of the stomach into the chest cavity with the pylorus near the esophageal hiatus and the loss of coordinated antroduodenal function as a result of vagotomy combine to increase reflux of bile into the stomach. Because gastric emptying occurs more slowly in patients without a pyloroplasty, especially at night in the supine position when bile reflux is most common, even occasional episodes of bile reflux may be associated with prolonged bile exposure and increased injury. Further studies, ideally incorporating prokinetic therapy, will be required to clarify this particular issue.

References

1. Dragstedt LR, Shafer PW. Removal of the vagus innervation of the stomach in gastroduodenal ulcer. *Surgery* 1945;17:742–749.
2. Dragstedt LR, Camp EH. Follow-up of gastric vagotomy alone in the treatment of peptic ulcer. *Gastroenterology* 1948;11:460–465.
3. Bergin WF, Jordan PHJ. Gastric atonia and delayed gastric emptying after vagotomy for obstructing ulcer. *Am J Surg* 1959;98:612–616.
4. Hagen JA, DeMeester TR. *En bloc* oesophagectomy for cancer of the distal oesophagus, cardia and proximal stomach. In: Jamieson GG, Debas HT, eds. *Surgery of the Upper Gastrointestinal Tract.* 5th ed. London: Chapman & Hall Medical; 1994:214–229.
5. Orringer MB. Transhiatal oesophagectomy. In: Jamieson GG, Debas HT, eds. *Surgery of the Upper Gastrointestinal Tract.* 5th ed. London: Chapman & Hall; 1994:196–210.
6. Angorn IB. Oesophagogastrostomy without a drainage procedure in oesophageal carcinoma. *Br J Surg* 1975;62:601–604.
7. Logan A. The surgical treatment of carcinoma of the esophagus and cardia. *J Thorac Cardiovasc Surg* 1963;46:150–161.
8. Collis JL. Surgical treatment of carcinoma of the oesophagus and cardia. *Br J Surg* 1971;58:801–804.
9. Ludwig DJ, Thirlby RC, Low DE. A prospective evaluation of dietary status and symptoms after near-total esophagectomy without gastric emptying procedure. *Am J Surg* 2001;181:454–458.
10. Burt M, Scott A, Williard WC, et al. Erythromycin stimulates gastric emptying after esophagectomy with gastric replacement: a randomized clinical trial. *J Thorac Cardiovasc Surg* 1996;111:649–654.
11. Nakabayashi T, Mochiki E, Garcia M, et al. Gastropyloric motor activity and the effects of erythromycin given orally after esophagectomy. *Am J Surg* 2002;183:317–323.
12. Hill AD, Walsh TN, Hamilton D, et al. Erythromycin improves emptying of the denervated stomach after oesophagectomy. *Br J Surg* 1993;80:879–881.
13. Bemelman WA, Brummelkamp WH, Bartelsman JF. Endoscopic balloon dilation of the pylorus after esophagogastrostomy without a drainage procedure. *Surg Gynecol Obstet* 1990;170:424–426.
14. Mannell A, McKnight A, Esser JD. Role of pyloroplasty in the retrosternal stomach: results of a prospective, randomized, controlled trial. *Br J Surg* 1990;77:57–59.
15. Urschel JD, Blewett CJ, Young JE, Miller JD, Bennett WF. Pyloric drainage (pyloroplasty) or no drainage in gastric reconstruction after esophagectomy: a meta-analysis of randomized controlled trials. *Dig Surg* 2002;19:160–164.
16. Fok M, Cheng SW, Wong J. Pyloroplasty versus no drainage in gastric replacement of the esophagus. *Am J Surg* 1991;162:447–452.
17. Velanovich V. Esophagogastrectomy without pyloroplasty. *Dis Esophagus* 2003;16:243–245.
18. Golematis BC, Delikaris PG, Bonatsos GN, Douzinas MC, Kambyssi S. Is a gastric drainage procedure necessary after proximal gastrectomy or esophagogastrectomy and esophagogastrostomy? *Mt Sinai J Med* 1982;49:418–420.
19. Mannell A, Hinder RA, San-Garde BA. The thoracic stomach: a study of gastric emptying, bile reflux and mucosal change. *Br J Surg* 1984;71:438–441.
20. Wang LS, Huang MH, Huang BS, Chien KY. Gastric substitution for resectable carcinoma of the esophagus: an analysis of 368 cases. *Ann Thorac Surg* 1992;53:289–294.
21. Chattopadhyay TK, Gupta S, Padhy AK, Kapoor VK. Is pyloroplasty necessary following intrathoracic transposition of stomach? Results of a prospective clinical study. *Aust N Z J Surg* 1991;61:366–369.
22. Cheung HC, Siu KF, Wong J. Is pyloroplasty necessary in esophageal replacement by stomach? A prospective, randomized controlled trial. *Surgery* 1987;102:19–24.
23. Huang GJ, Zhang DC, Zhang DW. A comparative study of resection of carcinoma of the esophagus with and without pyloroplasty. In: DeMeester TD, Skinner DB, eds. *Esophageal Disorders.* New York: Raven Press; 1985:383–388.
24. Finley FJ, Lamy A, Clifton J, Evans KG, Fradet G, Nelems B. Gastrointestinal function following esophagectomy for malignancy. *Am J Surg* 1995;169:471–475.
25. Kao CH, Chen CY, Chen CL, Wang SJ, Yeh SH. Gastric emptying of the intrathoracic stomach as oesophaged replacement for oesophageal carcinomas. *Nucl Med Commun* 1994;15:152–155.
26. Hinder RA. The effect of posture on the emptying of the intrathoracic vagotomized stomach. *Br J Surg* 1976;63:581–584.

27. Gutschow CA, Collard JM, Romagnoli R, Michel JM, Salizzoni M, Holscher AH. Bile exposure of the denervated stomach as an esophageal substitute. *Ann Thorac Surg* 2001;71:1786–1791.

28. Chattopadhyay TK, Shad SK, Kumar A. Intragastric bile acid and symptoms in patients with an intrathoracic stomach after oesophagectomy. *Br J Surg* 1993;80:371–373.

29. Gupta S, Chattopadhyay TK, Gopinath PG, Kapoor VK, Sharma LK. Emptying of the intrathoracic stomach with and without pyloroplasty. *Am J Gastroenterol* 1989;84:921–923.

30. Bemelman WA, Taat CW, Slors JF, van Lanschot JJ, Obertop H. Delayed postoperative emptying after esophageal resection is dependent on the size of the gastric substitute. *J Am Coll Surg* 1995;180:461–464.

31
Posterior Mediastinal or Retrosternal Reconstruction Following Esophagectomy for Cancer

Lara J. Williams and Alan G. Casson

Despite recent advances in multimodality therapy, the mainstay of therapy for esophageal carcinoma remains surgical resection. Following esophagectomy, there are a number of options to restore continuity of the upper gastrointestinal tract. Important considerations for reconstruction include: choice of conduit (e.g., stomach, colon, jejunum); technique of conduit construction (e.g., whole stomach vs. gastric tube, left vs. right colon, etc.); location of anastomosis (i.e., intrathoracic vs. cervical); need for gastric drainage procedures (pyloroplasty, pyloromyotomy, or no drainage); and the route of reconstruction (posterior mediastinal, retrosternal, transpleural, subcutaneous).[1] Each of these factors may have a significant impact on postoperative morbidity and long-term function.

Specifically, the route of alimentary reconstruction remains controversial, reflecting advantages and disadvantages of the two most commonly employed options: the posterior mediastinal (orthotopic, prevertebral) route and the retrosternal (anterior mediastinal, heterotopic) route. As the vast majority of published literature pertains to gastric transposition, this chapter will critically evaluate the optimal route (posterior mediastinal vs. retrosternal) for reconstruction using a gastric conduit following esophagectomy for cancer.

The reported advantages of using the posterior mediastinal (PM) route for reconstruction include:

1. Lower incidence of operative mortality.[2]
2. Less cardiac and pulmonary morbidity.[3,4]
3. Lower incidence of cervical esophagogastric anastomotic leaks.[5,6]
4. Shorter distance for reconstruction (implying less anastomotic tension).[7]
5. Better long-term function (i.e., swallowing function, gastric emptying).[1]
6. Avoidance of foregut angulation which may lead to difficulties performing esophageal dilatation.[1]
7. Lack of interference with subsequent access for cardiac surgery.[1]
8. Preservation of the thoracic inlet structures.[8]

Reported disadvantages to the PM route include:

1. Possibility of tumor recurrence within the conduit, especially following incomplete resection of the primary tumor when lateral margins are positive.[9]
2. Potential damage to the gastric conduit if radiation therapy is used to treat residual disease in the posterior mediastinum.[1]

These disadvantages have prompted some surgeons to advocate an alternate route of reconstruction, namely the retrosternal (RS) approach. Proponents of this route suggest the following additional advantages[1]:

1. Ease and efficiency of drainage of anastomotic leaks.
2. Ease of reoperation for anastomotic stricture.
3. Feasibility of gastrostomy tube insertion (suprasternal or xiphisternal).

In order to objectively define the optimal route of upper gastrointestinal reconstruction, it is helpful to systematically assess all clinically relevant and measurable outcomes. These may be considered as two broad categories: early (in hospital); and late (following discharge from hospital). The following sections of this chapter will discuss the available published literature in an outcome-based manner. An overview of selected randomized clinical trials included in this review of the literature is summarized in Table 31.1.

31.1. Early Outcomes

There are a number of important early perioperative outcomes that can be quantitated following esophageal resection and reconstruction. These outcomes include: operative mortality, pulmonary and cardiac morbidity, and anastomotic leaks.

31.1.1. Operative Mortality

To date, discussion surrounding operative mortality have focused more on the choice of conduit than the route of reconstruction. One large retrospective review of esophagectomy and reconstruction for benign disease showed no association between route of reconstruction and operative mortality.[6] Three small randomized, controlled trials (RCTs) have looked specifically at this issue with regards to "curative" resection and reconstruction for malignant disease.[2,10,11] Two of these trials showed a trend towards lower operative mortality for patients who underwent PM reconstruction.[2,10] One study showed no difference in mortality rates when either the PM or RS route was used,[11] but when subjected to meta-analysis, no significant difference in mortality rate between the PM and RS route of reconstruction was identified.[12] Relative risk (RR), expressed as PM versus RS route, was 0.56 [95% confidence interval (95% CI), 0.17–1.82; $p = 0.34$]. It is important to note, however, that these small studies were underpowered to detect subtle differences in mortality rates between the two groups.

31.1.2. Pulmonary Complications

A number of pulmonary complications (aspiration, atelectasis, and pneumonia) may follow esophageal resection, and may be related to the route of reconstruction.[3] A multivariate analysis by Tsutsui and colleagues indicated that the RS route was a significant factor predisposing to postoperative atelectasis.[4] Another retrospective study identified RS reconstruction as a risk factor for postoperative complications causing death.[3] In this study, however, two groups from different time periods were compared and exhibited important and possibly confounding differences in perioperative management.

In one RCT, right to left intrapulmonary shunt was measured and found to be markedly increased in both groups.[2] Respiratory function, however, was less compromised in patients following PM reconstruction. A meta-analysis by Urschel and coworkers compared pulmonary morbidity using the results of three RCTs.[12] Again, the point estimates indicated a trend towards the PM route having fewer pulmonary complications, but statistical significance was not reached (RR = 0.67; 95% CI, 0.34–1.33; $p = 0.260$).

31.1.3. Cardiac Complications

Cardiac complications following esophagectomy include arrhythmia, myocardial infarction, and congestive heart failure. It has been suggested that placement of the conduit in the anterior mediastinum may compromise cardiac function by obstruction of the right ventricle or by causing paradoxical movements of the septum.[13] Indeed, Bartels and associates found a significantly lower cardiac index in patients following RS reconstruction, primarily due to a reduction in stroke volume index. These results correlated clinically to a slightly higher (but not statistically significant) rate of cardiac complications in patients who underwent RS reconstruction. Although meta-analysis did not show any significant difference in cardiac mortality between the two routes, there was a trend towards increased morbidity when the RS approach was used (RR = 0.43; 95% CI, 0.17–1.12; $p = 0.08$).[12] Again, these results may be difficult to interpret given the possibility that small differences were missed due to a small number of patients and trials included in this meta-analysis.

TABLE 31.1. Summary of randomized, controlled trials comparing posterior mediastinal (PM) and retrosternal (RS) reconstruction following esophagectomy.

Study author, year	Type of study	Number of patients	Early outcomes				Late outcomes			
			Operative mortality	Pulmonary morbidity	Cardiac morbidity	Anastomotic leaks	Anastomotic stricture	Gastric emptying	Swallowing function	Quality of life
Bartels[2] 1993	RCT	96	RR = 0.45 (0.09, 2.22)[a] p = 0.31[b]	RR = 0.65 (0.20, 2.07) p = 0.46	RR = 0.23 (0.03, 1.87) p = 0.13	RR = 1.13 (0.35, 3.66) p = 0.83	na	na	na	na
Zieren[15,c] 1993	RCT	107	na	na	na	RR = 0.32 (0.14, 0.74) p < 0.05	RR = 0.69 (0.43, 1.11) p = 0.13	na	na	na
Coral[16] 1995	RCT	15	na	na	na	na	na	Similar	na	na
Imada[17] 1998	RCT	38	na	na	na	na	na	Similar	na	na
van Lanschot[11] 1999	RCT	60	RR = 1.00 (0.07, 15.26) p = 1.00	RR = 0.57 (0.19, 1.75) p = 0.32	RR = 0.20 (0.01, 4.00) p = 0.24	RR = 1.33 (0.53, 3.38) p = 0.54	RR = 1.20 (0.61, 2.34) p = 0.59	Delayed in RS (<30 min)	Similar	na
Gawad[10] 1999	RCT	26	RR = 0.58 (0.06, 5.66) p = 0.64	RR = 0.88 (0.24, 3.16) p = 0.84	RR = 0.58 (0.18, 1.85) p = 0.34	RR = 4.67 (0.60, 36.29) p = 0.09	na	Delayed in RS (@1 min)	Similar	Similar
Urschel[12] 2001	Meta-analysis	342	RR = 0.56 (0.17, 1.82) p = 0.34	RR = 0.67 (0.34, 1.33) p = 0.26	RR = 0.43 (0.17, 1.12) p = 0.08	RR = 1.01 (0.35, 2.94) p = 0.98	na	Similar	Similar	na

Abbreviations: na, information not available; RCT randomized, controlled trial.

[a]RR, relative risk (95% confidence interval), expressed as posterior mediastinal (PM) vs. retrosternal (RS) route of reconstruction.

[b]$p < 0.05$ considered significant.

[c]Study was randomized for type of cervical esophagogastroanastomosis, not for route of reconstruction.

31.1.4. Anastomotic Leaks

Leakage at the esophagogastric anastomosis remains a significant early complication of esophageal reconstruction. Comparative anatomical studies have shown that the RS route is up to 2.5 cm longer than the PM route.[14] This longer distance underlies anecdotal reports that the longer RS route is associated with increased anastomotic tension and a higher leak rate. A review of multiple case series revealed anastomotic leak rates for RS reconstruction from 0% to 47%.[5] A retrospective multivariate analysis of postoperative complications following esophageal resection for cancer identified the RS route as a statistically significant, independent risk factor predisposing to anastomotic leakage.[4] Another retrospective study of resection for benign disease identified a statistically significant higher incidence of anastomotic leak for extra-anatomic routes of reconstruction.[6]

Four different RCTs were included in a meta-analysis to evaluate the outcome of anastomotic leak.[2,10–12,15] Criteria for diagnosing anastomotic leaks varied between the four trials and included both clinical and/or radiographic evidence of a leak. Although most studies showed a trend towards increased anastomotic leak rate with the PM route of reconstruction, none reached statistical significance. This is in contrast to anecdotal reports suggesting that the RS reconstruction is associated with higher leak rates. The only study that suggested a trend towards higher leak rates following RS reconstruction evaluated groups that were randomized primarily to technique (one-layer vs. two-layer anastomosis), not for route of reconstruction.[15]

31.1.5. Other Perioperative Outcomes

A number of other important perioperative outcomes have been used to compare PM and RS routes of reconstruction. They include duration of operation, blood loss, duration of postoperative mechanical ventilation, and length of hospital stay. A comparison of a number of trials shows no differences for any of these outcomes.[2,10,11]

31.2. Late Outcomes

There are a number of late outcomes following esophagectomy that may reflect the route of reconstruction. Dysphagia may have an anatomic (e.g., stricture, tumor recurrence) or functional basis, and other clinically relevant variables include gastric emptying, quality of life, and pulmonary aspiration resulting from duodenogastroesophageal reflux.

31.2.1. Anastomotic Stricture

According to published reports, the prevalence of benign cervical anastomotic stricture ranges from 3% to 50%.[8] There are few studies that have specifically compared anastomotic stricture rates between PM and RS reconstruction. In one RCT, no differences were found in stricture rates between the groups.[11] In another study, results were difficult to interpret because of the confounding variable of one- versus two-layer anastomosis.[15] Although anecdotal reports suggest it is more difficult to perform esophageal dilatation for stricture after RS reconstruction, published data on this matter is scarce.

31.2.2. Tumor Recurrence in the Conduit

There is a paucity of information regarding the incidence of dysphagia secondary to loco-regional tumor recurrence based on route of reconstruction. One retrospective study evaluated patients who underwent potentially curative esophageal resection with PM reconstruction.[9] The outcome of interest was intrathoracic tumor recurrence, as this patient group potentially may benefit from esophageal reconstruction away from the original tumor bed. Overall, 35% of patients ($n = 209$) had loco-regional recurrence. As expected, the most important predictors of recurrence included N1 and M1 disease (i.e., positive celiac nodes). Recurrence caused upper gastrointestinal symptoms in 22% of patients, and in 59% of this subset of patients the recurrence was intrathoracic. The authors estimated that in 13% of all patients undergoing curative esophagectomy, dysphagia from recurrent disease could have been prevented by using the RS route of reconstruction. They suggested RS reconstruction be considered after incomplete resection (R1 or R2), or in the presence of positive celiac nodes.[9]

31.2.3. Gastric Emptying

One of the major goals of esophageal reconstruction is to create a conduit that closely resembles physiological foregut function. A number of studies have evaluated gastric emptying as an indirect measure of function of the transposed conduit.[10,11,16–18] The most frequently utilized method for measuring gastric emptying has been radionuclide scintigraphy. In a prospective study of 35 patients with PM reconstruction, transit times for radiolabelled solids and liquids suggested that the transposed stomach retained its gastric identity, rather than acting as an inert conduit.[18] In most RCTs, gastric emptying was generally delayed more in patients who were reconstructed using the RS route[10,11,16] although it is unclear whether or not these subtle differences are clinically significant.

31.2.4. Swallowing Function

A variety of techniques have been used to assess swallowing as an objective outcome, and an attempt has been made to correlate results with body weight and scintigraphic studies of gastric emptying. Overall, no differences in swallowing have been demonstrated objectively when the route of reconstruction is considered.[10,11]

31.2.5. Quality of Life

Relatively few studies have specifically addressed quality of life for patients following esophagectomy.[10,19] In one retrospective study, no association between route of reconstruction and quality of life was identified,[19] although this study did not evaluate patients with malignant disease. One RCT evaluating patients treated for esophageal malignancy reported the global quality of life score was slightly lower in patients who were reconstructed using the PM route, although this did not reach statistical significance.[10]

31.2.6. Duodenogastroesophageal Reflux

The role of duodenogastroesophageal reflux (DGR) as a risk factor for development of a columnar epithelium-lined esophagus is well docu-

mented.[20–22] After esophagectomy and gastric transposition, reflux of duodenal and gastric contents may contribute to the development of intestinal metaplasia in the gastric conduit. This may have important consequences for selected patients with favorable prognosis after esophageal resection for cancer or for benign disease.

In a prospective, but nonrandomized study, Katsoulis and colleagues evaluated the effect of reconstruction route on DGR.[23] Patients who underwent PM reconstruction had an increased percentage of reflux time and an increased number of reflux episodes regardless of body position or temporal relation to food ingestion. Exposure to bile was highest in patients with a PM reconstruction, and lowest when a RS route was used. The authors suggested consideration of RS reconstruction for patients predicted to have a long life expectancy in order to avoid the detrimental effects of DGR.

31.3. Impact on Clinical Practice

Based on published data, and as summarized in Table 31.2, there does not appear to be any convincing superiority of the PM route of

TABLE 31.2. Levels of evidence and grades of recommendation for posterior mediastinal or retrosternal reconstruction following esophagectomy for cancer.

Statement	Level of evidence	Grade of recommendation
There is no difference in operative mortality between the two routes	1a−	C
There is no difference in cardiopulmonary morbidity between the two routes	1a−	C
There is no difference in anastomotic leak rates between the two routes	1a−	C
There is no difference in anastomotic stricture rate between the two routes	1b−	C
There is no difference in late foregut function between the two routes	1a	A
There is no difference in quality of life between the two routes	1b	A

−, indicates inconclusive evidence based on wide confidence intervals which failed to exclude clinically important benefit or harm.

reconstruction over the RS route, or vice versa. There are some limitations, however, in drawing conclusions based on this literature. In terms of assessing early outcomes, most of the RCTs reviewed were small and underpowered to detect potentially relevant differences between the two groups. Even when subjected to meta-analysis, the number of trials and patients was insufficient to specifically answer questions regarding the effect of route of reconstruction on perioperative complications.[12] Despite the fact that the relative risk point estimates tended to favor the PM route for some important outcomes, such as operative mortality and cardiac and pulmonary morbidity, the confidence intervals were wide and failed to exclude clinically important benefit or harm. The same holds true for the complication of anastomotic leak, in which the point estimates favored RS reconstruction. It is for these reasons that only grade D recommendations could be assigned to these early outcome measures. Similarly, the overall grade D recommendation surrounding anastomotic stricture rates reflects small patient numbers and wide confidence intervals. The literature reviewed, however, does provide more definitive information with respect to the effect of route of reconstruction on other important late outcomes. Systematic qualitative review appears to indicate that both the PM and RS routes provide similar late foregut function and quality of life, reflected in an overall grade A recommendation.[12]

> The posterior mediastinal and retrosternal routes are associated with similar rates of immediate postoperative complications (level of evidence 1a– to 1b–; recommendation grade C).
>
> The posterior mediastinal and retrosternal routes are associated with similar long-term outcomes in relation to survival and quality of life (level of evidence 1a to 1b; recommendation grade A).

31.4. Personal View

As reported, our preference is to use the PM route for immediate reconstruction after esophageal resection, utilizing a narrow gastric tube based on the right gastroepiploic artery, and performing a cervical esophagogastric anastomosis using a left neck incision.[24] Functional studies have consistently demonstrated satisfactory swallowing long term with this technique of reconstruction.[18,25] We currently reserve the RS route for delayed reconstruction of the upper gastrointestinal tract when access to the posterior mediastinum is technically not possible. When using the RS approach, we feel it is essential to resect a portion of manubrium, left medial clavicle, and first rib to ensure there is no compression on the transposed conduit at the thoracic inlet. In highly selected patients, we have had success utilizing a subcutaneous route to restore swallowing, with surprisingly good functional results. To date, we have no experience using the transpleural route of reconstruction.

References

1. Urschel, JD. Does the interponat affect outcome after esophagectomy for cancer? *Dis Esophagus* 2001;14:124–130.
2. Bartels, H, Thorban S, Siewert J. Anterior versus posterior reconstruction after transhiatal oesophagectomy: a randomized controlled trial. *Br J Surg* 1993;80:1141–1144.
3. Nishi M, Hiramatsu Y, Hioki K, et al. Pulmonary complications after subtotal oesophagectomy. *Br J Surg* 1988;75:527–530.
4. Tsutsui S, Moriguchi S, Morita M, et al. Multivariate analysis of postoperative complications after esophageal resection. *Ann Thorac Surg* 1992;53:1052–1056.
5. Orringer MB. Substernal gastric bypass of the excluded esophagus – results of an ill-advised operation. *Surgery* 1984;96:467–470.
6. Young MM, Deschamps C, Trastek VF, et al. Esophageal reconstruction for benign disease: early morbidity, mortality, and functional results. *Ann Thorac Surg* 2000;70:1651–1655.
7. Ngan SY, Wong J. Lengths of different routes for esophageal replacement. *J Thorac Cardiovasc Surg* 1986;91:790–792.
8. Horvath OP, Lukacs L, Cseke L. Complications following esophageal surgery. *Recent Results Cancer Res* 2000;155:161–173.
9. van Lanschot JJ, Hop WC, Voormolen MH, et al. Quality of palliation and possible benefit of extra-anatomic reconstruction in recurrent dysphagia after resection of carcinoma of the esophagus. *J Am Coll Surg* 1994;179:705–713.

10. Gawad KA, Hosch SB, Bumann D, et al. How important is the route of reconstruction after esophagectomy: a prospective randomized study. *Am J Gastroenterol* 1999;94:1490–1496.

11. van Lanschot JJ, van Blankenstein M, Oei HY, et al. Randomized comparison of prevertebral and retrosternal gastric tube reconstruction after resection of oesophageal carcinoma. *Br J Surg* 1999;86:102–108.

12. Urschel JD, Urschel DM, Miller JD, et al. A meta-analysis of randomized controlled trials of route of reconstruction after esophagectomy for cancer. *Am J Surg* 2001;182:470–475.

13. Niederle B, Burghuber OC, Roka R, et al. Influence of transthoracic and transmediastinal esophagectomy and of various degrees of gastric filling on cardiopulmonary function. In: Siewert JR, Hölscher AH, eds. *Diseases of the Esophagus.* Berlin: Springer; 1987:237–244.

14. Coral RP, Constant-Neto M, Silva S, et al. Comparative anatomical study of the anterior and posterior mediastinum as access routes after esophagectomy. *Dis Esophagus* 2003;16:236–238.

15. Zieren HU, Müller JM, Pichlmaier H. Prospective randomized study of one- or two-layer anastomosis following oesophageal resection and cervical oesophagogastrostomy. *Br J Surg* 1993;80:608–611.

16. Coral RP, Constant-Neto M, Velho AV, et al. Scintigraphic analysis of gastric emptying after esophagogastroanastomosis: comparison of the anterior and posterior mediastinal approaches. *Dis Esophagus* 1995;8:61–63.

17. Imada T, Ozawa Y, Minamide J, et al. Gastric emptying after gastric interposition for esophageal carcinoma: comparison between the anterior and posterior mediastinal approaches. *Hepatogastroenterology* 1998;45:2224–2227.

18. Casson AG, Powe J, Inculet RI, et al. Functional results of gastric interposition following total esophagectomy. *Clin Nuclear Med* 1991;12:918–922.

19. Young MM, Deschamps C, Allen MS, et al. Esophageal reconstruction for benign disease: self-assessment of functional outcome and quality of life. *Ann Thorac Surg* 2000;70:1799–1802.

20. Dresner SM, Griffin SM, Wayman J, et al. Human model of duodenogastro-oesophageal reflux in the development of Barrett's metaplasia. *Br J Surg* 2003;90:1120–1128.

21. de Martinez Haro L, Ortiz A, Parrilla P, et al. Intestinal metaplasia in patients with columnar lined esophagus is associated with high levels of duodenogastroesophageal reflux. *Ann Surg* 2001;233:34–38.

22. Byrne JP, Attwood SE. Duodenogastric reflux and cancer. *Hepatogastroenterology* 1999;46:74–85.

23. Katsoulis IE, Robotis I, Kouraklis G, et al. Duodenogastric reflux after esophagectomy and gastric pull-up: the effect of route of reconstruction. *World J Surg* 2005;29:174–181.

24. Casson AG, Porter GA, Veugelers PJ. Evolution and critical appraisal of anastomotic technique following resection of esophageal adenocarcinoma. *Dis Esophagus* 2002;15:296–302.

25. Koh PS, Turnbull G, Attia E, et al. Functional assessment of the cervical esophagus after gastric transposition and cervical esophagogastrostomy. *Eur J Cardiothorac Surgery* 2004;25:480–485.

32
Postoperative Adjuvant Therapy for Completely Resected Esophageal Cancer

Nobutoshi Ando

The standard procedure for esophageal cancer resection among surgeons in Japan has been a transthoracic esophagectomy with lymphadenectomy. Since the late 1980s, a three-field lymphadenectomy including dissection in the neck, mediastinum, and abdomen for patients with cancer of the thoracic esophagus has become popular among Japanese esophageal surgeons seeking a more curative intent. The rationale for an extensive three-field lymphadenectomy[1] is based on the empirical intelligence accumulated from a conventional two-field lymphadenectomy, namely a relatively high incidence of cervical nodal metastases and cervical nodal recurrences. Therefore, cervical lymphadenectomy was added and an upper mediastinal lymphadenectomy was performed thoroughly in keeping with the new philosophy regarding aggressive surgical therapy.

Nonetheless, the 5-year survival rate of the patients with pathological stage IIa to IV squamous cell carcinoma of the thoracic esophagus remains relatively modest at less than 40%.[2] The surgical invasiveness of this procedure is approaching the limits of tolerability for patients, precluding even more aggressive surgery. Therefore, to improve outcome for esophageal cancer patients, the development of effective multimodality treatment is urgently required. In Western countries, preoperative (neoadjuvant) chemotherapy or chemoradiotherapy[3,4] predominates. Japanese surgeons historically have preferred to wait until after surgery to avoid increasing operative morbidity, considering the invasiveness of transthoracic esophagectomy with extensive lymphadenectomy.

32.1. Growth of Surgical Adjuvant Therapy for Resected Esophageal Cancer in Japan

Since 1978, the Japan Esophageal Oncology Group (JEOG), a subgroup of the Japan Clinical Oncology Group (JCOG),[5] has been developing adjuvant therapies for esophageal squamous cell carcinoma (ESCC) using prospective, randomized, controlled trials. Regarding the histology of the tumors, squamous cell carcinoma comprises more than 90% of the patients with esophageal cancer in Japan. The second phase III study (JCOG8201[6] 1981–1984) revealed that the 5-year survival in the postoperative irradiation group (50 Gy) was significantly higher than that in the preoperative plus postoperative irradiation (30 + 24 Gy) group (level of evidence 1b). The third phase III study (JCOG8503[7] 1984–1987) was designed to compare postoperative irradiation (50 Gy) and postoperative combination chemotherapy with cisplatin and vindesine. This study revealed that there was no significant difference in survival between the two groups (level of evidence 1b). Although these results suggest that chemotherapy had an effect on survival equivalent to postoperative irradiation, the results could also have been interpreted as demonstrating that neither postoperative chemotherapy nor irradiation had an impact on survival when compared to surgery alone. Even though the postoperative irradiation regimen in the second and third studies were the same, the 5-year survival in the postoperative irradiation group in the third study

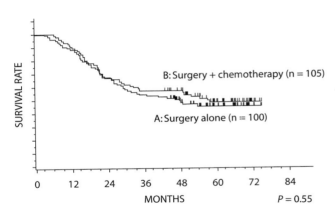

FIGURE 32.1. Overall survival curves of all registered patients randomized to surgery alone or surgery and postoperative chemotherapy with cisplatin and vindesine. The 5-year overall survival was 45% in patients with surgery alone and 48% in patients with surgery plus chemotherapy ($p = 0.55$).

(44%) was better than that in the second study (33%). This may be explained by improvements in the cervico-upper mediastinal lymphadenectomy, which was developed during the period of the third study.

Following the surgical improvements, it again became important to study whether adjuvant chemotherapy following optimal surgery had any additional impact on survival. The fourth phase III study (JCOG8806[8]) was thus designed to compare surgery alone with surgery plus postoperative chemotherapy with cisplatin and vindesine.

32.2. Postoperative Adjuvant Chemotherapy with Cisplatin and Vindesine for Resected Esophageal Squamous Cell Carcinoma

In JCOG8806, a total of 205 patients with stage I to IV esophageal squamous cell carcinoma underwent transthoracic esophagectomy with lymphadenectomy between December 1988 and July 1991 at 11 institutions. These patients were randomized into a surgery alone group (100 patients) and a surgery plus chemotherapy group (105 patients). The surgery plus chemotherapy group received two courses of cisplatin (70mg/m^2) and vindesine (3mg/m^2). This is the same postoperative chemotherapy regimen used in the third phase III study. While the chemotherapy doses were low by Western standards, there was only one treatment-related death in the surgery plus chemotherapy group. Therefore, the chemotherapy dose was consistent with general policies in Japan.

The 5-year survival rate was 45% with surgery alone, and 48% with surgery plus chemotherapy (Figure 32.1). There were no statistically significant differences in survival between two groups (log-rank, $p = 0.55$), even with lymph node stratification, pN0 or pN1. Based on these data, it was concluded that postoperative adjuvant chemotherapy using cisplatin and vindesine has no additive effect on survival in patients with ESCC compared to surgery alone (level of evidence 1b).

32.3. Postoperative Adjuvant Chemotherapy with Cisplatin and Fluorouracil for Resected Esophageal Squamous Cell Carcinoma

The JEOG phase II study of cisplatin and vindesine for patients with advanced esophageal cancer (JCOG8703)[9] suggested that the chemotherapy used in the above JCOG 8806 study had only a modest effect (level of evidence 3b). In contrast, a JEOG phase II study (JCOG8807)[10] of cisplatin and 5-fluorouracil demonstrated a promising response rate of 36% (level of evidence 3b). We therefore initiated a randomized, controlled trial (JCOG9204)[11] to determine whether postoperative adjuvant chemotherapy using a combination of cisplatin and 5-fluorouracil has an additive effect on disease-free survival and overall survival in patients with stage IIa, IIb, III, or IV due to M1 esophageal squamous cell carcinoma.

Patients undergoing transthoracic esophagectomy with lymphadenectomy between July 1992 and January 1997 at 17 institutions were random-

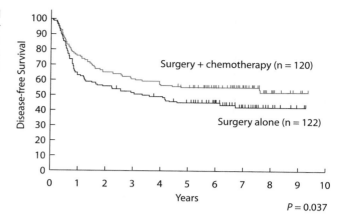

FIGURE 32.2. Disease-free survival curves of all registered patients randomized to surgery alone or surgery and postoperative chemotherapy with cisplatin and 5-fluorouracil. The 5-year disease-free survival was 45% in patients with surgery alone and 55% in patients with surgery plus chemotherapy ($p = 0.037$).

ized to receive surgery alone or surgery plus chemotherapy. Chemotherapy included two courses of cisplatin (80mg/m^2/1 day) and 5-fluorouracil (800mg/m^2/5 days) within 2 months after surgery. Eligible patients were stratified according to lymph node status (pN0 vs. pN1). The primary endpoint was disease-free survival. Of the 242 patients, 122 were assigned to surgery alone, and 120 to surgery plus chemotherapy. In the surgery plus chemotherapy group, 91 patients (75%) received both full courses of chemotherapy; grade 3 or 4 hematologic or nonhematologic toxicities were limited. The 5-year disease-free survival rate was 45% with surgery alone, and 55% with surgery plus chemotherapy (one-sided log-rank, $p = 0.037$; Figure 32.2). In the pN0 subgroup, the 5-year disease-free survival was 76% in surgery alone group and 70% in surgery plus chemotherapy group ($p = 0.433$). In the pN1 subgroup, it was 38% in surgery alone group and 52% in surgery plus chemotherapy group ($p = 0.041$; Figure 32.3). Mortality risk reduction by postoperative chemotherapy was remarkable in the subgroup with

lymph node metastases. The 5-year overall survival rates were 52% and 61% respectively ($p = 0.13$; Figure 32.4).

We found that disease-free survival in the surgery-plus-chemotherapy arm was superior to that with surgery alone with marginal statistical significance even though no difference was shown for overall survival. We can offer two hypotheses to explain the divergence between disease-free survival and overall survival. One is the effect of imbalance in extent of lymphadenectomy between the arms. The other is the sham of overall survival data. We believe that the difference in disease-free survival between the two study arms probably resulted from eradication of intranodal and perinodal micrometastatic disease by chemotherapy. The benefit of chemotherapy for overall survival was diluted by subsequent therapy given after recurrence, for example, chemoradiotherapy or extirpation of lymph nodes. We favor this second hypothesis and consider disease-free survival prolongation by adjuvant chemotherapy to reflect the true patient benefit.

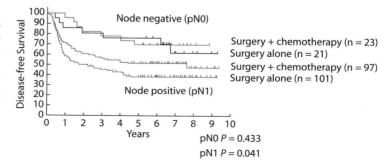

FIGURE 32.3. Disease-free survival curves of all registered patients randomized to surgery alone or surgery and postoperative chemotherapy with cisplatin and 5-fluorouracil. stratified by nodal status. In the pN0 subgroup, the 5-year disease-free survival was 76% in surgery alone group and 70% in surgery plus chemotherapy group ($p = 0.433$). In the pN1 subgroup, it was 38% in surgery alone and 52% in surgery plus chemotherapy ($p = 0.041$).

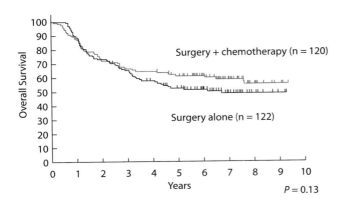

FIGURE 32.4. Overall survival curves of all registered patients, disease-free survival curves of all registered patients randomized to surgery alone or surgery and postoperative chemotherapy with cisplatin and 5-fluorouracil. The 5-year overall survival was 52% in patients with surgery alone and 61% in patients with surgery plus chemotherapy ($p = 0.13$).

On the basis of these data, we concluded that postoperative adjuvant chemotherapy with cisplatin and 5-fluorouracil has a detectable preventive effect on relapse in patients with ESCC compared with surgery alone. Accordingly, the present standard modality for stage II and III ESCC in Japan is transthoracic esophagectomy with extensive lymphadenectomy followed by chemotherapy with cisplatin and fluorouracil (level of evidence 1b; recommendation grade A). In the future we need to know the optimal time for giving effective adjuvant chemotherapy, and a randomized, controlled trial comparing postoperative adjuvant chemotherapy with neoadjuvant chemotherapy using cisplatin and 5-fluorouracil is ongoing (JCOG9907).

> The present standard modality for stage II and III esophageal squamous cell cancer in Japan is transthoracic esophagectomy with extensive lymphadenectomy followed by chemotherapy with cisplatin and fluorouracil (level of evidence 1b; recommendation grade A).

32.4. Study of Adjuvant Chemotherapy Reported from Western Countries

As mentioned before, preoperative (neoadjuvant) chemotherapy or chemoradiotherapy predominates in the Western countries, and only the following studies regarding postoperative adjuvant chemotherapy are available from a literature-based review. The French Association for Surgical Research performed a randomized controlled trial[12] comparing surgery alone with postoperative adjuvant chemotherapy using cisplatin and 5-fluorouracil for patients with ESSC. Before randomization, they stratified 120 patients into two strata, curative complete resection and palliative resection leaving macroscopic or microscopic tumor tissue. Chemotherapy consisted of a maximum of eight courses (minimum six courses) of cisplatin ($80 \, \mathrm{mg/m^2}$/1 day or $30 \, \mathrm{mg/m^2}$/5 days) and 5-fluorouracil ($1000 \, \mathrm{mg/m^2}$/5 days) within 1.5 months after surgery. Overall survival was similar between two groups with almost identical medians of 13 months in adjuvant chemotherapy group (52 patients) and 14 months in surgery alone group (68 patients). The survival curves with and without chemotherapy were similar in stratum of curative resection, with identical median of 20 months, and in stratum of palliative resection, with identical median of 9 months. On the basis of these data, they concluded that cisplatin and 5-fluorouracil are not useful for patients with ESCC who have not undergone curative resection (level of evidence 1b).

Armanios and colleagues carried out a multicenter phase II trial[13] of postoperative paclitaxel and cisplatin in patients with R0 resected, pathological T2N1 to T3–4 Nany adenocarcinoma of the distal esophagus, gastro-esophageal junction, or gastric cardia. Postoperative chemotherapy consisted of four cycles of paclitaxel ($175 \, \mathrm{mg/m^2}$) followed by cisplatin ($75 \, \mathrm{mg/m^2}$) every 21 days. Fifty-nine patients were recruited from 20 centers. Two-year survival was 60%, and they compared this with their historic control value with surgery alone of 38%. They concluded that adjuvant paclitaxel and cisplatin may improve survival in completely resected patients with locally advanced adenocarcinoma of the distal esophagus, GE junction, and cardia (level of evidence 3).

32.5. Postoperative Radiotherapy

Preoperative radiotherapy had been the standard treatment for patients with ESSC until the early 1980s in Japan. Based on the result of an above-mentioned randomized controlled trial, in which the 5-year survival rate of postoperative irradiation (50Gy) group was significantly higher than that in the preoperative plus postoperative irradiation (30 + 24Gy) group, thereafter postoperative radiotherapy took the place of preoperative radiotherapy. In order to determine whether postoperative radiotherapy had an additive effect on survival of patients who underwent esophagectomy, randomized, controlled trials were carried out. French Associations for Surgical Research performed a randomized, controlled trial[14] comparing surgery alone with surgery followed by radiotherapy of 45 to 55 Gy for patients with ESSC. The median survival time was almost identical to 13 months in surgery alone group (119 patients) and in postoperative radiotherapy group (102 patients). They concluded that postoperative radiotherapy did not improve survival, and this lack of improvement in survival was present regardless of lymph node status (level of evidence 1b). In another randomized, controlled trial[15] comparing surgery alone with surgery (followed) by radiotherapy for patients with both ESSC and adenocarcinoma, 130 patients were stratified into two subgroups: resection (60 patients) and palliative resection (70 patients). Radiation dose to the target volume was 49Gy after curative resection and 52.5 Gy after palliative resection. The median survival time in postoperative radiotherapy group (65 patients) was 8.7 months, which was shorter than 15.2 months for surgery alone group (65 patients). On the basis of these data, they concluded that the role of postoperative radiotherapy is limited to a specific group of patients with residual tumor in the mediastinum after operation (level of evidence

1b). Postoperative radiation therapy is appropriate in the specific group of patients with an R0 resection of squamous cell esophageal cancer with a T4 tumor invading the tracheobronchial tree or the aorta and with bulky N1 disease abutting neighboring structures (recommendation grade A).

Invasive preoperative explorations are recommended in order to achieve a more accurate selection of patients for resection after induction therapy (level of evidence 2++; grade of recommendation B).

In well-identified subgroups, such as patients with mediastinal downstaging to N0-1 status, the benefits of surgery are more significant (level of evidence 2+; grade of recommendation C).

References

1. Akiyama H, Tsurumaru M, Udagawa H, et al. Radical lymph node dissection for cancer of the thoracic esophagus. *Ann Surg* 1994;220:364–373.
2. Ando N, Ozawa S, Kitagawa Y, et al. Improvement in the results of treatment of advanced squamous esophageal carcinoma over fifteen consecutive years. *Ann Surg* 2000;232:225–232.
3. Bosset JF, Gignoux M, Triboulet JP, et al. Chemoradiotherapy followed by surgery compared with surgery alone in squamous-cell cancer of the esophagus. *N Engl J Med* 1997;337:161–167.
4. Urba SG, Orringer MB, Turrisi A, et al. Randomized trial of preoperative chemoradiation versus surgery alone in patients with locoregional esophageal carcinoma. *J Clin Oncol* 2001;19:305–313.
5. Shimoyama M, Fukuda H, Saijo N, et al. Japan Clinical Oncology Group (JCOG) *Jpn J Clin Oncol* 1998;28:158–162.
6. Iizuka T, Kakegawa T, Ide H, et al. Preoperative radioactive therapy for esophageal carcinoma: randomized evaluation trial in eight institutions. *Chest* 1988;93:1054–1058.
7. Japan Esophageal Oncology Group. A comparison of chemotherapy and radiotherapy as adjuvant treatment to surgery for esophageal carcinoma. *Chest* 1993;104:203–207.
8. Ando N, Iizuka T, Kakegawa T, et al. A randomized trial of surgery with and without chemotherapy for localized squamous carcinoma of the thoracic esophagus: The Japan Clinical Oncology

Group study. *J Thorac Cardiovasc Surg* 1997;114:205–209.

9. Iizuka T, Kakegawa T, Ide H, et al. Phase II evaluation of cisplatin and vindesine in advanced squamous cell carcinoma of the esophagus: Japan Esophageal Oncology Group Trial. *Jpn J Clin Oncol* 1991;21:176–179.

10. Iizuka T, Kakegawa T, Ide H, et al. Phase II evaluation of cisplatin and 5-fluorouracil in advanced squamous cell carcinoma of the esophagus: Japan Esophageal Oncology Group Trial. *Jpn J Clin Oncol* 1992;22:172–176.

11. Ando N, Iizuka T, Ide H, et al. Surgery plus chemotherapy compared with surgery alone for localized squamous cell carcinoma of the thoracic esophagus: A Japan Clinical Oncology Group Study-JCOG9204. *J Clin Oncol* 2003;21:4592–4596.

12. Pouliquen X, Levard H, Hay JM, et al. 5-fluorouracil and cisplatin therapy after palliative surgical resection of squamous cell carcinoma of the esophagus. A multicenter randomized trial. French Associations for Surgical Research. *Ann Surg* 1996;223:127–133.

13. Armanios MA, Xu R, Forastiere AA, et al. Adjuvant chemotherapy for resected adenocarcinoma of the esophagus, gastro-esophageal junction, and cardia: phase II trial (E8296) of the Eastern Cooperative Oncology Group. *J Clin Oncol* 2004;22:4495–4499.

14. French University Association for Surgical Research, Teniere P, Hay J, Fingerhut A, et al. Postoperative radiation therapy does not increase survival after curative resection for squamous cell carcinoma of the middle and lower esophagus as shown by a multicenter controlled trial. *Surg Gynecol Obstet* 1991;173:123130.

15. Fok M, Sham ST, Choy D, et al. Postoperative radiotherapy for carcinoma of the esophagus: a prospective, randomized controlled study. *Surgery* 1993;113:138–147.

33
Celiac Lymph Nodes and Esophageal Cancer

Thomas W. Rice and Daniel J. Boffa

Celiac lymph nodes are considered a distant metastatic site (M1) in esophageal cancer. The M1a subclassification is recommended for distal thoracic esophageal cancer metastatic to celiac lymph nodes.[1] This suggests that although these cancers are beyond cure, they are different from esophageal cancers with other sites of distant metastases (M1b). Of 46 disease sites for which the American Joint Committee on Cancer (AJCC) has staging recommendations, only 7 (15%) require subdivision of M1: 2 with 3 subclassifications (M1a, M1b and M1c) – cutaneous melanoma and prostate; and 5 with 2 subclassifications (M1a and M1b) – bone, retinoblastoma, testis, gestational trophoblastic tumor, and esophagus. Only prostate, testis, and esophagus designate nonregional nodes as M1a. However, 12 (26%) disease sites have stage IV subgroupings: lip and oral cavity, pharynx, larynx, nasal cavity and paranasal sinuses, major salivary glands, thyroid, vulva, vagina, cervix, corpus uteri, gestational trophoblastic tumor, and esophagus. Lymph node metastases are designated as stage IVA for head and neck cancers (regional), vulva (regional), and esophagus (nonregional). Are these unique subclassifications and subgroupings warranted for esophageal cancer?

These staging dichotomies in esophageal cancer patients with the worst prognosis are considered needless and counterproductive by many physicians. Yet, some highly selected M1a (stage IVA) patients respond to treatment and are cured. Thus, there is considerable controversy surrounding the clinical importance of celiac lymph node status in esophageal cancer. Currently, there is no consensus regarding evaluation of celiac lymph nodes, their influence on management, or their impact on survival. The literature contains only retrospective reports of clinical experiences (level of evidence 2– or 3). Does the literature support the M1a classification for esophageal cancer?

33.1. Celiac Lymph Nodes and Their Identification

The celiac artery arises from the anterior wall of the aorta as the aorta exits the aortic hiatus to enter the abdomen. It lies just below the esophageal hiatus at the superior border of the pancreas. This stubby, retroperitoneal artery, or celiac trunk, is 1 cm to 2 cm long and arises as a single artery in more than 98% of patients. Celiac lymph nodes lie around the celiac artery, deeply buried in an almost tunnel-like retroperitoneal location high in the epigastrium (Figure 33.1). Their location makes accessibility difficult, particularly in the obese patient.

The celiac artery, or celiac axis, immediately trifurcates into left gastric, hepatic, and splenic arteries in more than 85% of patients. Each has associated regional lymph nodes. This close, compact anatomy of arteries and lymph nodes and difficult celiac lymph node accessibility may result in misidentifying a left gastric lymph node (station 17, N1 classification) or a splenic or hepatic lymph node (station 18 and 19, M1b classification) as a celiac lymph node (station 20, M1a classification) or vice versa (Figure 33.2). The lesser and greater omentum and transverse

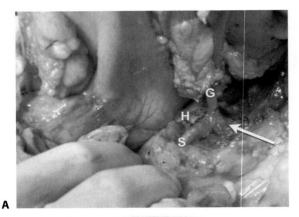

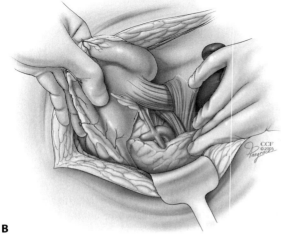

FIGURE 33.1. (A) The celiac artery (*arrow*) exposed via a left-thoracoabdominal incision. The stomach is retracted superiorly after mobilization of the greater curve and the pancreas retracted inferiorly. The left gastric (G), splenic (S), and hepatic (H) arteries are dissected and their associated regional lymph nodes removed. Celiac lymph nodes lie about the short retroperitoneal celiac artery. (B) Graphic depiction of the anatomy. Reprinted with permission of the Cleveland Clinic Foundation.

mesocolon lie close to or over the celiac artery. Layering of these fatty planes on the celiac artery allows regional gastric or colonic lymph nodes to be situated near celiac lymph nodes, potentiating misidentification. Problems with location and identity may occur at laparotomy, laparoscopy, or endoscopic ultrasonography. The relationship between nodal stations can be altered with patient positioning, noninvasive staging technique, surgical approach, or routine handling of the resection specimen in the pathology laboratory. The anatomy of the celiac region facilitates inconsis-

tent identification of celiac lymph nodes. When making comparison between reports of staging modalities, treatment protocols, and outcome of therapy it is important to keep in mind that reported differences may be due to misidentification or incorrect staging of celiac lymph nodes.

Misclassification can occur due to inconsistencies in staging guidelines for distal esophageal and proximal gastric cancers and difficulties identifying the origin of a tumor. It may be problematic to determine if a cancer involving the esophagogastric junction is a proximal gastric cancer or a distal esophageal cancer. For lesser curve gastric cancers, celiac lymph nodes are region lymph nodes. Depending on the number of metastatic regional nodes, a patient with a high lesser curve gastric cancer with esophageal invasion and celiac lymph node metastasis may have N1 (depending upon T and M, stage grouping IB, II, or IIIA), N2 (depending upon T and M, stage grouping II, IIIA, or IIIB), or N3 (stage grouping IV) cancer.[1] If this tumor is misinterpreted as distal thoracic esophageal cancer, it is an M1a (stage grouping IVA) cancer.

With careful dissection around the celiac artery, one to three celiac lymph nodes and two to three left gastric nodes can be retrieved.[2,3] Reported in surgical series, overall prevalence of celiac lymph node metastases is between 15% and 20%.[2,4-8] Several factors influence the likelihood of finding celiac lymph nodes metastases at resection. Cancer location within the esophagus is

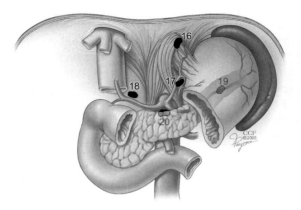

FIGURE 33.2. The celiac artery, its branches, and associated lymph nodes: 16 paracardial, 17 left gastric, 18 hepatic, 19 splenic, and 20 celiac. Reprinted with permission of the Cleveland Clinic Foundation.

important. For squamous cell carcinomas in the middle esophagus, the prevalence is 4.4% and increases to 21.2% for tumors of the distal esophagus.[9] As with regional nodal beds, more advanced T classification (≥T3) is associated with a higher prevalence of celiac lymph node metastases.[6,10,11] In patients with adenocarcinoma, the prevalence of celiac lymph node metastases increases with the number of regional lymph node metastases, reaching 65% in patients with six or more positive regional nodes.[12] Celiac lymph node metastases in the absence of regional lymph node metastases is uncommon, skip metastases occurring in about 5% of patients.[12] Of 70 patients undergoing esophagectomy with radical lymphadenectomy, 76% recurred but only 5% developed celiac lymph node recurrences.[3]

33.2. Staging Celiac Lymph Nodes

Computerized tomography (CT) relies on lymph node size to diagnose metastases (Figure 33.3). Clinical staging of celiac lymph nodes by helical CT scanning is reported to be 53% sensitive [95% confidence interval (95% CI), 28%–79%], 86% specific (95% CI, 73%–99%), 67% positively predictive (95% CI, 40%–93%), and 77% negatively predictive (95% CI, 63%–92%).[13] Sensitivity of CT for celiac lymph node metastases has been reported as low as 8%.[14] For celiac lymph nodes

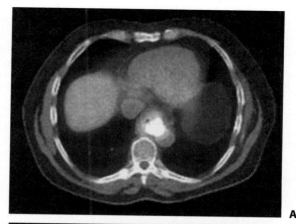
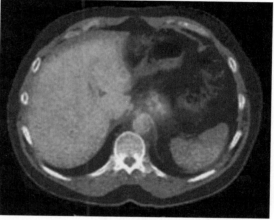

FIGURE 33.4. Computed tompgraphy PET demonstrates (A) a hypermetabolic mass at the esophagogastric junction and (B) a hypermetabolic celiac lymph node which is difficult to differentiate from the primary tumor.

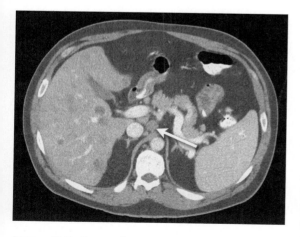

FIGURE 33.3. Computed tomography of the abdomen demonstrates an large celiac lymph node (*arrow*). Multiple hepatic metastases are also seen.

this clinical staging tool is both insensitive in screening and of poor positive predictive value in clinical decision making. Despite its poor performance in assessment of celiac lymph nodes, CT is an integral part of clinical staging of esophageal cancer, particularly when fused with positron emission tomography (PET).

Positron emission tomography is superior to CT in detecting distant metastases in patients with esophageal cancer; however, assessing celiac lymph nodes is problematic because of proximity of the primary tumor to the celiac lymph nodes, despite the "distant" staging status of these nodes (Figure 33.4). In 42 clinically staged operable patients with adenocarcinoma of the esophagus or esophagogastric junction, 4 patients were found to have metastases to celiac lymph nodes and 2 to para-aortic lymph nodes that were not detected by PET.[15] This finding prompted the authors to conclude that "the diagnostic value of PET in staging of adenocarcinoma of the esophagus and esophagogastric junction is limited because of low accuracy in staging para-tumoral and distant lymph node metastases."

Endoscopic esophageal ultrasound (EUS) is useful in staging celiac lymph nodes because it can provide both clinical and pathologic staging. At EUS evaluation, metastatic lymph nodes typically appear as large (>1cm in diameter), round, well demarcated, homogeneously hypoechoic, and in close proximity to the primary tumor (Figure 33.5). Using the first four of these criteria,

EUS was 83% sensitive, 98% specific, 91% positively predictive, and 97% negatively predictive in 149 patients with pathological confirmation of celiac nodal status.[16] Eloubeidi and colleagues[17] reported that EUS in 211 patients was 77% (95% CI, 67–88) sensitive, 85% (95% CI, 74–96) specific, 89% (95% CI, 81–97) positively predictive, and 71% (95% CI, 58–84) negatively predictive in detecting celiac lymph node metastases. Tumor location may play a role in the ability of EUS to detect celiac nodal metastases. Heeren and colleagues[18] reported that EUS assessment of celiac lymph node metastases was better in esophageal tumors than esophagogastric junctional tumors (93% vs. 63%, $p < 0.001$).

Endoscopic evaluation of celiac lymph nodes has prognostic significance. The ability to detect

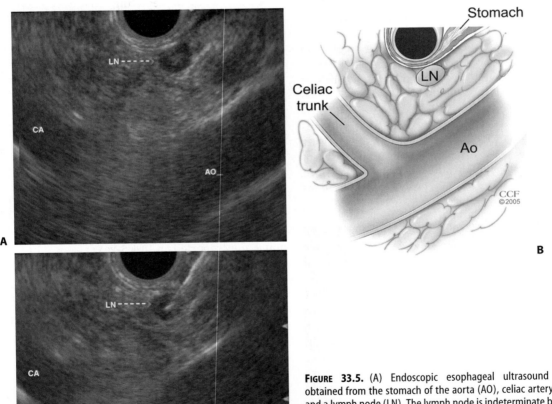

FIGURE 33.5. (A) Endoscopic esophageal ultrasound view obtained from the stomach of the aorta (AO), celiac artery (CA), and a lymph node (LN). The lymph node is indeterminate by EUS. Although it is round, well demarcated, and hypoechoic, it is small (<1cm in diameter). (B) Graphic depiction of the anatomy. (C) EUS-FNA of the lymph node (?, celiac lymph node). The fine needle can be seen entering the lymph node, the aspirate was cytologically diagnostic for metastatic adenocarcinoma. Reprinted with permission of the Cleveland Clinic Foundation.

a celiac lymph node (any node >5mm) by EUS was associated with a poorer outcome: 13% (95% CI, 5%-21%) 5-year survival in patients with a detectable celiac lymph node versus 30% (95% CI, 21%-40%; $p = 0.007$) in those without.[19] Size of celiac lymph nodes measured at EUS is also predictive of survival. Median survival of patients with celiac lymph nodes >2cm was 13.5 months compared to 7 months for nodes >2cm.[20]

Endoscopic esophageal ultrasound – directed fine-needle aspiration (EUS-FNA) differs from CT and PET, which are purely clinical staging tools. If performed correctly, that is, location and technique (a clean biopsy channel and an uncontaminated needle passed into the lymph node in an area removed from the tumor; Figure 33.5), a pathological assessment of celiac lymph nodes can be obtained. Eloubeidi and colleagues[19] reported EUS-FNA possible in 94% of patients with EUS-identified celiac lymph nodes. EUS-FNA was 98% (95% CI, 90–100) accurate, 98% (95% CI, 88–99) sensitive, 100% (95% CI, 48–100) specific, 100% (95% CI, 92–100) positively predictive, and 83% (95% CI, 36–99) negatively predictive for celiac lymph node metastases. Univariable risk factors for celiac lymph node metastases were (1) EUS detection of cT3 or cT4 cancer with 4.8 (95% CI, 1.8–12.6) times the risk of cT1 or cT2 tumors; (2) need for dilation to permit EUS examination with 2.6 (95% CI, 0.95–7.3) times the risk of patients not requiring dilation; (3) EUS detection of cN1 with 2.43 (95% CI, 1.03–5.74) times the risk of cN0; and (4) African-American patients with 1.38 (95% CI, 1.03–1.86) times the risk of white patients. However, multivariable analysis only identified increasing cT associated with celiac lymph node metastases.

Parmar and colleagues[21] have used EUS-FNA to direct therapy. Twenty-three of 40 patients (58%) had at least one EUS characteristic of a positive celiac lymph node. In 18 of 20 patients, EUS-FNA of the celiac axis was positive. The two patients who were negative underwent surgery and were confirmed M0; the 18 patients diagnosed M1a received definitive chemoradiotherapy. Computed tomography scan detected only 6 of the 20 (30%) EUS-detected celiac lymph nodes. Of these, 5 were M1a and 1 was M0.

Minimally invasive staging of esophageal cancer using video-assisted thoracic surgery (VATS) and laparoscopy has been technically feasible in over 70% of patients.[22] In a population containing roughly two thirds adenocarcinomas and one third squamous cell carcinomas, celiac nodal metastases were identified in 27% of patients. In an earlier study, the sensitivity of laparoscopy for celiac lymph node metastases was 14%, specificity was 100%, and overall accuracy 94%.[9] Considerations with laparoscopy are time and cost. A laparoscopic assessment in combination with a thoracoscopic evaluation is 2 to 3 hours.[8,9] Cost of the procedure depends on number of biopsies and length of hospital stay. Average cost is between $20,000 to $25,000.[23]

Because celiac lymph nodes are not easily accessible at laparoscopy, Stein and colleagues[24] used laparoscopic ultrasound (LUS) in clinical staging. They reported 67% sensitivity and 92% specificity of LUS in predicting celiac lymph node metastases. Loss of pathological staging and need for laparoscopy to perform ultrasound make this procedure unattractive.

33.3. Treatment for Celiac Lymph Node Metastases

The published results of treatment of esophageal cancer with celiac lymph node metastases demonstrate the poor outcome with surgery. Akiyama and colleagues[5] were the first to bring attention to the importance of celiac lymph node metastases in planning treatment of esophageal cancer patients. In patients with squamous cell carcinoma, they reported an 18% 5-year survival in 31 patients with celiac lymph node metastases treated with resection and three-field lymphadenectomy and 49% in 162 patients without celiac lymph node metastases ($p < 0.001$; level of evidence 3). Using en bloc esophagectomy in 16 patients with adenocarcinoma of the esophagus and celiac lymph node metastases, Hagan and colleagues[6] reported a 28% 5-year survival (level of evidence 3). Hulsher and colleagues[4] treated patients with both adenocarcinoma and squamous cell carcinoma of the esophagus with transhiatal esophagectomy and no formal lymph node dissection. They reported a median survival of 1.5 years (95% CI, 0.5–2.5), however, lymph nodes within 1cm of the origin of the left gastric artery were considered to be celiac lymph nodes (level of evidence 3). Clark and associates[2] reported that survival of nine patients with celiac lymph node metastases was not different from those without, but 67% had cancer recurrence at 18 months. These findings led them to conclude that "although most patients with celiac node metastases have recurrences, celiac metastases did not preclude long-term survival, as two patients survived 56 and 68 months" (level of evidence 3).

Frizzell and colleagues[25] reported treating 13 patients with distant metastases limited to celiac lymph nodes. Five received definitive chemoradiotherapy, five received induction chemoradiotherapy followed by surgery, and three received combined preoperative and postoperative chemotherapy and radiotherapy. One and 2-year survival in this group was 85% and 55%, respectively. In this small group of patients early survival was not different from their 11 N0M0 and 23 N1M0 patients treated predominately with definitive chemoradiotherapy (level of evidence 3).

Our experience at the Cleveland Clinic Foundation with esophageal carcinoma patients with celiac lymph node metastases has been disappointing.[26] In 36 patients with M1a esophageal carcinoma, 32 (92%) of whom had distal esophageal adenocarcinoma, median and 5-year survival was 11 months and 6%. Although this outcome was statistically better than patients with M1B disease (5 months and 2%, $p = 0.001$), it was clinically insignificant (level of evidence 3). No difference was noted in patients with celiac lymph node metastases whether or not they underwent surgery ($p = 0.02$). Patients receiving chemotherapy and/or radiotherapy did 2.2 times better than those who did not ($p < 0.001$). With no survival in 26 patients with celiac lymph node metastases at 5 years after esophagectomy, we proposed that the current M1a subclassification was not warranted (level of evidence 3).[27] Patients with celiac lymph node metastases have the poorest survival of any resected stage grouping and carry a prognosis not different from those patients with other distant metastatic disease (M1b), three or more regional lymph node metastases (proposed N2), or T4N1M0 cancers.[27]

33.4. Conclusions and Recommendations

This literature does not support the M1a classification for esophageal cancer with celiac lymph node metastases. Therefore, the unique subclassification M1a and subgroupings IVA are not warranted (evidence level 2– to 3; recommendation grade D).

Clinical staging of all patients with esophageal cancer should include CT/PET and EUS. Any accessible, abnormal lymph node identified by EUS evaluation should be subject to EUS-FNA. All suspicious celiac lymph nodes must be aspirated transgastrically. It is the endoscopist's and surgeon's responsibility to assure that the node sampled is truly a celiac node.

The clinical or pathological finding of celiac lymph node metastases is ominous. Rarely will a patient be cured with surgery alone. Chemoradiotherapy is crucial for improved survival. In a protocol setting, this may be administered preoperatively followed by surgery, but the patient must be aware that the treatment is experimental. If unsuspected celiac lymph node metastases are found at surgery and the cancer is otherwise resectable, the operation should be completed and the patient considered for postoperative adjuvant chemoradiotherapy (level of evidence 3; recommendation grade D).[28–30]

The unique subclassification M1a and subgroupings IVa and IVb are not warranted (level of evidence 2– to 3; recommendation grade D).

The finding of celiac lymph node metastases is ominous and chemoradiotherapy is crucial for improved survival. This may be administered preoperatively followed by surgery, but this treatment is experimental. If unsuspected celiac lymph node metastases are found at surgery and the cancer is otherwise resectable, the operation should be completed and the patient considered for postoperative adjuvant chemoradiotherapy (level of evidence 3; recommendation grade D).

References

1. *AJCC Cancer Staging Manual*. 6th ed. New York: Springer; 2002.
2. Clark GW, Peters JH, Ireland AP, et al. Nodal metastasis and sites of recurrence after en bloc esophagectomy for adenocarcinoma. *Ann Thorac Surg* 1994;58:646–653; discussion 53–54.
3. Fujita H, Kakegawa T, Yamana H, et al. Lymph node metastasis and recurrence in patients with a carcinoma of the thoracic esophagus who underwent three-field dissection. *World J Surg* 1994;18: 266–272.
4. Hulscher JB, Buskens CJ, Bergman JJ, Fockens P, Van Lanschot JJ, Obertop H. Positive peritruncal nodes for esophageal carcinoma. not always a dismal prognosis. *Dig Surg* 2001;18:98–101.
5. Akiyama H, Tsurumaru M, Udagawa H, Kajiyama Y. Radical lymph node dissection for cancer of the thoracic esophagus. *Ann Surg* 1994;220:364–372; discussion 72–73.
6. Hagen JA, DeMeester SR, Peters JH, Chandrasoma P, DeMeester TR. Curative resection for esophageal adenocarcinoma: analysis of 100 en bloc esophagectomies. *Ann Surg* 2001;234:520–530; discussion 30–31.
7. Hulscher JB, Van Sandick JW, Offerhaus GJ, Tilanus HW, Obertop H, Van Lanschot JJ. Prospective analysis of the diagnostic yield of extended en bloc resection for adenocarcinoma of the oesophagus or gastric cardia. *Br J Surg* 2001;88:715–719.
8. Sannohe Y, Hiratsuka R, Doki K. Lymph node metastases in cancer of the thoracic esophagus. *Am J Surg* 1981;141:216–218.
9. Akiyama H, Tsurumaru M, Kawamura T, Ono Y. Principles of surgical treatment for carcinoma of the esophagus: analysis of lymph node involvement. *Ann Surg* 1981;194:438–446.
10. Igaki H, Kato H, Tachimori Y, Sato H, Daiko H, Nakanishi Y. Prognostic evaluation for squamous cell carcinomas of the lower thoracic esophagus treated with three-field lymph node dissection. *Eur J Cardiothorac Surg* 2001;19:887–893.
11. Baba M, Aikou T, Yoshinaka H, et al. Long-term results of subtotal esophagectomy with three-field lymphadenectomy for carcinoma of the thoracic esophagus. *Ann Surg* 1994;219:31–36.
12. Feith M, Stein HJ, Siewert JR. Pattern of lymphatic spread of Barrett's cancer. *World J Surg* 2003;27: 1052–1057.
13. Romagnuolo J, Scott J, Hawes RH, et al. Helical CT versus EUS with fine needle aspiration for celiac nodal assessment in patients with esophageal cancer. *Gastrointest Endosc* 2002;55:648–654.
14. Reed CE, Mishra G, Sahai AV, Hoffman BJ, Hawes RH. Esophageal cancer staging: improved accuracy by endoscopic ultrasound of celiac lymph nodes. *Ann Thorac Surg* 1999;67:319–321; discussion 322.
15. Rasanen JV, Sihvo EI, Knuuti MJ, et al. Prospective analysis of accuracy of positron emission tomography, computed tomography, and endoscopic ultrasonography in staging of adenocarcinoma of the esophagus and the esophagogastric junction. *Ann Surg Oncol* 2003;10:954–960.
16. Catalano MF, Alcocer E, Chak A, et al. Evaluation of metastatic celiac axis lymph nodes in patients with esophageal carcinoma: accuracy of EUS. *Gastrointest Endosc* 1999;50:352–356.
17. Eloubeidi MA, Wallace MB, Reed CE, et al. The utility of EUS and EUS-guided fine needle aspiration in detecting celiac lymph node metastasis in patients with esophageal cancer: a single-center experience. *Gastrointest Endosc* 2001;54:714–719.
18. Heeren PA, van Westreenen HL, Geersing GJ, van Dullemen HM, Plukker JT. Influence of tumor characteristics on the accuracy of endoscopic ultrasonography in staging cancer of the esophagus and esophagogastric junction. *Endoscopy* 2004;36:966–971.
19. Eloubeidi MA, Wallace MB, Hoffman BJ, et al. Predictors of survival for esophageal cancer patients with and without celiac axis lymphadenopathy: impact of staging endosonography. *Ann Thorac Surg* 2001;72:212–219; discussion 919–920.
20. Marsman WA, van Wissen M, Bergman JJ, et al. Outcome of patients with esophageal carcinoma and suspicious celiac lymph nodes as determined by endoscopic ultrasonography. *Endoscopy* 2004; 36:961–965.
21. Parmar KS, Zwischenberger JB, Reeves AL, Waxman I. Clinical impact of endoscopic ultrasound-guided fine needle aspiration of celiac axis lymph nodes (M1a disease) in esophageal cancer. *Ann Thorac Surg* 2002;73:916–920; discussion 920–921.
22. Krasna MJ, Reed CE, Nedzwiecki D, et al. CALGB 9380: a prospective trial of the feasibility of thoracoscopy/laparoscopy in staging esophageal cancer. *Ann Thorac Surg* 2001;71:1073–1079.
23. Luketich JD, Schauer P, Landreneau R, et al. Minimally invasive surgical staging is superior to endoscopic ultrasound in detecting lymph node metastases in esophageal cancer. *J Thorac Cardiovasc Surg* 1997;114:817–821; discussion 821–823.

24. Stein HJ, Kraemer SJ, Feussner H, Fink U, Siewert JR. Clinical value of diagnostic laparoscopy with laparoscopic ultrasound in patients with cancer of the esophagus or cardia. *J Gastrointest Surg* 1997;1:167–173.

25. Frizzell B, Sinha D, Williams T, Reed CE, Sherman CA, Turrisi A. Influence of celiac axis lymph nodes in the definitive treatment of esophageal cancer. *Am J Clin Oncol* 2003;26:215–220.

26. Christie NA, Rice TW, DeCamp MM, et al. M1a/M1b esophageal carcinoma: clinical relevance. *J Thorac Cardiovasc Surg* 1999;118:900–907.

27. Rice TW, Blackstone EH, Rybicki LA, et al. Refining esophageal cancer staging. *J Thorac Cardiovasc Surg* 2003;125:1103–1113.

28. Macdonald JS, Smalley SR, Benedetti J, et al. Chemoradiotherapy after surgery compared with surgery alone for adenocarcinoma of the stomach or gastroesophageal junction. *N Engl J Med* 2001;345:725–730.

29. Bedard EL, Inculet RI, Malthaner RA, Brecevic E, Vincent M, Dar R. The role of surgery and postoperative chemoradiation therapy in patients with lymph node positive esophageal carcinoma. *Cancer* 2001;91:2423–2430.

30. Rice TW, Adelstein DJ, Chidel MA, et al. Benefit of postoperative adjuvant chemoradiotherapy in locoregionally advanced esophageal carcinoma. *J Thorac Cardiovasc Surg* 2003;126:1590–1596.

34
Partial or Total Fundoplication for Gastroesophageal Reflux Disease in the Presence of Impaired Esophageal Motility

Jedediah A. Kaufman and Brant K. Oelschlager

Anti-reflux surgery has evolved greatly in the last 15 years as a durable, viable, and safe option for treatment of gastroesophageal reflux disease (GERD), mainly due to the advent of minimally invasive techniques. The debate regarding partial fundoplication (PF) versus total fundoplication (TF) for patients with defective peristalsis and GERD has evolved as well. Nissen fundoplication is by far the most common fundoplication technique used for many decades. However, many surgeons prefer a PF in patients with defective peristalsis. This tailored approach developed due to the logical, but unproven, theory that dysphagia is more likely when impaired esophageal peristalsis fails to propel a swallowed bolus across a 360° fundoplication (or TF). Recent literature has challenged this notion, suggesting that TF is not more likely to cause dysphagia than PF. Moreover, there is evidence that PF provides inferior control of reflux compared with TF, thus tailoring may be to the detriment of reflux control.

We will consider the evidence for performing a partial fundoplication in patients with impaired peristalsis, as well as any differences in postoperative dysphagia and the ability of TF or PF to control GERD.

34.1. Detailed Review of Key Studies

The literature on anti-reflux surgery for patients with defective peristalsis has several inherent problems. There are no standard definitions for defective and normal peristalsis, and techniques and types of TF and PF vary widely. Large, prop-

erly powered randomized trials differentiating outcomes for patients undergoing fundoplication in the setting of impaired esophageal peristalsis do not exist. Objective data is also missing in most studies. Postoperative manometry and pH studies are rarely performed in sufficient numbers for adequate comparison, and are more often done in patients with recurrent or persistent problems, thus potentially skewing the results. Still, there are some good studies published recently that can help answer the question: partial or total fundoplication for GERD in the presence of impaired esophageal motility?

Oleynikov and others compared PF and TF outcomes in patients with defective peristalsis [defined as distal esophageal amplitude (DEA) <40mmHg in >70% of swallows].[1] Eighty-six patients were studied, 39 underwent PF and 57 underwent TF. No patient in the TF group developed new dysphagia. In fact, preoperative dysphagia among all TF patients greatly improved. There were inferior results in the PF group, as existing dysphagia failed to significantly improve after operation. Heartburn improved after both PF and TF, although TF provided much better control of reflux. While both groups experienced a significant improvement in the objective control of GERD, there were lower levels of acid exposure in the TF group on pH monitoring. The DeMeester scores in the TF group decreased from a median of 57.1 preoperatively to 6.3 postoperatively, compared to 72.3 preoperatively to 11.3 postoperatively for the PF group. Interestingly, postoperative manometry demonstrated a significant increase in amplitude of esophageal peristalsis in the TF

group from 30.6 mmHg to 49.0 mmHg postfundoplication. While the peristaltic amplitudes
increased in the PF patients (27.7 mmHg to
35.6 mmHg, p = ns), this change was not statistically significant. The sample size in this study is
moderate, but the results are compelling. The
study looks at specific outcomes of laparoscopic
partial versus total fundoplication to answer specific questions regarding dysphagia, GERD symptoms, and requirements for invasive or operative
treatment for complications or recurrence of
symptoms. The study suggests that TF be used in
all patients regardless of peristaltic quality (level
of evidence 4). However, patients with true aperistalsis, such as those with scleroderma, may still
be candidates for partial fundoplication.

Patti and others compared their experience
with a tailored approach (1992–1999) to their
more recent nontailored approach (2000–2002).[2]
With the tailored approach they had more reflux
(15% TF vs. 33% PF) and the same amount of
dysphagia (11% TF vs. 8% PF). In patients with
defective peristalsis (55), early dysphagia occurred
in 5 (9%), resolving in 3 patients after an average
of 5 months (3–6 months) and after dilation in 2
patients. No patient in either group required
operation or had residual dysphagia after dilation. There was no difference in rates of dysphagia, dysphagia scores, lower esophageal sphincter
(LES) length, amplitude of peristaltic waves,
medication requirements, or re-operations
between TF and PF. There were differences in the
competency of the cardia, as TF resulted in better
relief of heartburn, increased LES pressure, and
lower DeMeester scores. In the subsequent period
of time when the tailored approach was abandoned, routine TF resulted in superior objective
and subjective control of GERD, while dysphagia
rates did not increase. The authors suggest that a
tailored approach should be abandoned in favor
of routine TF (level of evidence 4). The large
sample size and excellent comparison of both
defective peristalsis patients undergoing PF and
TF as well as normal peristalsis patients undergoing TF allows proper analysis of outcomes of new
dysphagia and recurrent GERD symptoms.

Rydberg and others randomized one hundred
and six patients to PF or TF irrespective of their
preoperative esophageal peristalsis characteristics.[3] Sixty-seven patients had defective peristal-

sis (defined as DEA ≤30 mmHg, failed primary
peristalsis, or >20% simultaneous contractions).
Of the patients with defective peristalsis, 34
underwent TF and 33 PF. Follow-up for these
patients was at least 3 years. Overall, dysphagia
incidence decreased from 20% preoperatively
to 8% postoperatively at a minimum of 3-year
follow-up. No difference in symptoms was found
postoperatively between those receiving PF and
TF. There were fewer patients with hyperflatu-
lence after PF than TF (23 vs. 58). The authors
concluded that tailoring antireflux surgery based
on preoperative esophageal motor function was
not supported (level of evidence 2b). This is a
well-designed trial with 3 years minimum follow-
up. Although only a small sample size was
reported, the results are reproducible in many
other similar-sized studies. The authors specifically analyzed their data utilizing several methods
and were still unable to find correlations between
outcomes, peristalsis, and type of fundoplication. The length of follow-up strengthens the conclusions that tailoring anti-reflux surgery to
peristaltic quality is unfounded.

In a well-designed, short-term prospective,
randomized trial, Zornig and others evaluated
200 consecutive patients undergoing anti-reflux
surgery.[4] They were not selected according to
their esophageal motility; however, patient outcomes were analyzed according to motility post
hoc. Patients were randomly assigned TF or PF.
Defective peristalsis was defined as mean DEA
<40 mmHg and/or failed primary peristalsis in
>40% of 10 wet swallows. Results were analyzed
at 1 week and 4 months postoperatively only, thus
long-term results are not available. This negatively affects the impact of this study. Patients
with early dysphagia, even after only 1 week,
underwent early endoscopic evaluation and dilation. At four months, 41 patients had dysphagia
(57 had dysphagia preoperatively), and of these
41, 19 had normal peristalsis and 22 had defective
peristalsis preoperatively. The incidence of dysphagia increased in the TF group (from 24 to 30
patients) while decreasing in the PF group (from
33 to 11 patients). New dysphagia was found in 24
patients, equally distributed between patients
with normal and defective peristalsis. Fourteen
patients required redo fundoplication (13 TF, 1
PF), 10 for recurrent reflux with esophagitis and

mild dysphagia, and 4 for severe dysphagia. Of these 14 redo patients, 10 TF patients herniated their intact wrap above the diaphragm, a known anatomical cause of dysphagia postfundoplication. Therefore, it is possible that poor construction and not the 360° nature of the TF caused these failures. In the defective peristalsis group, no significant difference in dysphagia was seen based on operation performed, with seven undergoing TF and five with PF.

Technical aspects of anti-reflux surgery are no doubt important in avoiding dysphagia and control of GERD after fundoplication. The authors concluded that PF is superior to TF in prevention of postoperative complications such as dysphagia (level of evidence 2b), although the very high incidence of recurrent hiatal hernia casts doubt on this conclusion. The authors also pursued an unorthodox approach of early dilation for dysphagia within the first few weeks, a practice that has been associated with fundoplication disruption. Finally, dysphagia after TF is common 3 to 6 months following surgery, and most surgeons do not intervene as it usually resolves. The extremely short follow-up of this study severely detracts from the ability to generalize its findings.

The small randomized, prospective trial by Chrysos and others evaluates 33 patients with defective peristalsis (defined as DEA <35 mmHg) comparing TF (Nissen–Rossetti) with PF (Toupet) and found no differences in dysphagia at 12 month follow-up.[5] In the short term (3-month follow-up), TF was associated with more dysphagia (57% TF vs. 16% PF); however, by 1 year only 14% of TF patients and 16% of PF patients reported mild dysphagia. No patient had severe dysphagia at 1 year. In a similar pattern, gas-bloat syndrome occurred more often in the TF at 3 months, but this difference was not apparent at 1 year when 21% of TF and 16% of PF patients reported bloating symptoms. Postoperative LES pressures were significantly improved in all patients, with no difference between TF and PF. Total fundoplication and PF equally controlled reflux with postoperative DeMeester scores decreasing to 12 in PF and 14 in TF. The authors recommended TF in patients with defective peristalsis due to literature indicating it as a superior long-term barrier of reflux compared to PF (level of evidence 2b).

This is a small study without the appropriate power to determine whether TF or PF is superior; however, it was properly randomized and double blinded. The results concur with large studies regarding TF in patients with defective peristalsis.

The study by Ludemann and others evaluates long-term follow-up of a randomized, double-blinded trial between laparoscopic TF versus anterior 180° PF.[6] Although patients with motility problems were not included, this well-designed and executed paper is an excellent comparison between PF and TF. At 5 years, 101/107 (98%) patients were included, with 51 undergoing TF and 50 undergoing PF. There were no significant differences between the groups with regards to control of heartburn, patient satisfaction, or use of proton-pump inhibitors. Dysphagia for solids, bloating, inability to belch, and flatulence were more common after TF. Recurrent reflux was more common after PF. Re-operation was required for three patients with TF for dysphagia and three patients with PF for recurrent reflux. Few studies have 5-year follow-up, with 98% response in a moderate-sized patient group (level of evidence 2b). In addition, the researchers remained blinded initially and at 5 years, eliminating reporter bias. The main weakness is that results are based solely on questionnaire answers of patients and no objective data is reported. However, at 6 months, the same patient group underwent manometry, pH monitoring, and clinical evaluation. Results showed that both operations normalized esophageal acid exposure, TF improved LES pressures compared to PF, and a higher incidence of dysphagia at 3 months was seen with TF. This increase disappeared at 6-month follow-up.[7] The authors concluded that anterior PF was as effective as TF for long-term GERD symptom control. However, a higher risk of recurrent GERD symptoms was seen with PF.

The available quality of evidence throughout the literature is comprised of predominantly case series of small-to-moderate numbers of patients. The vast number of technical differences found in anti-reflux procedures and the subtle differences in definitions of motility disorders often hampers proper comparison of studies and techniques. Without larger, significantly powered studies with definitions that are agreed upon for accurate patient comparison, specific guidelines are difficult to create. Based on the available data and substantial experience utilizing both a tailored and nontailored approaches to anti-reflux surgery, we find little to support PF for patients with poor motility (level of evidence 2b; recommendation grade B). Although a few large case series show PF does improve reflux (although less than TF), and although TF may have higher rates of early complications, no convincing evidence supports the tailored approach. Evidence continues to mount showing PF is inferior for reflux control and a properly constructed TF causes little significant dysphagia or decreased quality of life beyond 3 to 6 months from surgery.

34.2. Impact on Clinical Practice

Application of the literature to determine the correct approach for patients with defective peristalsis depends on its interpretation. One must apply knowledge of the key technical aspects of fundoplication construction and look critically at causes of dysphagia and poor reflux control. It is clear that there is not a degree of impaired peristalsis, as determined by manometry, which consistently results in a greater rate of postoperative dysphagia if a TF is performed.[8] Therefore, for most abnormalities of peristalsis, a TF can be safely performed. Partial fundoplication does not appear to reliably decrease the incidence of dysphagia either in patients with or without defective peristalsis. No properly weighted and designed study yet demonstrates true correlation between preoperative factors and the development of postoperative dysphagia.[9] The literature currently supports that patients with defective peristalsis undergoing TF have more early (6–12 weeks) dysphagia than those undergoing PF; however, this seems to be transient and no difference between TF and PF remains at 1 year and beyond. In fact, esophageal motility tends to improve after TF, perhaps due to better control of GERD, reducing esophageal inflammation and injury.[1,3,10,11] The compilation of long-term data seems to suggest that preoperative motor function does not predict postoperative dysphagia,[3,12,13] but that operative technique is more likely the culprit than preoperative variables. Anatomical

causes such as tight, twisted, or slipped fundoplications and use of the stomach body rather than the fundus to create the wrap, essentially causing a bilobed, obstructed, or inefficient wrap, all significantly effect postoperative dysphagia and GERD control.[4,14–17] New or worsening dysphagia occurs after fundoplication in 2% to 14% of patients.[3,18] Barring significant technical errors, unexplained dysphagia, with a normal fundoplication, decreases to around 1% to 2%.

With a few notable exceptions, the literature currently supports that patients with defective peristalsis and TF have better control of GERD than those undergoing PF.[1,2,8,19–26] Most studies show inferior results of PF, both in patients with and without defective peristalsis. In most surgeons' hands, PF does not provide as reliable control of GERD as a TF. There are, however, some exceptions as shown in the articles reviewed. Thus, the best way to prevent dysphagia and control reflux is a well constructed fundoplication. Tailoring the fundoplication, based solely on the peristalsis measured by manometry, is not supported by data, and the approach should be abolished.

34.3. Opinion Statement

We perform TF for all patients with defective peristalsis except in those patients who have essentially no peristaltic activity (i.e., aperistalsis). We feel that our experience and the evidence suggest that this provides the best combination of reflux control while limiting side effects. We perform preoperative manometry with impedance on all patients to (1) properly identify the LES for accurate pH probe placement, (2) provide objective information about the physiology of GERD in each patient (LES function, esophageal clearance, etc.), and (3) regularly identify patients with achalasia and other primary esophageal motility disorders that affect management.

We place great importance on certain technical aspects of the Nissen fundoplication in order to relieve GERD and avoid dysphagia.[27] These steps include:

1. Mobilization of the distal esophagus adequately into the mediastinum to obtain 3 to 4 cm

of intra-abdominal esophageal length to prevent recurrent hernia. Results of studies examining outcomes of patients with extensive mediastinal dissection show that lengthening procedures such as the Collis gastroplasty are rarely needed, even with large paraesophageal hernias.[28,29]

2. Complete gastric fundus mobilization, including all short gastric vessels to avoid torque or angulation. A few studies refute division of the short gastric vessels, however an abstract by Jones and colleagues showed significant decrease in dysphagia with complete fundal mobilization.[30] Experienced clinicians find that leaving these fundic and body attachments increases torque and angulation of the gastroesophageal junction and potentially increases postoperative dysphagia.[31]

3. Creation of a 360° fundoplication over a bougie 52 to 60 Fr to help assure a very floppy fundoplication. Although disagreement over the appropriate size bougie or whether to use one at all still exists, the loss of palpation of the esophagus and wrap looseness supports the idea of using multiple methods to avoid creating too tight a wrap. Most accepted technique for this includes use of a larger bougie, especially with dysmotility.[32]

4. Careful construction of the wrap with equal portions of posterior and anterior fundus, avoiding errors such as using the body of the stomach or leaving redundant fundus behind the wrap.[33] By utilizing equal portions of the anterior and posterior fundus, the esophagus is imbricated into a neutral fundus, preventing torque and minimizing angulation.

Although we can hope for larger, randomized studies, with long-term clinical and objective results to more definitively end this debate, the existing evidence does not support the construction of a PF because of impaired esophageal peristalsis. Rather, it suggests that the surgeon perform the best fundoplication he/she can in terms of controlling reflux and avoiding complications. This opinion is based on level 2b evidence and should only be applied specifically to the techniques described. Several pitfalls exist in interpreting this data, pitfalls we have found ameliorated by very careful techniques that, although may not prevent all complications, cer-

tainly minimized postoperative dysphagia. Sufficiently powered studies to prove these techniques do not exist, and yet our investigations have shown that overall technical aspects of the operation are more often the cause of dysphagia than quality of peristalsis.

> The existing evidence does not support the construction of a partial fundoplication in the management of GERD because of impaired esophageal peristalsis (level of evidence 2b; recommendation grade B).

References

1. Oleynikov DET, Oelschlager BK, Pellegrini CA. Total fundoplication is the operation of choice for patients with gastroesophageal reflux and defective peristalsis. *Surg Endosc* 2002;16:909–913.
2. Patti MG, Robinson T, Galvani C, Gorodner MV, Fisichella PM, Way LW. Total fundoplication is superior to partial fundoplication even when esophageal peristalsis is weak. *J Am Coll Surg* 2004;198:863–869; discussion 869–870.
3. Rydberg L, Ruth M, Abrahamsson H, Lundell L. Tailoring antireflux surgery: a randomized clinical trial. *World J Surg* 1999;23:612–618.
4. Zornig C, Strate U, Fibbe C, Emmermann A, Layer P. Nissen vs Toupet laparoscopic fundoplication. *Surg Endosc* 2002;16:758–766.
5. Chrysos E, Tsiaoussis J, Zoras OJ, et al. Laparoscopic surgery for gastroesophageal reflux disease patients with impaired esophageal peristalsis: total or partial fundoplication? *J Am Coll Surg* 2003;197:8–15.
6. Ludemann R, Watson DI, Jamieson GG, Game PA, Devitt PG. Five-year follow-up of a randomized clinical trial of laparoscopic total versus anterior 180 degrees fundoplication. *Br J Surg* 2005;92:240–243.
7. Lundell L, Abrahamsson H, Ruth M, Sandberg N, Olbe LC. Lower esophageal sphincter characteristics and esophageal acid exposure following partial or 360 degrees fundoplication: results of a prospective, randomized, clinical study. *World J Surg* 1991;15:115–120; discussion 121.
8. Beckingham IJ, Cariem AK, Bornman PC, Callanan MD, Louw JA. Oesophageal dysmotility is not associated with poor outcome after laparoscopic Nissen fundoplication. *Br J Surg* 1998;85:1290–1293.

9. Wills VL, Hunt DR. Dysphagia after antireflux surgery. *Br J Surg* 2001;88:486–499.

10. Heider TR, Farrell TM, Kircher AP, Colliver CC, Koruda MJ, Behrns KE. Complete fundoplication is not associated with increased dysphagia in patients with abnormal esophageal motility. *J Gastrointest Surg* 2001;5:36–41.

11. Heider TR, Behrns KE, Koruda MJ, et al. Fundoplication improves disordered esophageal motility. *J Gastrointest Surg* 2003;7:159–163.

12. Mughal MM, Bancewicz J, Marples M. Oesophageal manometry and pH recording does not predict the bad results of Nissen fundoplication. *Br J Surg* 1990;77:43–45.

13. Hakanson BS, Thor KB, Pope CE 2nd. Preoperative oesophageal motor activity does not predict postoperative dysphagia. *Eur J Surg* 2001;167:433–437.

14. Watson DI, Jamieson GG, Mitchell PC, Devitt PG, Britten-Jones R. Stenosis of the esophageal hiatus following laparoscopic fundoplication. *Arch Surg* 1995;130:1014–1016.

15. Horgan S, Pohl D, Bogetti D, Eubanks T, Pellegrini C. Failed antireflux surgery: what have we learned from reoperations? *Arch Surg* 1999;134:809–815; discussion 815–817.

16. Soper NJ, Dunnegan D. Anatomic fundoplication failure after laparoscopic antireflux surgery. *Ann Surg* 1999;229:669–676; discussion 676–677.

17. Hunter JG, Smith CD, Branum GD, et al. Laparoscopic fundoplication failures: patterns of failure and response to fundoplication revision. *Ann Surg* 1999;230:595–604; discussion 606.

18. Wetscher GJ, Glaser K, Gadenstaetter M, Profanter C, Hinder RA. The effect of medical therapy and antireflux surgery on dysphagia in patients with gastroesophageal reflux disease without esophageal stricture. *Am J Surg* 1999;177:189–192.

19. Eubanks TR, Omelanczuk P, Richards C, Pohl D, Pellegrini CA. Outcomes of laparoscopic antireflux procedures. *Am J Surg* 2000;179:391–395.

20. Jobe BA, Wallace J, Hansen PD, Swanstrom LL. Evaluation of laparoscopic Toupet fundoplication as a primary repair for all patients with medically resistant gastroesophageal reflux. *Surg Endosc* 1997;11:1080–1083.

21. Farrell TM, Archer SB, Galloway KD, Branum GD, Smith CD, Hunter JG. Heartburn is more likely to recur after Toupet fundoplication than Nissen fundoplication. *Am Surg* 2000;66:229–236; discussion 236–237.

22. Pessaux P, Arnaud JP, Ghavami B, et al. Laparoscopic antireflux surgery: comparative study of Nissen, Nissen–Rossetti, and Toupet fundoplication. Societe Francaise de Chirurgie Laparoscopique. *Surg Endosc* 2000;14:1024–1027.

23. Bell RC, Hanna P, Mills MR, Bowrey D. Patterns of success and failure with laparoscopic Toupet fundoplication. *Surg Endosc* 1999;13:1189–1194.

24. Horvath KD, Jobe BA, Herron DM, Swanstrom LL. Laparoscopic Toupet fundoplication is an inadequate procedure for patients with severe reflux disease. *J Gastrointest Surg* 1999;3:583–591.

25. Livingston CD, Jones HL Jr, Askew RE Jr, Victor BE, Askew RE Sr. Laparoscopic hiatal hernia repair in patients with poor esophageal motility or paraesophageal herniation. *Am Surg* 2001;67:987–991.

26. Baigrie RJ, Cullis SN, Ndhluni AJ, Cariem A. Randomized double-blind trial of laparoscopic Nissen fundoplication versus anterior partial fundoplication. *Br J Surg* 2005;92:819–823.

27. Pellegrini CA. Therapy for gastroesophageal reflux disease: the new kid on the block. *J Am Coll Surg* 1995;180:485–487.

28. O'Rourke RW, Khajanchee YS, Urbach DR, et al. Extended transmediastinal dissection: an alternative to gastroplasty for short esophagus. *Arch Surg* 2003;138:735–740.

29. Horvath KD, Swanstrom LL, Jobe BA. The short esophagus: pathophysiology, incidence, presentation, and treatment in the era of laparoscopic antireflux surgery. *Ann Surg* 2000;232:630–640.

30. Jones DBDD, Soper NJ. Dysphagia after laparoscopic fundoplication is diminished by dividing short gastric vessels. *Gastroenterology* 1995;4(suppl 3):A1224.

31. Hunter JG, Swanstrom L, Waring JP. Dysphagia after laparoscopic antireflux surgery. The impact of operative technique. *Ann Surg* 1996;224:51–57.

32. Limpert PA, Naunheim KS. Partial versus complete fundoplication: is there a correct answer? *Surg Clin North Am* 2005;85:399–410.

33. Oelschlager BK, Pellegrini CA. Minimally invasive surgery for gastroesophageal reflux disease. *J Laparoendosc Adv Surg Tech A* 2001;11:341–349.

35
Botox, Balloon, or Myotomy: Optimal Treatment for Achalasia

Lee L. Swanstrom and Michelle D. Taylor

Achalasia is a primary and profound esophageal motility disorder with an unclear etiology and which is, to date, incurable. In spite of its rare occurrence in the population (1:100,000), it stimulates large amounts of research and commentary by gastrointestinal (GI) physicians and surgeons, in large part due to ongoing controversy over the optimal treatment of these patients. When analyzing treatment options it is critical to keep in mind that all treatments are palliative in nature and are primarily aimed at relief of dysphagia and regurgitation. Normal esophageal function is almost never restored, and even a patient with an excellent result will not have completely normal swallowing.

Definitions: For the purpose of this review the terms used are defined as follows:

- *Achalasia*: A primary motility disorder of the esophagus characterized by complete absence of antegrade peristalsis in the smooth muscle body; either due to total noncontractility or simultaneous contraction (vigorous achalasia) and by abnormalities in the receptive relaxation function of the lower esophageal sphincter (LES).
- *Botox*: Flexible endoscopic injection of purified *Botulinum* toxin (a potent neurotoxin) into the musculature of the LES. Typically 100 units of the toxin are injected into at least four quadrants of the sphincter.
- *Balloon dilation*: Rapid dilation of the LES, usually under fluoroscopic or endoscopic visualization, with a large-caliber (3 or 4 cm) rigid balloon to achieve disruption of the circular fibers of the LES.
- *Myotomy*: Surgical division of all muscle layers of the lower esophageal sphincter mechanism, extending from the dilated portion of the esophageal body well onto the anterior gastric wall to insure complete disruption of the contractile mechanism.

35.1. Data Review

This review will cover four main controversies:

- Balloon dilatation vs. myotomy as initial treatment.
- The role of Botox in the treatment of achalasia.
- The superiority of open or laparoscopic myotomy.
- Should minimally invasive myotomy be performed through the chest or the abdomen?

While other controversies still exist regarding achalasia treatment, for the sake of this review, several controversies will be considered resolved, including: the size and type of dilating balloon (large and rigid), the role of medical therapy (only for symptomatic spasm), the treatment of failed myotomy or dilatation (repeat myotomy or esophagectomy), the extent of the myotomy (long), and the best treatment for mega or sigmoid esophagus (myotomy or esophagectomy).

35.2. Balloon Dilation, Botox, or Myotomy as Initial Treatment

This question has definite clinical impact as it effectively determines which specialty should primarily treat the achalasia patient. The outcomes to be considered are not only efficacy of the intervention but also relative morbidities and cost effectiveness. Supporting data ranges from a few level 1 randomized, prospective trials to level 5 data based on opinion or animal models. Numbers in clinical studies are small because of the relative rarity of achalasia and pooled data (level of evidence 3) provides the best generalizable data. Where possible, studies using large diameter balloon (vs. small balloon or rigid dilators) dilatation and laparoscopic/thoracoscopic (vs. open) myotomy were used.

Botox injection is an easy-to-administer outpatient treatment with a good safety profile.

Early dysphagia relief is achieved in up to 66% of cases.[1] Level 1 evidence would indicate that even these good early results are poorer than those seen with surgical intervention. Zaninotto and colleagues have reported a prospective, randomized trial comparing Botox injection with laparoscopic myotomy in 80 patients. At 12-month follow-up, these comparable groups showed an 88% rate of dysphagia relief with surgery versus a 60% rate with Botox[2] (Figure 35.1). Objective follow-up (pH and motility) was the same at 6 months.

The neurotoxicity of *Botulinum* toxin is a transient phenomenon and there is a progressive failure rate with time. This is confirmed by the long-term results of the randomized, controlled trial (RCT) by Costantini and colleagues (level of evidence 1) showing a 65% rate of dysphagia at

2-year follow-up versus an 18% rate with laparoscopic myotomy and fundoplication.[3] Case series reports also indicate that this failure is progressive with time and that eventually almost all patients will have recurrent problems.[4,5]

Level 3 evidence also indicates that the best results postachalasia treatment result when the LES pressure falls beneath 10 mmHg.[6] Follow-up testing in cohort series also indicates that Botox does not decrease sphincter pressures significantly[2,7] and this leaves concern that the Botox-treated esophagus will have progressive dilation with time rather than the decrease in diameter seen after successful surgery.[8] Finally, other evidence (level of evidence 3–5) supports the concept that definitive treatment (myotomy) is more difficult and subjects the patient to a higher perforation rate following Botox treatment, although the end result appears to be the same.[9,10]

We conclude that surgical myotomy is superior to initial treatment with Botox for management of achalasia.

> Surgical myotomy is superior to initial treatment with Botox for management of achalasia (level of evidence 1; recommendation grade A).

Balloon dilation and surgical myotomy are both longstanding and effective treatments for achalasia. Because they are typically used by different specialties, comparative studies are rare. The literature has a single published RCT that offers a direct, prospective comparison.[11] This 1989 study had 81 patients who were well matched and randomized to dilation with a 3-cm balloon versus a Heller myotomy (with no fundoplication) done by thoracotomy. The surgery patients had 95% near complete symptom relief compared to 51% with dilation at 5-year follow-up. The morbidity was higher in the balloon group as well, primarily a 5.4% incidence of esophageal perforation. Repeat dilation was performed in 16% of the patients.

More recent comparative case series (level of evidence 3–4) also support the efficacy of myotomy over balloon dilation. Patti and coworkers present a nonrandomized, retrospective study comparing outcomes between large-caliber balloon dilation (19 patients) and a thoracoscopic

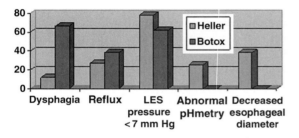

FIGURE 35.1. Outcomes of a randomized, prospective trial comparing Botox to Heller myotomy for achalasia.[2]

myotomy (30 patients). In this study, the long-term outcomes were markedly better for the thoracoscopic approach (87% relief of dysphagia vs. 26%).[12] Another retrospective study looked at the outcomes of 61 patients after balloon dilation with a crossover strategy of surgical myotomy in case of treatment failure. The study had a rather high perforation rate of 14% with another 14% of patients having no improvement in dysphagia after dilation. Both of these groups were treated with a surgical myotomy. On long-term follow-up (mean 5 years), this intervention cohort had a 61% failure rate following successful dilation and a 7% failure rate after myotomy. This particular study, although a level 2 prospective cohort study, has been criticized for its high perforation and failure rate in the dilatation arm.[13]

Finally, the relative effectiveness of Botox, balloon, or laparoscopic myotomy as initial treatment strategies for achalasia were compared using a Markov modeling strategy (level of evidence 3).[14] One of the conclusions of this analysis was that Botox had the lowest efficacy as an initial treatment in elective cases [quality-adjusted life-years (QALY) = 7.33]. Both dilation and laparoscopic myotomy were comparable and acceptable initial treatments (QALY = 7.40 for dilation and 7.41 for myotomy) as long as the perforation rate of balloon dilation was less than 3.8% and the success rate was at least 90%, while the mortality and failure rate of myotomy were less than 7% and 10%, respectively (Figure 35.2) Repeat dilations, however, were not indicated in this analysis, and patients who failed their first dilation should be offered laparoscopic surgery.

We conclude that surgical myotomy is superior to balloon dilation for the initial management of achalasia.

> Surgical myotomy is superior to balloon dilation for the initial management of achalasia (level of evidence 1 to 3; recommendation grade B).

Laparoscopic myotomy was first described in 1991[15] and since then has become progressively more popular. It now is performed more often than open procedures done either through the chest or the abdomen. While this is true for many procedures now done laparoscopically, it doesn't necessarily follow that the laparoscopic approach is superior. However, in the case of open versus laparoscopic myotomy, there is at least level 2 to 3 evidence to support the superiority of the less invasive approach. Table 35.1 summarizes the outcomes of these various studies. Overall, the studies reported similar outcomes. In all four studies described, it should be noted that the dysphagia outcomes and postoperative reflux complaints were universally similar or slightly better for the laparoscopic groups. Likewise, operative complications were the same for laparoscopic and open approaches, but blood loss and hospital stay were markedly less for the laparoscopic approach. A uniform negative for the laparoscopic cohorts was a significantly increased operative time, but this was counterbalanced by a more rapid return to normal activity in the one study that recorded this parameter.[16] It is unfortunate that there are no randomized, prospective comparisons between laparoscopic and open

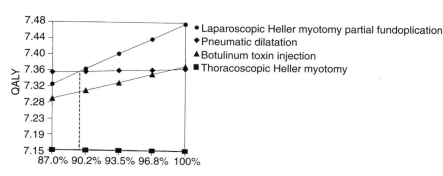

Figure 35.2. Results of Markov modeling of initial treatment strategies for achalasia. One-way sensitivity analysis shows that laparoscopic Heller myotomy with partial fundoplication is the most effective treatment as long as the success rate for dysphagia relief is greater than 89.7%.[14]

TABLE 35.1. Case comparisons between laparoscopic and open Heller myotomy.

Author	Study type	Number	Excellent/good result % (dysphagia)	Reflux %	Patient satisfaction	Operation time (min)	Blood loss (cc)	LOS days
Ancona[21]	Retrospective case-matched	17 open	100	6	–	125	–	10
		17 laparoscopic	94	0	–	178	–	4
Collard[22]	Retrospective series comparison	8 open	75	10	–	–	–	–
		12 laparoscopic	84	0	–	–	–	–
Dempsey[16]	Retrospective case-matched	10 open	90	40	80	122	220	8.8
		12 laparoscopic	92	25	84	137	50	2.7
Douard[23]	Prospective series nonrandomized	30 open	93	7	83	120	120	7.5
		52 laparoscopic	92	10	83	145	145	4

myotomy, but at this point it is unlikely that there ever will be. However, the strong, consistent and statistically significant outcomes in nonrandomized studies, as well as the factor of patient demand, define the minimally invasive approach to myotomy as the gold standard. We conclude that laparoscopic myotomy is superior to open myotomy for surgical management of achalasia.

> Laparoscopic myotomy is superior to open myotomy for surgical management of achalasia (level of evidence 2 to 3; recommendation grade B).

There is no level 1 evidence, but level 3 to 5 data strongly supports the superiority of laparoscopic over thoracoscopic esophageal myotomy for achalasia. Because open myotomy was frequently done via thoracotomy, it is not surprising that the first reports of a minimally invasive treatment replicated this approach. The thoracoscopic approach quickly lost favor, partly because of its technical difficulty, complex anesthesia requirements, and, most importantly, because of its poor results in most series. One of the first reports describing a minimally invasive approach for esophageal myotomy was the 1992 report by Pellegrini and associates, which described early results for 17 thoracoscopic myotomies and 2 laparoscopic myotomies. This report mentions the technical difficulties involved, including the difficulty in accessing the anterior gastric wall through the hiatus and the awkwardness of

performing a myotomy with the perpendicular approach provided by thoracoscopic access.[17] While this report described an 82% rate of good-to-excellent dysphagia relief (level of evidence 3), follow-up was quite short and a subsequent report in 1995 indicated a 60% incidence of significant acid reflux on pH study in 60% of the thoracoscopic patients even though only one of six of these patients was symptomatic.[18] In 1998 the same authors performed a case-matched analysis of the two groups and found that the laparoscopic approach was superior to the thoracoscopic in most parameters [length of stay (LOS) and postoperative reflux rates in particular][19] (Table 35.2). One retrospective study, which had 88 laparoscopic repairs with fundoplications compared to 14 thoracoscopic with no fundoplication, found no significant difference between the two approaches although there was a trend towards lower complications and faster recovery with the laparoscopic approach.[20] On the other hand, a similar retrospective (level of evidence 3) study comparing 16 thoracoscopic to 17 laparoscopic

TABLE 35.2. Results of a case-matched comparison of laparoscopic and thoracoscopic Heller myotomy.

30 THM vs. 30 LHM (+Dor)[a]			
–	LOS	THM = 6 days	LHM = 3.5 days
–	Dysphagia	THM = 13%	LHM = 10%
–	Reflux (pH)	THM = 60%	LHM = 10%

Abbreviations: LHM, laparoscopic Heller myotomy; THM, thorascopic Heller myotomy.
[a]Case matched.
Source: Patti et al.[19]

myotomies with partial fundoplications showed uniform superiority of the laparoscopic approach (Table 35.3).[24] We conclude that laparoscopic myotomy is superior to thoracoscopic or transthoracic approaches for surgical management of achalasia.

> Laparoscopic myotomy is superior to thoracoscopic or transthoracic approaches for surgical management of achalasia (evidence level 3 to 5; recommendation grade C).

35.3. Clinical Implications

Because of the relative rarity of the disease and the fact that achalasia patients are seen by both gastroenterologists and surgeons, many questions regarding the treatment of achalasia remain only partially answered. On the other hand, the clinical realities of achalasia practice are obvious: laparoscopic myotomy is the current gold standard for treatment. Transthoracic approaches, in spite of their primacy in the past, simply do not work as well as laparoscopic myotomy. This is particularly true of thoracoscopic approaches, which have been calculated to be the least cost-effective treatment available.[14] In most institutions, balloon dilation, though not a bad treatment, has been largely abandoned. This is due partly to the excellent efficacy of laparoscopic myotomy (89%–98% good-to-excellent results) but perhaps even more to the risk aversion of gastroenterologists who are reluctant to deal with the 2% to 6% perforation rate of most series. Botox, on the other hand, remains sporadically popular and still fairly widely practiced. This is in spite of its poor long-term success, low cost effectiveness, and risk of creating problems for

definite treatment in the form of a surgical myotomy. Its use is probably driven mostly by its ease of application, good safety profile, and immediate gratification factor.[1]

35.4. Current Practice

Clinical practice will often ignore the facts as presented in the medical literature, either from ignorance, because it goes against the practitioner's training, institutional bias, or for financial reasons. In the case of achalasia, it would seem that the majority of institutions treat patients more or less in line with the weight of the scientific evidence. Our current practice is to establish the diagnosis of achalasia with a barium swallow and esophageal manometry in all cases. The patient must have an upper endoscopy to exclude pseudoachalasia as a cause for symptoms or other findings. In cases where the patient presents with nutritional compromise and near or complete esophageal outlet obstruction, treatment with Botox injection and small-caliber balloon dilation is done to temporize until more definitive treatment can be arranged. Repeat Botox injections are never offered unless the patient is too morbid for any other care.

Patients are not typically risk stratified for treatment otherwise, as the morbidity and mortality of either balloon dilation or laparoscopic myotomy are equal. Patients are counseled about their disease and the need for lifelong follow-up after any treatment. They are given the choice of either balloon dilation or a laparoscopic myotomy with the benefits and drawbacks of each being carefully defined. Balloon treatment is described as convenient, safe (<0.1% morbidity, 5% perforation rate, and a 2% emergency intervention

TABLE 35.3. Retrospective comparison of the results of laparoscopic myotomy and partial fundoplication compared to thoracoscopic myotomy without a wrap.[24]

	Operative time (min)	LOS (days)	Late dysphagia (%)	Reflux (%)	Final LES pressure (mm Hg)	Reduction LES diameter at 2-year follow-up (%)
Thoracoscopic myotomy	222	2	37.5	25	15.3	27
Laparoscopic Myotomy + Dor	148	5	5	10	10.4	50
	$p = 0.0001$	$p = 0.0001$	$p = 0.01$	$p = 0.0001$	$p = 0.0001$	$p = 0.0001$

incidence), and relatively effective (around a 65% initial relief or dramatic improvement in dysphagia). It is mentioned that around 20% of patients will subsequently require medication for acid reflux and that there is a progressive failure rate over the first 5 years, with only 30% to 40% of patients free from dysphagia at 5 years. Laparoscopic myotomy is described as highly effective (88%–92% relief of dysphagia over 3 years), but we stress that it requires a true operation including a general anesthetic and a 24- to 48-hours hospital stay. With the addition of a partial fundoplication, acid reflux rates are described as being between 10% and 15%. Mortality rates are also quoted as 0.1% and acute reinterventions as being necessary 2% of the time. In our experience, even though the dilations and myotomies are done by the same team, 90% of patients decide on the surgical myotomy – most often saying that the higher initial success rate is their primary consideration and the fear of perforation the next concern.

All myotomies are done laparoscopically unless the patient has a hostile abdomen and all are accompanied by a partial wrap if at all possible. We will attempt a laparoscopic myotomy on a massively dilated or sigmoid esophagus but do cite a higher failure rate in such a case. Failure of a myotomy is treated with a balloon dilation and, if that fails, by a second laparoscopic myotomy without a fundoplication. Second failures, or failures with mega-esophagus, are encouraged to consider a minimally invasive esophagectomy.

After therapy, patients are sent home on a pureed diet for 2 weeks. All patients are requested to undergo repeat manometry and a 24-hour pH test. Decision to place the patient on acid-suppressive medication is only based on the result of the postoperative testing as we have found symptoms after surgery to have almost no correlation with objective findings. Upper endoscopy is performed every 5 years for the slightly increased risk of malignancy due to the stasis.

34.5. Conclusion

The relative rarity of achalasia and its poorly understood etiology means that there is a relative lack of high-quality literature to base treatment recommendations on. This is further complicated by the fact that there are three fairly good therapies for this incurable disease and that it is rare for a single practitioner to offer all three. In actuality, there is undoubtedly a place for all three in a comprehensive treatment algorithm, and it is hoped that initial treatment will be based on medical evidence and not expedience or personal bias.

References

1. Storr M, Born P, Frimberger E, et al. Treatment of achalasia: the short-term response to botulinum toxin injection seems to be independent of any kind of pretreatment. *Gastroenterology* 2002;2:19–27.
2. Zaninotto G, Annese V, Costantini M, et al. Randomized controlled trial of botulinum toxin versus laparoscopic heller myotomy for esophageal achalasia. *Ann Surg* 2004;239:364–370.
3. Costantini M, Zaninotto G, Guirroli E, et al. The laparoscopic Heller–Dor operation remains an effective treatment for esophageal achalasia at a minimum 6-year follow-up. *Surg Endosc* 2005;19: 345–351.
4. Zaninotto G, Vergadoro V, Annese V, et al. Botulinum toxin injection versus laparoscopic myotomy for the treatment of esophageal achalasia: economic analysis of a randomized trial 43. *Surg Endosc* 2004;18:691–695.
5. Kolbasnik J, Waterfall WE, Fachnie B. Long-term efficacy of Botulinum toxin in classical achalasia. *Am J Gastroenterol* 1999;94:3434–3438.
6. Diener U, Patti MG, Molena D, et al. Laparoscopic Heller myotomy relieves dysphagia in patients with achalasia and low LES pressure following pneumatic dilatation. *Surg Endosc* 2001;15:687–690.
7. Andrews CN, Anvari M, Dobranowski J. Laparoscopic Heller's myotomy or botulinum toxin injection for management of esophageal achalasia. Patient choice and treatment outcomes. *Surg Endosc* 1999;13:742–746.
8. Anselmino M, Zaninotto G, Costantini M, et al. One-year follow-up after laparoscopic Heller–Dor operation for esophageal achalasia. *Surg Endosc* 1997;11:3–7.
9. Patti MG, Feo CV, Arcerito M, et al. Effects of previous treatment on results of laparoscopic Heller myotomy for achalasia. *Dig Dis Sci* 1999;44:2270–2276.
10. Richardson WS, Willis GW, Smith JW. Evaluation of scar formation after botulinum toxin injection

or forced balloon dilation to the lower esophageal sphincter. *Surg Endosc* 2003;17:696–698.

11. Csendes A, Braghetto I, Henriquez A, Cortes C. Late results of a prospective randomised study comparing forceful dilatation and oesophagomyotomy in patients with achalasia. *Gut* 1989;30:299–304.

12. Patti MG, Pellegrini CA, Arcerito M, Tong J, Mulvihill SJ, Way LW. Comparison of medical and minimally invasive surgical therapy for primary esophageal motility disorders. *Arch Surg* 1995;130:609–615.

13. Anselmino M, Perdikis G, Hinder RA, et al. Heller myotomy is superior to dilatation for the treatment of early achalasia. *Arch Surg* 1997;132:233–240.

14. Urbach DR, Hansen PD, Khajanchee YS, Swanstrom LL. A decision analysis of the optimal initial approach to achalasia: laparoscopic Heller myotomy with partial fundoplication, thoracoscopic Heller myotomy, pneumatic dilatation, or botulinum toxin injection. *J Gastrointest Surg* 2001;5:192–205.

15. Shimi S, Nathanson LK, Cuschieri A. Laparoscopic cardiomyotomy for achalasia. *J R Coll Surg Edinb* 1991;36:152–154.

16. Dempsey DT, Kalan MM, Gerson RS, Parkman HP, Maier WP. Comparison of outcomes following open and laparoscopic esophagomyotomy for achalasia. *Surg Endosc* 1999;13:747–750.

17. Pellegrini C, Wetter LA, Patti M, et al. Thoracoscopic esophagomyotomy. Initial experience with a new approach for the treatment of achalasia. *Ann Surg* 1992;216:291–296.

18. Patti MG, Arcerito M, Pellegrini CA. Thoracoscopic and laparoscopic Heller's myotomy in the treatment of esophageal achalasia. *Ann Chir Gynaecol* 1995;84:159–164.

19. Patti MG, Arcerito M, De PM, et al. Comparison of thoracoscopic and laparoscopic Heller myotomy for achalasia. *J Gastrointest Surg* 1998;2:561–566.

20. Raftopoulos Y, Landreneau RJ, Hayetian F, et al. Factors affecting quality of life after minimally invasive Heller myotomy for achalasia. *J Gastrointest Surg* 2004;8:233–239.

21. Ancona E, Anselmino M, Zaninotto G, et al. Esophageal achalasia: laparoscopic versus conventional open Heller–Dor operation. *Am J Surg* 1995;170:265–270.

22. Collard JM, Romagnoli R, Lengele B, Salizzoni M, Kestens PJ. Heller–Dor procedure for achalasia: from conventional to video-endoscopic surgery. *Acta Chir Belg* 1996;96:62–65.

23. Douard R, Gaudric M, Chaussade S, Couturier D, Houssin D, Dousset B. Functional results after laparoscopic Heller myotomy for achalasia: A comparative study to open surgery. *Surgery* 2004;136:16–24.

24. Ramacciato G, Mercantini P, Amodio PM, et al. The laparoscopic approach with antireflux surgery is superior to the thoracoscopic approach for the treatment of esophageal achalasia. Experience of a single surgical unit. *Surg Endosc* 2002;16:1431–1437.

36
Fundoplication after Laparoscopic Myotomy for Achalasia

Fernando A. Herbella and Marco G. Patti

Esophageal achalasia is a primary esophageal motility disorder of unknown origin characterized by lack of esophageal peristalsis and inability of the lower esophageal sphincter (LES) to relax properly in response to swallowing. The goal of treatment is to relieve the functional obstruction caused by the LES, therefore allowing emptying of food into the stomach by gravity. However, the elimination of the LES may be followed by reflux of gastric contents into the aperistaltic esophagus, with slow clearance of the refluxate and the risk of developing esophagitis, strictures, Barrett's esophagus, and even adenocarcinoma.[1-4]

The following chapter reviews the results of surgery for achalasia, describing what is considered today the best procedure to achieve the goal of relieving dysphagia while avoiding development of reflux.

36.1. Treatment of Esophageal Achalasia: The Open Era

During the 1970s and 1980s, pneumatic balloon dilatation was considered the primary form of treatment for achalasia. During that period, only an average 1.5 Heller myotomies were performed each year in our tertiary care hospital as well as in other centers, mostly for patients whose dysphagia did not improve with balloon dilatation or whose esophagus was perforated during a balloon dilation.[5] We followed Ellis' technique and used a left trans-thoracic approach to perform a Heller myotomy which extended for

only 5mm onto the gastric wall.[2] The rationale for this approach (followed by most surgeons in North America) was to make the myotomy long enough to relieve dysphagia but short enough to avoid reflux and therefore the need for a fundoplication. The results published by Ellis seemed to confirm the soundness of this approach: in a review of his 22-year experience with 197 patients he documented symptomatic reflux in only 9 (5%) of them.[2] The problem with his analysis, however, was that it was based on symptom evaluation only (presence of heartburn) rather than objective evaluation of the reflux status by pH monitoring. Many studies have, in fact, shown that most patients who develop reflux after a Heller myotomy do not experience heartburn, so that the symptomatic evaluation usually underestimates the real incidence of reflux.[6,7] As a matter of fact, when the same author used manometry and pH monitoring to objectively assess gastroesophageal reflux after short myotomy, he found abnormal esophageal acid exposure in 29% of patients.[8]

Contrary to the trans-thoracic approach used in North America, surgeons in Europe[9] and South America[10] traditionally used a transabdominal approach, performing a longer myotomy onto the gastric wall in combination with an anti-reflux procedure. For instance, in 1992 Bonavina and colleagues reported the long-term results of myotomy and Dor fundoplication in 206 patients with achalasia operated between 1976 and 1989. Excellent or good results were obtained in 94% of patients while the rate of postoperative reflux measured by pH monitoring was 8.6% only.[9]

36.2. Treatment of Esophageal Achalasia: The Minimally Invasive Surgery Era

Shimi and Cuschieri first reported in 1991 the performance of a Heller myotomy for esophageal achalasia by minimally invasive techniques.[11] In 1992 we described our initial experience with a thoracoscopic Heller myotomy.[12] We initially used the technique developed by Cuschieri,[11] which we modified as we gained experience, and performed a left thoracoscopic myotomy (with the guidance of intraoperative endoscopy) which extended for only 5mm onto the gastric wall. The long-term follow-up in the first 30 patients who underwent a left thoracoscopic Heller myotomy confirmed the excellent outcome of the initial report: almost 90% of patients had relief of dysphagia, the hospital stay was short, the postoperative discomfort was minimal, and the recovery was fast. However, some shortcomings of the thoracoscopic technique soon became apparent, particularly when compared to the laparoscopic approach[13]:

- Poor exposure of the gastroesophageal junction, particularly important when trying to extend the myotomy onto the gastric wall for 5mm only. Excellent exposure by the laparoscopic approach.
- Cumbersome intraoperative management (double lumen endotracheal tube, right lateral decubitus position, intraoperative endoscopy). Very simple for the laparoscopic approach.
- Postoperative discomfort due to the chest tube.
- High incidence of postoperative reflux and inability to correct preexisting reflux from pneumatic dilatation. We found that a thoracoscopic myotomy was associated to reflux in 60% of patients studied postoperatively by pH monitoring. We also encountered patients who already had abnormal reflux secondary to dilatation even though they still experienced dysphagia. Some of these patients had very low LES pressure.[14]

These were probably the key reasons that made us switch to a laparoscopic myotomy and Dor fundoplication as suggested by Ancona and colleagues,[15] in the attempt to find a balance between relieving dysphagia and avoiding postoperative reflux. Similar findings about postoperative reflux after transthoracic myotomy and the decision to switch to a laparoscopic myotomy and fundoplication were reported by others.[16,17]

36.3. Laparoscopic Heller Myotomy: Is a Fundoplication Necessary?

It is generally accepted that a fundoplication is necessary to prevent reflux after a laparoscopic Heller myotomy, by either performing a Dor fundoplication,[18-24] a Toupet fundoplication,[25-28] or a Nissen fundoplication.[29-31]

This approach is based on some retrospective studies and two prospective, randomized trials comparing laparoscopic myotomy alone versus myotomy and fundoplication. Kjellin and colleagues found abnormal reflux by pH monitoring in 8 of 14 (57%) patients after laparoscopic myotomy without fundoplication.[32] Five of the 8 patients (62%) were asymptomatic. Similarly, Burpee and colleagues documented reflux (by pH monitoring or endoscopy) in 18 of 30 patients (60%) after laparoscopic Heller myotomy without fundoplication.[33] Thirty-nine percent of patients with reflux were asymptomatic. Gupta and colleagues reported heartburn after laparoscopic myotomy in 80% of their patients. They felt that it was not a problem as symptoms were well controlled with medications.[34]

The observation of a very high incidence of reflux after laparoscopic myotomy alone has also been confirmed by two prospective and randomized trials. In 2003, Kalkenback and colleagues reported the results of a prospective, randomized trial comparing myotomy alone versus myotomy and Nissen fundoplication.[29] Postoperative reflux was present in 25% of patients who had a myotomy and fundoplication but in 100% of patients who had a myotomy alone. Twenty percent of the patients in the latter group developed Barrett's esophagus. In 2004, Richards and colleagues reported the results of a prospective, randomized trial comparing laparoscopic myotomy alone versus laparoscopic myotomy and Dor fundoplication.[24] Postoperative ambulatory pH monitoring showed reflux in 48% of patients after myotomy alone but in only 9% of patients when a Dor fundoplication was added to the myotomy. The incidence and the score of postoperative dysphagia were similar in the two groups.

These data can be summarized as follows:

- Myotomy alone is followed by a high incidence of postoperative reflux, which is asymptomatic in most cases.
- A fundoplication prevents reflux in the majority of patients.
- It is dangerous to claim that postoperative reflux does not matter and that nothing should be done to prevent it. Today we are operating on many young patients[35] who may develop severe esophageal damage if exposed to years of reflux.[1-4]

Based on these data we feel that a fundoplication should be performed after a laparoscopic Heller myotomy (level of evidence 1+ to 3; recommendation grade B).

A fundoplication should be performed after a laparoscopic Heller myotomy (level of evidence 1+ to 3; recommendation grade B).

36.4. Which Fundoplication? Partial Versus Total Fundoplication

It has been shown that a laparoscopic total (360º) fundoplication is the procedure of choice in patients with gastroesophageal reflux disease. When compared to a partial fundoplication, a total fundoplication determines a better control of reflux without a higher incidence of postoperative dysphagia, even when esophageal peristalsis is weak.[36] In esophageal achalasia, however, the pump action of the esophageal body is completely missed, as there is no peristalsis. Therefore, a total fundoplication might determine too much of a resistance at the level of the gastroesophageal junction, impeding the emptying of food from the esophagus into the stomach by gravity, and eventually causing persistent or recurrent dysphagia. Albeit some groups still claim good results adding a total fundoplication after a myotomy,[29-31] others have abandoned this approach and switched to a partial fundoplica-

tion. This decision was based on the results of long-term studies which showed that esophageal decompensation and recurrence of symptoms eventually occurs in most patients.[37-41] For instance, Duranceau and colleagues initially reported excellent results with a Heller myotomy and total fundoplication.[39] Ten years later, however, they noted that symptoms had recurred in 14 of 17 patients (82%), five of whom required a second operation.[40] They felt that over time the total fundoplication determines a progressive increase in esophageal retention with poor emptying and recurrence of symptoms. They were able to correct this problem by switching to a partial fundoplication.[41]

Today a laparoscopic Heller myotomy with partial fundoplication is considered the procedure of choice for esophageal achalasia, as it attains the best balance between relief of dysphagia and prevention of reflux.[42]

Based on these data we feel that a partial rather than a total fundoplication should be performed after a laparoscopic Heller myotomy (level of evidence 2++ to 4; recommendation grade C).

A partial fundoplication is superior to a total fundoplication after a laparoscopic Heller myotomy (level of evidence 2++ to 4; recommendation grade C).

36.5. Partial Fundoplication: Anterior Versus Posterior

There are no published prospective, randomized trials comparing a partial posterior (Toupet) versus an anterior (Dor) fundoplication in association to a Heller myotomy in patients with achalasia. Some groups feel that a posterior fundoplication is better as it keeps the edges of the myotomy separated and it is a more effective anti-reflux operation.[25-28] Others, however, feel that a Dor fundoplication is simpler to perform as it does not need posterior dissection, and it adds the advantage of covering the exposed mucosa.[18-24]

Our philosophy at the University of California, San Francisco during the last 12 years has been to perform a laparoscopic Heller myotomy and

Dor fundoplication.[43] The myotomy is about 9 cm in length and extends for about 2 cm onto the gastric wall. Intraoperative endoscopy is helpful at the beginning of a surgeon's experience to gauge the extent of the myotomy onto the gastric wall in respect to the squamous–columnar junction, as seen by endoscopy. However, once the surgeon has gained experience with the anatomy from a laparoscopic perspective, it can be omitted. After the short gastric vessels are divided, an anterior 180° fundoplication (Dor) is performed. There are two rows of sutures, one right and one left. The left row has three stitches: the first stitch incorporates the stomach, the esophagus, and the left pillar of the crus. The second and the third stitch incorporate only the stomach and the esophageal wall. Subsequently, the fundus is folded over the exposed mucosa, so that the greater curvature of the stomach is next to right pillar of the crus. Similar to the left the row, the right row has three stitches and only the uppermost stitch incorporates the fundus, the esophagus, and the right pillar of the crus. Finally, two additional stitches (apical stitches) are placed between the anterior rim of the esophageal hiatus and the superior aspect of the fundoplication. After laparoscopic Heller myotomy and Dor fundoplication, excellent or good results for dysphagia were obtained in 91% of patients, with a 15% incidence of postoperative reflux.[43]

Based on the available data, it is not possible to give a recommendation regarding the type of partial fundoplication (anterior vs. posterior) to be added after a laparoscopic Heller myotomy for achalasia.

> There is insufficient data to give a recommendation regarding the type of partial fundoplication (anterior vs. posterior) to be added after a laparoscopic Heller myotomy for achalasia.

36.6. Conclusions

The last decade has witnessed radical changes in the treatment of esophageal achalasia due to the adoption of minimally invasive techniques. The high success rate of laparoscopic Heller myotomy has brought a radical shift in practice, as surgery has become the preferred treatment modality of most gastroenterologists and other referring physicians. During the last 5 years, we have noted a 15-fold increase in the number of patients referred for surgery every year. In addition, the gradual increase in the number of referred patients has been paralleled by an increase in the number of patients referred without previous treatment.[44] This remarkable change has followed documentation that laparoscopic myotomy outperforms balloon dilatation and botulinum toxin injection.[45,46]

References

1. Ellis FH Jr, Crozier RE, Gibb SP. Reoperative achalasia surgery. J Thorac Cardiovasc Surg 1986;92:859–865.
2. Ellis FH Jr. Oesophagomyotomy for achalasia: a 22-year experience. Br J Surg 1993;80:882–885.
3. Malthaner RA, Todd TR, Miller L, Pearson FG. Long-term results in surgically managed esophageal achalasia. Ann Thorac Surg 1994;58:1343–1347.
4. Devaney EJ, Iannettoni MD, Orringer MB, Marshall B. Esophagectomy for achalasia: patient selection and clinical experience. Ann Thorac Surg 2001;72:854–858.
5. Sauer L, Pellegrini CA, Way LW. The treatment of achalasia. A current perspective. Arch Surg 1989;124:929–932.
6. Shoenut JP, Duerksen D, Yaffe CS. A prospective assessment of gastroesophageal reflux before and after treatment of achalasia patients. Pneumatic dilation versus transthoracic limited myotomy. Am J Gastroenterol 1997;92:1109–1112.
7. Patti MG, Arcerito M, Tong J, et al. Importance of preoperative and postoperative pH monitoring in patients with esophageal achalasia. J Gastrointest Surg 1997;1:505–510.
8. Streitz JM, Ellis FH Jr, Williamson WA, et al. Objective assessment of gastroesophageal reflux after short esophagomyotomy for achalasia with the use of manometry and pH monitoring. J Thorac Cardiovasc Surg 1996;111:107–113.
9. Bonavina L, Nosadini A, Bardini R, et al. Primary treatment of esophageal achalasia. Long-term results of myotomy and Dor fundoplication. Arch Surg 1992;127:222–226.
10. Pinotti HW, Habr-Gama A, Cecconello I, et al. The surgical treatment of mega esophagus and mega colon. Dig Dis 1993;11:206–215.

11. Shimi S, Nathason LK, Cuschieri A. Laparoscopic cardiomyotomy for achalasia. *J R Coll Surg Edinb* 1991;36:152–154.

12. Pellegrini CA, Wetter LA, Patti MG, et al. Thoracoscopic esophagomyotomy. Initial experience with a new approach for the treatment of achalasia. *Ann Surg* 1992;216:291–296.

13. Patti MG, Arcerito M, De Pinto M, et al. Comparison of thoracoscopic and laparoscopic Heller myotomy for achalasia. *J Gastrointest Surg* 1998; 2:561–566.

14. Diener U, Patti MG, Molena D, et al. Laparoscopic Heller myotomy relieves dysphagia in patients with achalasia and low LES pressure following pneumatic dilatation. *Surg Endosc* 2001;15:687–690.

15. Ancona E, Anselmino M, Zaninotto G, et al. Esophageal achalasia: laparoscopic versus conventional Heller-Dor operation. *Am J Surg* 1995; 170:265–270.

16. Lindenmann J, Maier A, Eherer A, et al. The incidence of gastroesophageal reflux after transthoracic esophagocardio-myotomy without fundoplication: a long term follow-up. *Eur J Cardiothorac Surg* 2005;27:357–360.

17. Stewart KC, Finley RJ, Clifton JC, et al. Thoracoscopic versus laparoscopic modified Heller myotomy for achalasia: efficacy and safety in 87 patients. *J Am Coll Surg* 1999;189:164–170.

18. Zaninotto G, Costantini M, Molena D, et al. Treatment of esophageal achalasia with laparoscopic Heller myotomy and Dor partial fundoplication: prospective evaluation of 100 consecutive patients. *J Gastrointest Surg* 2000;4:282–289.

19. Yamamura MS, Gilster JC, Myers BS, et al. Laparoscopic Heller myotomy and anterior fundoplication for achalasia results in a high degree of patient satisfaction. *Arch Surg* 2000;135:902–906.

20. Patti MG, Molena D, Fisichella PM, et al. Laparoscopic Heller myotomy and Dor fundoplication for achalasia: analysis of successes and failures. *Arch Surg* 2001;136:870–877.

21. Finley RJ, Clifton JC, Stewart KC, et al. Laparoscopic Heller myotomy improves esophageal emptying and the symptoms of achalasia. *Arch Surg* 2001;136:892–896.

22. Ackroyd R, Watson DI, Devitt PG, Jamieson GG. Laparoscopic cardiomyotomy and anterior partial fundoplication for achalasia. *Surg Endosc* 2001;15: 683–686.

23. Chapman JR, Joehl RJ, Murayama KM, et al. Achalasia treatment: improved outcome of laparoscopic myotomy with operative manometry. *Arch Surg* 2004;139:508–513.

24. Richards WO, Torquati A, Holzman MD, et al. Heller myotomy versus Heller myotomy with Dor fundoplication for achalasia: a prospective randomized double-blind clinical trial. *Ann Surg* 2004;240:405–412.

25. Swanstrom LL, Pennings J. Laparoscopic esophagomyotomy for achalasia. *Surg Endosc* 1995;9: 286–292.

26. Hunter JG, Trus TL, Branum GD, Waring JP. Laparoscopic Heller myotomy and fundoplication for achalasia. *Ann Surg* 1997;225:655–664.

27. Vogt D, Curet M, Pitcher D, et al. Successful treatment of esophageal achalasia with laparoscopic Heller myotomy and Toupet fundoplication. *Am J Surg* 1997;174:709–714.

28. Oelschlager BK, Chang L, Pellegrini CA. Improved outcome after extended gastric myotomy for achalasia. *Arch Surg* 2003;138:490–495.

29. Falkenback D, Johansson J, Oberg S, et al. Heller's esophagomyotomy with or without a 360 degrees floppy Nissen fundoplication for achalasia. Long-term results from a prospective randomized study. *Dis Esophagus* 2003;16:284–290.

30. Frantzides CT, Moore RE, Carlson MA, et al. Minimally invasive surgery for achalasia: a 10-year experience. *J Gastrointest Surg* 2004;8:18–23.

31. Rossetti G, Brusciano L, Amato G, et al. A total fundoplication is not an obstacle to esophageal emptying after Heller myotomy for achalasia: results of a long-term follow up. *Ann Surg* 2005;241:614–621.

32. Kjellin AP, Granqvist S, Ramel S, Thor KBA. Laparoscopic myotomy without fundoplication in patients with achalasia. *Eur J Surg* 1999;165:1162–1166.

33. Burpee SE, Mamazza J, Schlachta CM, et al. Objective analysis of gastroesophageal reflux after laparoscopic Heller myotomy: an anti-reflux procedure is required. *Surg Endosc* 2005;19:9–14.

34. Gupta R, Sample C, Bamehriz F, et al. Long-term outcomes of laparoscopic Heller cardiomyotomy without an anti-reflux procedure. *Surg Laparosc Endosc Percutan Tech* 2005;15:129–132.

35. Patti MG, Albanese CT, Holcomb GW, et al. Laparoscopic Heller myotomy and Dor fundoplication for esophageal achalasia in children. *J Pediatr Surg* 2001;36:1248–1251.

36. Patti MG, Robinson T, Galvani C, et al. Total fundoplication is superior to partial fundoplication even when esophageal peristalsis is weak. *J Am Coll Surg* 2004;198:863–869.

37. Donahue PE, Schlesinger PK, Sluss KF, et al. Esophagocardiomyotomy-floppy Nissen fundoplication effectively treats achalasia without causing

esophageal obstruction. *Surgery* 1994;116:719–724.

38. Donahue PE, Horgan S, Liu KJ, Madura JA. Floppy Dor fundoplication after esophagocardiomyotomy for achalasia. *Surgery* 2002;132:716–722.
39. Duranceau A, LaFontaine ER, Vallieres B. Effects of total fundoplication on function of the esophagus after myotomy for achalasia. *Am J Surg* 1982;143:22–28.
40. Topart P, Deschamps C, Taillefer R, Duranceau A. Long-term effect of total fundoplication on the myotomized esophagus. *Ann Thorac Surg* 1992;54:1046–1051.
41. Chen LQ, Chugtai T, Sideris L, et al. Long-term effets of myotomy and partial fundoplication for esophageal achalasia. *Dis Esophagus* 2002;15:171–179.

42. Wills VL, Hunt DR. Functional outcome after Heller myotomy and fundoplication for achalasia. *J Gastrointest Surg* 2001;5:408–413.
43. Patti MG, Gorodner MV, Galvani C, et al. Spectrum of esophageal motility disorders. Implications for diagnosis and treatment. *Arch Surg* 2005;140:442–449.
44. Patti MG, Fisichella PM, Perretta S, et al. Impact of minimally invasive surgery on the treatment of esophageal achalasia. A decade of change. *J Am Coll Surg* 2003;196:698–703.
45. Eckardt VF, Gockel I, Bernhard G. Pneumatic dilation for achalasia: late results of a prospective follow up investigation. *Gut* 2004;53:629–633.
46. Zaninotto G, Annese V, Costantini M, et al. Randomized controlled trial of botulinum toxin versus laparoscopic Heller myotomy for esophageal achalasia. *Ann Surg* 2004;239:364–370.

37
Primary Repair for Delayed Recognition of Esophageal Perforation

Cameron D. Wright

Delayed recognition of esophageal perforation occurs due to the rarity of this problem and the protean manifestations of its presentation. The great majority of reports indicate delayed diagnosis of a perforated esophagus leads to more morbidity and mortality and greater length of stay when compared to those diagnosed less than 24 hours after perforation. Earlier reports and recommendations suggested that late recognition of an esophageal perforation mandated treatment other than primary repair.[1] Grillo was one of the first to promote the concept of primary repair even in patients who were diagnosed late with an esophageal perforation.[2] Most recent reports confirm the safety and efficacy of primary repair regardless of time of perforation.[1] No randomized clinical trials have been performed of treatment options in esophageal perforations.

37.1. Published Data

37.1.1. Standard Repair

There is a relative paucity of reports of primary repair of esophageal perforations older than 12 to 24 hours from which to glean information. In Table 37.1 there are only 108 patients reported from nine papers over a 12-year period. All reports are uncontrolled case series with an evidence level of 4. There is a consensus among experts that there are three factors which most influence the success of treatment of an esophageal perforation: (1) etiology of perforation with emetogenic (spontaneous, or Boerhaave's syn-

drome) worse than the more common instrumental perforation; (2) location of perforation with thoracic worse than cervical; and (3) time to diagnosis and treatment, with a delay of more than 24 hours being worse. This report is focused on thoracic perforations that are diagnosed late so two of these variables are eliminated from concern. A recent review reported a combined mortality of only 19% from instrumental perforations, whereas the mortality was 36% from emetogenic perforations. It is important to identify the number of emetic perforations in an individual series when looking at the results as the particular case mix of a series could skew the results regardless of the treatment. The same review confirmed the greater mortality of thoracic perforations compared with cervical (27% vs. 6%) and the greater mortality of delayed treatment beyond 24 hours (27% vs. 14%). Most surgeons have strong biases as to how perforations should be treated, so comparison of series and patients with others is fraught with confounding bias.

Salo and colleagues reported on 34 patients with a delayed diagnosis, of which 19 had primary repair and 15 had esophagectomy (Tables 37.1, 37.2).[3] Six of 19 patients had the primary repair covered by a pleural flap. Only six patients survived primary repair (68% mortality). There were eight leaks from the primary repair (42%). The most common cause of death was sepsis with multisystem organ failure (MOF). The authors concluded that because their mortality for esophagectomy was only 13% that primary repair should not be done for delayed diagnosis of thoracic perforations.

TABLE 37.1. Recent reports of delayed primary repair of thoracic esophageal perforations.

Author	Year	Patients	Evidence level	Emetic %	Morbidity	Mortality	Leak %	LOS
Salo[3]	1993	19	4	68%	67%	68%	42%	ns
Ohri[4]	1993	5	4	20%	40%	20%	30%	38
Wright[5]	1995	13	4	50%	85%	31%	54%	47
Whyte[6]	1995	9	4	22%	ns	5%	25%	21
Wang[7]	1996	7	4	50%	86%	14%	83%	45
Lawrence[8]	1999	12	4	100%	ns	8%	25%	14
Port[9]	2003	6	4	8%	38%	8%	17%	ns
Jougon[10]	2004	16	4	100%	ns	13%	8%	63
Richardson[11]	2005	21	4	38%	ns	3%	16%	ns

Abbreviations: LOS, length of stay; ns, not stated.

Ohri and colleagues reported on five patients with a delayed diagnosis that had primary repair (Table 37.1).[4] The mortality was 20% and leaks developed in 30%. Two leaks healed without further intervention and one required drainage of a mediastinal abscess. The authors concluded that primary repair is the procedure of choice for a thoracic esophageal perforation whether diagnosed early or late.

Wright and colleagues reported 13 patients with late thoracic esophageal perforations (Table 37.1).[5] Fifty percent were emetogenic perforations. Leaks developed in 54% of patientsand preoperative sepsis was found to be a risk factor for leak. The mortality was 31% with two patients dying of MOF and two of unrelated causes. The repair was buttressed in all patients. All leaks were without symptoms; four healed without further intervention and two became controlled fistulas. The authors concluded that primary repair remained the procedure of choice irregardless of the time of diagnosis. Use of a tissue buttress was stressed to contain any possible postoperative leak.

Whyte and colleagues reported nine patients with late esophageal perforations (Table 37.1).[6] Most were iatrogenic. The perforation was closed by a linear stapler over a bougie followed by sutured muscle closure. About one third of repairs were buttressed. Leaks occurred in 20% and all healed with drainage (two chest tubes and two rib resections for drainage). The mortality was only one patient who died of an arrhythmia with an intact repair. The authors concluded that primary repair should be undertaken in the absence of cancer or a nonsalvagable esophagus (tight stricture, end-stage achalasia) regardless of when the injury occurred.

Wang and colleagues reported on seven patients that had a late diagnosis of a thoracic esophageal perforation (Table 37.1).[7] Half the leaks were emetogenic. The leak rate was quite high at 83%, but the death rate was low at 14%. Two leaks healed without further intervention, three patients required further drainage, and one patient was diverted. Six patients had their repairs buttressed. The authors concluded that primary repair should be performed in all repairable patients, even if diagnosed late.

TABLE 37.2. Recent reports of esophagectomy in the treatment of thoracic esophageal perforation with a delayed diagnosis.

Author	Year	Patients	Evidence level	Emetic %	Morbidity	Leak %	LOS
Attar[12]	1990	9	4	17%	22%	ns	ns
Orringer[13]	1990	22	4	9%	13%	5%	22
Port[9]	2003	2	4	100%	0	0	ns
Gupta[14]	2004	33	4	6%	6%	26%	14
Richardson[11]	2005	14	4	ns	0	0	ns

Abbreviations: LOS, length of stay; ns, not stated.

Lawrence and colleagues reported on 12 patients, all of whom had Boerhaave's syndrome and a late diagnosis (Table 37.1).[8] The repairs were not buttressed and the leak rate was low at 25%. All leaks healed with observation only. The mortality was low at 14%. The authors concluded that primary repairs of emetogenic perforations can be performed at any time period.

Port and colleagues reported on six patients with a late diagnosis of a thoracic esophageal perforation (Table 37.1).[9] Most of the perforations were iatrogenic. The leak rate was low at 17% and the mortality was also low at 8%. The two postoperative leaks healed without further intervention. The authors concluded that primary repair was advantageous regardless of the time to presentaion and that esophagectomy should be reserved for cancer or extensive necrosis.

Jougon and colleagues reported on 16 patients who had a late diagnosis of an emetogenic perforation (Table 37.1).[10] The leak rate and mortality were low. Some of the patients had a tissue buttress. The authors concluded that primary repair should be undertaken in Boerhaave's syndrome whatever the delay in diagnosis is.

Richardson reported a personal series of 21 patients with a late diagnosis of a thoracic esophageal perforation (Table 37.1).[11] The majority were iatrogenic. The leak rate and mortality were quite low. All repairs were buttressed (the majority with a diaphragm flap). All leaks healed with observation. The author concluded that primary repair (in the absence of cancer or a severely diseased esophagus) was the technique of choice.

The morbidity is high in patients treated with primary repair of late esophageal perforations and the mortality is quite significant with a mean of 20% (3%–68%). Postoperative leaks that complicate management, delay oral intake, and increase length of stay occurred on the average in 33% (8%–83%) of patients. Collectively, these series demonstrate it is feasible to close perforations despite a late diagnosis but there is still substantial morbidity, especially related to leaks associated with the repair. Only one report found that primary repair is ill advised and favored esophagectomy. The results from this one series are quite poor and stand out from all other series. The vast majority of the postoperative leaks

are handled as controlled fistulas that heal with conservative therapy. Good results have been reported with and without a tissue buttress. The length of stay (LOS) is quite long with a mean LOS of 38 days (14–63 days). This prolonged LOS illustrates just how complex and demanding these patients are to care for.

37.1.2. Esophagectomy for Management of Esophageal Perforation

An alternative to primary repair is esophagectomy for the management of thoracic esophageal perforations that are diagnosed late. Five relatively recent series have enough patients to examine (Table 37.2). Most reports do not segregate out early from late patients, so for these series the patients represent a mix of both. Attar and colleagues reported on nine patients who had an esophgectomy for their perforation.[12] Three had a severe stricture, three had cancer, and three had a caustic ingestion. Six patients had an immediate reconstruction. Leaks were not reported. Three patients subsequently had a colon bypass. The mortality was 22%. The authors concluded that the esophagus should be preserved whenever possible but that esophagectomy was favored when cancer or severe intrinsic disease was present.

Orringer and Stirling reported on 22 patients with thoracic esophageal perforation of which 11 were treated beyond 24 hours.[13] Most perforations were iatrogenic. Thirteen patients had immediate reconstruction with only 1 postoperative anastomotic leak. The mortality was only 13%. The authors concluded that the sickest patients with a thoracic perforation were the ones most likely to benefit from an esophageactomy rather than a more conservative procedure.

Port and colleagues reported two patients who had esophagectomy to manage a thoracic perforation.[9] Both patients had an emetogenic perforation and both survived. One patient had immediate reconstruction without an anastomotic leak.

Gupta reported 33 personal patients managed by esophagectomy of which 25 were diagnosed late. Most patients had a severe stricture (16) or cancer (11), while four had achalasia and only two were emetogenic.[14] The mortality was low at 6%.

Only two patients had transhiatal esophagectomy without reconstruction. Twenty-six percent of patients developed an anastomotic leak but all healed with observation. The LOS was quite low. The author concluded that perforations in the diseased esophagus should be treated by transhiatal esophagectomy with a cervical anastomosis but that late diagnosed perforations should be treated by nonoperative therapy in the intrinsically normal esophagus.

Richardson reported a personal series of 14 patients who had an esophagectomy to manage a thoracic perforation.[11] Nine patients had cancer. Thirteen patients had immediate reconstruction and there were no postoperative leaks. There were no deaths. The author concluded that esophagectomy was appropriate for cancer or a severe stricture.

Esophagectomy can be carried out as an emergency procedure with surprisingly low mortality in patients with thoracic esophageal perforations. Immediate reconstruction can be carried out in most patients who present early, especially those that have a transhiatal esophagectomy. Most authors reserve esophagectomy for cancer, severe stricture, or a nonrepairable perforation. It is important to note that the majority of reported cases of esophagectomy for perforation have been done in early patients so the results are not directly comparable to primary repair of late perforations. Most late perforations are treated with esophagectomy without reconstruction so the morbidity and mortality are often underestimated as a second major reconstructive operation must be done.

37.1.3. Nonoperative Therapy for Esophageal Perforation

Another alternative to primary repair of late perforations is nonoperative treatment with aggressive treatment of collections. The ability to accurately drain collections and perforations has been markedly enhanced with the advent of interventional radiology. Three recent reports illustrate current results with nonoperative therapy (Table 37.3). Altorjay and colleagues reported on 10 patients with thoracic perforations treated nonoperatively.[15] They selected these patients from a larger group of 86 patients who otherwise had surgery for the perforation. Seventy percent of perforations were transmural and 25% were intramural. Only 30% were diagnosed late. Three patients required operative intervention (drainage in two and esophagectomy in one). There was one death for a mortality of 10%. Interventional radiology drainage was not used in these patients. The mortality of the nonoperative group (10%) was similar to that of their patients treated with surgery (14%). The authors concluded that nonoperative therapy was proper in intramural perforations and carefully selected transmural perforations (well-encapsulated perforation, drains back into esophagus, minimal symptoms, no cancer, or obstruction).

Hasan and colleagues reported on 17 patients with iatrogenic thoracic perforations.[16] Only 15% were diagnosed late. Fifteen of the perforations were caused by dilation. Most patients did not have any drainage procedures performed. Interventional radiology drainage was not used. Eight patients had leaks into the pleural space and four of these died. The mortality was 24% but two of the four deaths were in patients with advanced perforated cancers. The authors concluded that most clean, iatrogenic perforations can be treated without operation, even in the presence of cancer or stricture.

Vogel and colleagues reported a very interesting series of 37 thoracic perforations of which 28 had nonoperative treatment.[17] Most of the

TABLE 37.3. Recent reports of nonoperative treatment of thoracic esophageal perforations.

Author	Year	Patients	Evidence level	Emetic %	Morbidity	Mortality	Leak %	LOS
Altorjay[15]	1997	10	4	0	70%	20%	10%	15
Hasan[16]	2005	17	4	0	100%	>46%	24%	ns
Vogel[17]	2005	28	4	50%	ns	ns	0	26

Abbreviations: LOS, length of stay; ns, not stated.

patients had a late diagnosis of their perforation (62%). Fifty percent of patients had an emetogenic perforation. Interventional radiology techniques were used to drain all collections and pleural fluid with careful attention to accurate placement of drains. Frequent contrast studies and CT scans were done to ensure proper drainage. Four patients required limited thoracotomy for better drainage. All esophageal fistulas healed with drainage. There were no deaths in the nonoperative patients and the LOS was reasonable at 26 days. The authors concluded that with aggressive treatment of sepsis and radiologically guided drainage of esophageal leaks and pleural collections that surgery can be avoided in most patients with an esophageal perforation.

Another minimally invasive method of treatment of esophageal perforations that has been utilized with increasing frequency is the placement of self-expanding covered stents to seal the leak. Small case series and individual case reports have been published such that the evidence quality is again low at 3. Gelbmann and colleagues reported on four patients treated with an expandable plastic stent [Rusch (Kernan, Germany) Polyflex stent] for thoracic esophageal perforations.[18] Three were iatrogenic and one was emetogenic. The iatrogenic perforations all were treated early while the Borhaave's perforation was treated at 22 days. Three of the stents were removed at 32, 74, and 242 days after insertion with confirmation of esophageal healing. One patient with perforated cancer died with an intact stent in place of progressive cancer. Stents were found to be easily removable and, in the absence of a stricture, tended to migrate. The authors concluded that these plastic stents were reasonable treatment options for esophageal perforations, particularly in patients with extensive comorbidities.

Ferri and colleagues reported two patients with thoracic esophageal perforations successfully treated with self-expanding metallic covered stents.[19] Both patients had advanced cancers with spontaneous perforations. Insertion of a metallic self-expanding covered stent (Ultraflex, Boston Scientific, Newton, MA) controlled the leaks and allowed oral intact and further therapy.

37.2. Clinical Practice Based on Published Data

The published data provide only weak evidence as to the proper treatment of esophageal perforations with a delayed diagnosis. There are numerous deficiencies in the data we do have that form the basis of treatment recommendations for thoracic esophageal perforations with a delayed diagnosis. These include a relative paucity of reported patients which are typically collected from a 10- to 20-year experience with obvious changes in patient care during that period. Most centers have a strong bias toward one approach such that a relatively favorable experience is reported with one method while another has poor results but with unfavorable patients selected for the nonfavored approach. Some centers report a poor result with a method while numerous others report much more favorable results; this may be due to unrecognized failure to properly perform a technique or to adequately care for these complex patients. Series are frequently compared with one another but the patient mix may be very dissimilar in important prognostic factors such as time delay, location, symptom status, whether sepsis is present, whether the perforation is contained or leaks into the pleural space, the cause of the perforation, comorbidites, etc. Putting all these concerns in perspective, it is impossible to be dogmatic about the proper treatment of thoracic esophageal perforation. A case can be made that primary repair (with or without a tissue buttress), esophagectomy, or nonoperative treatment (with radiologically directed drainage or stent insertion if needed) are reasonable treatment options for thoracic esophageal perforation with a delayed diagnosis. The consensus opinion among most recent papers and reviews (which is only level 4 evidence) is that primary repair should be undertaken no matter what time interval has elapsed if

---

Primary repair should be undertaken for management of esophageal perforation no matter what time interval has elapsed if the underlying esophagus is relatively normal (level of evidence 4; recommendation grade C).

the underlying esophagus is relatively normal (no cancer, severe stricture, or distal obstruction that is not easily fixed) (recommendation grade C).

37.3. Personal View of the Data

I believe the data we do have is fraught with bias and that we are left with decision making in the end based on personal experience and expert opinion. There is no study of such quality that leads me to be dogmatic about a particular treatment option. Every case must be individualized to a degree so that all potential factors that might mitigate for success are considered. All patients require antibiotics, nutritional support, and vigorous supportive care. The expertise at the treating institution must be factored into the decision making with consideration of the quality of patient monitoring and radiologic support if a nonoperative approach is chosen. If an operative approach is chosen, the skill of the surgeon, especially if esophagectomy is to be done, along with the skill of the anesthesia team is important to consider. What might be possible in one center might be very difficult to duplicate in another if a critical skill set is missing. Based on a review of the data and my own experience, I favor primary repair of most thoracic esophageal perforations regardless of the time the diagnosis is made. It is intuitive to close a gastrointestinal (GI) perforation and cleanse the local area to help the body deal with a septic insult, but I recognize the absence of data that confirms the absolute necessity of that approach. I cover the repair with a tissue buttress (an intercostal muscle, a pericardial fat pad, omentum, a diaphragmatic flap) with the idea that my repair has a relatively high risk of leak (especially if the diagnosis was late or sepsis was present) and I want to try to contain it and prevent an esophagopleural fistula. I place a suction drain immediately adjacent to the repair, suture it in place, and leave it in until a barium swallow confirms a healed repair. I perform esophagectomy if there is a resectable cancer, severe stricture, end-stage esophagus (old corrosive injury, sigmoid esophagus from achalasia, etc.), necrotizing infection of the esophageal muscle, or for a previous failed repair. I place

covered stents in patients with unresectable cancers and those with severe comorbidites and drain the mediastinum or pleural space as dictated by computed tomography (CT) imaging. I am intrigued by the recent publication of Vogel and colleagues that reports a very high success rate with aggressive but nonoperative management of esophageal perforations with radiologically guided drainage of collections.[17] This approach has proven successful in the abdomen and appears to be promising in the chest with the esophagus. The results appear to be improved over older results with unguided drainage. We need further reports from other centers to see if this result is reproducible.

Due to the rarity of esophageal perforation I do not see a randomized trial ever being carried out to compare treatment options. Case series could be enhanced by more uniform reporting of important prognostic data that would aid in assessing treatment and comparing results. Important data to be collected include location, time to diagnosis and treatment, extent of symptoms, presence of the sepsis syndrome, extent of leakage, cause of the perforation, the status of the underlying esophagus, comorbidities, the precise surgical techniques used, any complications after treatment including further leaks, any further treatments needed, length of stay, length of intensice care unit (ICU) stay, cost, ability to swallow, death rate, and cause of death.

References

1. Brinster CJ, Singhal S, Lee L, et al. Evolving options in the management of esophageal perforation. *Ann Thorac Surg* 2004;77:1475–1483.
2. Grillo HC, Wilkens EW. Esophageal repair following late diagnosis of intrathoracic perforation. *Ann Thorac Surg* 1975;20:387–399.
3. Salo JA, Isolauri JO, Heikkila LJ, et al. Management of delayed esophageal perforation with mediastinal sepsis. *J Thorac Cardiovasc Surg* 1993;106:1088–1091.
4. Ohri SK, Liakakos TA, Pathi V, et al. Primary repair of iatrogenic thoracic esophageal perforation and Boerhaaves syndrome. *Ann Thorac Surg* 1993;55:603–606.
5. Wright CD, Mathisen DJ, Wain JC, et al. Reinforced primary repair of thoracic esophageal perforation. *Ann Thorac Surg* 1995;60:245–249.

6. Whyte RI, Iannettoni MD, Orringer MB. Intrathoracic esophageal perforation. The merit of primary repair. *J Thorac Cardiovasc Surg* 1995;109:140–146.

7. Wang N, Razzouk AJ, Safavi A, et al. Delayed primary repair of intrathoracic esophageal perforation: Is it safe? *J Thorac Cardiovasc Surg* 1996;111:114–122.

8. Lawrence DR, Ohri SK, Moxon RE, et al. Primary esophageal repair for Boerhaaves syndrome. *Ann Thorac Surg* 1999;67:818–820.

9. Port JL, Kent MS, Korst RJ, et al. Thoracic esophageal perforations; a decade of experience. *Ann Thorac Surg* 2003;75:1071–1074.

10. Jougon J, Mc Bride T, Delcambre F, et al. Primary repair for Boerhaaves syndrome what ever the free interval between perforation and treatment. *Eur J Cardiothorac Surg* 2004;25:475–479.

11. Richardson JD. Management of esophageal perforations: the value of aggressive surgical treatment. *Am J Surg* 2005;190:161–165.

12. Attar S, Hankins JR, Suter CM, et al. Esophageal perforation: a theraputic challenge. *Ann Thorac Surg* 1990;50:45–51.

13. Orringer MB, Stirling MC. Esophagectomy for esophageal disruption. *Ann Thorac Surg* 1990;49:35–43.

14. Gupta NM, Kaman L. Personal management of 57 consecutive patients with esophageal perforation. *Am J Surg* 2004;187:58–63.

15. Altorjay A, Kiss J, Voros A, et al. Nonoperative management of esophageal perforations. Is it justified? *Ann Surg* 1997;225:415–421.

16. Hasan S, Jilaihawi AN, Prakash D. Conservative management of iatrogenic oesophageal perforations-a viable option. *Eur J Cardiothorac Surg* 2005;28:7–10.

17. Vogel SB, Rout WR, Martin TD, et al. Esophageal perforation in adults. Aggressive, conservative treatment lowers morbidity and mortality. *Ann Surg* 2005;241:1016–1023.

18. Gelbmann CM, Ratiu NL, Rath HC, et al. Use of self-expandable plastic stents for the treatment of esophageal perforations and symptomatic anastomotic leaks. *Endoscopy* 2004;36:695–699.

19. Ferri L, Lee JKT, Law S, et al. Management of spontaneous perforation of esophageal cancer with covered self expanding metallic stents. *Dis Esophagus* 2005;18:67–69.

38
Lengthening Gastroplasty for Managing Gastroesophageal Reflux Disease and Stricture

Sandro Mattioli and Maria Luisa Lugaresi

A lengthening gastroplasty consists of the formation of a gastric tube by vertically stapling the proximal stomach from the angle of His parallel to the lesser gastric curvature. This procedure is designed to elongate the esophageal tube as part of surgical treatment of complicated cases of gastroesophageal reflux disease (GERD) in which the esophagus is irreversibly shortened, thus the gastroesophageal (GE) junction cannot be repositioned into the abdomen without excessive tension.

This technique was proposed in 1957 by J.L. Collis for the treatment of complicated cases of GERD as an alternative to esophageal resection.[1,2] A few years later, Collis, after following up the patients operated upon, reported 59% with GERD at barium swallow and 50% with specific symptoms.[3] In 1971, Pearson, Langer, and Henderson published the results of a series of 24 patients in whom a Collis gastroplasty had been performed in combination with a modified Belsey anti-reflux procedure.[4] The concept of the Pearson operation was to elongate the esophagus in order to perform an effective intra-abdominal anti-reflux fundoplication, avoiding any tension on the sutures placed through the distal esophagus, the gastric fundus, and the diaphragmatic hiatus. Based on the same concept, the combination of a Collis gastroplasty with the Nissen fundusplication was proposed by Orringer and Sloan (transthoracic Collis–Nissen).[5] Details of the Collis–Nissen operation were successively modified by Demos[6] and Cameron[7] (uncut Collis–Nissen; thoracic and abdominal approaches) and Steichen[8] (abdominal Collis–Nissen). Innovative laparoscopic and laparothoracoscopic techniques for lengthening gastroplasty associated with a fundoplication have been designed in order to replace the open procedures.[6,9–11] Techniques of laparoscopic tubularization of the lesser gastric curvature by a wedge resection of the gastric fundus have also been published.[12–14]

With the lack of tactile appreciation of the viscera, laparoscopic surgery has increased the need to identify the anatomy of the GE junction and more precisely its position with respect to the diaphragmatic hiatus. Minimally invasive surgery has revitalized the debate regarding the diagnosis and treatment of short esophagus and stricture; today, as in the past, even the very existence of the short esophagus is discussed. Many surgeons currently recognize cases of short esophagus that are managed with dedicated surgical techniques[9,10,12,13,15–26]; others deny it is a clinical entity or state they have not seen one, even in large case series.[27–59] Traditionally, the short esophagus was coupled with pan mural esophagitis and stricture[4,14,60–64] in patients affected by severe GERD and mucosal esophagitis. Recent data indicate a decreasing frequency of peptic stenosis in the GERD population,[65–67] but also the not uncommon existence of true short esophagus in the absence of esophageal stricture.[12,13,26,68,69] Further knowledge has been acquired on the negative role of hiatus hernia,[70–72] and particularly regarding the effect of a permanent intrathoracic location of the lower esophageal sphincter (LES)[73–76] on the gastroesophageal anti-reflux barrier. The conceptual differentiation between the intrathoracic position of the GE junction, generally diagnosed by barium swallow, and the true short esophagus unequivocally ascertained only in the operating room,[9,25,26,77-79] may be a significant step of the clarification of controversies.

The consideration of factors predicting the existence of true esophageal shortening,[17,23-26,68,77,80] the precise intraoperative localization of the position of cardia with respect to diaphragmatic hiatus,[14,68,77,81] the knowledge of surgical physiology of anti-reflux operations, the correct choice and performance of the surgical technique, and adequate experience in open and minimally invasive esophageal surgery are at the present time the key factors in the surgical therapy of complicated cases of GERD in whom the lengthening gastroplasty may be indicated. The above-mentioned issues are discussed in this chapter.

38.1. The Short Esophagus: Definition, Predictors, Diagnosis, Surgical Techniques, and Results

38.1.1. Definition

The definition of short esophagus was firstly adopted by radiologists to describe the intrathoracic position of the GE junction and to classify this condition among the various types of hiatus hernia, taking into consideration the morphology of the thoracic esophagus (straight or redundant) and of the gastric fundus (axial displacement, funnel type, paraesophageal).[82-87] Surgeons generally base the diagnosis of short esophagus on the inability to reduce the GE junction below the diaphragm intraoperatively. Other surgeons deny the existence of short esophagus, stating they always are able to reposition the GE junction below the diaphragm.[88-91] Data related to the prevalence of short esophagus in open surgery case series, mainly expressed in terms of nonreducibility, range widely from 0% to 60% (Table 38.1). The scattering of data strongly suggests that the clinical research was biased by methodological errors such as the subjective identification of the GE junction and the equally subjective quantification of the tension needed to be applied to the distal esophagus in order to reposition an

TABLE 38.1. Incidence of short esophagus in the surgical literature 1964–1995.

Reference	Year	No. Patients	Surgery	Short Esophagus (%)
Nygard[122]	1964	102	Open	40.2%
Collis[123]	1968	420	Open	18%
Hill[88]	1970	36	Open	0
Gatzinsky[124]	1979	140	Open	37%
Maillet[125]	1980	800	Open	10%
Moghissi[126]	1983	245	Open	39.2%
Pearson[115]	1987	430	Open	60%
Kauer[97]	1995	104	Open	9.6%
Mattioli[26]	2004[a]	149	Open	29%

Abbreviation: nr, not reported.
[a]1980–1991.

adequate segment into the abdomen.[14,26,77,80,81,92] In the last decade, the widespread diffusion of minimally invasive surgery has again produced controversial effects on the perception of surgeons with respect to short esophagus: besides a generalized attitude to ignore the problem within the rush of new operative techniques,[80,93] an increasing interest has become evident among surgeons who pay specific attention to the issue (Table 38.2). The recent literature unequivocally tries to overcome the low grade of reliability of the historical data, instead referring to more objective methods aimed at localizing precisely the GE junction.[26,68,77,81] The current definition of short esophagus accepted by the majority of the groups interested in the argument,[9,10,14,17,26,92-96] includes several major concepts: (1) the short esophagus is diagnosed only intraoperatively; (2) only after extensive mobilization of the mediastinal esophagus[9-14,17,23-26,68,77,80,81,92,93,97,98]; and (3) when the intra-abdominal portion of the esophagus is shorter than 2 to 3 cm with no downward tension applied.[9,11,13,14,17,23-26,68,77,80,81,92,98] Horwath and coworkers[77] subdivide short esophagus in: (1) true, nonreducible short esophagus; (2) true but reducible short esophagus; and (3) apparent short esophagus. Preoperative radiologic and endoscopic studies in the three groups placed the GE junction across or above the hiatus. In the first category the GE junction cannot be reduced for at least 2.5 to 3 cm below the diaphragm, while in the second category this length of the intra-

TABLE 38.2. Incidence of short esophagus in the surgical literature 1996–2004.

Reference	Year	No. Patients	Surgery	Short Esophagus (%)
Swanstrom[9]	1996	238	Mini-invasive	14%
Csendes[33]	1998	152	Open	0
Anvari[27]	1998	381	Mini-invasive	0
Dallemagne[35]	1998	622	Mini-invasive	0
Eshraghi[37]	1998	157	Mini-invasive	0
Kiviluoto[42]	1998	200	Mini-invasive	0
Landreneau[44]	1998	150	Mini-invasive	0
Lefebvre[45]	1998	100	Mini-invasive	0
Patti[50]	1998	201	Mini-invasive	0
Meyer[48]	1998	224	Mini-invasive	0
Peters[52]	1998	100	Mini-invasive	0
McKernan[15]	1998	968	Mini-invasive	1.9%
Johnson[10]	1998	220	Mini-invasive	4%
Jobe[16]	1998	580	Mini-invasive	2.5%
El-Serag[36]	1999	1147	Open	0
Rydberg[53]	1999	106	Open	0
Arnaud[28]	1999	1470	Mini-invasive	0
Barrat[29]	1999	150	Mini-invasive	0
Champault[32]	1999	156	Mini-invasive	0
Coelho[34]	1999	503	Mini-invasive	0
Johanet[40]	1999	335	Mini-invasive	0
Klinger[43]	1999	102	Mini-invasive	0
Loustarinen[47]	1999	127	Mini-invasive	0
Soper[55]	1999	292	Mini-invasive	0
Watson[56]	1999	107	Mini-invasive	0
Gastal[17]	1999	236	Mini-invasive	15.6%
Bohmer[31]	2000	106	Open	0
Basso[30]	2000	135	Mini-invasive	0
Farrell[38]	2000	669	Mini-invasive	0
Kamolz[41]	2000	175	Mini-invasive	0
Leggett[46]	2000	239	Mini-invasive	0
O'Boyle[49]	2000	511	Mini-invasive	0
Pessaux[51]	2000	1470	Mini-invasive	0
Ross[54]	2000	200	Mini-invasive	0
Yau[58]	2000	757	Mini-invasive	0
Eubanks[18]	2000	228	Mini-invasive	0.8%
Zaninotto[19]	2000	621	Mini-invasive	0.9%
Luketich[127]	2000	100	Mini-invasive	27%
Kleimann[21]	2001	255	Mini-invasive	2%
Terry[22]	2001	1000	Mini-invasive	1.5%
Awad[23]	2001	260	Mini-invasive	5%
Urbach[24]	2001	153	Mini-invasive	13%
O'Rourke[25]	2003	487	Mini-invasive	19%
Lin[13]	2004	1579	Mini-invasive	4.3%
Terry[12]	2004	143	Mini-invasive	11.2%
Mattioli[26]	2004[a]	170	Open, mini-invasive	23%

[a] 1992–2003.

abdominal esophagus is achieved. In the third category, the esophagus has a normal length but is accordioned into the distal mediastinum.[77]

38.1.2. Predictive Factors

Among patients undergoing surgery for GERD, up to 40% have developed complications such as macroscopic esophagitis, Barrett's esophagus, peptic esophageal stricture, or acquired short esophagus.[14,60–62] Esophageal stricture is the clinical finding most commonly related with esophageal shortening[14,24,68,80]; it may occur in 1% to 5%[14,63,64] of patients with longstanding severe esophagitis. Other abnormalities that should raise the suspicion of a short esophagus include the radiologic diagnosis of a large, nonreducible hiatal hernia in the upright position, a hiatal hernia larger than 5 cm, or an esophageal length of less than 35 cm from the incisors as determined by endoscopy.[13,17,77] The presence of a paraesophageal hiatal hernia is considered to be highly predictive of the presence of short esophagus.[24,78,80] Maziak and colleagues[99] reported that 80% (75/94) of patients with a large paraesophageal hernia required a lengthening procedure for short esophagus. Of lesser importance, but still thought to play a role, is a history of severe esophagitis or Barrett's esophagus.[80] The incidence of reoperative surgery has been shown to be significantly increased in patients with esophageal stricture following standard Belsey and Nissen repairs.[100,101] The risk of gastroplasty was increased 3.8-fold [95% confidence level (95% CI), 1.0–15.0] in the presence of esophageal stricture in the study of Urbach and colleagues,[24] and by a factor of 7.5 (95% CI, 3.3–16.7) according to Gastal.[17] Urbach observed that for paraesophageal hernia the risk of gastroplasty was increased 4.5-fold (95% CI, 1.4–14.6), 4.3-fold for Barrett's esophagus (95% CI, 1.3–14.3), and 11.6-fold for reoperative surgery (95% CI, 2.8–48.4).[24] Mittal[68] found that, although the presence of Barrett's esophagus or an esophageal stricture was associated with the need for esophageal lengthening, the presence of a large hiatal hernia on barium studies and the preoperative manometric length of the esophagus did not appear to be a statistically significant factor. Preoperative esophagraphy, endoscopy, and esophageal manometric length assessment are useful, though not ideal, for identifying patients in need of an esophageal lengthening procedure.[17,23,24,68] However, it has been shown that neither a single preoperative diagnostic test nor any combination of tests is completely accurate in making the diagnosis.[23] The combination of two or more tests resulted in a specificity ranging from 63% to 100% but a low sensitivity (28%–42%).[23]

In a study on the outcomes of the surgical treatment of GERD in 319 patients, the preoperative factors predictive of the need for an esophageal lengthening procedure were evaluated.[26] The multivariate analysis showed the following preoperative factors as predicting the need of a Collis procedure: radiologic classification [$p = 0.005$; odds ratio (OR) 20.53; 95% CI, 2.47–170.15), manometry in the upright position performed after the standard recording in the supine position ($p = 0.038$; OR 5.26; 95% CI, 1.09–25.41), and the presence of peptic stenosis ($p = 0.015$; OR 5.18; 95% CI, 1.38–19.44). The radiologic classification adopted for the study was based on the assessment of the position of the GE junction with respect to the hiatus and not on the size of the hernia. Three grades of orad migration of the GE junction were considered: hiatal insufficiency, concentric hiatus hernia, and short esophagus. The classification had been validated with a manometric–radiologic study, which demonstrated that the distance (in centimeters) from the LES inferior margin to the diaphragm was significantly different in healthy volunteers versus the three grades of migration and between each contiguous grade.[75] Although the combination of endoscopy, radiology, and manometry has been shown to be associated with a high positive predictive value for short esophagus, the sensitivity and negative predictive value for the combination of these tests are low, and no single criterion has been shown to be associated with a high specificity or predictive value.[23,25]

38.1.3. Intraoperative Diagnosis

In course of laparoscopic surgery for GERD, the surgeon may underestimate the presence of esophageal shortening because of a number of contributing factors. Complete dissection of the fat pad overlying the GE junction is necessary to identify the true GE junction, but this is not routinely described in laparoscopic reports.[92] The presence of pneumoperitoneum elevates the diaphragm significantly and may give the false impression that an adequate length of intra-abdominal esophagus is achieved.[26,92,102] In some reports, a Penrose drain is placed around the distal esophagus and downward tension is applied during the dissection and wrap; this apparent intra-abdominal segment of esophagus may later retract back up into the thoracic cavity when the Penrose drain is removed.[92] Finally, many laparoscopic surgeons routinely place a weighted bougie into the esophagus, and the downward pressure from the bougie pushes the esophagus distally for a distance up to 2 to 3 cm.[92] During laparoscopy it is possible to miss the exact position of the GE junction because the proximal stomach, attracted upward, acquires a funnel like form after years of herniation, the serosa loses brightness, and the wall thins.[26] The tubularized proximal stomach is hardly distinguishable from the distal esophagus.[98,103] One or more of these factors can lead the surgeon to overestimate the length of intra-abdominal esophagus.

Recently, intraoperative endoscopy has been proposed in order to identify the GE junction in relation to the hiatus.[26,68,81,103] The reference to the gastric folds as an anatomical–endoscopic landmark of the GE junction[104,105,106] helps to eliminate the subjective component of the evaluation in the presence of short and long Barrett's esophagus.[23,26,107] As the gastric folds are normally located at or few millimeters below the Z line, this anatomical reference also eliminates the risk of overdiagnosing the condition of short esophagus.[26,103] After the endoscopist has placed the tip of the fiberscope at the level of the gastric folds, the surgeon recognizes the point of passage between the tubular esophagus and the stomach by means of transillumination[68] or by localizing the tip of the scope with a grasping forceps. As the length of the open jaws of the forceps is known, the distance between the hiatus and the GE junction can be estimated.[81]

The gold standard for determination of short esophagus is intraoperative esophageal mobilization followed by assessment of length.[68] As described by Collis,[1] there is a large subset of patients who have true but moderate esophageal shortening, which can be treated by an extended mediastinal dissection. Recently, O'Rourke and coworkers[25] proposed an extended laparoscopic transmediastinal dissection in patients with moderately short esophagus. These authors defined an esophageal dissection less than 5cm into the mediastinum as type I, and an esophageal dissection greater than or equal to 5cm into the mediastinum as type II. On average, a type II dissection was carried up between 7 and 10cm into the mediastinum. In cases in which type II dissection failed to release intra-abdominally an adequate segment of tension-free esophagus, a thoracoscopic-assisted Collis gastroplasty was performed.[25] A concern associated with type II dissection is the potential for occult injury to the vagus nerves.[25] The decision to measure the length of the intra-abdominal esophagus after isolation without tension has the advantage of overcoming the totally subjective concepts of moderate or reasonable or adequate tension applied to pull downward the stomach. Any modality of objective measurement of the applied tension, although feasible with a dynamometer, would be unacceptably cumbersome. It is gener-

ally agreed that if a minimum of 2.5 to 3 centimeters of tension–free intra-abdominal esophagus are not obtained after adequate mobilization, a lengthening gastroplasty should be added to the fundoplication.[9,11,13,23,25,26,68,77,92,95,102]

38.1.4. Surgical Techniques

The techniques of transthoracic and transabdominal lengthening gastroplasty, associated with a total or partial fundoplication, are familiar to thoracic and esophageal surgeons who have an adequate training. These procedures remain the cornerstones of anti-reflux surgery, especially for complicated cases and re-operative surgery. The minimally invasive Collis–Nissen has gained popularity, mainly in tertiary reference centers via laparoscopic or combined thoracolaparoscopic approaches. In the mid 1990s, two techniques of thoracoscopic gastroplasty and laparoscopic fundoplication were published.[9,108] Swanstrom performed a lengthening gastroplasty by introducing an endostapler through the right chest [Figure 38.1(A)].[9] In 1998, Johnson,

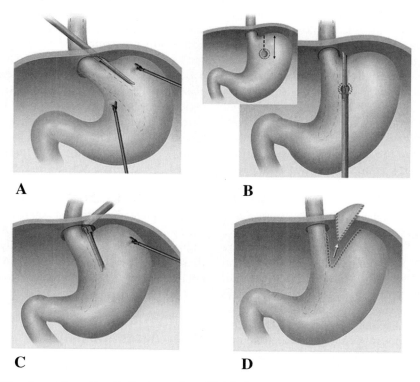

A   **B**

C   **D**

FIGURE 38.1. Mini invasive esophageal lengthening gastroplasty: (A) right thoracoscopic approach, (B) laparoscopic approach, (C) left thoracoscopic approach, and (D) laparoscopic stapled wedge gastroplasty.

Oddostir, and Hunter[10] proposed a laparoscopic technique that reproduced the open one promoted by Steichen [Figure 38.1(B)]. The authors intended to avoid a "double cavity procedure" and its potential complications. Awad has preferred the left thoracoscopic approach for introducing the articulated endostapler [Figure 38.1(C)].[11] The most recent modification of the Collis gastroplasty is the stapled wedge gastroplasty published in 2004 by Tierry, Vernon, and Hunter,[12] Lin and associates,[13] and Hoang and coworkers.[14] This technique is performed laparoscopically, and requires the resection of a wedge of gastric fundus in order to staple the lesser curvature vertically [Figure 38.1(D)]. The wedge gastroplasty has been developed because, with the fully laparoscopic technique [Figure 38.1(B)], the apex of the tubularized fundus could become ischemic.[12]

38.1.5. Results

With regard to the transthoracic Collis–Belsey and Collis–Nissen operations, Pearson and Orringer reported an operative mortality of 0.5% to 1.1%.[109–111] Other authors achieved analogous results.[6,112–114] Complications related to the lengthening gastroplasty included leaks and fistulas, which occurred in 10% or fewer patients.[77] Pearson reported good long-term results in 84.5% and fair/poor results in 15.5%,[115] and Orringer observed good results in 89%.[110,111] The long-term results of the open Collis procedure associated with anti-reflux surgery are not uniform, and satisfactory results vary from 59%[107,116] to 80%.[26]

With regard to the minimally invasive Collis–Nissen, the early results are satisfactory and compare favorably with previous open surgery series. Mean operative time for Hunter's series was 294 min,[10] and for Swanstrom's series, it was 257 min.[16] The average length of stay has been 2 to 3 days.[10,11,16,92] No operative mortalities were reported.[10,11,12,14,16,92,117] Complications ranged from 0% to 50%.[10–12,14,16,92,117] Postoperative functional assessment at 12 months for Hunter's series revealed that 11% of patients complained of reflux symptoms and 11% had dysphagia.[10] Short-term follow-up in Swanstrom's series revealed no evidence of recurrent reflux.[9] However in medium-term follow up, 14% of patients complained of reflux symptoms and 14% had dysphagia.[16] No wrap failures or mediastinal herniations were observed.[16] Awad and coworkers reported similar outcome data at a mean follow-up of 17 months: 9% of patients complained of reflux symptoms and 9% had dysphagia.[23] They objectively documented a 9% wrap failure rate and a 9% mediastinal herniation rate.[23] Pierre and colleagues[118] reported on a group of 112 patients with paraesophageal hernia who underwent a laparoscopic Collis–Nissen procedure. At a median of 18 months of follow-up, the patients satisfaction rate was 93%, 16% required, at least occasionally, anti-secretory medications, and 6% had dysphagia warranting dilation. Recurrent hiatal hernias were observed in 2.7%.[118]

The Collis gastroplasty is a suitable procedure also in case of re-operation after a failed anti-reflux procedure, as performed in open surgery by Deschamps in 62.7% of cases[119] and recently in minimally invasive surgery by Luketich in 52.5%.[120] Two specific causes of malfunction of the lengthening gastroplasty have been identified. The neoesophagus' lack of motility may predispose to dilation of the tube or contribute to postoperative dysphagia.[13,14,77] Of more potential concern is the production of acid within the neoesophagus producing localized esophagitis, as was observed in open Collis procedures.[13,14,77,107] Jobe and coworkers[16] performed an objective follow-up in 15 patients after laparoscopic lengthening gastroplasty and anti-reflux fundoplication: in 7 of 15 patients the neoesophagus above the wrap was found to contain parietal cells that continued to secrete acid. This was indicated by an abnormal postoperative DeMeester score and it was confirmed by positive Congo red testing of the suspected mucosa. In order to avoid leaving parietal cells above the fundoplication, Hunter suggests placing the highest stitch of the fundoplication on the native esophagus.[13] Although the Collis gastroplasty is conceptually appealing, these problems call into question the liberal application of this technique during anti-reflux surgery.[13]

38.2. Recommendations

All the data of the past and present literature originate from single center reports; no study was randomized; the criteria for inclusion of patients were not defined; the indications for surgical therapy of GERD were not specified; and the methods for studying the patients were neither standardized nor uniform. The surgical techniques adopted in the last 10 years are substantially different and have been applied to relatively small numbers of patients. In consequence, the quality of data of the body of literature available regarding the arguments treated in the present chapter is unfortunately low (level of evidence 3 to 4). Nevertheless, every day patients affected by GERD undergo surgical therapy. It is imperative to draw empirical guidelines for the management of these patients.

Authors who believe that the lengthening gastroplasty is still the only way to manage true short esophagus and other complex situations agree on the following concepts: (1) the preoperative evaluation offers the clinician positive elements of suspicion on the eventual complexity of the case, but the diagnosis of short esophagus can be made only in the operating room with a combined surgical and endoscopic measurement of the distance between the GE junction and the diaphragm; (2) only after extensive mobilization of the mediastinal esophagus; and (3) when the intra-abdominal portion of the esophagus is shorter than 2 to 3 cm with no downward tension applied. With regard to the surgical techniques, many insist on the utility of performing the fundoplication around the proximal neo-esophagus.

> The diagnosis of short esophagus can be made only in the operating room with a combined surgical and endoscopic measurement of the distance between the GE junction and the diaphragm, and only after extensive mobilization of the mediastinal esophagus. When these conditions are met and the intra-abdominal portion of the esophagus is shorter than 2 to 3 cm with no downward tension applied, it is appropriate to perform a Collis gastroplasty (level of evidence 3 to 4; recommendation grade C).

38.3. Our Approach

The 25 years of clinical research of the Bologna group on anti-reflux surgery, specifically on diagnosis, pathophysiology, and treatment of short esophagus, and the continuous attention paid to the work of others, has led us to progressively mature and share the above-mentioned principles according to our experience. We have adopted a series of technical details with the intention of eliminating the reasons for failure, still certainly not negligible, of the Collis procedure associated with anti-reflux surgery.[26] At the present time, we believe that the only alternative to a lengthening gastroplasty for true short esophagus, with or without stricture or paraesophageal hernia, is long-term medical therapy, with the consequences already depicted.[76] The preoperative barium swallow and the radiologic classification in three steps of cranial migration of the GE junction[75] provide enough information to adequately inform the patient and to plan the operative procedure.

When a concentric hiatus hernia or short esophagus are diagnosed radiologically, we place the patient in the 45° left lateral position on the operating table [Figure 38.2(A)]. Rotating the bed on the left or on the right, the surgeon can comfortably perform laparoscopy or laparoscopy-left thoracoscopy; the 10-mm optic port is placed at least 5 cm above the standard umbilicus position [Figure 38.2(A)]. The left thoracoscopic approach [Figure 38.2(B)] has been preferred because it permits effective control of the otherwise blind passage of the endostapler into the mediastinum and upper abdomen (if a second optic is not used). The tip of the stapler is clearly visible while walking the stapler tip along the left diaphragm. Moreover, with the left thoracic approach, the lower esophagus and hiatus are well displayed. The routine marking by clips of the GE junction with the help of the fiberscope is useful in placing the fundoplication in the correct position around the esophagus or the neo-esophagus. Intraoperative endoscopy requires a few technical details to precisely measure the length of the intraabdominal esophagus: (1) deflate the stomach to avoid distension of the fundus and the consequent shortening of the submerged esophageal segment; (2) mark the level of the gastric folds while

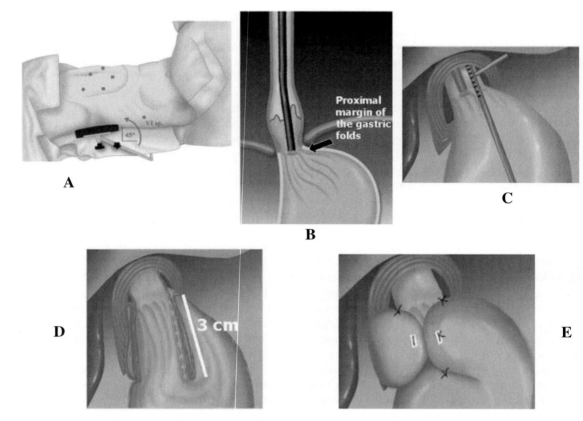

FIGURE 38.2. Left thoracoscopic–laparoscopic Collis–Nissen procedure: (A) position of the patient on the operative bed, the chest is rotated 45° to the right side, the optic port is placed 5 cm above the ombilicus in the mid line, the thoracoscopic port (12 mm) is placed in the posterior axillary line 5th to 7th interspace according to the size of the chest; (B) the tip of the fiberscope is in correspondence of the gastric folds; (C) the L-shaped ruler; (D) the neoesophagus, and (E) the floppy Nissen is anchored to the esophagus at the level of the native GE junction.

withdrawing the instrument [Figure 38.2(B,C)] measure the distance between the anterior apex of the hiatus (which is more cranial than the posterior aspect) and the clips. For measuring the distance between the clips and the apex of the diaphragm, we have created an L-shaped ruler which eliminates the perspective errors caused by the bidimensional video image [Figure 38.2(C)]. In order to avoid the formation of an amotile acid secreting pouch above the upper margin of the fundoplication, we consider it crucial that the neoesophagus is not longer than 3 cm [Figure 38.2(D)]. With the thoracoscopic approach, the lengthening achieved with one application of the roticulator endostapler cannot exceed 3 cm. It is therefore always possible to include the entire neo-esophagus in the 360° fundoplication. To date, the neo-esophagus and the fundoplication always have been placed below the diaphragm without tension.

The importance of preserving a soft, balloon-shaped gastric fundus to wrap smoothly around the neo-esophagus has been clearly pointed out in the past.[121] With the EEA laparoscopic gastroplasty (same for the open Collis–Nissen), a long stiff fundus is frequently obtained that cannot softly cover the whole length of the neo-esophagus. We believe that this was the main reason for some of the poor long-term results we obtained with the abdominal Collis–Nissen with respect to the Pearson operation, in the absence of ischemia of the stapled gastric remnant and of anatomical relapse.[26] We extend this concern to the stapled wedge Collis gastroplasty techniques[12-14] which drastically reduce the volume of the gastric fundus. To prevent the formation of a gastric pouch above the fundoplication we fix the wrap laterally to the native cardia with two stitches placed at the apex of the gastroplasty [Figure 38.2(E)]. To avoid the intraoperative splitting of the endosuture,[26] we currently use a 46 Maloney bougie to calibrate the gastroplasty. We have not yet registered any cases of troubling dysphagia.

In summary, when treating complex cases of GERD, surgeons must optimize the pre- and intra-operative recognition of the anatomical and pathophysiological situation and must possess the experience and skill necessary to adequately perform very complex surgical procedures.

References

1. Collis JL. An operation for hiatus hernia with short oesophagus. *Thorax* 1957;12:181–188.
2. Collis JL. An operation for hiatus hernia with short esophagus. *J Thorac Surg* 1957;34:768–778.
3. Collis JL. Review of surgical results in hiatus hernia. *Thorax* 1961;16:114.
4. Pearson FG, Langer B, Henderson MB. Gastroplasty and Belsey hiatal hernia repair: an operation for the management of peptic stricture with acquired short esophagus. *J Thorac Cardiovasc Surg* 1971;61:50–63.
5. Orringer MB, Sloan H. Complications and failings of the combined Collis–Belsey operation. *J Thoracic Cardiovasc Surg* 1977;74:726–735.
6. Demos NJ. Stapled, uncut gastroplasty for hiatal hernia: 12-year follow-up. *Ann Thorac Surg* 1984;38:393–399.
7. Cameron BH, Cochran WJ, McGill CW. The uncut Collis–Nissen fundoplication: results for 79 consecutively treated high-risk children. *J Pediatr Surg* 1997;32:887–891.
8. Steichen FM. Abdominal approach to the Collis gastroplasty and Nissen fundoplication. *Surg Gynecol Obstet* 1986;162:272–274.
9. Swanstrom LL, Marcus DR, Galloway GQ. Laparoscopic Collis gastroplasty is the treatment of choice for the shortened esophagus. *Am J Surg* 1996;171:477–481.
10. Johnson AB, Oddsdottir M, Hunter JG. Laparoscopic Collis gastroplasty and Nissen fundoplication: a new technique for the management of esophageal foreshortening. *Surg Endosc* 1998;12:1055–1060.
11. Awad ZT, Filipi CJ, Mittal SK, et al. Left side thoracoscopically assisted gastroplasty: a new technique for managing the shortened esophagus. *Surg Endosc* 2000;14:508–512.
12. Terry ML, Vernon A, Hunter JG. Stapled-wedge Collis gastroplasty for the shortened esophagus. *Am J Surg* 2004;188:195–199.
13. Lin E, Swafford V, Chadalavada R, et al. Disparity between symptomatic and physiologic outcomes following esophageal lengthening procedures for antireflux surgery. *J Gastrointest Surg* 2004;8:31–39.
14. Hoang CD, Koh PS, Maddaus MA. Short esophagus and esophageal stricture. *Surg Clin North Am* 2005;85:433–451.
15. McKernan JB, Champion JK. Minimally invasive antireflux surgery. *Am J Surg* 1998;175:271–276.
16. Jobe BA, Horvath KD, Swanstrom LL. Postoperative function following laparoscopic Collis gastroplasty for shortened esophagus. *Arch Surg* 1998;133:867–874.
17. Gastal OL, Hagen JA, Peters JH, et al. Short esophagus: analysis of predictors and clinical implications. *Arch Surg* 1999;134:633–638.
18. Eubanks TR, Omelanczuk P, Richards C, et al. Outcomes of laparoscopic antireflux procedures. *Am J Surg* 2000;179:391–395.
19. Zaninotto G, Molena D, Ancona E. A prospective multicenter study on laparoscopic treatment of gastroesophageal reflux disease in Italy: type of surgery, conversions, complications, and early results. Study Group for the Laparoscopic Treatment of Gastroesophageal Reflux Disease of the Italian Society of Endoscopic Surgery (SICE). *Surg Endosc* 2000;14:282–288.
20. Luketich JD, Raja S, Fernando HC, et al. Laparoscopic repair of giant paraesophageal hernia: 100 consecutive cases. *Ann Surg* 2000;232:608–618.
21. Kleimann E, Halbfass HJ. The "short esophagus problem" in laparoscopic anti-reflux surgery. *Chirurgie* 2001;72:408–413.
22. Terry M, Smith CD, Branum GD, et al. Outcomes of laparoscopic fundoplication for gastroesophageal reflux disease and paraesophageal hernia. *Surg Endosc* 2001;15:691–699.
23. Awad ZT, Mittal SK, Roth TA, et al. Esophageal shortening during the era of laparoscopic surgery. *World J Surg* 2001;25:558–561.
24. Urbach DR, Khajanchee YS, Glasgow RE, et al. Preoperative determinants of an esophageal lengthening procedure in laparoscopic antireflux surgery. *Surg Endosc* 2001;15:1408–1412.
25. O'Rourke RW, Khajanchee YS, Urbach DR, et al. Extended transmediastinal dissection: an alter-

native to gastroplasty for short esophagus. *Arch Surg* 2003;138:735–740.

26. Mattioli S, Lugaresi ML, Di Simone MP, et al. The surgical treatment of the intrathoracic migration of the gastro-oesophageal junction and of short oesophagus in gastro-oesophageal reflux disease. *Eur J Cardiothorac Surg* 2004;25:1079–1088.

27. Anvari M, Allen C. Laparoscopic Nissen fundoplication. Two-year comprehensive follow-up of a technique of minimal paraesophageal dissection. *Ann Surg* 1998;227:25–32.

28. Arnaud JP, Pessaux P, Ghavami B, et al. Fundoplicature laparoscopique pour reflux gastrooesophagien. E´ tude multicentrique de 1470 cas. *Chirurgie* 1999;124:516–522.

29. Barrat C, Cueto-Rozon R, Catheline JM, et al. Influence de l'apprentissage et de l'expérience dans le traitement laparoscopique du reflux gastro-oesophagien. *Chirurgie* 1999;124:675–680.

30. Basso N, De Leo A, Genco A, et al. 360° laparoscopic fundoplication with tension-free hiatoplasty in the treatment of symptomatic gastroesophageal re.ux disease. *Surg Endosc* 2000;14:164–169.

31. Bohmer RD, Roberts RH, Utley RJ. Open Nissen fundoplication and highly selective vagotomy as a treatment for gastro-oesophageal reflux disease. *Aust N Z J Surg* 2000;70:22–25.

32. Champault GG, Barrat C, Rozon RC, et al. The effect of the learning curve on the outcome of laparoscopic treatment for gastroesophageal reflux. *Surg Laparosc Endosc* 1999;9:375–381.

33. Csendes A, Braghetto I, Burdiles P, et al. Longterm results of classic antireflux surgery in 152 patients with Barrett's esophagus: clinical, radiologic, endoscopic, manometric, and acid reflux test analysis before and late after operation. *Surgery* 1998;123:645–657.

34. Coelho JCU, Wiederkehr JC, Campos ACL, et al. Conversions and complications of laparoscopic treatment of gastroesophageal reflux disease. *J Am Coll Surg* 1999;189:356–361.

35. Dallemagne B, Weerts JM, Jeahes C, et al. Results of laparoscopic Nissen fundoplication. *Hepatogastroenterology* 1998;45:1338–1343.

36. El-Serag HB, Sonnenberg A. Outcome of erosive reflux esophagitis after Nissen fundoplication. *Am J Gastroenterol* 1999;94:1771–1776.

37. Eshraghi N, Farahmand M, Soot SJ, et al. Comparison of outcomes of open versus laparoscopic Nissen fundoplication performed in a single practice. *Am J Surg* 1998;175:371–374.

38. Farrell TM, Archer SB, Galloway KD, et al. Heartburn is more likely to recur after Toupet fundoplication than Nissen fundoplication. *Am Surg* 2000;66:229–237.

39. Franzen T, Bostrom J, Tibbling Grahn L, Johansson K. Prospective study of symptoms and gastro-oesophageal reflux 10 years after posterior partial fundoplication. *Br J Surg* 1999;86:956–960.

40. Johanet H, Bellouard A, Bokobza B. Cure de reflux gastrooesophagien par coelioscopie. Résultats d'une étude multicentrique. *Ann Chir* 1999;53:382–386.

41. Kamolz T, Bammer T, Wykypiel H Jr, et al. Quality of life and surgical outcome after laparoscopic Nissen and Toupet fundoplication: one-year follow-up. *Endoscopy* 2000;32:363–368.

42. Kiviluoto T, Sirén J, Färkkilä M, et al. Laparoscopic Nissen fundoplication. A prospective analysis of 200 consecutive patients. *Surg Laparosc Endosc* 1998;8:429–434.

43. Klinger PJ, Hinder RA, Cina RA, et al. Laparoscopic antireflux surgery for the treatment of esophageal strictures refractory to medical therapy. *Am J Gastroenterol* 1999;94:632–636.

44. Landreneau RJ, Wiechmann RJ, Hazelrigg SR, et al. Success of laparoscopic fundoplication for gastroesophageal reflux disease. *Ann Thorac Surg* 1998;66:1886–1893.

45. Lefebvre JC, Belva P, Takieddine M, et al. Laparoscopic Toupet fundoplication. Prospective study of 100 cases. Results at one year and literature review. *Acta Chir Belg* 1998;98:1–4.

46. Leggett PL, Bissell CD, Churchman-Winn R, et al. A comparison of laparoscopic Nissen fundoplication and Rossetti's modification in 239 patients. *Surg Endosc* 2000;14:473–477.

47. Loustarinen MES, Isolauri JO. Surgical experience improves the long-term results of Nissen fundoplication. *Scand J Gastroenterol* 1999;34:117–120.

48. Meyer C, Firtion O, Rohr S, et al. Résultats de la fundoplicature par voie laparoscopique dans le traitement de reflux gastro-oesophagien. Á propos de 224 cas. *Chirurgie* 1998;123:257–262.

49. O'Boyle CJ, Heer K, Smith A, et al. Iatrogenic thoracic migration of the stomach complicating laparoscopic Nissen fundoplication. *Surg Endosc* 2000;14:540–542.

50. Patti MG, Arcerito M, Feo CV, et al. An analysis of operations for gastroesophageal reflux disease. *Arch Surg* 1998;133:600–607.

51. Pessaux P, Arnaud JP, Ghavami B, et al. Laparoscopic antireflux surgery: comparative study of Nissen, Nissen-Rossetti, and Toupet fundoplication. *Surg Endosc* 2000;14:1024–1027.

52. Peters JH, DeMeester TR, Crookes P, et al. The treatment of gastroesophageal reflux disease with laparoscopic Nissen fundoplication. Prospective evaluation of 100 patients with typical symptoms. *Ann Surg* 1998;228:40–50.

53. Rydberg L, Ruth M, Abrahamsson H, et al. Tailoring antireflux surgery: a randomized clinical trial. *World J Surg* 1999;23:612–618.

54. Ross S, Ramsay CR, Watson AJM, et al. Symptomatic outcome following laparoscopic anterior partial fundoplication. Follow-up of a series of 200 patients. *J R Coll Surg Edinb* 2000;45:363–365.

55. Soper NJ, Dunnegan D. Anatomic fundoplication failure after laparoscopic antireflux surgery. *Ann Surg* 1999;229:669–677.

56. Watson DI, Jamieson GG, Pike GK, et al. Prospective randomized double-bind trial between laparoscopic Nissen fundoplication and anterior partial fundoplication. *Br J Surg* 1999;86:123–130.

57. Windsor JA, Yellapu S. Laparoscopic anti-reflux surgery in New Zealand: a trend towards partial fundoplication. *Aust N Z J Surg* 2000;70:184–187.

58. Yau P, Watson DI, Devitt PG, et al. Laparoscopic antireflux surgery in the treatment of gastroesophageal reflux in patients with Barrett esophagus. *Arch Surg* 2000;135:801–805.

59. Nguyen NT, Schauer PR, Hutson W, et al. Preliminary results of thoracoscopic Belsey Mark IV antireflux procedure. *Surg Laparosc Endosc* 1998;8:185–188.

60. Stein HJ, Barlow AP, DeMeester TR, et al. Complications of gastroesophageal refux disease. Role of the lower esophageal sphincter, esophageal acid and acid/alkaline exposure, and duodenogastric reflux. *Ann Surg* 1992;216:35–43.

61. Richter JE. Peptic strictures of the esophagus. *Gastroenterol Clin North Am* 1999;28:875–891.

62. Bremner RM, Crookes PF, DeMeester TR, et al. Concentration of refluxed acid and esophageal mucosal injury. *Am J Surg* 1992;164:522–527.

63. Ben Rejeb M, Bouche O, Zeitoun P. Study of 47 consecutive patients with peptic esophageal stricture compared with 3880 cases of refux esophagitis. *Dig Dis Sci* 1992;37:733–736.

64. Loof L, Gotell P, Elfberg B. The incidence of refux oesophagitis. A study of endoscopy reports from a defined catchment area in Sweden. *Scand J Gastroenterol* 1993;28:113–118.

65. Johanson JF. Epidemiology of esophageal and supraesophageal reflux injuries. *Am J Med* 2000; 108(suppl 4a):99S–103S.

66. Sonnenberg A. Esophageal diseases. In: Everhart JE, ed. *Digestive Diseases in the United States: Epidemiology and Impact*. US Department of Health and Human Services, Public Health Service, National Institutes of Health, National Institute of Diabetes and Digestive and Kidney Disease. NIH publication no. 94–1447. Washington, DC: US Government Printing Office, 1994:300–355.

67. Spechler SJ. Esophageal complications of gastroesophageal reflux disease: presentation, diagnosis, management, and outcomes. *Clin Cornerstone* 2003;5:41–50.

68. Mittal SK, Awad ZT, Tasset M, et al. The preoperative predictability of the short esophagus in patients with stricture or paraesophageal hernia. *Surg Endosc* 2000;14:464–468.

69. Legare JF, Henteleff HJ, Casson AG. Results of Collis gastroplasty and selective fundoplication, using a left thoracoabdominal approach, for failed antireflux surgery. *Eur J Cardiothorac Surg* 2002;21:534–540.

70. Mittal RK. Hiatal hernia. Myth or reality? *Am J Med* 1997;103:33S–39S.

71. Murray JA, Camilleri M. The fall and rise of the hiatal hernia. *Gastroenterology* 2000;119:1779–1781.

72. Penagini R, Carmagnola S, Cantu P. Gastrooesophageal reflux disease – pathophysiological issues of clinical relevance. *Aliment Pharmacol Ther* 2002;16(suppl 4):65–71.

73. Sloan S, Kahrilas PJ. Impairment of esophageal emptying with hiatal hernia. *Gastroenterology* 1991;100:596–605.

74. Kahrilas PJ, Lin S, Chen J, et al. The effect of hiatus hernia on gastro-oesophageal junction pressure. *Gut* 1999;44:476–482.

75. Mattioli S, D'Ovidio F, Di Simone MP, et al. Clinical and surgical relevance of the progressive phases of intrathoracic migration of the gastroesophageal junction in gastroesophageal reflux disease. *J Thorac Cardiovasc Surg* 1998;116: 267–275.

76. Mattioli S, Lugaresi ML, Di Simone MP, et al. Review article: indications for anti-reflux surgery in gastro-oesophageal reflux disease. *Aliment Pharmacol Ther* 2003;17(suppl 2):60–67.

77. Horvath KD, Swanstrom LL, Jobe BA. The short esophagus: pathophysiology, incidence, presentation, and treatment in the era of laparoscopic antireflux surgery. *Ann Surg* 2000;232:630–640.

78. Bremner RM, Bremner CG, Peters HJ, et al. Fundamentals of antireflux surgery. In: Peters JH, DeMeester TR, eds. *Minimally Invasive Surgery of the Foregut*. St. Louis: Quality Medical Publishing; 1994:119–143.

79. Richardson JD, Richardson RL. Collis–Nissen gastroplasty for shortened esophagus: long-term evaluation. *Ann Surg* 1998;227:735–742.

80. Low DE. The short esophagus-recognition and management. *J Gastrointest Surg*. 2001;5:458–461.

81. Awad ZT, Dickason TJ, Filipi CJ, et al. A combined laparoscopic-endoscopic method of assessment to prevent the complications of short esophagus. *Surg Endosc* 1999;13:626–627.

82. Akerlund AKE. I. hernia diapragmatica hiatus oesophagei vom anatomischen und rontgenogischen gesichtspunkt. *Acta Radiol* 1926;6:3–22.

83. Wolf BS. Roentgen features of the normal and herniated oesophago-gastric region: problems in terminology. *Am J Digest Dis* 1960;5:751–758.

84. Wolf BS, Lazar HP. Inflammatory lesions of the esophagus – reflux esophagitis. In: Vantrappen G, Hellemans J, eds. *Diseases of the Esophagus*. Berlin: Springer-Verlag; 1974:493–524.

85. Pringot J, Ponette E. Radiological examination of the esophagus. In: Vantrappen G, Hellemans J, eds. *Diseases of the Esophagus*. Berlin: Springer-Verlag; 1974:154–156.

86. Rex JC, Andersen HA, Bartholomew LG, et al. Esophageal hiatal hernia: a 10-year study of medically treated cases. *JAMA* 1961;178:271–274.

87. Nissen R, Rossetti M, Siewert R. *Fundoplication und Gastropexie bei Refluxkrankheit und Hiatushernie. Indikation, Technik und Ergebnisse.* Stuttgart: Georg Thieme Verlag; 1981.

88. Hill L, Gelfand M, Bauermeister D. Simplified management of reflux esophagitis with stricture. *Ann Surg* 1970;172:638–651.

89. Boherema I. Hiatal hernia: gastropexia anterior geniculata. In: Nyhus L, Harkins H, eds. *Hernia*. Philadelphia: Lippincott; 1964:500.

90. Lam C, Gahagan T. The myth of the short oesophagus. In: Nyhus L, Harkins H, eds. *Hernia*. Philadelphia: Lippincott; 1964:450.

91. Nyhus LM, Harkins HN. The treatment of hiatal hernia and esophageal reflux by fundoplication. In: Nyhus L, Harkins H, eds. *Hernia*. Philadelphia: Lippincott; 1964.

92. Luketich JD, Grondin SC, Pearson FG. Minimally invasive approaches to acquired shortening of the esophagus: laparoscopic Collis–Nissen gastroplasty. *Semin Thorac Cardiovasc Surg* 2000;12: 173–178.

93. Low DE. Surgery for hiatal hernia and GERD. Time for reappraisal and a balanced approach? *Surg Endosc* 2001;15:913–917.

94. Peters JH, Heimbucher J, Kauer WK, et al. Clinical and physiologic comparison of laparoscopic and open Nissen fundoplication. *J Am Coll Surg* 1995;180:385–393.

95. Hinder RA, Filipi CJ, Wetscher G, et al. Laparoscopic Nissen fundoplication is an effective treatment for gastroesophageal reflux disease. *Ann Surg* 1994;220:472–483.

96. Cadiere GB, Houben JJ, Bruyns J, et al. Laparoscopic Nissen fundoplication: technique and preliminary results. *Br J Surg* 1994;81:400–403.

97. Kauer WK, Peters JH, DeMeester TR, et al. A tailored approach to antireflux surgery. *J Thorac Cardiovasc Surg* 1995;110:141–147.

98. Demeester SR, Demeester TR. Editorial comment: the short esophagus: going, going, gone? *Surgery* 2003;133:364–367.

99. Maziak DE, Todd TR, Pearson FG. Massive hiatus hernia: evaluation and surgical management. *J Thorac Cardiovasc Surg* 1998;115:53–60.

100. Skinner DB, Belsey RHR. Surgical management of esophageal reflux and hiatus hernia: Long-term results with 1030 patients. *J Thorac Cardiovasc Surg* 1967;53:33–54.

101. Hunter JG, Smith CD, Branum GD, et al. Laparoscopic fundoplication failures: Patterns of failure and response to fundoplication revision. *Ann Surg* 1999;230:595–606.

102. Rice TW. Why antireflux surgery fails. *Dig Dis* 2000;18:43–47.

103. Mattioli S, Di Simone MP, D'Ovidio F, et al. Surgical approaches for various grades of axial migration of the GEJ in GERD. Available at: CTS Net. The Society of Thoracic Surgeons. http://www.sts.org/ (accessed Aug. 29, 2006).

104. Sharma P, Morales TG, Sampliner RE. Short segment Barrett's esophagus. The need for standardization of the definition and of endoscopic criteria. *Am J Gastroenterol* 1998;93: 1033–1036.

105. McClave SA, Boyce HW Jr, Gottfried MR. Early diagnosis of columnar-lined esophagus: a new endoscopic diagnostic criterion. *Gastrointest Endosc* 1987;33:413–416.

106. Chandrasoma P, Makarewicz K, Wickramasinghe K, et al. A proposal for a new validated histological definition of the gastroesophageal junction. *Hum Pathol* 2006;37:40–47.

107. Chen LQ, Nastos D, Hu CY, et al. Results of the Collis-Nissen gastroplasty in patients with Barrett's esophagus. *Ann Thorac Surg* 1999;68:1014–1021.

108. Demos NJ, Kulkarni VA, Arago A. Video-assisted transthoracic hiatal hernioplasty using stapled, uncut gastroplasty and fundoplication. *Surg Rounds* 1994;XX:427–436.

109. Pearson FG, Cooer JD, Nelems JM. Gastroplasty and fundoplication in the management of complex reflux problems. *J Thorac Cardiovasc Surg* 1978;76:665–672.

110. Orringer MB, Orringer JS. The combined Collis-Nissen operation: early assessment of reflux control. *Ann Thorac Surg* 1982;33:534–539.

111. Stirling MC, Orringer MB. Continued assessment of the combined Collis-Nissen operation. *Ann Thorac Surg* 1989;47:224–230.

112. Urschel HC, Razzuk MA, Wood RE, et al. An improved surgical technique for the complicated hiatal hernia with gastroesophageal reflux. *Ann Thorac Surg* 1973;15:443–451.

113. Evangelist FA, Taylor FH, Alford JD. The modified Collis–Nissen operation for control of gastroesophageal reflux. *Ann Thorac Surg* 1978;26:107–111.

114. Mustard RA. A survey of techniques and results of hiatus hernia repair. *Surg Gynecol Obstet* 1970;130:131–136.

115. Pearson FG, Cooper JD, Patterson GA, et al. Gastroplasty and fundoplication for complex reflux problems. Long-term results. *Ann Surg* 1987;206:473–481.

116. Trastek VF, Deschamps C, Allen MS, et al. Uncut Collis-Nissen fundoplication: learning curve and long-term results. *Ann Thorac Surg* 1998;66:1739–1744.

117. Mattioli S, Lugaresi ML, Di Simone MP, et al. Laparoscopic and left thoracoscopic Collis-Nissen procedure: technique and short term results. *Chir Ital* 2005;57:183–191.

118. Pierre AF, Luketich JD, Fernando HC, et al. Results of laparoscopic repair of giant paraesophageal hernias: 200 consecutive patients. *Ann Thorac Surg* 2002;74:1909–1915.

119. Deschamps C, Trastek VF, Allen MS, et al. Long-term results after reoperation for failed antireflux procedures. *J Thorac Cardiovasc Surg* 1997;113:545–551.

120. Luketich JD, Fernando HC, Christie NA, et al. Outcomes after minimally invasive reoperation for gastroesophageal reflux disease. *Ann Thorac Surg* 2002;74:328–331.

121. Reilly KM, Jeyasingham K. A modified Pearson gastroplasty. *Thorax* 1984;39:67–69.

122. Nygaard K, Linaker O, Helsingen N, Jr. Esophageal hiatus hernia: a follow-up study. *Acta Chir Scand* 1964;128:293–302.

123. Collis JL. Surgical control of reflux in hiatus herina. *Am J Surg* 1968;115:465–471.

124. Gatzinsky P, Bergh NP. Hiatal hernia and shortened oesophagus. *Acta Chir Scand* 1979;145:159–166.

125. Maillet P, Boulez J, Baulieux J, Peix JL, Donne R. Peptic stenosis or esophageal carcinoma: difficulties of the pre-operative diagnostic and value of the surgical exploration (author's transl). *Chirurgie* 1980;106:719–721.

126. Moghissi K. Intrathoracic fundoplication for reflux stricture associated with short oesophagus. *Thorax* 1983;38:36–40.

127. Luketich JD, Grondin SC, Pearson FG. Minimally invasive approaches to acquired shortening of the esophagus: laparoscopic Collis-Nissen gastroplasty. *Semin Thorac Cardiovasc Surg* 2000;12:173–178.

39
Lengthening Gastroplasty for Managing Giant Paraesophageal Hernia

Kalpaj R. Parekh and Mark D. Iannettoni

The herniation of stomach into the thorax has been classified into four major types. The sliding hiatus hernia (type I), which is the commonest type and accounts for 95% of all cases, has the gastroesophageal (GE) junction as the leading point of the hernia.[1] The GE junction is herniated into the thorax in this type of hernia. The pure paraesophageal hernia (type II), which is extremely rare, is characterized by a GE junction that maintains its intra-abdominal position while the fundus herniates into the chest through the anterolateral hiatus. The majority of the paraesophageal hernias (type III) are a combination of the above two types, in which the GE junction is herniated along with the fundus into the thorax. Finally, type IV hernias are those in which other organs like colon, small intestine, and spleen are also present in the sac.

Paraesophageal hernias are likely to incarcerate or strangulate and may also present with a volvulus of the stomach, and hence often need to be operated on electively when diagnosed. Controversy exists about the role of surgery, the approach (transthoracic or transabdominal), and the need for esophageal lengthening during repair. Esophageal shortening is a result of long-standing gastroesophageal reflux disease wherein chronic irritation and injury leads to fibrosis and scarring of the esophagus.[2] This results in a relative shortening of the esophagus that cannot be reduced intra-abdominally at the time of repair, thereby precluding a tension-free repair. In this chapter we will review the incidence, preoperative and intra-operative evaluation of esophageal shortening, and the role of lengthening gastro-plasty in the management of giant paraesophageal hernias.

39.1. Preoperative Evaluation

The true incidence of the short esophagus in a giant paraesophageal hernia remains unknown. This is mainly because there is no single test that can accurately assess the degree of esophageal shortening preoperatively. Mittal and colleagues[3] analyzed the accuracy of preoperative assessment in predicting the true incidence of short esophagus at the time of surgery. The criteria used for diagnosis of short esophagus preoperatively in their study included (1) hiatal hernia 5cm or larger on upright esophagogram, (2) large paraesophageal hernia (>5cm), (3) stricture formation or Barrett's esophagus as evaluated by endoscopy, and (4) manometric esophageal length two standard deviations below their laboratory mean for height. Using these criteria they identified 39 patients as having a preoperative diagnosis of short esophagus. However, intraoperatively, only eight patients required an esophageal lengthening procedure. The remaining 31 patients did not require an esophageal lengthening procedure, and intra-operative mobilization was sufficient to allow the gastroesophageal junction to lie below the diaphragmatic crus. They concluded that, in their experience, the most sensitive preoperative test was an endoscopic finding of either a stricture or Barrett's esophagus for predicting the need for lengthening. Another study from the same institution showed similar results, with the sensitivity of 61% for an endoscopy in predicting esophageal shortening.[4]

Altorki and colleagues demonstrated that 77% of their patients had the gastroesophageal junction in the mediastinum, based on a preoperative barium swallow. However, none of their patients required a lengthening gastroplasty. In contrast, Maziak and colleagues[5] noted that 91 of their 94 patients had their gastroesophageal junction in the thorax and 75 of their patients ended up requiring a lengthening gastroplasty. The authors used manometry to measure the length of the esophagus between the upper and lower sphincters in 13 patients and found that the mean length in patients with giant paraesophageal hernias was significantly lower compared to matched normal controls.

In summary, all patients with giant paraesophageal hernias should have a barium swallow and esophagoscopy prior to hernia repair. Manometry and acid testing are not very reliable in this group of patients. However, the most accurate way of determining esophageal shortening is in the operating room at the time of repair.

39.2. Lengthening Gastroplasty: Is It Necessary? What Is the Ideal Technique?

The role of esophageal lengthening gastroplasty remains a controversial point among clinicians as the true incidence of shortening is unknown. While there are no prospective, randomized, controlled trials comparing the outcomes with or without lengthening gastroplasty in patients with giant paraesophageal hernias, there are several reports of retrospective single-institution experiences.

The lengthening Collis gastroplasty is seeing an increasing application in the management of giant paraesophageal hernias in order to decrease the incidence of recurrent herniation. While there is consensus among most surgeons about the importance of adequate esophageal mobilization, there is no consensus about the role of lengthening gastroplasty.

Traditionally, the majority of the paraesophageal hernia repairs were open repairs either via a transabdominal or transthoracic approach. In recent years laparoscopic repairs of these hernias have shown mixed outcomes. Experienced centers have good results with this technique, while others report a high recurrence rate.

Maziak and colleagues, using an open transthoracic approach, added a lengthening gastroplasty in 80% of their patients and had a very low recurrence rate of 2% over a median follow-up of 72 months. In another large open transthoracic series ($n = 240$) from the University of Michigan, Patel and associates reported an addition of lengthening gastroplasty in the majority of their patients (96%) and reported an anatomical recurrence in 7.9% of the patients. These two retrospective reviews set a benchmark for outcomes following repairs of paraesophageal hernia as they have a large number of patients and a good follow-up. In contrast, there are two reviews where a lengthening gastroplasty was not routinely used in an open repair. Low and coworkers report their experience with 72 patients where a lengthening gastroplasty was not added in any patient and had a recurrence rate of 18% after a mean follow-up of 30 months. Similarly, Williamson and colleagues report a recurrence of 11% after a median follow-up of 61 months. There is one report by Geha and colleagues where a lengthening gastroplasty was added in only 2% of the patients and on a routine postoperative swallow no recurrences were identified. However, there is no long-term follow-up available in these patients and the timing of obtaining the barium swallow is not clear. Based on these results it is fair to say that addition of lengthening gastroplasty is associated with a lower rate of anatomical recurrences following paraesophageal hernia repair. Table 39.1 summarizes results of open technique for the repair.

These results are corroborated in the technically challenging laparoscopic approach for paraesophageal hernia repair. The University of Pittsburgh experience published by Pierre and coworkers[6] sets the standard for the laparoscopic technique. The authors reported their experience on 200 patients with a recurrence rate of 2.5% after a median follow-up of 18 months. They performed a lengthening gastroplasty on 56% of their patients using a laparoscopic approach. Several other series reported a high rate of

TABLE 39.1. Outcomes of paraesophageal hernia repairs following open technique.

Reference	Year	N	Lengthening gastroplasty	Anatomical recurrence	Follow-up	Level of evidence
Williamson[13]	1993	119	1 (0.8%)	11%	61 months (median)	3
Allen[14]	1993	124	81 (68%)	na	42 months (median)	3
Maziak[5]	1998	94	75 (80%)	2 (2%)	72 months (median)	3
Altorki[15]	1998	47	0 (0%)	3 (6.3%)	45 months (median)	3
Geha[16]	2000	100	2 (2%)	0 (0%)	na	3
Patel[1]	2004	240	231 (96%)	19 (7.9%)	42 months (median)	3
Low[17]	2005	72	0 (0%)	11 (18%)	30 months (mean)	3

Abbreviation: na, not available.

recurrence using the laparoscopic approach[7-11] when a lengthening gastroplasty was not routinely used for esophageal shortening. Table 39.2 summarizes the results following the laparoscopic technique of paraesophageal hernia repair. Andujar and colleagues in their experience with the laparoscopic technique report a 5% incidence of anatomical recurrence for the paraesophageal hernia; however, they also report a 20% incidence of a recurrent sliding hernia in their follow-up swallows. True paraesophageal hernias are rare and most of them are a combination of sliding and paraesophageal hernias. Although some authors argue about the clinical significance of asymptomatic anatomical recurrences on postoperative barium swallow, there is no long-term follow-up available on these asymptomatic anatomical recurrences. There is only one report, by Hashemi and associates,[12] which compares the open techniques with laparoscopic techniques. They performed a lengthening gastroplasty in only one of their 54 patients. In their experience laparoscopic technique had a higher rate of recurrence (42% vs. 15%) compared to open technique.

Thus, published data suggests that addition of a lengthening gastroplasty is associated with a lower incidence of recurrent herniation by open or laparoscopic technique. The evidence (level of

TABLE 39.2. Outcomes of paraesophageal hernia repair following laparoscopic technique.

Author	Year	N	Lengthening gastroplasty	Anatomical recurrence	Follow-up	Level of evidence
Trus[18]	1997	76	6 (7.9%)	9 (11%)		3
Dahlberg[9]	2001	37	1 (2.7%)	4 (13%)	15 months (median)	3
Wiechmann[11]	2001	60	0 (0%)	3/44 (9%)	6 months	3
Mattar[7]	2002	136	6 (5%)	14/32 (43%)	40 months (mean)	3
Pierre[6]	2002	203	112 (56%)	5 (2.5%)	18 months (median)	3
Jobe[8]	2002	52	0 (0%)	11/34 (32%)	37 months (mean)	3
Diaz[10]	2003	116	6 (5%)	21 (32%)		3
Andujar[19]	2004	166	0 (0%)	6 (5%)[a]	15 months (mean)	3
				24 (20%)[b]		

[a]Recurrent paraesophageal hernias.
[b]Recurrent sliding hernias.

evidence 3) suggests that all patients with giant paraesophageal hernia repair should have an open repair (recommendation grade C) and a lengthening gastroplasty should be added if there is any question of esophageal shortening (recommendation grade C). Laparoscopic repairs can be performed with good results in experienced hands.

> Addition of a lengthening gastroplasty is associated with a lower incidence of recurrent herniation after repair of giant paraesophageal hernia by open or laparoscopic technique. A lengthening gastroplasty should be added if there is any question of esophageal shortening (level of evidence 3; recommendation grade C).

At our institution, we evaluate all patients with paraesophageal hernia with a barium swallow and an endoscopy at the time of the operation. Manometry is not routinely performed on these patients. Intraoperatively we perform the repair via a left thoracotomy and routinely perform a Collis gastroplasty along with a Nissen fundoplication on majority of our patients.

In summary, the incidence of esophageal shortening in giant paraesophageal hernia is unknown. There is no single preoperative investigation that can identify all patients with true esophageal shortening and the most definitive way of determining shortening is intraoperatively. The data suggests that the recurrence rate following repair is higher if a lengthening gastroplasty is not used routinely in cases of esophageal shortening.

References

1. Patel HJ, Tan BB, Yee J, Orringer MB, Iannettoni MD. A 25-year experience with open primary transthoracic repair of paraesophageal hiatal hernia. *J Thorac Cardiovasc Surg* 2004;127:843–849.

2. Mattioli S, D'Ovidio F, Di Simone MP, et al. Clinical and surgical relevance of the progressive phases of intrathoracic migration of the gastroesophageal junction in gastroesophageal reflux disease. *J Thorac Cardiovasc Surg* 1998;116:267–275.

3. Mittal SK, Awad ZT, Tasset M, et al. The preoperative predictability of the short esophagus in patients with stricture or paraesophageal hernia. *Surg Endosc* 2000;14:464–468.

4. Awad ZT, Mittal SK, Roth TA, Anderson PI, Wilfley WA Jr, Filipi CJ. Esophageal shortening during the era of laparoscopic surgery. *World J Surg* 2001;25:558–561.

5. Maziak DE, Todd TR, Pearson FG. Massive hiatus hernia: evaluation and surgical management. *J Thorac Cardiovasc Surg* 1998;115:53–60; discussion 61–62.

6. Pierre AF, Luketich JD, Fernando HC, et al. Results of laparoscopic repair of giant paraesophageal hernias: 200 consecutive patients. *Ann Thorac Surg* 2002;74:1909–1915; discussion 1915–1916.

7. Mattar SG, Bowers SP, Galloway KD, Hunter JG, Smith CD. Long-term outcome of laparoscopic repair of paraesophageal hernia. *Surg Endosc* 2002;16:745–749.

8. Jobe BA, Aye RW, Deveney CW, Domreis JS, Hill LD. Laparoscopic management of giant type III hiatal hernia and short esophagus. Objective follow-up at three years. *J Gastrointest Surg* 2002; 6:181–188; discussion 188.

9. Dahlberg PS, Deschamps C, Miller DL, Allen MS, Nichols FC, Pairolero PC. Laparoscopic repair of large paraesophageal hiatal hernia. *Ann Thorac Surg* 2001;72:1125–1129.

10. Diaz S, Brunt LM, Klingensmith ME, Frisella PM, Soper NJ. Laparoscopic paraesophageal hernia repair, a challenging operation: medium-term outcome of 116 patients. *J Gastrointest Surg* 2003; 7:59–66; discussion 67.

11. Wiechmann RJ, Ferguson MK, Naunheim KS, et al. Laparoscopic management of giant paraesophageal herniation. *Ann Thorac Surg* 2001;71:1080–1086; discussion 1086–1087.

12. Hashemi M, Peters JH, DeMeester TR, et al. Laparoscopic repair of large type III hiatal hernia: objective followup reveals high recurrence rate. *J Am Coll Surg* 2000;190:553–560; discussion 560–561.

13. Williamson WA, Ellis FH Jr, Streitz JM Jr, Shahian DM. Paraesophageal hiatal hernia: is an antireflux procedure necessary? *Ann Thorac Surg* 1993;56:447–451; discussion 451–452.

14. Allen MS, Trastek VF, Deschamps C, Pairolero PC. Intrathoracic stomach. Presentation and results of operation. *J Thorac Cardiovasc Surg* 1993;105:253–258; discussion 258–259.

15. Altorki NK, Yankelevitz D, Skinner DB. Massive hiatal hernias: the anatomic basis of repair. *J Thorac Cardiovasc Surg* 1998;115:828–835.

16. Geha AS, Massad MG, Snow NJ, Baue AE. A 32-year experience in 100 patients with giant paraesophageal hernia: the case for abdominal approach and selective antireflux repair. *Surgery* 2000;128:623–630.

17. Low DE, Unger T. Open repair of paraesophageal hernia: reassessment of subjective and objective outcomes. *Ann Thorac Surg* 2005;80:287–294.

18. Trus TL, Bax T, Richardson WS, et al. Complications of laparoscopic paraesophageal hernia repair. *J Gastrointest Surg* 1997;1:221–228.

19. Andujar JJ, Papasavas PK, Birdas T, et al. Laparoscopic repair of large paraesophageal hernia is associated with a low incidence of recurrence and reoperation. *Surg Endosc* 2004;18:444–447.

40
Management of Zenker's Diverticulum: Open Versus Transoral Approaches

Douglas E. Paull and Alex G. Little

Pharyngoesophageal (Zenker's) diverticulum is a false diverticulum of the cervical esophagus. This pulsion diverticulum is composed of mucosa, covered by thin areolar tissue, herniating at Killian's triangle between the obliquely positioned inferior constrictor muscle and the transversely oriented cricopharyngeus muscle. Pharyngoesophageal diverticulum was first described by Abraham Ludlow in 1764[1] as a "bag formed in pharynx." Friedrich Albert Zenker in 1867 described the clinicopathological characteristics of 23 previous cases and 5 of his own cases in *Kraukenheiten Des Oesophagus*.[1,2] The pathophysiology of Zenker's diverticulum has been attributed to functional abnormalities of the upper esophageal sphincter zone created by the cricopharyngeus muscle. Cricopharyngeal spasm and achalasia, cricopharyngeal incoordination, impaired upper esophageal sphincter opening, and structural changes of the cricopharyngeal muscle have all been implicated in the etiology of Zenker's diverticulum.[3,4]

The incidence of Zenker's diverticulum is 2 per 100,000/year and it is more common in men than women.[5] Patients mainly present in the seventh and eighth decades of life. The disease is rare in patients before the age of 40.[6,7] Patients may have symptoms for years prior to the diagnosis. Typical symptoms include dysphagia and regurgitation. Patients may also complain of halitosis, choking, cough, weight loss, and/or hoarseness. Aspiration of food may lead to pneumonia and lung abscess. Massive bleeding from ulcers in the diverticulum is unusual, but may require urgent intervention.[8] Cancer in the diverticulum is rare, but symptoms that suggest such a possibility include hemoptysis/hematemesis, complete esophageal obstruction, and a sudden increase in chronic symptoms.[9] The only physical finding of Zenker's diverticulum is Boyce's sign, the gurgling sensation and noise generated beneath the examiner's fingertips as the neck mass is compressed.[5]

Zenker's diverticulum is easily identified on barium swallow and video fluoroscopy. Unless signs or symptoms suggest the rare malignancy, most authors do not recommend preoperative endoscopy given the hazard of perforation. Although the diverticulum originates posteriorly, it usually projects to the patient's left neck and inferiorly, towards the mediastinum. The diverticulum can be staged according to size using either the Brombart or Lahey classifications.[10,11] Diverticular size is defined as small (<2 cm), medium (2–4 cm), or large (>4 cm). Diverticular size plays an important role in the selection of therapy.

There is no viable medical treatment option for Zenker's diverticulum, although esophageal dilation and Botox injection have been utilized with poor results. The surgical treatment options are of two types: open and transoral endoscopic procedures. Open procedures include (1) myotomy alone for small diverticula; (2) myotomy and diverticulectomy; and (3) myotomy and diverticulopexy. Endoscopic procedures include (1) the Dohlman procedure utilizing diathermy or laser and (2) endoscopic stapling. The purpose of this chapter is to compare and contrast the techniques, complications, and results of open versus endoscopic procedures. Level of evidence and grade of recommendation for the procedures are provided in the concluding summary.

40.1. Open Approaches

40.1.1. Open Techniques

Although myotomy alone has been accomplished under local anesthesia, the majority of patients undergoing an open procedure will benefit from general anesthesia for comfort and to prevent aspiration.[12] A left lateral cervical incision along the anterior border of the sternocleidomastoid muscle is the most common approach. The carotid sheath is gently retracted laterally, the larynx retracted medially, and the omohyoid muscle either divided or retracted inferiorly. The middle thyroid vein and inferior thyroid artery are divided. The diverticulum is carefully dissected free from its attachments to surrounding tissues. Placement of a 28F to 50F bougie in the esophagus facilitates the dissection and prevents compromise of the esophageal lumen at diverticulectomy. Most authors believe myotomy is the indispensable component of an operation for Zenker's diverticulum. Cricopharyngeal myotomy is performed posterolaterally, avoiding any injury to the recurrent laryngeal nerve. (See Figure 40.1)

Following the myotomy, in all but patients with small diverticula, either diverticulectomy or diverticulopexy is performed. Recent experiences utilizing endoscopic staplers for diverticulectomy, especially with 3.5-mm staples, report a low leak rate and early resumption of oral diet compared to results after excision and suturing.[13] Publications on patients undergoing myotomy and stapled diverticulectomy have reported resumption of liquid diet on postoperative day 1 and discharge to home by postoperative day 3.[14]

Proponents of diverticulopexy claim a lower rate of fistula, mediastinitis, and stricture; a quicker resumption of diet; and shorter hospital stay when compared to diverticulectomy. After the sac is dissected, it is oriented superiorly, and sewn to the prevertebral fascia. The sac then empties by gravity into the esophagus. Bremner recommends using diverticulum size to select patients and employs diverticulectomy for sacs

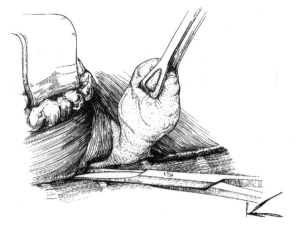

FIGURE 40.1. Open procedure. Approach is via a left cervical incision. The thyroid and larynx are gently retracted medially, the carotid sheath laterally. Diverticulum has been completely dissected from surrounding tissues. Cricopharyngeal myotomy is shown being performed posterolaterally, avoiding the recurrent laryngeal nerve. The diverticulum is subsequently either resected or suspended as described in the text.

more than 5cm and diverticulopexy for sacs less than 5cm.[15] Diverticulopexy has been suggested to be the preferred treatment of debilitated patients with concurrent illness to avoid the risk of a suture/staple line leak.

40.1.2. Results of Open Operation

By far the largest reported series of open diverticulectomy, which included patients with and without myotomy, for Zenker's diverticulum is by Payne at the Mayo Clinic in 1983.[16] In this landmark study of 888 patients, 93% of patients were improved at a follow-up of 14 years. Operative mortality was 1.2%, and recurrence occurred in 3.6% of patients. Allen, reporting in 1995 on a subset of the same patients, noted a fistula rate of 3% and vocal cord dysfunction in 3.1%.[17] Barthlen (1990) reviewed 43 patients with Zenker's diverticulum undergoing open procedures, of whom 32 were treated by myotomy and diverticulectomy.[6] There was no mortality, no recurrence, and 82% of postoperative patients were completely asymptomatic. Crescenzo (1998) studied 75 patients treated with an open procedure, 57 undergoing myotomy and diverticulectomy.[18] There were no deaths, a 5.3% fistula rate was reported, the hospital stay averaged 5 days, and 94% of patients were significantly improved. The most common cause of late death was coronary artery disease.

Alternative open procedures have excellent results as well. Laccoudeye (1994), Fraczek (1998), and Konowitz (1989) all demonstrated fewer leaks and shorter hospital stay for their diverticulopexy patients compared to their diverticulectomy patients.[19-21] Schmit (1992) reported on 48 patients with small diverticula undergoing myotomy alone under local anesthesia.[12] Mortality was 2.1%, hospital stay was 2.7 days, and 70% of patients had good to excellent results.

Manometric abnormalities generally improve following myotomy and diverticulectomy. Preoperative versus postoperative findings include pharyngoesophageal dyscoordination in 45% versus 8%, late relaxation of the upper esophageal sphincter in 50% versus 8%, and incomplete relaxation in 38% versus 8%.[6] Normal manometric findings are present in only 40% of preoperative patients and this increases to 92% of patients postoperatively. Postoperative barium swallow studies may show a residual diverticulum, cricopharyngeal bar, indentation, or aspiration.[22] However, multiple studies have demonstrated no correlation between these postoperative radiographic abnormalities and the presence or absence of recurrent symptoms.

As shown in Table 40.1, open myotomy and diverticulectomy is a time-tested operation for Zenker's diverticulum. Meticulous surgical technique results in low mortality in an elderly patient population with multiple comorbidities. Success rates are outstanding and enduring. The primary disadvantages of open procedures include significant complication rates and relatively long hospital stays; the more serious complications of fistula and vocal cord paralysis are relatively infrequent. Open diverticulopexy, compared to diverticulectomy, appears to have similar outcomes with a low risk of complications, earlier resumption of diet, and shorter hospital stays. One advantage of open diverticulectomy over endoscopic stapling or open diverticulopexy is the removal of the sac. Carcinoma has been reported in 0.4% to 3.7% of Zenker's diverticula.[23] For this reason, even some proponents of endoscopic stapling suggest a role for open diverticulectomy and myotomy in younger patients.[24]

In summary, the results of open procedures for Zenker's diverticulum can be characterized as demonstrating: (1) a high degree of success; (2) low mortality; (3) a low recurrence rate; and (4) durable results upon long-term follow-up. This is accomplished with a complication rate of approximately 10%, although most complications are of a minor nature.[6,7,16,18-21,25]

TABLE 40.1. Open procedures for Zenker's diverticulum.

Study (year)	Operation	No. patients	Complications[a]	Mortality	Success[b]	Recurrence[c]	Follow-up (months)
Payne[16] (1983)	D + M	888	6.1%	1.2%	93%	3.6%	60–168
Konowitz[19] (1989)	D,P + M	32	18%	0%	100%	0%	5–60
Barthlen[6] (1990)	D + M	43	9.3%	0%	82%	0%	25
Laccourreye[20] (1994)	D,P + M	43	30%	2.3%	100%	0%	6–24
Bonafede[7] (1997)	D + M	87	24%	3.4%	90%	1%	7.5
Fraczek[21] (1998)	D,P + M	37	46%	0%	95%	0%	1–228
Crescenzo[18] (1998)	D + M	75	11%	0%	94%	5.3%	40
Feeley[25] (1999)	D + M	24	37%	0%	100%	0%	18
Total/weighted average		1186	11%	1.0%	92%	3%	95[d]

Abbreviations: D + M, majority of patients in study underwent diverticulectomy and myotomy; D,P + M, patients underwent diverticulopexy or diverticulectomy and mytomy.
[a]Complications include aspiration, fistula, hematoma, mediastinitis, myocardial infarction, pneumonia, stricture, wound infection, urinary tract infection, and vocal cord paralysis.
[b]Success defined as good-to-excellent result with either no symptoms or improved symptoms postoperatively.
[c]Recurrence defined as recurrent symptoms requiring a second operation.
[d]Total number of follow-up months /1186 total patients.

40.2. Endoscopic Approaches

40.2.1. Background

Transoral endoscopic surgery, dividing the crico-pharyngeal bar between the sac and the esophagus, was first performed by Mosher in 1917.[26] Dohlman, in 1935, introduced a specialized diverticuloscope and cautery into the endoscopic armamentarium and reported on a series of 100 patients so treated in 1960.[27] Overbeek further refined the endoscopic approach with the use of a 400-mm-lens operating microscope, allowing more precise division of the common wall.[28] In 1993, Collard introduced the use of the linear stapler to divide the tissue bridge to obtain a secure closure, reducing the risk of mediastinitis and bleeding.[29]

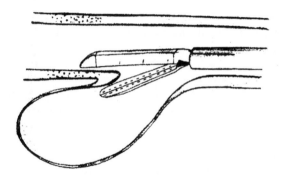

FIGURE 40.2. Endoscopic stapling. Via the Weerda diverticuloscope, not shown, the endoscopic stapler is inserted, with the stapler cartridge in the esophageal lumen and the cutting platform blade in the diverticulum. Firing the stapler creates a V-shaped opening between the sac and esophagus, forming a common cavity. Depending on the size of the pouch, more than one stapling application may be required.

40.2.2. Endoscopic Techniques

General anesthesia is employed and the patient is placed in the supine position with the neck extended. A dental guard helps prevent tooth injuries from the rigid diverticuloscope. A Weerda diverticuloscope is inserted transorally with the long tip placed in the esophagus and the shorter tip in the sac. The instrument is gently spread, exposing the bar of tissue separating the posterior sac lumen from the anterior esophageal lumen. The scope is held in place with the aid of a chest support. A telescope with an attached camera and monitor provide excellent exposure. The pouch is inspected, debris is removed, and cancer is excluded. An endoscopic linear cutting stapler is used to divide the exposed bridge of tissue. A V-shaped opening between the sac and esophagus is created, forming a common cavity. Endoscopic sutures may be placed for traction prior to application of the stapler. Depending on the size/length of the pouch, a second, and rarely a third, stapling application may be required. A small residual spur often results, but it is safer to under divide than risk perforation and mediastinitis. (See Figure 40.2)

When perforation does occur, it is usually detected intraoperatively and can be treated with endoscopic suture, conversion to an open procedure, or conservative treatment with antibiotics and nothing by mouth.[30] The postoperative care

of the uneventful endoscopic stapling usually includes a liquid diet within 6 to 12h and discharge by postoperative day 1 or 2. While a chest X ray is often routinely performed to exclude cervical/subcutaneous/mediastinal emphysema; a postoperative barium swallow study is not usually obtained.

There are other endoscopic techniques besides stapling. The Dohlman procedure is similar to the stapling approach but either a carbon dioxide (CO_2) laser or electrocautery are utilized to divide the tissue between the diverticulum and the esophagus to create a common cavity. In an effort to avoid general anesthesia altogether, a number of authors have reported the use of a soft diverticuloscope and flexible endoscopy, with division of the tissue bar utilizing a needle knife papillotome or argon plasma coagulator.[31]

40.2.3. Results of Endoscopic Techniques

A review of over 29 papers involving patients undergoing endoscopic stapling by Sen revealed that: general anesthesia was applied in all cases; 80% of the cases were performed in Europe; endoscopic stapling was abandoned in 0% to 30% of patients because of limited neck extension, prominent incisors, a small diverticulum, or a mucosal tear; patients resumed a diet within 24h postoperatively; and the hospital length of stay was 2 to 3 days.[32] Complications occurred in 0%

to 17% of patients, and mortality was 0.43%. In short-term follow-up, 53% to 100% of patients had complete resolution of symptoms. Postma, in a review of five series totaling 230 patients undergoing endoscopic stapling, reported a complication rate of only 0% to 3%.[33]

Complications such as vocal cord paralysis, an occasional complication of open procedures, are exceedingly rare after endoscopic stapling.[34] As shown in Table 40.2, advantages of endoscopic stapling include (1) shortened operating/anesthesia time; (2) early resumption of oral intake; (3) short hospital stay; (4) few complications and low mortality; (5) ease of application in open failures; and (6) excellent symptom relief.[25,35–49] Manometric studies following endoscopic stapling have consistently demonstrated a reduction of intrabolus pressure and upper esophageal sphincter pressures.[35,40]

Possible disadvantages of endoscopic stapling include: (1) difficulty in managing small (<2 cm) diverticula; (2) stapling difficulty due to exposure problems secondary to cervical arthritis or craniofacial abnormalities; (3) relatively high symptom recurrence rates; (4) residual pouch; (5) persistence of sac and possibilities of future cancer; and (6) lack of information on long-term outcomes because of relatively short follow-up.

Proponents of endoscopic stapling point out that recurrent symptoms are rather easily handled by a second, or in some cases, a third stapling. Small sacs can be treated utilizing traction sutures or converted to endoscopic laser treatment. Studies document a residual pouch in nearly 100% of patients undergoing endoscopic stapling.[50] This is in contrast to the much lower incidence in postoperative open procedure patients. However, the presence of a small pouch distal to the cricopharyngeus appears to have no correlation to symptoms.

Von Doersten reviewed 40 cases of the Dohlman procedure in which electrocautery was utilized to divide the tissue bridge.[51] Operative time was 41 min. Average hospital stay was 4.5 days. There were no postoperative deaths. Pneumomediastinum occurred in 4 (10%) of patients, but all responded to conservative treatment without reoperation. Thirty-seven (92%) of the 40 patients

TABLE 40.2. Endoscopic stapling for Zenker's diverticulum.

Study (year)	No. patients	Converted to open[a]	Complications[b]	Mortality	Success[c]	Recurrence[d]	Follow-up (months)
Baldwin[38] (1998)	51	2%	2%	0%	100%	0%	15.5
Scher[49] (1998)	36	5%	3%	0%	89%	5%	9.3
Peracchia[35] (1998)	95	3%	0%	0%	98%	5%	23
Narne[40] (1999)	102	4%	0%	0%	100%	4%	16
Omote[42] (1999)	21	0%	5%	5%	95%	0%	12
Cook[39] (2000)	74	8%	3%	0%	96%	9%	17
Phillipsen[44] (2000)	14	14%	7%	0%	100%	14%	na
Luscher[37] (2000)	23	0%	4%	0%	96%	4%	12
Sood[41] (2000)	44	0%	22%	2%	95%	9%	na
Jaramillo[43] (2001)	32	16%	4%	0%	87%	7%	24
Thaler[45] (2001)	23	30%	0%	0%	87%	13%	1–24
Raut[47] (2002)	25	8%	8%	0%	61%	35%	24–60
Stoeckli[36] (2002)	30	10%	27%	0%	96%	4%	13
Chiari[48] (2003)	46	15%	10%	0%	85%	11%	na
Chang[46] (2003)	159	6%	7%	0%	98%	11%	32
Total/weighted Average	798	7%	6%	0.2%	92%	8%	21[e]

Abbreviation: na, not applicable.
[b]Complications including aspiration, bleeding, cervical emphysema, cervical spine irritation, dental injury, mediastinitis, myocardial infarction, pharyngeal perforation, pneumonia, postoperative fever, urinary tract infection, and vocal cord paralysis.
[a]Converted to an open procedure because of insufficient exposure (limited neck extension, retrognathia, etc.) or mucosal tear.
[c]Success defined as good-to-excellent result with either no symptoms or improved symptoms postoperatively.
[d]Recurrence defined as recurrent symptoms requiring a second operation.
[e]Total number of follow-up months/798 total patients.

TABLE 40.3. Open versus endoscopic procedures for Zenker's diverticulum: retrospective studies.

Study (year)	Operation	No.	OR (min)		LOS (days)		Complications (%)		Mortality (%)		Success[a] (%)	
			Open	Endoscopic	Open	Endoscopic	Open	Endoscopic	Open	Endoscopic	Open	Endoscopic
Van Eeden[55] (1999)	O vs. ES	37	na	na	4.0	2.3	23	6	0	0	70	88
Zbaren[60] (1999)	O vs. D	97	na	na	11.4	8	15	6.4	1.5	0	94	97
Smith[56] (2002)	O vs. ES	16	88	25	5.2	1.3	0	6	0	0	100	100
Mirza[57] (2002)	O vs. ES	43	na	na	8.5	3.0	13	15	0	0	91	55
Zaninotto[58] (2003)	O vs. ES	58	80	20	9	5	9	0	0	0	100	87
Safdar[59] (2004)	O vs. ES	19	105	25	10	3.9	22	0	0	0	100	100
Chang[61] (2004)	O vs. D	49	107	47	5	4	14	8	0	0	100	90
Total/average		319	95	29	7.6	3.9	13.7	5.9	0.2	0	94	88

Abbreviations: D, majority of endoscopic patients having Dohlman procedure; Endo, endoscopic procedure; ES, majority of endoscopic patients having endoscopic stapling; LOS, length of hospital stay postoperatively; na, not applicable; O/open, open diveticulectomy and myotomy group; OR, operating room.
[a]Success defined as good-to-excellent result with either no symptoms or improved symptoms postoperatively.

were asymptomatic at an average follow-up of 42 months.

The results of treatment of Zenker's diverticulum using the endoscopic CO_2 laser to divide the tissue bridge are also favorable. In one study of 119 patients treated with CO_2 laser, there were no cases of postoperative mediastinitis, and 90% of patients were asymptomatic at 1-to 3-year follow-up.[52] Nyrop reported on 61 patients endoscopically treated with the CO_2 laser.[53] Eight percent had postoperative emphysema in the neck and 3% of patients developed evidence of mediastinitis; all of the latter were successfully treated with antibiotics and nasogastric feeding. Ninety-two percent of patients were satisfied with the result, and 70% were asymptomatic at a median follow-up of 37 months.

40.2.4. Open Verus Endoscopic Approaches: Retrospective Studies

Seventy-five percent of surgeons perform fewer than three operations for Zenker's diverticulum per year. The choice of open procedure or endoscopic stapling varies. Endoscopic stapling is the procedure of choice among 83% of British surgeons but is less commonly performed in the United States.[54] Otolaryngologists are more likely to favor endoscopic stapling.

Unfortunately, there is no randomized, controlled trial of open procedures versus endoscopic stapling for Zenker's diverticulum. There have been a number of retrospective studies directly

comparing the results of the two techniques. Several literature reviews from 1990–2002 have been conducted specifically comparing open to endoscopic procedures for Zenker's diverticulum, as seen in Table 40.3.[55-61] Endoscopic stapling has a shorter operative duration, lower complication rate, lower mortality rate, shorter hospital stay, and shorter time to oral intake than open procedures. Both endoscopic stapling and open procedure patients provide good relief of symptoms. However, long-term follow-up is lacking for endoscopic stapling, whereas open procedures have known, durable results. Furthermore, recent studies of open procedures using endoscopic staplers have demonstrated hospital stays of 2 days, rivaling that for endoscopic stapling.[14]

40.3. Recurrent Zenker's Diverticulum

Re-operative diverticulectomy and myotomy for recurrent Zenker's diverticulum following a failed open procedure is typically successful, albeit with a higher mortality and morbidity rate. Huang (1984) reported on open diverticulectomy for 31 recurrent patients.[62] Six of 31 developed a postoperative fistula, and altogether 35% patients had postoperative complications. Of 28 evaluable patients, 27 had a good to excellent result. Payne (1992) reported a mortality of 3% and a morbidity of 51% in a large series of patients undergoing redo open operation.[63]

Scher published the outcomes of 18 patients with recurrent Zenker's diverticulum treated with endoscopic stapling.[64] The primary operation was an open procedure in nine cases and endoscopic stapling in nine cases. There were no perioperative complications and all patients were discharged by postoperative day 2. Symptom relief occurred in 16 of 18 patients.

40.4. Conclusions

Based on our review, the following observations can be made[65]:

1. Both open and endoscopic approaches provide equivalent early results in experienced hands (level of evidence 2+; recommendation grade B).

2. Since longer follow-up is available with the open approach, it remains the standard. However, intermediate follow-up of endoscopically treated patients with stapling and longer term follow-up with the Dohlman procedure suggest similar outcomes. Endoscopic approaches may eventually prove to be preferable in the majority of patients, especially the elderly, with medium-sized pouches. Complications are minimal, and relief of symptoms is high. Patients who have limitation of neck extension, retrognathia, goiters, or other exposure problems prohibiting stapler use may undergo either an open procedure or endoscopic laser treatment depending on the surgeon's preference and skill (level of evidence 2++; recommendation grade B).

3. Patients with a small diverticulum, less than 2 cm, should undergo open myotomy (level of evidence 2++; recommendation grade B).

4. Patients who develop a mucosal tear during endoscopic stapling may be repaired endoscopically, treated conservatively, or converted to an open procedure depending on the particular clinical circumstance (level of evidence 2++; recommendation grade B).

5. Patients with recurrent pouch after previous open procedure are probably best approached by endoscopic stapling given the high complication rate associated with redo open procedures (level of evidence 3; recommendation grade D).

6. Patients with suspected cancer in the pouch based on symptoms, barium studies, or endoscopy should undergo open diverticulectomy and myotomy (level of evidence 3; recommendation grade D).

> Both open and endoscopic approaches provide equivalent early results in experienced hands (level of evidence 2++; recommendation grade B).
>
> Patients with a small diverticulum (<2 cm) should undergo open myotomy (level of evidence 2++; recommendation grade B).
>
> Patients with a recurrent pouch after previous open procedure are best approached by endoscopic stapling (level of evidence 3; recommendation grade D).

References

1. Ferguson MK. Evolution of therapy for pharyngoesophageal (Zenker's) diverticulum. *Ann Thorac Surg* 1991;51:848–852.
2. Aly A, Devitt PG, Jamieson GG. Evolution of surgical treatment for pharyngeal pouch. *Br J Surg* 2004;91:657–664.
3. Knuff TE, Benjamin SB, Castell DO. Pharyngoesophageal (Zenker's) diverticulum: a reappraisal. *Gastroenterology* 1982;82:734–736.
4. Zaninotto G, Costantini M, Boccu C, et al. Functional and morphological study of the cricopharyngeal muscle in patients with Zenker's diverticulum. *Br J Surg* 1996;83:1263–1267.
5. Siddiq MA, Sood S, Strachan D. Pharyngeal pouch (Zenker's diverticulum). *Postgrad Med J* 2001;77:506–511.
6. Barthlen W, Feussner H, Hannig C, et al. Surgical therapy of Zenker's diverticulum: low risk and high efficiency. *Dysphagia* 1990;5:13–19.
7. Bonafede JP, Lavertu P, Wood BG, et al. Surgical outcome in 87 patients with Zenker's diverticulum. *Laryngoscope* 1997;107:720–725.
8. Kensing KP, White JG, Korompai F, et al. Massive bleeding from a Zenker's diverticulum. *South Med J* 1994;87:1003–1004.
9. Johnson JT, Curtin HD. Carcinoma associated with Zenker's diverticulum. *Ann Otol Rhinol Laryngol* 1985:94:324–325.
10. Colombo-Benkmann M, Unruh V, Krieglstein C, et al. Cricopharyngeal myotomy in the treatment

of Zenker's diverticulum. *J Am Coll Surg* 2003;196: 370–378.

11. Ponette E, Coolen J. Radiological aspects of Zenker's diverticulum. *Hepatogastroenterology* 1992;39:115–122.

12. Schmit PJ, Zuckerbraun L. Treatment of Zenker's diverticula by cricopharyngeus myotomy under local anesthesia. *Am Surg* 1992;58:710–716.

13. Spiro SA, Berg HM. Applying the endoscopic stapler in excision of Zenker's diverticulum: a solution for two intraoperative problems. *Otolaryngology* 1994;110:603–604.

14. Busaba NY, Ishoo E, Kieff D. Open Zenker's diverticulectomy using stapling techniques. *Ann Otol Rhinol Laryngol* 2001;110:498–501.

15. Bremner CG. Zenker diverticulum. *Arch Surg* 1998;133:1131–1133.

16. Payne WS, King RM. Pharyngoesophageal (Zenker's) diverticulum. *Surg Clin North Am* 1983;63:815–824.

17. Allen MS. Pharyngoesophageal diverticulum: technique of repair. *Chest Surg Clin North Am* 1995;5:449–458.

18. Crescenzo DG, Trastek VF, Allen MS, et al. Zenker's diverticulum in the elderly: is operation justified? *Ann Thorac Surg* 1998;66:347–350.

19. Konowitz PM, Biller HF. Diverticulopexy and cricopharyngeal myotomy: treatment for the high-risk patient with a pharyngoesophageal (Zenker's) diverticulum. *Otolaryngol Head Neck Surg* 1989;100:146–152.

20. Laccourreye O, Menard M, Cauchois R, et al. Esophageal diverticulum: diverticulopexy versus diverticulectomy. *Laryngoscope* 1994;104:889–892.

21. Fraczek M, Karwowski A, Krawczyk M, et al. Results of surgical treatment of cervical esophageal diverticula. *Dis Esophogus* 1998;11:55–57.

22. Witterick IJ, Gullane PJ, Yeung E. Outcome analysis of Zenker's diverticulectomy and cricopharyngeal myotomy. *Head Neck* 1995;17:382–388.

23. Kerner MM, Bates ES, Hernandez F, et al. Carcinoma-in-situ occurring in a Zenker's diverticulum. *Am J Otolaryngol* 1994;15:223–226.

24. Bradley PJ, Kochaar A, Quraishi MS. Pharyngeal pouch carcinoma: real or imaginary risks? *Ann Otol Laryngol* 1999;108:1027–1032.

25. Feeley MA, Righi PD, Weisberger EC, et al. Zenker's diverticulum: analysis of surgical complications from diverticulectomy and cricopharyngeal myotomy. *Laryngoscope* 1999;109:858–861.

26. Burstin PP, Merry D. Endoscopic stapling treatment of pharyngeal pouch. *Aust N Z J Surg* 1998;68:532–535.

27. Van Overbeek JJM. Pathogenesis and methods of treatment of Zenker's diverticulum. *Ann Otol Rhinol Laryngol* 2003;112:583–593.

28. Van Overbeek JJM. Meditation on the pathogenesis of hypopharyngeal (Zenker's) diverticulum and a report of endoscopic treatment in 545 patients. *Ann Otol Rhinol Laryngol* 1994;103:178–185.

29. Collard JM, Otte JB, Kestens PJ. Endoscopic stapling technique of esophagodiverticulostomy for Zenker's diverticulum. *Ann Thorac Surg* 1993;56:573–576.

30. Mirza S, Dutt SN, Irving RM. Iatrogenic perforation in endoscopic stapling deverticulotomy for pharyngeal pouches. *J Laryngol Otol* 2003;117:93–98.

31. Hashiba K, de Paula AL, da Silva JGN, et al. Endoscopic treatment of Zenker's diverticulum. *Gastrointest Endosc* 1999;49:93–97.

32. Sen P, Bhattacharyya AK. Endoscopic stapling of pharyngeal pouch. *J Laryngol Otol* 2004;118:601–606.

33. Postma GN. Endoscopic diverticulotomy of Zenker's diverticulum: management and complications. *Dysphagia* 2003;18:227–228.

34. Thorne M, Harris P, Marcus K, et al. Bilateral vocal fold paresis after edoscopic stapling diverticulotomy for Zenker's diverticulum. *Head Neck* 2004;26:294–297.

35. Peracchia A, Bonavina L, Narne S, et al. Minimally invasive surgery for Zenker's diverticulum. *Arch Surg* 1998;133:695–700.

36. Stoeckli SJ, Schmid S. Endoscopic stapler-assisted diverticuloesophagostomy for Zenker's diverticulum: patient satisfaction and subjective relief of symptoms. *Surgery* 2002;131:158–162.

37. Luscher MS, Johansen LV. Zenker's diverticulum treated by the endoscopic stapling technique. *Acta Otolaryngol* 2000;543:235–238.

38. Baldwin DL, Toma AG. Endoscopic stapled diverticulotomy: a real advance in the treatment of hypopharyngeal diverticulum. *Clin Otolaryngol* 1998;23:244–247.

39. Cook RD, Huang PC, Richstmeier WJ, et al. Endoscopic staple-assisted esophagodiverticulostomy: an excellent treatment of choice for Zenker's diverticulum. *Laryngoscope* 2000;110:2020–2025.

40. Narne S, Cutrone C, Chella B, et al. Endoscopic diverticulotomy for the treatment of Zenker's diverticulum: results in 102 patients with staple-assisted endoscopy. *Ann Otol Rhinol Laryngol* 1999;108:810–815.

41. Sood S, Newbegin CJR. Endoscopic stapling of pharyngeal pouches in patients from the Yorkshire region. *J Laryngol Otol* 2000;114:853–857.

42. Omote K, Feussner H, Stein HJ, et al. Endoscopic stapling diverticulostomy for Zenker's diverticulum. *Surg Endosc* 1999;13:535–538.

43. Jaramillo MJ, McLay KA, McAteer D. Long-term clinico-radiological assessment of endoscopic stapling of pharyngeal pouch: a series of cases. *J Laryngol Otol* 2001;115:462–466.

44. Phillipsen LP, Weisberger EC, Whiteman TS, et al. Endoscopic stapled diverticulotomy: treatment of choice for Zenker's diverticulum. *Laryngoscope* 2000;110:1283–1286.

45. Thaler ER, Weber RS, Goldberg AN, et al. Feasibility and outcome of endoscopic staple-assisted esophagodiverticulosotomy for Zenker's diverticulum. *Laryngoscope* 2001;111:1506–1508.

46. Chang CY, Payyapilli RJ, Scher RL. Endoscopic staple diverticulostomy for Zenker's diverticulum: review of literature and experience in 159 consecutive cases. *Laryngoscope* 2003;113:957–965.

47. Raut VV, Primrose WJ. Long-term results of endoscopic stapling diverticulotomy for pharyngeal pouches. *Otolaryngol Head Neck Surg* 2002;127:225–229.

48. Chiari C, Yeganehfar W, Scharitzer M, et al. Significant symptomatic relief after transoral endoscopic staple-assisted treatment of Zenker's diverticulum. *Surg Endosc* 2003;17:596–600.

49. Scher RL, Richtsmeier WJ. Long-term experience with endoscopic staple-assisted esophagodiverticulostomy for Zenker's diverticulum. *Laryngoscope* 1998;108:200–205.

50. Ong CC, Elton PG, Mitchell D. Pharyngeal pouch endoscopic stapling-are post-operative barium swallow radiographs of any value? *J Laryngol Otol* 1999;113:233–236.

51. Von Doersten PG, Byl FM. Endoscopic Zenker's diverticulotomy (Dohlman procedure): Forty cases reviewed. *Otolaryngol Head Neck Surg* 1997;116:209–212.

52. Hoffman M, Rudert HH, Scheunemann D, Maune S. Zenker's diverticulotomy with the carbon dioxide laser: perioperative management and long term results. *Ann Otol Rhinol Laryngol* 2003;112:202–205.

53. Nyrop M, Svendstrup F, Jorgensen KE. Endoscopic CO_2 laser therapy of Zenker's diverticulum-experience from 61 patients. *Acta Otolaryngol* 2000;(suppl 543):232–234.

54. Siddiq MA, Sood S. Current management in pharyngeal pouch surgery by UK otorhinolaryngologists. *Ann R Coll Surg Engl* 2004;86:247–252.

55. van Eeden S, Lloyd RV, Tranter RM. Comparison of the endoscopic stapling technique with more established procedures for pharyngeal pouches: results and patient satisfaction survey. *J Laryngol Otol* 1999;113:237–240.

56. Smith SR, Genden EM, Urken ML. Endoscopic stapling technique for the treatment of Zenker's diverticulum vs. standard open-neck technique. *Arch Otolaryngol Head Neck Surg* 2002;128:141–144.

57. Mirza S, Dutt SN, Minhas SS, et al. A retrospective review of pharyngeal pouch surgery in 56 patients. *Ann R Coll Surg Engl* 2002;84:247–251.

58. Zaninotto G, Narne S, Costantini M, et al. Tailored approach to Zenker's diverticula. *Surg Endosc* 2003;17:129–133.

59. Safdar A, Curran A, Timon CV. Endoscopic stapling vs. conventional methods of surgery for pharyngeal pouches: results, benefits and modifications. *Irish Med J* 2004;97:75–76.

60. Zbaren P, Schar P, Tschopp L, et al. Surgical treatment of Zenker's diverticulum: Transcutaneous diverticulectomy versus microendoscopic myotomy of the cricopharyngeal muscle with the CO_2 laser. *Otolaryngol Head Neck Surg* 1999;121:482–487.

61. Chang CWD, Burkey BB, Netterville JL, et al. Carbon dioxide laser endoscopic diverticulotomy versus open diverticulectomy for Zenker's diverticulum. *Laryngoscope* 2004;114:519–527.

62. Huang B, Payne WS, Cameron AJ. Surgical management for recurrent pharyngoesophageal (Zenker's) diverticulum. *Ann Thorac Surg* 1982;37:189–191.

63. Payne WS. The treatment of pharyngoesophageal diverticulum: the simple and complex. *Hepatogastroenterology* 1992;39:109–114.

64. Scher RL. Endoscopic staple diverticulostomy for recurrent Zenker's diverticulum. *Laryngoscope* 2003;113:63–67.

65. Harbour R, Miller J. A new system for grading recommendations in evidence based guidelines. *BMJ* 2001;323:334–336.

41
Management of Minimally Symptomatic Pulsion Diverticula of the Esophagus

Giovanni Zaninotto and Giuseppe Portale

Diverticula of the esophageal body are protrusions or outpouchings of the esophageal lumen. They are usually classified according to their anatomical relationship with the esophagus and/or mechanism of formation: diverticula originating close to the middle third of the esophagus, 4 to 5cm from the carina, are defined as midthoracic or parabronchial diverticula; diverticula close to the diaphragm are named epiphrenic diverticula. Midthoracic diverticula have been seen as the consequence of chronic inflammatory processes starting from the mediastinal lymph nodes (usually from granulomatous disease, as in tuberculosis) and involving the esophageal wall; they have also been called traction diverticula, according to Rokitansky.[1] An abnormal esophageal motility, generating high intraluminal pressures in short segments of the gullet, with or without esophageal wall weakness, can lead to mucosal herniation[2] and the development of pulsion diverticula. Epiphrenic diverticula are generally considered secondary to abnormal motility.

Such anatomical and pathogenic considerations have been challenged, however. According to Jordan, small diverticula can originate anywhere in the distal half of the esophagus and when they become larger, approaching the diaphragm, they acquire the status of epiphrenic diverticula.[3] Some authors believe that traction diverticula are nonexistent, or extremely rare, and the underlying mechanism is really always an abnormal esophageal motility; others claim that esophageal abnormalities are not always identifiable (and/or demonstrable) in all epiphrenic diverticula.

Midthoracic diverticula account for 10% to 17% of all esophageal diverticula (14 tuberculosis-associated midthoracic esophageal diverticula were found in 15,000 autopsies[4]). Radiological studies (contrast esophagograms) have shown a prevalence of epiphrenic diverticula of around 0.015% in the United States, and up to 0.77% in Japan and 2% in Europe.[5-7] The true prevalence of epiphrenic diverticula remains unknown, however. Trastek[8] estimated the ratio of epiphrenic to Zenker's diverticula at 1:5, and, because it is generally assumed that the incidence of Zenker's diverticula is less than 1/100,000/year, the estimated incidence of epiphrenic diverticula is approximately 1/500,000/year; these figures gives us an idea of just how rare diverticula of the thoracic esophagus are.

The clinical questions to address when dealing with diverticula of the thoracic esophagus are:

1. Do they need treatment?
2. If surgery is warranted, should only a diverticulectomy be performed, or do we need to routinely perform a myotomy to deal with the underlying esophageal motor disorder?
3. Which is the best approach: open or minimally invasive?
4. Which is the best route: transthoracic or transabdominal?

The aim of this chapter is to review the current medical literature for evidence to support decisions on these issues. The disease is so rare that only cohort studies or case series with a low level of evidence (2+ to 3) have been published in the medical literature. The overall grade of the evidence upon which our recommendations are made is thus C.

41.1. Do All Esophageal Thoracic Diverticula Need Treatment?

This statement from Orringer is quoted in many articles addressing this issue: "A masterful inactivity in asymptomatic or mildly disturbing diverticula is a good practice even if, in this time of mini-invasive surgery and stapling device, an esophageal diverticulectomy may represent a tempting trophy for a hyperactive surgeon."[9] This is a wise attitude to take because the mere presence of a diverticulum in the thoracic esophagus is not, per se, an indication for surgery and the decision whether to operate or not depends on the patient's symptoms, the risk of complications from the diverticulum, and the surgery-related risks.

41.1.1. Symptoms

Dysphagia, regurgitation, and respiratory symptoms are commonly associated with esophageal body diverticula. Chest pain has occasionally been reported and may be a sign of inflammation and/or ulceration,[10] or more likely of the underlying esophageal motor disorder. The proportion of asymptomatic diverticula patients is disputed: the percentage reported to have symptoms insufficient to warrant treatment ranges from 0% to 60%. Thomas and colleagues[4] recently published a review that also mentioned a large series of 121 diverticula patients, 97 (80%) of them asymptomatic, in a paper published in 1956.

41.1.2. Risk of Complications

Perforations or rupture of diverticula in the mediastinum (spontaneous or after diagnostic maneuvers, such as endoscopy), carcinoma in the diverticulum, lung abscess, and recurrent aspiration pneumonia are the most common complications. The pulmonary complications were emphasized by Altorki, who reported on 3 of 20 patients having severe respiratory problems (two cases of aspiration pneumonia and one of tracheo-esophageal fistula) due to esophageal body diverticula.[11] Apart from this and other similar anecdotal reports,[12–14] the natural history of asymptomatic or mildly symptomatic patients is difficult to predict. It has been estimated that less than 5% of patients will develop symptoms (or complications) from their diverticula. Conversely, the disease tends to progress in symptomatic patients followed up for years, even with a fatal outcome in some instances (a patient in the Nehra[15] series died of aspiration pneumonia before surgery could be performed; Table 41.1).

41.1.3. Surgical Risk

Surgery for esophageal diverticula carries a high risk of complications and even mortality. Table 41.2 shows the mortality and morbidity rates for 170 patients operated for esophageal diverticula. The most common complication is leakage from the suture line after diverticulectomy, accounting for one third of all postoperative deaths. The overall mortality rate (5%) for diverticulectomy is even higher than after esophagectomy for benign diseases.[23]

In summary, if we compare the surgical complications with the fate of unoperated patients – in the mid-term at least – surgery can only be justified when patients suffer from severe, incapacitating symptoms such as dysphagia, regurgitation, and aspiration, and/or have existing or impending complications. Patients with minimal or no symptoms should be managed conservatively.

> Surgery can only be justified when patients suffer from severe, incapacitating symptoms such as dysphagia, regurgitation, and aspiration, and/or have existing or impending complications; patients with minimal or no symptoms should be managed conservatively (level of evidence 3; recommendation grade C).

TABLE 41.1. Natural history of epiphrenic diverticula.

Reference	No. patients	Clinical condition	Diameter (cm)	Follow-up (years)[a]	Evidence Stable	Evidence Progression
Altorki[11] (1993)	3	3 symptomatic	≥3.5	–	1 (liquid diet)	1 MI (†) 1 asp pn (†)
Benacci[16] (1993)	42	35 asymptomatic/mild	–	7	35	0
		7 symptomatic referred to surgery		5	0	7
Nehra[15] (2002)	3[b]	1 symptomatic	–	–	0	1 asp pn (†)[e]
Jordan[3] (1999)	6[c]	5 asymptomatic 1 unfit for surgery[c]	–	6	1 asymptomatic 2 mild	2 referred to surgery
Castrucci[17] (1998)	16[d]	16 asymptomatic	≥1.5	5.3	13	0
Klaus[18] (2003)	5[c]	5 asymptomatic/mild[c]	≤2	–	2 asymptomatic 2 mild	0
All authors	68[b,c,d]	57 asymptomatic/mild 11 symptomatic	–	–	55 (96.5%) 1 (9%)	2 (3.5%) 10 (91%)

[a]Data are expressed as median.
[b]Two patients refused surgery, lost to follow-up.
[c]One patient lost to follow-up.
[d]Three patients lost to follow-up.
[e]One patient died while waiting for surgery.
asp pn: aspiration pneumonia.

41.2. Is Myotomy Always Mandatory when Surgery for Esophageal Diverticula Is Planned?

The aims of surgery for esophageal diverticula are: (1) to eliminate the diverticulum and prevent food retention, food and saliva regurgitation, and the risk of perforations and malignancies; and (2) to treat any underlying esophageal motor disorder. The vast majority of surgeons consider diverticulectomy necessary, though their reasons are frequently not specified.[4] Diverticulopexy, or inversion of the diverticulum, is only recom-

mended for small diverticula (<2 cm).[18] The advantages of a selective resection policy, reserving resection for large diverticula, is a lower risk of suture line leaks, but there are no clear data in the literature to support one choice or the other. In this era of minimally invasive surgery, all authors but one report diverticulectomies: when using endostapler devices through laparoscopic or thoracoscopic approaches, diverticulectomy is probably more practical to achieve than pexy or inversion of the diverticulum.

Tables 41.3 and 41.4 show the results of simple diverticulectomy and diverticulectomy plus myotomy. When the two options are compared,

TABLE 41.2. Morbidity and mortality following surgery for esophageal diverticula.

Reference	Level of evidence	No. patients	Mortality[a]	Leaks[a]	Morbidity[a]
Streitz[19] (1992)	2+	13	0	1 (7.7)	1 (7.7)
Altorki[11] (1993)	2+	17	1 (5.9)	0	0
Benacci[16] (1993)	2+	33	3 (9)	6 (18)	11 (33)
Nehra[15] (2002)	2+	18	1 (5.5)	1 (5.5)	2 (11)
Jordan[3] (1999)	2+	19	0	1 (5.3)	1 (5.3)
Castrucci[17] (1998)	2+	27	2 (7)	2 (7)	3 (11)
Rosati[20] (2001)	3	11	0	1 (9)	1 (9)
Klaus[18] (2003)	3	11	0	1 (9)	2 (18)
Costantini[21] (2004)	3	8	0	3 (37.5)	4 (50)
Del Genio[22] (2004)	3	13	1 (7.7)	3 (23)	4 (31)
All authors		170	8 (4.7)	19 (11.1)	29 (17.1)

[a]Data are expressed as n (%).

TABLE 41.3. Results following diverticulectomy alone for esophageal diverticula.

Reference	No. patients	Mortality[a]	Leaks[a]	Persistent/recurrent symptoms[a]	Recurrence of diverticulum[a]
Streitz[19] (1992)	3	0	1 (33.3)	0	0
Benacci[16] (1993)	7	0	0	1 (14.3)	0
Jordan[3] (1999)	6	0	1 (16.7)	1 (16.7)	0
Castrucci[17] (1998)	5	1 (20)	1 (20)	0	–
Klaus[18] (2003)	1	0	1 (100)	–	–
All authors	22	1 (4.5)	4 (18.2)	2 (9.2)	0

[a]Data are expressed as n (%).

the rate of leakage from the diverticulectomy suture line, the incidence of persistent or recurrent symptoms, and the rate of recurrent diverticulum are clearly higher after diverticulectomy without myotomy. Stationary manometry reveals motor abnormalities in 75% to 90% of patients with epiphrenic diverticula.[17,19] The most common motor abnormalities found in these patients are achalasia and diffuse esophageal spasm (DES). When esophageal motor disorders could not be demonstrated by ordinary means (i.e., stationary esophageal manometry), Nehra and coworkers reported a 30% diagnostic yield using 24-h ambulatory manometry.[15] The most consistent finding of ambulatory manometry was a higher percentage of simultaneous esophageal body contractions of high amplitude and duration during meals, findings that small bolus wet swallows normally used to elicit peristalsis during esophageal manometry were unable to pinpoint. Based on these findings, Nehra suggested the routine

use of myotomy when operating on epiphrenic diverticula.

A selective use of myotomy, that is, only when hypertonic esophageal motor disorders have been demonstrated, is recommended by Castrucci,[17] Jordan,[3] and Streitz.[19] Because the rationale for myotomy is to reduce the endoluminal esophageal pressure, these authors do not recommend it for cases of nonspecific esophageal motor disorder (NSEMD) or akinesia characterized by hypotonic motility patterns, because adding an esophageal body myotomy will lead to impaired peristalsis in such patients. Myotomy of the cardia is not warranted in patients with a normally relaxing lower esophageal sphincter for the same reasons: adding a cardiomyotomy in such patients could induce severe gastroesophageal reflux without offering any benefit. When the outcomes of routine and selective myotomy are compared, no differences emerge in terms of complications and late results.

TABLE 41.4. Results following diverticulectomy and myotomy for esophageal diverticula.

Reference	No. patients	Mortality[a]	Leaks[a]	Persistent/recurrent symptoms[a]	Recurrence of diverticulum[a]
Streitz[19] (1992)	13	0	0	0	0
Altorki[11] (1993)	14	0	0	1 (7.1)	0
Benacci[16] (1993)	22	3 (13.6)	6 (27.2)	3 (13.6)	0
Nehra[15] (2002)	13	1 (7.7)	1 (7.7)	–	–
Jordan[3] (1999)	9	0	0	0	1 (11.1)
Castrucci[17] (1998)	12	1 (8.3)	1 (8.3)	1 (9)	–
Rosati[20] (2001)	11	0	1 (9)	0	1 (9)
Klaus[18] (2003)	5	0	0	–	–
Costantini[21] (2004)	8	0	3 (37.5)	0	0
Del Genio[22] (2004)	13	1 (7.7)	3 (23)	0	0
All authors	120	6 (5)	15 (12.5)	5 (4.2)	2 (1.7)

[a]Data are expressed as n (%).

The extent of the myotomy and the use of an anti-reflux procedure are still a matter of debate. No reliable data are available in the medical literature to support either a long, indiscriminate esophagomyotomy extending from the aortic arch to below the cardia,[11] or a myotomy limited to the manometric region of dysmotility or to the level of the diverticulum. Most authors agree that the myotomy should be performed on the side opposite the diverticulum. When achalasia is the underlying abnormality, the myotomy should include the cardia region, extending 1.5 to 2 cm onto the gastric wall, as in simple achalasia. If a spastic motor disorder is diagnosed (DES), it seems reasonable to perform the myotomy starting at least at the inferior lip of the diverticulum, accepting the notion that a pulsion diverticulum forms just proximal to an obstruction, and that a subdiverticular myotomy is the best treatment for the condition.[4]

It is not uncommon to find gastroesophageal reflux disease, with or without a hiatal hernia, associated with an esophageal diverticulum. Benacci[16] reported on a sliding hiatal hernia diagnosed by barium swallow in 48% of 33 patients operated at the Mayo Clinic; concomitant hernia repair was performed in 6 patients. A randomized trial showing that fundoplication reduces postoperative gastroesophageal reflux in achalasia patients undergoing laparoscopic cardiomyotomy, without any negative effect on the relief of dysphagia, has recently added to the debate.[24] It seems reasonable to follow the same logic when treating epiphrenic diverticula requiring cardiomyotomy. Though there is no strong evidence in favor of a complete or partial fundoplication, the consensus is towards a partial repair, given the fear that a more obstructive one might be implicated in suture line leaks.

In conclusion, esophageal motor abnormalities should be carefully investigated in patients with intrathoracic esophageal diverticula, even with the aid of sophisticated techniques such as ambulatory manometry. When a motor disorder is demonstrated, myotomy should be considered a fundamental step in the procedure and, if the cardia is dyschalasic, the myotomy should include this region. As for achalasia, an anti-reflux repair should be added whenever a cardiomyotomy is performed.

> Myotomy should be considered a fundamental step in the management of a pulsion diverticulum; if the cardia is dyschalasic, the myotomy should include this region (level of evidence 2+ to 3; recommendation grade B).

41.3. Open or Minimally Invasive Surgery?

Minimal access surgery has become popular for treating a range of different benign esophageal diseases. In the last 5 years, most articles on the treatment of intrathoracic esophageal diverticula were reports on small numbers of patients, focusing more on the novelty and feasibility of the minimally invasive approach than on the pathogenesis of this disease and the different treatment options. The first minimally invasive approach to be used was the thoracoscopic – a logical consequence of the traditional transthoracic route. The first and, so far, largest series has been described by the Milan group, with eight patients treated. The operation was completed thoracoscopically in six patients, with one leak[25]. A Dutch team reported on their experience with five patients operated with no mortality and one suture line leak.[26]

The laparoscopic approach to epiphrenic diverticula appears to be more popular, but it is worth emphasizing that the largest reported series contains only 13 patients. Table 41.5 summarizes the outcome of minimally invasive surgery for esophageal intrathoracic diverticula. The vast majority of authors routinely include myotomy of the cardia and an anti-reflux procedure. The clinical results of minimally invasive surgery seem to be as good as after open surgery, and the risk of leakage from the suture line is also similar. No deaths related to suture line leakage were reported, however. It is not clear whether this remarkable difference is due to the different approach (abdominal instead of thoracic), the use of minimally invasive surgery, a better management of leaks by these particular authors, or mere chance. The perceived (but not yet demonstrated) advantages of minimally invasive techniques are a lower wound-related morbidity and better

TABLE 41.5. Laparoscopic treatment of epiphrenic diverticula: results.

Reference[a]	No. patients	Type of surgery	Mortality[b]	Leaks[b]	Good/excellent outcome[b]
Rosati[20] (2001)	11	Diverticulectomy + myotomy + fundoplication	0	1 (9)	100
Raakow[27] (2002)	3	Diverticulectomy + myotomy + fundoplication	0	0	100
Neoral[28] (2002)	3	Myotomy + fundoplication	0	0	100
		4 diverticulectomy + myotomy			
		1 diverticulectomy			
Klaus[18] (2003)	10	3 diverticulectomy included into fundoplication	0	1 (10)	–
		2 diverticulectomy inverted + myotomy			
Fraiji[29] (2003)	5	Diverticulectomy + myotomy + fundoplication	0	1 (20)	100
Matthews[30] (2003)	4	Diverticulectomy + myotomy + fundoplication	0	0	100
Pitchford[31] (2003)	1	Diverticulectomy + myotomy + fundoplication	0	0	100
Costantini[21] (2004)	8	Diverticulectomy + myotomy + fundoplication	0	3 (37.5)	75
Del Genio[22] (2004)	13	Diverticulectomy + myotomy + fundoplication	1 (7.7)	3 (23)	100
Muller[32] (2004)	4	Myotomy + fundoplication	1 (25)	0	100
All authors	62	–	2 (3.2)	9 (14.5)	–

[a]All references are level of evidence 3.
[b]Data are expressed as n (%).

recovery rates. The laparoscopic approach avoids problems related to single-lung ventilation, but giant diverticula or those well above the epiphrenic region are still best approached thoracoscopically. The dissection of large or adherent diverticula may be more of a challenge using minimally invasive procedures, but excisions of diverticula up to 7 to 10 cm in size have been reported.[18,21]

In summary, the early experience with minimal access surgery for treating intrathoracic esophageal diverticula points to a potential benefit with no fallout on effectiveness and safety. The indications for and principles of such surgery remain the same as in the case of the open approach. Minimal access surgery has the potential to become the standard approach for this condition.[4]

> The early experience with minimal access surgery for treating intrathoracic esophageal diverticula points to a potential benefit with no fallout on effectiveness and safety. Minimal access surgery has the potential to become the standard approach for this condition (level of evidence 3; recommendation grade C).

41.4. Transthoracic or Transabdominal Approach?

For many years, the approach to intrathoracic diverticula was transthoracic, usually through a left thoracotomy. This allowed for both the management of the diverticulum and the treatment of the underlying motor disorder. Few authors used a transabdominal approach before the advent of minimally invasive techniques, but the attitude changed when the opportunity arose to treat epiphrenic diverticula laparoscopically, thanks to a better visualization using the laparoscope and the introduction of an endostapler capable of transecting the neck of the diverticulum while remaining parallel to the esophageal axis. The advantage of the transabdominal approach is more evident when hiatal hernia or achalasia are associated with the epiphrenic diverticulum. The transabdominal approach may be limited by the distance of the diverticulum from the hiatus, the size of the diverticulum, or severe inflammation and adhesions between the wall of the diverticulum and the mediastinal pleura. One problem to bear in mind in the choice of approach is the size of the diverticulum's neck. When the neck is very broad, it may need two or more cartridges of endostapler to cut and close it, in which case the crossing of the suture lines becomes a potential site of leakage. When planning the treatment of large diverticula, a thoracotomy approach should be considered, so that a TA stapler can be used, inserted via a thoracotomy – or a mini-thoracotomy if the diverticulum is dissected thoracoscopically. The TA stapler has a longer jaw than the endostapler and thus enables the use of a single cartridge to secure the diverticulum's neck, avoiding the creation of a weak point at the crossing of the suture lines.

In summary, no standard approach can be recommended for intrathoracic diverticula on the basis of evidence; a pragmatic and eclectic attitude is necessary.

> No standard approach can be recommended for intrathoracic diverticula on the basis of existing evidence; a pragmatic approach and eclectic attitude is necessary.

References

1. Harrington SW. The surgical treatment of pulsion diverticula of the thoracic esophagus. *Ann Surg* 1949;129:606–618.

2. Cross FS. Esophageal diverticula related neuromuscular problems. *Ann Otol Rhinol Laryngol* 1968;77:914–926.

3. Jordan PH, Kinner BM. New look at epiphrenic diverticula. *World J Surg* 1999;23:147–152.

4. Thomas ML, Antony AA, Fosh BG, Finch JG, Maddern GJ. Oesophageal diverticula. *Br J Surg* 2001;88:629–642.

5. Wheeler D. Diverticula of the foregut. *Radiology* 1947;49:476–481.

6. Dobashi Y, Goseki N, Inutake Y, Kawano T, Endou M, Nemoto T. Giant epiphrenic diverticulum with achalasia occurring 20 years after Heller's operation. *J Gastroenterol* 1996;31:844–847.

7. Schima W, Schober E, Stacher G, et al. Association of midoesophageal diverticula with oesophageal motor disorders. Videofluoroscopy and manometry. *Acta Radiol* 1997;38:108–114.

8. Trastek VF, Payne WS. Esophageal diverticula. In: Shields TW, ed. *General Thoracic Surgery*. Philadelphia: Lea and Febiger; 1989:989–1001.

9. Orringer MB. Epiphrenic diverticula: fact and fable. *Ann Thorac Surg* 1993;55:1067–1068.

10. Mann NS, Borkar B, Mann SK. Phlegmonous esophagitis associated with epiphrenic diverticulum. *Am J Gastroenterol* 1978;70:510–513.

11. Altorki NK, Sunagawa M, Skinner DB. Thoracic esophageal diverticula. Why is operation necessary? *J Thorac Cardiovasc Surg* 1993;105:260–265.

12. Stalheim AJ. Spontaneous perforation of diverticulum of distal esophagus. *Minn Med* 1978;61:424–426.

13. Clark SC, Norton SA, Jeyasingham K, Ridley PD. Oesophageal epiphrenic diverticulum: an unusual presentation and review. *Ann R Coll Surg Engl* 1995;77:342–345.

14. Rigg KM, Walker RW. Tension pneumothorax secondary to ruptured esophageal diverticulum. *Br J Clin Pract* 1990;44:528–529.

15. Nehra D, Lord RV, DeMeester TR, et al. Physiologic basis for the treatment of epiphrenic diverticulum. *Ann Surg* 2002;235:346–354.

16. Benacci JC, Deschamps C, Trastek VF, Allen MS, Daly RC, Pairolero PC. Epiphrenic diverticulum: results of surgical treatment. *Ann Thorac Surg* 1993;55:1109–1014.

17. Castrucci G, Porziella V, Granone P, Picciocchi A. Tailored surgery for esophageal body diverticula. *Eur J Cardiothorac Surg* 1998;14:380–387.

18. Klaus A, Hinder RA, Swain J, Achem SR. Management of epiphrenic diverticula. *J Gastrointest Surg* 2003;7:906–911.

19. Streitz JM Jr, Glick ME, Ellis FH Jr. Selective use of myotomy for treatment of epiphrenic diverticula. Manometric and clinical analysis. *Arch Surg* 1992;127:585–587.

20. Rosati R, Fumagalli U, Bona S, et al. Laparoscopic treatment of epiphrenic diverticula. *JSLS* 2001;11:371–375.

21. Costantini M, Zaninotto G, Rizzetto C, Narne S, Ancona E. Oesophageal diverticula. *Best Pract Res Clin Gastroenterol* 2004;18:3–17.

22. Del Genio A, Rossetti G, Maffettone V, et al. Laparoscopic approach in the treatment of epiphrenic diverticula: long-term results. *Surg Endosc* 2004;18:741–745.

23. Devaney EJ, Iannettoni MD, Orringer MB, Marshall B. Esophagectomy for achalasia: patient selection and clinical experience. *Ann Thorac Surg* 2001;72:854–858.

24. Richards WO, Torquati A, Holzman MD, et al. Heller myotomy versus Heller myotomy with Dor fundoplication for achalasia: a prospective randomized double-blind clinical trial. *Ann Surg* 2004;240:405–412.

25. Peracchia A, Bonavina L, Rosati R, Bona S. Thoracoscopic resection of epiphrenic diverticula. In: Peters J, De Meester TR, eds. *Minimally Invasive Surgery of the Foregut*. St. Louis: QMP Inc.; 1994:110–116.

26. van der Peet DL, Klinkenberg-Knol EC, Berends FJ, Cuesta MA. Epiphrenic diverticula: minimally invasive approach and repair in five patients. *Dis Esophagus* 2001;14:60–62.
27. Raakow R, Schmidt S, Neuhaus P. Laparoscopic transhiatal approach to epiphrenic diverticula. *Chirurgie* 2002;73:46–49.
28. Neoral C, Aujesky R, Bohanes T, Klein G, Kral V. Laparoscopic transhiatal resection of epiphrenic diverticulum. *Dis Esophagus* 2002;15:323–325.
29. Fraiji E Jr, Bloomston M, Carey L, et al. Laparoscopic management of symptomatic achalasia associated with epiphrenic diverticulum. *Surg Endosc* 2003;17:1600–1603.
30. Matthews BD, Nelms CD, Lohr CE, Harold KL, Kercher KW, Heniford BT. Minimally invasive management of epiphrenic esophageal diverticula. *Am Surg* 2003;69:465–470.
31. Pitchford TJ, Price PD. Laparoscopic Heller myotomy with epiphrenic diverticulectomy. *JSLS* 2003;7:165–169.
32. Muller A, Halbfuss, HJ. Laparoscopic esophagotomy without diverticular resection for treating epiphrenic diverticulum in hypertonic lower esophageal sphincter. *Chirurgie* 2004;75:302–306.

Part 4
Diaphragm

42
Giant Paraesophageal Hernia: Thoracic, Open Abdominal, or Laparoscopic Approach

Glenda G. Callender and Mark K. Ferguson

Paraesophageal hernias represent approximately 5% of all hiatal hernias. The vast majority of hiatal hernias are type I, or sliding, hiatal hernias, which are characterized by a gastroesophageal junction that migrates through the hiatus. Paraesophageal hernias are commonly classified as type II or type III hiatal hernias. Type II hiatal hernias are true paraesophageal hernias in which the gastroesophageal junction maintains its normal anatomical position, whereas the fundus (and/or another organ) migrates through the hiatus. Type III, or mixed, hiatal hernias represent a combination of types I and II, in which the gastroesophageal junction and the fundus (and/or another organ) both herniate through the hiatal defect.

Giant paraesophageal hernias are distinguished by the presence of at least half of the stomach in an intrathoracic location. These hernias comprise a subset of paraesophageal hernias that is particularly challenging to manage for several reasons. First, the large crural defects that result are difficult to close without tension. Second, giant paraesophageal hernias are usually longstanding. If significant reflux has also been present, chronic inflammation may lead to cicatricial contracture of the tissues in the esophageal wall, and esophageal shortening may occur, which can also render a tension-free closure difficult. In addition, a stomach that has spent years in a rotated intrathoracic position may have a tendency to maintain this rotated position after reduction into the abdomen, thus retaining a risk for gastric volvulus even after repair of the hernia. Finally, giant paraesophageal hernias tend to occur in an elderly population with a frail constitution that does not tolerate a morbid operation well.

The purpose of this chapter is to review the published literature regarding the optimal approach for repair of the giant paraesophageal hernia. This operation has traditionally been performed through a thoracotomy or laparotomy. Since the early 1990s, laparoscopy has been used with increasing frequency. Controversy as to the optimal approach exists because the three approaches differ widely in their morbidity, technical difficulty, ability to offer adequate exposure should an esophageal lengthening procedure be necessary, and in reported recurrence and complication rates. This chapter will discuss these controversies in detail and will examine the available evidence for choosing a particular approach for repair of the giant paraesophageal hernia.

42.1. Thoracic Versus Open Abdominal Approach

One of the main benefits of the thoracic approach for repair of the giant paraesophageal hernia is that it permits complete esophageal mobilization. According to some experts, a foreshortened esophagus is the rule rather than the exception in the giant paraesophageal hernia, and extensive esophageal dissection or an esophageal lengthening procedure must be performed in order to reduce the risk of recurrence. (Please refer to Chapter 38 for a complete discussion of this topic.) Through a thoracic incision, the esophagus may be safely dissected to above the aortic arch, and the middle esophageal artery and esophageal branches of the left inferior bronchial artery may be divided if necessary. The thoracic approach also gives good exposure for creation of a Collis gastroplasty, if needed, for esophageal lengthening. In addition, resection of the hernia sac has been shown to reduce recurrence after paraesophageal hernia repair,[1] and this is easily accomplished via a thoracic incision.

A laparotomy offers a quicker and less painful approach to the giant paraesophageal hernia than a thoracotomy. For patients with limited cardiovascular and respiratory reserve, who may not tolerate collapse of a lung well, a laparotomy offers significantly less morbidity. The hernia is often easier to reduce because intraabdominal pressure is atmospheric during a laparotomy, whereas during a thoracotomy it may be necessary to attempt to reduce hernia contents against existing intraabdominal pressure. However, dissection of the hernia sac and the mediastinal esophagus are significantly more difficult through an open abdominal incision. The inability to visualize the mediastinal esophagus during dissection places many important structures, such as the vagus nerves, at risk.[2]

Very little objective evidence exists regarding the superiority of either the thoracic or open abdominal approaches to repair of the giant paraesophageal hernia. There are five major studies in the recent literature that specifically address one or both of these approaches in the context of giant paraesophageal hernia repair, and contain more than 30 patients.[3-7] All of these studies are retrospective case series, and hence are non-analytic studies with a level of evidence rating of 4.

One study[3] includes the patients presented in an earlier study[4]; therefore only the most recent and more complete study will be discussed in detail here. Table 42.1 lists these studies and their salient outcomes.

Geha and colleagues[5] present the largest and most recent series. It is perhaps the most helpful study in actually comparing the two approaches. The authors report 100 patients who underwent giant paraesophageal hernia repair between 1967 and 1999. Twenty patients underwent emergent operations; the rest were elective. A left thoracotomy was used in 18 patients and laparotomy was used in 82 patients. Thoracotomy was the approach of choice early in their experience, and for patients who demonstrated preoperative esophageal shortening and required Collis gastroplasty (two patients). The authors do not state why they preferred an open abdominal approach later in their experience. They had no hernia recurrences (follow-up time is not specified), and their overall mortality rate was 2% (both patients initially presented with acute gastric volvulus of several days' duration and sepsis; the operative approach for these two patients is not specified). There was a higher perioperative complication and re-operation rate in patients who underwent a thoracotomy, although statistical analysis was not performed. Two patients (11%) developed recurrent gastric volvulus and required re-operation after initial transthoracic hernia repair. In contrast, only four patients (4.8%) developed postoperative complications after open abdominal repair, and these did not require re-operation (two cases of delayed gastric emptying and two cases of mild pancreatitis, all self-limited). All surviving patients are reported to be symptom free, although the

TABLE 42.1. Thoracic and open abdominal approaches for giant paraesophageal hernia repair.

Reference	Type of study	Time frame	n	Thoracic	Abdominal	Complications	Reoperations	Mortality	Recurrence
Geha[5]	Retrospective case series	1967–1999	100	18	82	Thoracic: 11% Abdominal: 5%	Thoracic: 11% Abdomincal: 0%	2%	0%
Martin[6]	Retrospective case series	1977–1994	51	33	16	29%	2%	0%	4%
Altorki[7]	Retrospective case series	1988–1997	47	46	1	40%	Not stated	2%	6%
Maziak[3]	Retrospective case series	1960–1996	94	91	3	19%	5%	2%	2%

authors do not state specifically which symptoms were evaluated during follow-up. The authors advocate an open abdominal approach to giant paraesophageal hernia repair because they believe this approach allows for better reduction and fixation of the stomach, with reduced chance of recurrent volvulus.

Martin and colleagues[6] present the only other series that allows for comparison between the thoracic and open abdominal approaches. The authors report 51 patients who underwent giant paraesophageal hernia repair between 1977 and 1994. A transthoracic approach was used in 33 patients, and an open abdominal approach was used in 16 patients. Two patients underwent emergent operation, and one of the open abdominal cases was initially attempted laparoscopically. There were no deaths, and the hernia recurrence rate was 3.9% (mean follow-up was 27.1 months). One patient developed an acute recurrence on postoperative day 3 and required re-operation, and another patient was incidentally discovered to have a recurrence during a subsequent operation 11 months later. Postoperative complications developed in 29% of patients. The type of approach used in the patients who developed hernia recurrence or postoperative complications is not specified. However, a comparison is made between the percentage of patients in each group who experienced excellent and good results (no residual symptoms or one residual symptom) following their hernia repair. Excellent or good results were obtained in 84% of patients in the thoracic group and 88% of patients in the abdominal group; the difference was not statistically significant. The authors conclude that outcome is acceptable regardless of the approach.

Altorki and colleagues[7] and Maziak and colleagues[3] both report fairly large series of patients who underwent giant paraesophageal hernia repair primarily using a transthoracic approach. Altorki and colleagues report a series of 47 patients accrued between 1988 and 1997, who all underwent a thoracotomy except for one patient who had an attempted laparoscopic repair but required conversion to laparotomy. The authors report a mortality rate of 2% (one patient died of complications from antibiotic-associated pseudomembranous colitis) and a hernia recurrence

rate of 6.3% (median follow-up was 45 months). Postoperative complications occurred in 40% of patients, and a re-operation rate is not specified, although none of the postoperative complications reported appear to have required reoperation. At follow-up, 90% of their patients were symptom free or reported occasional symptoms. The authors prefer the transthoracic approach because they believe esophageal pseudoshortening is frequently encountered in patients with giant paraesophageal hernias, and adequate esophageal mobilization is needed to ensure a tension-free repair. Indeed, after extensive esophageal dissection, none of their patients required a Collis gastroplasty.

Maziak and coworkers also prefer the transthoracic approach, but in their opinion, most patients require a Collis gastroplasty, and they believe the transthoracic approach best facilitates this procedure. They report a series of 94 patients who underwent giant paraesophageal hernia repair between 1960 and 1996, all via thoracotomy except for three patients who underwent laparotomy because they had concomitant abdominal pathology requiring surgery. Through the 1960s, the authors did not routinely employ an esophageal lengthening procedure. However, in the 1970s they began performing a modified Collis gastroplasty as part of their standard repair because they found a high prevalence of significant distal esophageal scarring, thickening, and shortening, even in patients with no endoscopic evidence of severe active esophagitis.[4] The authors report a mortality rate of 2% (one patient experienced a severe aspiration event that led to respiratory failure, and one patient developed a free esophageal leak and died of septic shock) and a hernia recurrence rate of 2% (median follow-up was 72 months). The complication and re-operation rates were 19% and 5.3%, respectively. Excellent or good long-term results were obtained in 93% of patients. The authors ascribe their positive results to the routine addition of an esophageal lengthening procedure to their repair, and believe that this is easily accomplished via a thoracic approach. However, they suggest that if an adequate esophageal lengthening procedure could be performed laparoscopically, this approach could be potentially as effective with less morbidity.

42.2. Laparoscopic Approach

A laparoscopic approach for repair of the giant paraesophageal hernia provides some of the benefits of both thoracotomy and laparotomy, in that the hiatus may be easily accessed and the hernia sac and esophagus can be dissected under direct vision, while avoiding a morbid operation that involves collapse of a lung and a postoperative chest tube.[2] However, this is a technically challenging operation, and there have been some early reports of recurrence rates and intraoperative complication rates that appear unacceptably high.[8,9]

Two recent studies directly compare open versus laparoscopic paraesophageal hernia repair,[8,11] and these do not specifically address giant paraesophageal hernias. They are discussed here for background purposes only. Schauer and associates[10] published the first case series, which includes 95 patients who underwent paraesophageal hernia repair from 1990 to 1998. Laparoscopy was used in 67 patients, laparotomy in 19 patients, and thoracotomy in 4 patients. There was one death (mortality rate of 1%), which occurred in the laparoscopy group and involved an immunocompromised patient. The laparoscopic group experienced a statistically significant decrease in intensive care unit stay, time to oral intake, hospital length of stay, and narcotic requirement when compared to the open group (laparotomy and thoracotomy combined). Major complications were significantly less frequent in the laparoscopic group (10.5% vs. 48%), as were minor complications (10.5% vs. 60%). In addition, there were no hernia recurrences in the laparoscopic group (mean follow-up was 13 months) compared to a recurrence rate of 8% in the open group (mean follow-up was 48 months). Based on this study, laparoscopy appeared to hold great promise for paraesophageal hernia repair.

Hashemi and colleagues[8] published the only other series that directly compares laparoscopic versus open paraesophageal hernia repair (again, this does not apply specifically to giant paraesophageal hernias), and their results were less favorable. They report a case series of 54 patients who underwent paraesophageal hernia repair from 1985 to 1998. Laparoscopy was used in 27

patients, laparotomy in 13 patients, and thoracotomy in 14 patients. There was one death (mortality rate of 1.7%), which occurred in a patient who had undergone laparotomy and developed respiratory failure. There was no difference in major or minor complication rates between the laparoscopic group and the open group (laparotomy and thoracotomy combined), but there was a statistically significant decrease in the time of nasogastric intubation and length of hospital stay in the laparoscopic group. However, video esophagrams were obtained in 41 patients at a median of 27 months postoperatively for routine radiographic follow-up, and the laparoscopic group was found to have an alarming 42% radiographic recurrence rate compared to a 15% recurrence rate in the open group. The significance of this finding is unclear, because most of these recurrences were asymptomatic and would not have been recognized without routine radiographic follow-up, but it certainly calls into question the efficacy of laparoscopic paraesophageal hernia repairs.

To date, there have been no studies that directly compare laparoscopic versus open technique for giant paraesophageal hernia repair. However, five major studies have been published which report results of laparoscopic giant paraesophageal hernia repair and contain more than thirty patients.[9,11–14] Again, all are retrospective case series, except for one retrospective review of a prospectively gathered database.[13] Hence, all are non-analytic studies with a level of evidence rating of 3. Table 42.2 lists these studies and their results.

Watson and coworkers[11] present a series of 86 patients who underwent laparoscopic giant paraesophageal hernia repair between 1992 and 1998. Their report underscores the technical difficulty of a laparoscopic repair and highlights the nature of the learning curve. Their results are similar to others with the exception of a very high rate of conversions to open surgery (23%). Early in their experience, during the first 40 cases, they did not resect the hernia sac, which further contributed to the difficulty of the operation. They converted 16 of these first 40 cases to open (40%). Their subsequent 46 cases did include resection of the hernia sac and, combined with their greater level of experience, resulted in conversion of only 4 cases to open (9%).

TABLE 42.2. Laparoscopic approach for giant paraesophageal hernia repair.

Reference	Type of study	Time frame	n	Conversions	Intraoperative complications	Postoperative complications	Re-operation rate	Mortality	Recurrence
Watson[11]	Retrospective case series	1992–1998	86	20	2%	13%	5%	0%	3%
Andujar[12]	Retrospective case series	1996–2002	166	2	Not stated	8%	6%	Not stated	Type I: 20% PEH: 5%
Luketich[9]	Retrospective case series	1995–2000	100	3	12%	Minor: 12% Major: 16%	3%	1%	1%
Swanstrom[13]	Prospective case series	1994–1997	52	2	6%	6%	6%	0%	8%
Weichmann[14]	Retrospective case series	1993–1997	60	6	3%	Not stated	3%	2%	7%

Andujar and coworkers[12] report a large series of 166 patients who underwent giant paraesophageal hernia repair between 1996 and 2002. Their report reinforces the concerns discussed earlier regarding the very high hernia recurrence rate in patients who had undergone paraesophageal hernia repair and routine radiographic follow-up. They obtained a routine barium esophagram in 120 patients (72%) at a mean of 15 months postoperatively. Of these 120 patients, 20% had a recurrent type I hiatal hernia, and 5% had a recurrent paraesophageal hernia. Two patients with a recurrent type I hiatal hernia and two patients with a recurrent paraesophageal hernia underwent re-operation; the remainder were asymptomatic and were observed. As discussed earlier, Hashemi and associates[8] reported a 42% recurrence rate after laparoscopic paraesophageal hernia repair; they considered any migration of the gastroesophageal junction above the hiatus to be a recurrence, but did not specify how many of their recurrences were type I hiatal hernias.

Luketich and colleagues[9] describe a large series of 100 patients who underwent laparoscopic giant paraesophageal hernia repair between 1995 and 2000. Their recurrence rate was 1% (median follow-up was 12 months), but their patients were not routinely studied radiographically. The authors attribute their low recurrence rate in part to their performance of a laparoscopic Collis gastroplasty in 27% of their patients. Toward the end of their experience, they began to recognize a high prevalence of foreshortened esophagus, and began to perform a laparoscopic Collis gastroplasty almost routinely. This group, however, experienced a somewhat high rate of intraoperative complications, including two gastric perforations and five esophageal perforations. These were repaired primarily without conversion to open surgery.

Swanstrom and colleagues[13] and Weichmann and colleagues[14] also reported significant intraoperative complications in their series. Most were able to be repaired laparoscopically without further sequelae, but in one case, an esophageal perforation resulted in death of the patient. Again, these potentially catastrophic intraoperative complications emphasize the technical challenges of laparoscopic repair.

42.3. Evidence-Based Recommendations

Due to the limited data available and the quality of the evidence, no particular approach to giant paraesophageal hernia repair appears clearly superior to another. Only two studies[5,6] actually compare two different approaches (thoracic and open abdominal). One study did not include a statistical analysis,[5] and the other study demonstrated basically equivalent results using either approach.[6] No studies directly compare laparoscopic versus open techniques specifically for giant paraesophageal hernia repair.

The literature does demonstrate, however, that giant paraesophageal hernia repair via any of the three approaches can be performed safely and effectively, although more time is needed to evaluate the long-term results of the laparoscopic series.

The available evidence suggests that there is not a/no single optimal approach to giant paraesophageal hernia repair. All studies reviewed above had a level of evidence rating of 4; therefore, the recommendation grade is C.

> There is no single optimal approach to giant paraesophageal hernia repair (level of evidence 4; recommendation grade C).

42.4. Summary

Although the quality of the available data is limited and no definitive recommendations can be made regarding the optimal approach to giant paraesophageal hernia repair, common sense permits formulation of some guidelines that may be of use.

First, if concomitant abdominal or thoracic pathology exists, it makes sense to repair the giant paraesophageal hernia through the same incision that can be used to manage the coexisting problem. Conversely, if there is a compelling reason to avoid a particular approach (such as extensive prior abdominal or thoracic surgery), an alternate approach should be chosen. The published series demonstrate that this repair can be performed safely and effectively using any of the three approaches, so this allows for versatility when considering each patient on an individual basis.

Second, the issue of esophageal length must be carefully considered when evaluating each patient, and there should be a low threshold for selecting an approach that would facilitate extensive esophageal dissection or an esophageal lengthening procedure. At this time, it appears that the thoracic approach offers the best exposure for ensuring adequate esophageal length. However, laparoscopy also allows for excellent visualization of the hiatus and mediastinal esophagus, and a Collis gastroplasty can certainly be performed laparoscopically. If, over the next several years, the laparoscopic approach can be shown to be comparable to open techniques, specifically regarding recurrence rates, laparoscopy would be a very reasonable alternative to a thoracotomy.

Third, significant prior laparoscopic experience is mandatory before attempting laparoscopic giant paraesophageal hernia repair. The operation is technically difficult, as suggested by the frequency of intraoperative visceral injuries.[9,13,14] In addition, the 42% hernia recurrence rate[8] was reported by a group that performs this operation laparoscopically on a fairly routine basis. It seems logical that a surgeon who only occasionally encounters a giant paraesophageal hernia will have even less success. In fact, if one has extensive experience or has attained a comfort level with any one of the three approaches, this is probably the best approach for that particular surgeon to use.

Finally, there exists an obvious need for further studies in this area. Longer follow-up is imperative for the current laparoscopic series, and a randomized, controlled trial comparing the three approaches would be very helpful.

References

1. Edye MB, Canin-Endris J, Gattorno F, et al. Durability of laparoscopic repair of paraesophageal hernia. *Ann Surg* 1998;228:528–535.
2. Oelschlager BK, Pellegrini CA. Paraesophageal hernias: open, laparoscopic, or thoracic repair? *Chest Surg Clin North Am* 2001;11:589–603.
3. Maziak DE, Todd TRJ, Pearson FG. Massive hiatus hernia: evaluation and surgical management. *J Thorac Cardiovasc Surg* 1998;115:53–62.
4. Pearson FG, Cooper JD, Ilves R, et al. Massive hiatal hernia with incarceration: a report of 53 cases. *Ann Thorac Surg* 1983;35:45–51.
5. Geha AS, Massad MG, Snow NJ, et al. A 32-year experience in 100 patients with giant paraesophageal hernia: the case for abdominal approach and selective antireflux repair. *Surgery* 2000;128:623–630.
6. Martin TR, Ferguson MK, Naunheim KS. Management of giant paraesophageal hernia. *Dis Esophagus* 1997;10:47–50.
7. Altorki NK, Yankelevitz D, Skinner DB. Massive hiatal hernias: the anatomic basis of repair. *J Thorac Cardiovasc Surg* 1998;115:828–835.
8. Hashemi M, Peters JH, DeMeester TR, et al. Laparoscopic repair of large type III hiatal hernia: objective followup reveals high recurrence rate. *J Am Coll Surg* 2000;190:553–561.
9. Luketich JD, Raja S, Fernando HC, et al. Laparoscopic repair of giant paraesophageal hernia: 100 consecutive cases. *Ann Surg* 2000;232:608–618.

10. Schauer PR, Ikramuddin S, McLaughlin RH, et al. Comparison of laparoscopic versus open repair of paraesophageal hernia. *Am J Surg* 1998;176:659–665.

11. Watson DI, Davies N, Devitt PG, et al. Importance of dissection of the hernial sac in laparoscopic surgery for large hiatal hernias. *Arch Surg* 1999;134:1069–1073.

12. Andujar JJ, Papasavas PK, Birdas T, et al. Laparoscopic repair of large paraesophageal hernia is associated with a low incidence of recurrence and reoperation. *Surg Endosc* 2004;18:444–447.

13. Swanstrom LL, Jobe BA, Kinzie LR, et al. Esophageal motility and outcomes following laparoscopic paraesophageal hernia repair and fundoplication. *Am J Surg* 1999;177:359–363.

14. Wiechmann RJ, Ferguson MK, Naunheim KS, et al. Laparoscopic management of giant paraesophageal herniation. *Ann Thorac Surg* 2001;71:1080–1087.

43
Management of Minimally Symptomatic Giant Paraesophageal Hernias

David W. Rattner and Nathaniel R. Evans

Hiatal hernias are a common finding in patients undergoing imaging procedures for various abdominal and thoracic complaints. Most hiatal hernias do not cause symptoms per se. Hiatal hernias are categorized as type I to IV, with type I or sliding hernias being the most common type. Type II or true paraesophageal hernias are defined as having the gastroesophageal junction below the diaphragm in a normal anatomic position. Type II hernias are quite rare. In their review of 46,236 patients with hiatal hernia seen at the Mayo Clinic between 1980 and 1990, Allen and colleagues found only 51 patients with type II hernia defects.[1]

Most reports regarding minimally symptomatic paraesophageal hernias are comprised of patients with type III hiatal hernias. These are mixed hernias with features of both type I and type II such that both the cardia of the stomach and, to a lesser degree, the gastroesophageal junction has herniated into the chest. Finally, hernias in which visceral organs other than stomach (most commonly colon) reside in the chest are designated type IV. Hiatal hernias in which more than half of the stomach resides above the diaphragm have been referred to as giant paraesophageal hernias.

The true incidence of paraesophageal hernias (i.e., types II, III, and IV) is unknown. According to published patient series, it is estimated that they comprise 15% of all hiatal hernias and hence the incidence in the general population is in the range of 45 per 100,000. Based on data from the Agency of Healthcare Research and Quality,[2] it can be inferred that in 1997, there were approximately 90,000 patients with paraesophageal hernias in the United States. As the population ages and radiologic imaging tests are more frequently performed, both the incidence and the detection of such hernias will increase. These two factors will create a growing subset of patients with incidentally discovered paraesophageal hernias.

This chapter concerns the significant proportion of patients with large paraesophageal hernias that are asymptomatic or complain only of minor symptoms. The exact proportion of truly asymptomatic patients is difficult to determine. While it is our belief that most paraesophageal hernias are asymptomatic, Oddsdottir reported that up to 89% of patients denying symptoms, will actually describe some symptoms when questioned carefully.[3] In these patients, however, the reported symptoms are usually minor in nature (i.e., belching, mild occasional heartburn, and dyspepsia) and do not affect their quality of life. The typical patient with a paraesophageal hernia is in the sixth or seventh decade of life and has significant comorbid conditions. In most surgical series, the majority of patients are classified as American Society of Anesthesiologists (ASA) III status. Although operative repair has been shown to be safe and effective in relieving symptoms and preventing volvulus in symptomatic patients, the merits of surgical repair in minimally symptomatic or asymptomatic patients is subject to debate.

43.1. Published Data

In order to make recommendations for treatment of minimally symptomatic paraesophageal hernias it is important to understand both the natural history of the condition and the results of surgical intervention. Much of the current support for repair of all paraesophageal hernias regardless of symptoms is based on the influential studies of Belsey and Hill. These studies are now more than 30 years old. In his report of the 87 patients with parahiatal hernias, Belsey noted that 6/21 who were treated medically due to minimal symptoms died of complications from their hernias. He did not report the time interval between the discovery of the hernia and the complications in those patients. Based on the mortality rate of 28% in this subgroup, he and others have advocated repair of all paraesophageal hernias upon diagnosis to prevent catastrophic complications.[4]

In 1973, Hill reported the outcomes of 29 patients with paraesophageal hernias.[5] Ten developed incarceration. The majority of these patients had been known to have paraesophageal hernia for years prior to this event. Four of the patients with incarcerated hernias were unable to be decompressed and were operated on emergently. Two of four patients died. Based on this very small amount of data, Hill quoted an operative mortality of 50% for emergent repair of incarcerated paraesophageal hernias.[5]

In 1983, Tracey and Jamison reported their experience with selective conservative management of paraesophageal hernias.[6] In a retrospective review of 368 patients with hiatal hernias, 71 were found to have paraesophageal hernias (type II or III hernias). Twenty-nine of 70 patients were managed nonoperatively with a mean follow-up of 6 years (2–120 months). Thirteen of the conservatively managed patients eventually underwent surgical repair. However, none of them developed acute symptoms or required emergency intervention. They concluded that operative management should be reserved for "those patients in whom symptoms supervene." This was one of the first studies to call into question the longstanding belief that all paraesophageal hernias should be repaired.

In 1993, Allen and coworkers reported a large retrospective chart review series from the Mayo Clinic.[1] From a database of 46,238 patients, they identified 147 with greater than 75% of their stomach in the chest as documented by endoscopy, radiographic studies, or surgical exploration. Within this group of 147 patients, 23 patients were managed nonoperatively though the selection criteria for this group were not given. Nineteen of these patients did not develop progressive symptoms. Of the four who did progress, only one died of complications related to his hernia. Among the patients undergoing operative repair, the median length of time between diagnosis and operation was 60 months. There were three patients who developed acute gastric volvulus. Thus in the Mayo Clinic series the incidence of acute gastric volvulus was 1 per 245 patients per year. This is significantly lower than the 30% incidence of incarceration reported by Hill.

As the experience with paraesophageal hernia (PEH) has grown, catastrophic events have not been observed at the rate proposed in earlier studies. Thus, there is a growing belief that only symptomatic patients should undergo surgical repair.[7] One of the first series in the laparoscopic era that addressed this point was reported by Horgan and associates.[8] In this series, 4 of 45 patients did not undergo elective repair. All patients were evaluated with preoperative and postoperative questionnaires. Postoperative functional studies and radiographs were obtained when indicated. Surgery was successful in relieving symptoms, and seven of eight patients undergoing postoperative upper gastrointestinal series were shown to have intact repairs. The lone radiographic recurrence was asymptomatic and was not repaired. Horgan concluded that the incidence of truly life-threatening complications in patients with PEH was extremely low and advocated repair in PEH only in the setting of symptoms. This more conservative approach has gained favor over the last decade.

With the proliferation of laparoscopic paraesophageal herniorrhaphy, many have questioned whether the reduced morbidity of a minimally invasive approach should lower the threshold for recommending surgery. The largest series of laparoscopic repairs is from the University of Pittsburgh. Pierre and coworkers published the results of 203 consecutive repairs of giant PEH in 2002.[9]

They defined giant hernias as those having as at least one third of the stomach within the chest as determined by preoperative esophagram – a fairly liberal definition of the condition. In 203 patients they performed 103 Collis–Nissen fundoplications, 69 Nissen fundoplications, and 19 other procedures. Of note, 86 of the last 103 patients had Collis–Nissen fundoplications, this change reflected their belief in the importance of a shortened esophagus as a potential cause for recurrence. Five patients in their series were re-operated on for recurrent hernia (2.5% re-operation rate). Of those questioned (152) 92% reported good or excellent results.[9] The operative mortality rate was 0.5% (1 in 203) and the combined major and minor morbidity rate was 28%. Pierre and coworkers did not report on results of postoperative esophagrams. Thus, their rate of asymptomatic recurrence is not known.

Diaz and Andujar reported the two largest studies with radiographic follow-up of patients undergoing laparoscopic repair of PEH. Andujar reported no operative mortality and a complication rate of 8.4% among 166 patients undergoing laparoscopic PEH repair. Of the 120 patients who underwent postoperative esophagrams, 34 had abnormal studies and 10 of these patients eventually needed re-operation.[10]

Diaz reported the outcomes from 116 patients, who underwent laparoscopic repair of PEH with an operative morbidity 13% of and mortality of 1.7%. Sixty-six of these patients underwent postoperative esophagrams, of whom 21 had radiological recurrence. In spite of the high radiographic recurrence rate, only three patients (2.6%) were re-operated on for recurrent hernias.[11]

Table 43.1 summarizes the results of 10 recent reports of laparoscopic repair of PEH, in which patients had radiographic evaluations postoperatively. The data reveal an average morbidity rate of 15% (6.4%–28%), a mortality rate of 2.1% (0%–5.4%), a recurrence rate of 19% (0%–42%), and a re-operation rate of 3.2% (0%–6%).[10-19] These data suggest that while laparoscopic repair of PEH is feasible and safe, the recurrence rate, specifically the asymptomatic recurrence rate, is high enough to bring into question the concept of prophylactic repair of such hernias in asymptomatic patients. Furthermore, the mortality rate is not inconsequential, even in the best of hands, due to comorbid conditions that are prevalent in these patients.

All of the aforementioned publications are case reports or series. As such they cannot definitively answer the central questions necessary to develop guidelines for management of minimally symptomatic paraesophageal hernias. The recent availability of large administrative databases, however, provides the opportunity to get fairly reliable data on the natural history of this condition as well as results of surgical intervention in the entire surgical community rather than just tertiary care facilities. The Nationwide Inpatient Sample (NIS) is part of the Healthcare Cost and Utilization Project, a powerful database developed by the Agency of Healthcare Research and Quality (AHRQ). It is drawn from 22 states and contains information on all inpatient stays from over 1000 hospitals, totaling 7,148,420 records in 1997 (national weighted estimate 35,408,170 inpatient stays). A recent analysis by our group demonstrated that previously published mortality rates of emergency repair of hiatal hernia are outdated and should be considered invalid. According to the analysis of NIS, the mortality rate of emergency operation for hiatal hernias in the

TABLE 43.1. Morbidity, mortality, recurrence, and re-operation rates for laparoscopic repair of PEH.

Reference (year published)	N	Follow-up (months)	Morbidity (%)	Mortality (%)	Recurrence (%)	Re-operation (%)
Andujar[10] (2004)	166	15	8.4	0	5	6
Diaz[11] (2003)	116	15	13	1.7	32	2.6
Aly[19] (2005)	60	47	14	5	30	1.3
Jobe[14] (2002)	52	37	19	0	32	3.8
Wu[16] (1999)	38	24	19	5	28	3
Dahlberg[13] (2001)	37	165	20	5.4	13.6	9
Khaitan[18] (2002)	31	25	6.4	0	7	NR
Ponsky[15] (2003)	28	21	11	0	0	0
Hashemi[17] (2000)	27	18	24	3.7	42	NR
Athanasakis[12] (2001)	10	3	20	0	0	0

United States is 5.4% [95% confidence interval (95% CI), 4.9%–5.8%]. This value represents the actual nationwide estimate for the mortality of emergency paraesophageal hernia repair for the year 1997 and was based on 1,035 patients with paraesophageal hernias that were repaired emergently.

In order to help examine the merits of repairing paraesophageal hernias prophylactically, we used a decision-analysis model to test the hypothesis that elective laparoscopic repair should be routinely recommended to patients with asymptomatic or minimally symptomatic paraesophageal hernias.[20] For the decision analysis, a Markov Monte Carlo computer simulation model was developed to generate a large number of patients with asymptomatic or minimally symptomatic PEH and record the possible clinical outcomes associated with two treatment strategies. In the first treatment strategy all the patients were subjected to an elective laparoscopic hernia repair, whereas in the second treatment strategy the patients were managed conservatively unless they developed symptoms requiring elective laparoscopic operation or they developed acute symptoms requiring emergency operation. A decision tree was constructed that represented the logical sequence of the clinical events and complications emerging from each treatment strategy over time. The probability and the utility (a value that reflects the impact of a condition on a patient's quality of life) of each clinical event and complication were calculated. The end point of the simulation was the quality-adjusted life expectancy that was measured in quality-adjusted life-years (QALYs). The model showed that there was no gain in quality-adjusted life expectancy with elective laparoscopic repair compared to watchful waiting. In fact, elective laparoscopic repair resulted in a reduction of 0.13 QALYs (10.78 vs. 10.65). The model also predicted that watchful waiting was the optimal treatment strategy in 83% of the patients and elective laparoscopic hernia repair in the remaining 17%. The model was not capable of identifying a priori which patients would fall into the 17% receiving benefit from elective surgery. Thus, if laparoscopic repair is recommended routinely to all patients with asymptomatic or minimally symptomatic paraesophageal hernias, fewer than one of five 65-year-old patients will benefit more than if watchful

waiting had been chosen. The difference in the quality-adjusted life expectancy between the two treatment strategies becomes more pronounced as the age of the patient increases, and according to this model only 1 out of 10 asymptomatic 85-year-old patients will benefit from an elective laparoscopic hernia repair. Even in the hypothetical scenario that the mortality of emergency surgery was 17% (as suggested by the pre-1997 literature), elective laparoscopic repair would become the optimal treatment option only if the mortality rate for laparoscopic repair was less than 1%. Under the assumption that the mortality rate of emergency surgery is currently 5.4% (1997 nationwide estimate), the mortality rate of laparoscopic repair should not exceed 0.5% in order for elective repair to be the optimal treatment option; an estimate, which is not supported by existing data.

43.2. Influence of Data

Based on the data discussed in the previous section it is hard to justify repairing asymptomatic PEH. There is no level 1 or even level 2 evidence to support such an approach. There have been no prospective, randomized, controlled trials to compare surgery versus expectant management. The volume of operations for PEH is low and there is no standardized surgical repair. These factors preclude the development of even multicenter trials, as there is a large amount variability in each center's surgical approach. Hence all of the information regarding treatment of PEH is level 3 or level 4 evidence. Administrative databases, while useful, are limited in their utility. The analysis by our group using a Markov Monte Carlo simulation model is dependant on a number of assumptions used to construct the model as well as exactly how one defines the term *asymptomatic* – particularly when using quality of life as an outcome measure.

Recently, a number of studies have investigated objective measurements of surgical failure. These studies have shown the recurrence rate after laparoscopic repair of paraesophageal hernia to be between 5% and 30%. These recurrences are rarely symptomatic, and are often dismissed as insignificant, particularly in patients who had significant gastroesophageal reflux disease

(GERD) symptoms, or gastrointestinal (GI) bleeding, that are improved by surgery. However, in patients who were asymptomatic preoperatively, the rate of asymptomatic recurrence is an important factor. These patients are subjected to operative repair solely to prevent volvulus. In this patient population, an asymptomatic recurrence should be regarded as a failure of treatment.

The conventional wisdom that PEH should be repaired electively is based on 40-year-old data that suggested an incidence of incarceration in patients with known PEH was approximately 30%. This combined with the belief that the operative mortality for emergency repair was as high as 50% has led to the widely held belief that all PEH should be repaired to prevent catastrophic sequelae. More recent studies suggest that the classic reports by Skinner and Hill likely overestimated the frequency of these complications. While repair of such hernias is safe and effective in controlling symptoms, large studies have shown that the morbidity of the procedure is not trivial and more concerning that the asymptomatic recurrence rate of the hernia is significant. In reviewing Medicare databases we also found that the operative mortality for emergency PEH was significantly less than previously reported. Therefore, data from the current era suggest that the widely held belief that all paraesophageal hernias should be repaired prophylactically must be reconsidered. In the asymptomatic or minimally symptomatic patient, repair subjects them to a significant morbidity and mortality risk and does not necessarily prevent recurrent hernia and incarceration. With this in mind, most symptomatic patients are best managed with periodic follow-up and conservative nonoperative management. However, given the lack of level 1 data regarding the natural history or management of minimally symptomatic PEH of any size, this is a grade C recommendation.

> In the asymptomatic or minimally symptomatic patient, repair subjects them to a significant morbidity and mortality risk; most symptomatic patients are best managed with periodic follow-up and conservative nonoperative management (level of evidence 3 to 4; recommendation grade C).

43.3. Personal View

Lucius Hill and Ronald Belsey were certainly giants in the field of hiatal surgery and as such it is hard to dismiss their recommendations to repair all paraesophageal hernias upon diagnosis. However, it is important to note that few of their patients had hernias that were truly asymptomatic. Prior to the widespread (some might even say indiscriminate) use of computed tomography (CT) scans, barium radiographs were obtained in patients with upper gastrointestinal complaints and therefore few patients in their series truly had incidentally discovered paraesophageal hernias. Similarly the high mortality and morbidity rates they reported in their conservatively managed patients were based on a referral practice that was not representative of the population at large. Data obtained from NIS and from the large Mayo Clinic study provide much more robust information about the true risk of symptom progression. Furthermore, NIS data demonstrate that even under emergency circumstances, the modern surgeon and hospital do a better job of getting patients through difficult emergency surgical situations than was the case 30 years ago. Repair of a paraesophageal hernia can be quite challenging either via laparoscopy or laparotomy. Low-volume (esophageal) surgeons should be mindful of extrapolating results reported from experts in high-volume centers to their own practice. Because most patients with paraesophageal hernias are elderly and have significant comorbid conditions, surgery should be performed in patients with symptoms clearly caused by the hernia. These include postprandial pain, vomiting and dry heaves, pulmonary compromise, GI bleeding, and medically intractable GERD. Death related to surgical repair of hiatal hernias does occur and one must carefully weigh the risk of surgical complications against the benefits. It is a rare situation indeed where data would support surgical repair over expectant management in an asymptomatic patient with a PEH regardless of what the X ray looked like!

References

1. Allen MS, Trastek VF, Deschamps C, Pairolero PC. "Intrathoracic stomach: presentation of results

of operation. *J Thorac Cardiovasc Surg* 1993;105: 253–259.

2. Healthcare Cost and Utilization Project. *Nationwide Inpatient Sample (NIS) Release 6* [CD-ROM]. Rockville, MD: Agency for Healthcare Research and Quality; 1997.

3. Oddsdottir M. Paraesophageal hernia. *Surg Clin North Am* 2000;80:1243–1252.

4. Skinner D, Belsey R, Russell P. Surgical management of esophageal reflux and hiatus hernia. *J Thorac Cardiovasc Surg* 1967;53:33–54.

5. Hill L. Incarcerated paraesophageal hernia; a surgical emergency. *Am J Surg* 1973;126:286–291.

6. Tracey P, Jamieson G. An approach to the management of para-oesophageal hiatus hernias. *Aust N Z J Surg* 1987;57:813–817.

7. Floch N. Paraesophageal hernias: current concepts [editorial]. *J Clin Gastroent* 1999;29:6–7.

8. Horgan S, Eubanks TR, Jacobsen G, et al. Repair of paraesophageal hernias. *Am J Surg* 1999;177:354–358.

9. Pierre AF, Luketich JD, Fernando HC, et al. Results of laparoscopic repair of giant paraesophageal hernias: 200 consecutive patients. *Ann Thorac Surg* 2002;74:1909–1916.

10. Andujar P, Papasavas P, Birdas T, et al. Laparoscopic repair of large paraesophageal hernia is associated with a low incidence of recurrence and reoperation. *Surg Endosc* 2004;18:444–447.

11. Diaz S, Brunt M, Klingensmith M, et al. Laparoscopic paraesophageal hernia repair, a challenging operation: medium term outcomes of 166 patients. *J Gastrointest Surg* 2003;7:59–67.

12. Athanasakis A, Tzotzinis A, Tsiaoussis J, et al. Laparoscopic repair of paraersophageal hernia. *Endoscopy* 2001;33:590–594.

13. Dahlberg P, Dechamps C, Miller D, et al. Laparoscopic repair of large paraesophageal hiatal hernia. *Ann Thorac Surg* 2001;72:1125–1129.

14. Jobe B, Aye R, Deveney C, et al. Laparoscopic management of giant type III hiatal hernia and short esophagus: objecticve follow-up at 3 years. *J Gastrointest Surg* 2002;6:181–188.

15. Ponsky J, Rosen M, Fanning A, et al. Anterior gastropexy may reduce recurrence rate after laparoscopic paraesophageal hernia. *Surg Endosc* 2003;17: 1036–1041.

16. Wu J, Dunnegan N, Soper, N. Clinical and radiologic assessment of laparoscopic paraesophageal hernia repair. *Surg Endosc* 1999;13:497–502.

17. Hashemi M, Peters J, DeMeester TR, et al. Laparoscopic repair of large type III hiatal hernia: objective followup reveals high recurrence rate. *J Am Coll Surg* 2000;190:553–561.

18. Khaitan L, Houston H, Sharp K et al. Laparoscopic paraesophageal hernia repair has an acceptable recurrence rate. *Am Surg* 2002;68:546–552.

19. Aly A, Munt J, Jamieson G, et al. Laparoscopic repair of large paraesophageal hernias. *Br J Surg* 2005;92:648–653.

20. Stylopoulos N, Gazelle G, Rattner D. Paraesophageal hernias: operation or observation? *Ann Surg* 2002;236:492–501.

44
Plication for Diaphragmatic Eventration

Marco Alifano

Diaphragmatic eventration is an anomaly defined by the long-lasting or permanent elevation of an entire hemidiaphragm or a portion of it, without defects. The muscular insertions are normal, the normal apertures are sealed, and there is no interruption in pleural or peritoneal layer.[1] These characteristics allow distinction from diaphragmatic hernias. By contrast, the terms eventration and paralysis are often confused: paralysis may be the cause of an abnormal elevation of the diaphragm, whereas pure eventration is not associated with paralysis.[1] A marked decrease in muscular fibers is a characteristic of eventration, whereas in paralysis the diaphragm is still muscular, even if somewhat atrophic.[1] True eventration would be, in the opinion of most authors, the consequence of a congenital defect of one portion or the entire central part of the diaphragm, resulting from an incomplete migration of cervical somites into the pleuro-peritoneal membrane.[2] This would explain the membranous appearance of the central portion of the hemidiaphragm, in spite of a normal muscular appearance of the peripheral portion of the muscle.[1,3]

Acquired elevation of the diaphragm is also often termed, though less appropriately, eventration. Though exhaustive workup often allows recognition of a phrenic nerve dysfunction, cases with an intact phrenic nerve do exist.[1,4] In spite of several differences, both eventration and paralysis (both will be often termed "eventration" in the following part of this chapter) carry the same physiological consequences and share most symptoms. However the management may be substantially different.[1]

In adulthood both the presence of symptoms and the amount of functional impairment are largely variable. Dyspnea is frequently observed and is typically worse in the supine position.[5] Other presentations include chest pain, recurrent respiratory infections, palpitations, and dyspepsia,[1,6] but completely asymptomatic patients exist. Decompensation of respiratory status requiring mechanical ventilation has been reported[4,7]; in these cases diaphragmatic eventration represents a factor aggravating an underlying pulmonary or cardiac problem.

Elevation of the diaphragm in childhood generally carries more pronounced symptoms, especially in newborns. Paradoxical respiration is much more frequent because of the weakness of intercostals muscles, softness of thoracic cage, and important mobility of mediastinum. Increased abdominal pressure associated with the supine position further aggravates paradoxical respiration. As a consequence, respiratory distress is frequent and mechanical ventilation may be necessary. Furthermore, the frequently associated cardiac or pulmonary malformations (especially ipsilateral lung hypoplasia) may contribute to the gravity of the clinical picture.[1] Overall, congenital eventration is symptomatic in most patients, although it is believed that some cases may be recognized only in adulthood.[1]

Different surgical techniques have been proposed to treat diaphragmatic eventration.[1] Plication through standard thoracotomy is the more frequently employed technique, but less invasive approaches employing video-assisted technology have been developed.[4,8,9] In this chapter we will review indications, technical options, and results of surgical treatment of diaphragmatic eventration.

44.1. Indications for Plication

44.1.1. Childhood

There are several papers addressing the issue of indication for surgery in children with diaphragmatic elevation.[1,7,9–15] Most of available data concern patients with phrenic nerve injury, whereas indications for surgery in patients with congenital eventration have been less extensively studied.

44.1.1.1. Congenital Eventration

Knowledge about treatment of congenital eventration is mainly derived from case reports and relatively small retrospective series.[1,11,12] Patients were generally symptomatic and in most cases they presented with respiratory distress. There are no data comparing surgical treatment to conservative management and the timing of operation with respect to the onset of symptoms is generally not stated. In these patients, if there is no evidence of phrenic nerve injury, spontaneous recovery is unlikely, and surgical indication is probably indicated in every symptomatic patient. These babies are often severely ill because of frequently associated comorbidities, and diaphragm repositioning may help partially restore hypoplastic lung function.[1,11,12] Little is known about management of patients with few or no symptoms; though conservative management is probably sufficient, some authors advocate routine plication in order to maximize the development of the ipsilateral lung.[11]

The indication for plication exists in every symptomatic child with congenital eventration (level of evidence 4; recommendation grade C). Indication for plication in asymptomatic children with congenital eventration: insufficient data to provide level of evidence or grade of recommendation.

> Every symptomatic child with congenital eventration should undergo repair (level of evidence 4; recommendation grade C).
>
> There is insufficient data to provide level of evidence or recommendation grade for children with asymptomatic congenital eventration.

44.1.1.2. Phrenic Nerve Injury

Management of pediatric patients with phrenic nerve injury (postpartum or postoperative) has been much more extensively studied. The condition is generally suspected because of respiratory distress, failure to thrive, and, in operated patients, difficulties in weaning from mechanical ventilation. Upon suspicion, confirmation is obtained by chest X ray, fluoroscopy, and/or ultrasonography of the chest.[1,7,9–15]

The policies of different centers are quite variable in terms of indication and timing of surgery. In the retrospective surgical series by Tsugawa and colleagues,[11] including 50 patients aged 4 days to 7 years with diaphragmatic elevation of miscellaneous origin (but secondary to phrenic nerve injury in most cases), the indication for surgery was always respiratory distress. Ventilatory support was necessary in 10 of the patients for 2 to 6 weeks before plication. Unfortunately the number of patients managed conservatively during the time frame of the study (1971–1996) is not stated. This type of information can be derived by the retrospective experience (1996–2000) of Joho-Arreola and colleagues,[10] dealing with 43 pediatric patients with diaphragmatic paralysis complicating cardiac surgery. Twenty-nine patients underwent plication because of failure to wean from mechanical ventilation or respiratory distress. In the 14 patients treated conservatively, the mean assisted ventilation time after cardiac surgery was relatively short (5 days), but some patients were mechanically ventilated for several weeks (up to 49 days). Patients ultimately treated by plication received mechanical ventilation for a longer period (mean, 13 days) before the decision to perform plication. Similarly, in the retrospective series by de Vries Reilingh and coworkers,[14] 18 consecutive patients with obstetrical phrenic nerve injury were evaluated between 1986 and

1997. All required resuscitation immediately after birth and 14 of them received intubation and mechanical ventilation. Thirteen out of 18 patients were ultimately treated by plication (on average 100 days postpartum), whereas in the remaining 5 patients spontaneous clinical and radiological recovery was observed within 1 month.

The general idea that can be drawn from the analysis of literature is that conservative management was always attempted before indicating surgery in children with phrenic nerve injury. There is general agreement that surgery should be performed only after stabilization of the patient's clinical condition by gastric decompression, administration of supplemental oxygen, and, if necessary, mechanical ventilation, but the optimal time frame to perform plication is not known. In fact, nonoperative management allows restoration of diaphragmatic function if the phrenic nerve is not transected, but the time necessary can be so long (several weeks or several months) to expose patients to the unacceptable risks associated to prolonged mechanical ventilation. As a result, surgery should be proposed within a few weeks from diagnosis of postsurgical diaphragmatic paralysis. If phrenic nerve injury is recognized to have occurred during the initial cardiac or mediastinal operation, immediate plication should be performed.

Plication is indicated in every pediatric patient with phrenic nerve injury, after a reasonably long period (1–3 weeks) of respiratory support (level of evidence 4; recommendation grade C).

44.1.2. Adulthood

Experience about surgical treatment of eventration in adulthood is much more limited. Most of the experience is derived from case reports, a small number of retrospective series,[3,12,16,17] and few prospective studies.[4,18] Controversies exist about indications and optimal timing of surgery; in this context considerations about the natural history of diaphragmatic elevation are of paramount importance.

44.1.2.1. Natural History of Diaphragmatic Elevation in Adults

Information about spontaneous evolution of nontraumatic diaphragmatic paralysis can be derived by the large retrospective study by Piehler and colleagues[19] of 247 patients seen at the Mayo Clinic between 1960 and 1980. The cause of paralysis could be identified at initial evaluation in 105 patients, but remained obscure in the remaining 142 subjects who could be followed-up for a mean of 8.7 years, as surgical repair was not attempted. The etiology of paralysis became evident in only six patients during the follow-up. In the remaining 136 cases, the leading symptom (exertional dyspnea) improved in only 34% of cases, whereas improvement in the other manifestations (cough or chest wall pain) was observed in 78% and 82% of cases, respectively. On chest X ray the diaphragm returned to its normal position in only 12 out of 131 patients who had this examination available.

Efthimiou and associates[20] studied the evolution of postsurgical diaphragmatic paralysis. In a prospective, observational study enrolling 100 consecutive patients over a 6-month period, they reported a 32% incidence of unilateral paralysis among patients receiving ice/slush topical hypothermia during cardiac surgery, as compared to 2% among those not receiving topical hypothermia. All these patients were treated conservatively and paralysis regressed within 1, 6, and 12 months in 25%, 56%, and 69% of cases, respectively. At the 2-year follow-up the paralysis had regressed in all but one patient. Electromyography showed the absence of nerve conduction in all the patients within 1 week after cardiac surgery, but there was progressive reappearance of conduction in patients who experienced restoring of diaphragmatic function. Obviously, in these patients, the phrenic nerve had suffered a thermal injury, but had not been transected.

In the experience of Deng and coworkers,[21] derived from a retrospective analysis of a prospectively collected database of patients undergoing high free right internal mammary artery harvesting, the incidence of right-sided diaphragmatic paralysis was 4%. In this setting, the phrenic nerve can be either thermally injured (by the proximity of electrocautery dissection) or completely transected. Management included immediate diaphragmatic plication (i.e., during the sternotomy for cardiac surgery) if phrenic nerve transection was identified intraoperatively, or a middle-term observation for postoperatively evidenced paralysis. Conservative management was adopted for the first 3 months after cardiac surgery and plication was recommended in the absence of spontaneous regression of paralysis (apparently regardless of the presence of symptoms). Among the 26 patients with postoperative diaphragmatic paralysis, a spontaneous regression was observed in 14 cases and all the remaining 12 were finally operated on.

44.1.2.2. Indications for Plication in Adults

Information about the indications for plication can be derived from some retrospective surgical series evaluating the outcomes in adult patients with diaphragmatic eventration treated by surgery.[3,7,12,16,17] All these studies included patients with diaphragmatic paralysis secondary to different conditions and idiopathic forms. In almost all the instances the indication for surgery was based on the presence of respiratory symptoms (mainly dyspnea or orthopnea but also cough and chest wall pain) or, less commonly, digestive symptoms (dyspepsia or meteorism) that interfered with the patients' normal activities. The mere presence of an elevated diaphragm on X ray was generally (with some exceptions) not considered an indication for operation. In some cases plication was indicated in an effort to aid weaning from mechanical ventilation in patients with postsurgical diaphragmatic paralysis considered responsible of ventilatory failure. Due to the retrospective character of these surgical series, conservative management was not evaluated and the number (and relative proportion) of patients treated by a nonoperative approach in the same time frames in the different institutions is not stated.

In the recent prospective study by Mouroux and colleagues,[4] plication was performed in 12 patients with unilateral diaphragmatic elevation (9 post-traumatic, 1 post-tuberculosis, 1 due to Charcot–Marie disease, 1 idiopathic) over an 11-year period. In 10 of 12 cases, the surgical indication was established on the basis of persistent symptoms (mainly dyspnea), after a long period of conservative management. In the remaining two patients, a plication was performed to aid in weaning patients from mechanical ventilation. In the same period of the study, two other patients were managed conservatively and spontaneous regression of paralysis was observed.

It is generally believed that there is no indication for surgical treatment of diaphragmatic eventration when the condition is secondary to a neoplastic disease or in the absence of symptoms. If a neoplastic origin is excluded on clinical and radiologic grounds, the surgical indication has to be evaluated on the basis of clinical presentation and timing of onset of symptoms.[4] If the patient is symptomatic and the diaphragmatic eventration is long-lasting (more than 2 years), surgery is generally indicated; surgery is planned once clinical conditions have been optimized (e.g., treatment of respiratory infections, obesity, etc.). If the patient is symptomatic but the diaphragmatic eventration is recent, a period of observation (18–24 months) prior to recommending surgery should be advocated. In these patients serial diaphragmatic electromyographies may be suggested to identify possible recovery in phrenic nerve function. Finally, if the patient has no or few symptoms, he has to be strictly followed-up in order to identify even moderate deterioration of respiratory function, which is an indication for surgery. In fact, if significant respiratory impairment is already present, a modest chest trauma or a pulmonary infection may precipitate the clinical conditions and require mechanical ventilation.[4]

Plication is indicated in adult patients with long-lasting symptomatic diaphragmatic elevation (level of evidence 4; recommendation grade C).

> Plication is indicated in adult patients with long-lasting symptomatic diaphragmatic elevation (level of evidence 4; recommendation grade C).
>
> Plication is indicated in every pediatric patient with phrenic nerve injury, after a reasonably long period (1–3 weeks) of respiratory support (level of evidence 4; recommendation grade C).

44.2. Surgical Technique

Morrison published a report of the first surgical repair in 1923.[22] Since this initial description, different surgical techniques have been proposed. Plication can be carried out by thoracic or abdominal access; open surgery or video-assisted techniques have been proposed.

44.2.1. Open Approaches

It is generally believed that a phrenic nerve injury complicating cardiac surgery in children, if recognized intraoperatively, should prompt immediate plication through the sternotomy.[1,13] There is no consensus or sufficient data about plication in similar circumstances in adults. In any other setting sternotomy is obviously not an option.

A midline laparotomy has been employed in cases of bilateral diaphragmatic elevation or infracardiac involvement, although such an approach is occasionally employed in case of pure unilateral diaphragmatic elevation.[1] The exception is represented by patients with diaphragmatic eventration associated with an intra-abdominal disease requiring surgery. In these cases laparotomy is adequate in dealing with both conditions.[23]

Transthoracic plication has been generally performed by a standard posterolateral thoracotomy. Simple plication is generally employed because it is faster and avoids entry into the peritoneal cavity. The technique described by Schwartz and Filler[24] (sometimes slightly modified) is usually employed: the slack portion of the diaphragm is pulled in a radial direction and pleats are created by full-thickness nonabsorbable mattress sutures. The surgeon should aim at repositioning the dome of the diaphragm one or two intercostal spaces below where it should ultimately be located.

The more frequently employed alternative technique is represented by resection of the excess aponeurotic portion of the diaphragm with a two-layer overlapping approximation of peripheral muscle. This technique offers the advantage of avoiding inadvertent injury to abdominal organs but it involves the frequent section of phrenic nerve branches. Cases of suture dehiscence have been reported.[1]

Repair of congenital eventration in children may present some challenges: a possibly associated pulmonary sequestration should be resected and the possible absence of the medial component of the diaphragm may be corrected by using the diaphragmatic portion of the pericardium rather than a prosthetic material. Furthermore, if abdominal organs cannot be reduced in the peritoneal cavity, creation of a temporary ventral hernia may be performed.[1]

44.2.2. Video-Assisted Thoracic Surgery

In 1996, Mouroux and colleagues[18] proposed plication through a video-assisted thoracic surgery (VATS) approach. Two 5-mm thoracic ports and a 4-cm minithoracotomy in the ninth intercostal space were employed. In the majority of cases no rib retraction is necessary. The apex of the eventration is invaginated into the abdomen, thus creating a transverse fold from the periphery to the cardiophrenic angle behind the prenic nerve. This fold is closed by two superposed series of transverse back-and-forth continuous sutures with a nonresorbable material. This first suture allows the surgeon to maintain the excess of diaphragm within the abdomen; the second row of stitches is inserted through more peripheral portions of diaphragm in order to obtain the desired tension.

Since the initial publication of Mouroux and colleagues, other authors reported their experience with the same or very similar techniques.[25,26] Several reports and some series have reported on the experiences of different centers in both adult and pediatric patients. Van Smith[26] successfully treated a newborn weighting 3kg. Totally endoscopic approaches have also been described.[7,27] The obvious advantage of VATS methods over open surgery is the minimal invasiveness which would facilitate postoperative recovery and respiratory muscle retraining.

Plication should be carried out by transthoracic approach in the absence of indication for an abdominal approach (bilateral or infracardiac involvement, associated intra-abdominal disease; level of evidence 4; recommendation grade C). Plication for eventration is technically feasible by VATS; the operation is bloodless and rapid, and the desired tension can be applied to the plicated diaphragm (level of evidence 4).

Plication should be carried out by transthoracic approach in the absence of indication for an abdominal approach (bilateral or infracardiac involvement, associated intra-abdominal disease) (level of evidence 4; recommendation grade C).

Plication for eventration is technically feasible by VATS; the operation is bloodless and rapid, and the desired tension can be applied to the plicated diaphragm (level of evidence 4; recommendation grade C).

44.3. Results

The results expected from plication are obviously different depending on the clinical context. As stated earlier in this chapter, children often undergo plication because of congenital or acquired elevation of the diaphragm that is responsible for serious respiratory impairment, and the goal of the operation is in most cases weaning from mechanical ventilation. In adulthood, respiratory function is generally much less compromised, and surgery is indicated to improve dyspnea or digestive symptoms.

44.3.1. Childhood

44.3.1.1. Postoperative Outcome

There are several studies evaluating the outcome of pediatric patients treated by diaphragmatic plication, generally for phrenic nerve injury. They are summarized in Table 44.1. These studies

aimed at evaluating operative mortality, the impact of the procedure on weaning patients from respiratory support, and, in some cases, improvement in clinical and/or radiologic status. In the retrospective series by Tsugawa and colleagues[11] dealing with 25 children with phrenic nerve injury treated by thoracotomy and plication, weaning from respiratory support (mechanical ventilation or supplemental oxygen) was possible in a short period (0–6 days) in 15/17 patients; the two failures were managed by redo plication that was successful in one instance. In the same study, 25 other patients underwent plication for congenital eventration and 4 of them were mechanically ventilated prior to operation; weaning was possible in all the cases from 1 to 61 days postoperatively.

Similar results are reported in the retrospective study by Simansky and colleagues.[7] Among the 10 children with postsurgical phrenic nerve injury responsible for respiratory failure and treated by open plication, 7 could be weaned from mechanical ventilation (within 8 days in 6 cases). The remaining three died in spite of a radiographically successful plication, mainly because of intractable underlying cardiac disease. No deaths were reported in the series by Tonz and coworkers,[15] who operated on 11 out of 25 patients with postsurgical phrenic nerve injury (the remaining patients were managed nonoperatively), because of failure to wean from mechanical ventilation or respiratory distress after extubation. Weaning was possible in all the cases (in all but two patients within a week) and respiratory distress could be managed successfully in all the cases.

TABLE 44.1. Outcome of plication in children.

Reference	Year of publication	Period of study	Design of study	No. of patients	Overall operative mortality	Mortality related to plication	Duration of follow-up (years)	Weaning from respiratory support	Radiological improvement	Clinical improvement
Tonz[15]	1996	1983–1992	Retrospective	11	0/11	0/11	3.2 (mean)	11/11	10/11	9/9
Tzugawa[11]	1997	1971–1996	Retrospective	25	5/25	0/25	1–25	–	20/20	20/20
De Vries[14]	1998	1986–1997	Retrospective	14	0/14	0/14	–	9/9	–	14/14
De Leeuw[13]	1999	1985–1997	Retrospective	68	4/68	0/68	–	49/50	–	–
Simansky[7]	2002	1988–2000	Retrospective	10	3/10	0/10	–	7/7[a]	–	–
Hines[9]	2003	–	Retrospective	5	0/5	0/5	–	2/2	5/5	5/5
Joho-Arreola[10]	2005	1996–2000	Retrospective	29	8/29	0/29	1	–	13/21	–

[a]Not taking into account operative mortality.

A more consistent experience, albeit retrospective, can be drawn from the study by de Leeuw and associates,[13] also dealing with postsurgical phrenic nerve paralysis. In their experience 40% of 170 children with this condition underwent open plication. The indication for operation was respiratory insufficiency in almost all of the cases, with most patients being mechanically ventilated at the time of plication. The median time to final extubation after plication was 4 days, with a range of 1 to 65 days. Multivariate analysis showed that independent factors associated with a longer time to extubation were bilateral paralysis and a longer interval from the initial operation to diagnosis. There were 4 in-hospital deaths, but none of these was considered related to the procedure. As in all the other above-mentioned pediatric series, all the deaths were considered secondary to underlying diseases.

Further evidence that the plication per se is not associated with mortality or major morbidity is provided by the experience of de Vries Reillingh and colleagues,[14] who performed the operation with an open approach in 13 patients with phrenic nerve injury, in almost all the cases resulting from an obstetrical trauma (therefore with no associated cardiac or pulmonary malformations). Respiratory distress requiring mechanical ventilation was present in most cases. Dramatic improvement was observed in all the patients, with discontinuation of mechanical ventilation possible within a few days and return to normal gas values in all the cases.

A small series of diaphragmatic plication in children by VATS has been recently published.[9] The authors reported on five children weighing 3.2 to 13.2 kg with congenital or postsurgical diaphragmatic eventration responsible for respiratory insufficiency or recurrent respiratory infections. Satisfactory clinical and radiologic results were observed in all the cases. In particular, weaning from mechanical ventilation was achieved within 3 days in both patients undergoing surgery for this indication.

44.3.1.2. Long-term Outcome

In some surgical series of pediatric patients, information about long-term follow-up is available. Tonz and colleagues[15] reported no late death

related to diaphragmatic paralysis and good radiologic results in 10 out of 11 patients. No children had respiratory symptoms at late follow-up. Similarly, Tsugawa and coworkers[11] observed fully satisfactory clinical and radiologic results in all the patients available at follow-up after plication for either phrenic nerve injury or congenital eventration. On the other hand, in the study by Joho-Arreola and associates,[10] 6 out of 21 patients had elevated diaphragm at 1-year follow-up; unfortunately, the percentage of patients with respiratory symptoms in that study is not stated.

Overall, diaphragmatic elevation secondary to phrenic nerve injury in children may be satisfactorily managed by plication: in almost all the instances weaning from respiratory support is possible, in many instances within a short delay. Mortality is generally related to the underlying disease and not to the operation itself. Similarly, long-term outcome is fixed by the possibly associated comorbidities, as the operation allows a permanent improvement of respiratory function (level of evidence 4).

44.3.2. Adulthood

As adults with unilateral diaphragmatic elevation generally present with mild respiratory insufficiency, weaning from mechanical ventilation is a rare indication for plication. In the recent prospective study by Mouroux and coworkers,[4] the operation (by video-assisted surgery) was performed for this indication in only two patients and both were successfully weaned within 1 week. In contrast, only one among the four mechanically ventilated patients in the series by Simanski and colleagues[7] (dealing with patients with phrenic nerve injury) could be weaned.

When the operation is performed because of less severe respiratory symptoms or because of digestive problems, satisfactory results are uniformly observed (Table 44.2). In the above-mentioned retrospective study by Simanski and colleagues, all of the seven nonventilated patients experienced an improvement of ATS dyspnea score of 2 or 3 levels at their 3-month re-evaluation. At long-term follow-up (11–114 months), all were completely asymptomatic from a respiratory point of view [7].

TABLE 44.2. Outcome of plication in adults (nonventilated patients).

Reference	Year of publication	Period of study	Design of study	No. of patients	Operative mortality	Duration of follow-up (years)	Improvement		
							Clinical	Radiologic	Functional
Wright[3]	1985	–	Retrospective	7	0	0.3–4	7/7	7/7	7/7
Graham[17]	1990	1979–1989	Retrospective	17	0	5–7	6/6	6/6	6/6
Ribet[12]	1992	1968–1988	Retrospective	11	0/11	8.5 (mean)	9/11	6/11	5/5
Simansky[7]	2002	1988–2000	Retrospective	7	0/7	7.3 (mean)	7/7	7/7	7/7
Higgs[16]	2002	1983–1990	Retrospective	19	0/19	7–14 (n = 15)	14/15	14/15	15/15
Mouroux[4]	2005	1992–2003	Prospective	10	0/10	6.3 (mean)	10/10	10/10	10/10

In the experience of Graham and coworkers dealing with 17 patients treated by thoracotomy and plication between 1979 and 1989, improvement was observed in all the patients in both subjective (dyspnea score) and objective measurements. In particular, the operation resulted in significant improvement in terms of postoperative forced vital capacity (FVC), total lung capacity (TLC), diffusing capacity of carbon monoxide (DLCO), P_{O_2}, and P_{CO_2}. These satisfactory results were still present in all the six patients who could be reassessed at long-term (>5 years) follow-up.[17] In the retrospective study by Ribet and Linder,[12] 9 out of 11 patients were persistently asymptomatic after the operation (3 months–18 years follow-up), 1 was mildly dyspneic, and 1 had persistent digestive symptoms. Of note, chest X rays showed a persistently elevated (though at a lesser extent) diaphragm in five cases. In this study only five patients had both preoperative and postoperative functional assessment, and an improvement in both FVC and forced expiratory volume in 1s (FEV_1) was observed in all the cases.

In the prospective study of Nice University Hospital dealing with 12 adult patients treated by video-assisted plication for diaphragmatic elevation of miscellaneous origin (post-traumatic in most instances),[4] all the patients experienced a complete disappearance of symptoms shortly after the operation and no radiologic relapse was observed at a follow-up of more than 64 months. A significant improvement in both FEV_1 and FVC was observed at late spirometry in all the cases.

Regardless of the surgical technique, diaphragmatic plication in nonventilated adult patients carries a low morbidity and a very low, if any, mortality (level of evidence 4). Functional results are fully satisfactory in almost all the cases,

regardless of the surgical approach (level of evidence 4).

Plication by VATS achieved results similar to those obtained by conventional surgery.[4] Unfortunately the rarity of eventration precludes the possibility of performing randomized studies to enable accurate comparisons. This technique can be proposed as an alternative to conventional plication through standard thoracotomy.

References

1. Frechette E, Cloutier R, Deslauriers J. Congenital eventration and acquired elevation of the diaphragm. In: Shields TW, ed. *General Thoracic Surgery*. Chicago: Lippincott Williams & Wilkins; 2004:1537–1549.
2. Schumpelick V, Steinau G, Schluper I, Prescher A. Surgical embriology and anatomy of the diaphragm with surgical applications. *Surg Clin North Am* 2000;80:213–239.
3. Wright CD, Williams JG, Ogilvie CM, Donnelly RJ. Results of the diaphragm plication for unilateral diaphragmatic paralysis. *J Thorac Cardiovasc Surg* 1985;90:195–198.
4. Mouroux J, Venissac N, Leo F, Alifano M, Guillot F. Surgical treatment of diaphragmatic eventration using video-assisted thoracic surgery: a prospective study. *Ann Thorac Surg* 2005;79:308–312.
5. Clague HW, Hall DR. Effect of posture on lung volume: airway closure and gas exchange in hemidiaphragmatic paralysis. *Thorax* 1979;34:523–526.
6. Dor J, Richelme H, Aubert J, Boyer R. L'éventration diaphragmatique. *J Chir* 1969;97:399–432.
7. Simansky DA, Paley M, Refaely Y, Yellin A. Diaphragm plication following phrenic nerve injury: a comparison of paediatric and adult patients. *Thorax* 2002;57:613–616.
8. Huttl TP, Wichmann MW, Reichart B, Geiger TK, Schildberg FW, Meyer G. Laparoscopic diaphragmatic plication. *Surg Endosc* 2004;18:547–551.

9. Hines MH. Video-assisted diaphragm plication in children. *Ann Thorac Surg* 2003;76:234–236.

10. Joho-Arreola AL, Bauersfeld U, Stauffer UG, Baenziger O, Bernet V. Incidence and treatment of diaphragmatic paralyisis after cardiac surgery in children. *Eur J Cardiothorac Surg* 2005;27:53–57.

11. Tsugawa C, Kimura K, Nishijima E, Muraji T, Yamaguchi M. Diaphragmatic eventration in infants and children. Is conservative treatment justified? *J Pediatr Surg* 1997;32:1643–1644.

12. Ribet M, Linder JL. Plication of the diaphragm for unilateral eventration or paralysis. *Eur J Cardiothorac Surg* 1992;6:357–360.

13. de Leeuw M, Williams JM, Freedom RM, Williams WG, Shemie SD, McCrindle BW. Impact of diaphragmatic paralysis after cardiothoracic surgery in children. *J Thorac Cardiovasc Surg* 1999;118:510–517.

14. de Vries Reilingh TS, Koens BL, Vos A. Surgical treatment of diaphragmatic eventration caused by phrenic nerve injury in the newborn. *J Pediatr Surg* 1988;33:602–605.

15. Tonz M, von Segesser LK, Mihaljevic T, Arbenz U, Stauffer UG, Turina MI. Clinical implications of phrenic nerve injury after pediatric cardiac surgery. *J Pediatr Surg* 1996;31:1265–1267.

16. Higgs SM, Hussain A, Jackson M, Donnelly RJ, Berrisford RG. Long term results of diaphragmatic plication for unilateral diaphragmatic paralysis. *Eur J Cardiothorac Surg* 2002;21:294–297.

17. Graham DR, Kaplan D, Evans CC, Hind CRK, Donelly RJ. Diaphragm plication for unilateral diaphragmatic paralysis: a 10-year experience. *Ann Thorac Surg* 1990;49:248–252.

18. Mouroux J, Padovani B, Poirier NC, et al. Technique for the repair of diaphragmatic eventration. *Ann Thorac Surg* 1996;62:905–907.

19. Pielher JM, Pairolero PC, Gracey DR, Bernatz PE. Unexplained diaphragmatic paralysis: a harbinger of malignant disease? *J Thorac Cardiovasc Surg* 1982;84:861–864.

20. Efthimiou J, Butler J, Benson MK, Westaby S. Bilateral diaphragm paralysis after cardiac surgery with topical hypothermia. *Ann Thorac Surg* 1991;52:1005–1008.

21. Deng Y, Byth K, Paterson H. Phrenic nerve injury associated with high free right internal mammary artery harvesting. *Ann Thorac Surg* 2003;76:459–463.

22. Morrison JMW. Eventration of diaphragm due to unilateral phrenic nerve paralysis. *Arch Radiol Electrother* 1923;28:72–75.

23. Smyrniotis V, Arkadopoulos N, Kostopanagiotou G, Gamaletsos E, Pistioli L, Kostopanagiotou E. Combination of diaphragmatic plication with major abdominal surgery in patients with phrenic nerve palsy. *Surgery* 2005;137:243–245.

24. Schwartz MZ, Filler RM. Plication of the diaphragm for symptomatic phrenic nerve paralysis. *J Pediatr Surg* 1978;13:259–263.

25. Lai DTM, Paterson HS. Mini-thoracotomy for diaphragmatic plication with thoracoscopic assistance. *Ann Thorac Surg* 1999;68:2364–2365.

26. Van Smith C, Jacobs JP, Burke RP. Minimally invasive diaphragm plication in a infant. *Ann Thorac Surg* 1998;65:842–844.

27. Cherian A, Stewart RJ. Thoracoscopic repair of diaphragmlatic eventration. *Pediatr Surg Int* 2004;20:872–874.

45
Pacing for Unilateral Diaphragm Paralysis

Raymond P. Onders

Symptoms of unilateral diaphragmatic paralysis can range from sleep-related symptoms to exertional dyspnea or orthopnea. At times unilateral diaphragm paralysis is found on routine chest radiograph alone when an elevated hemidiaphragm is seen. Ventilatory failure will usually only result if there is bilateral diaphragmatic involvement. When diaphragmatic paralysis is suspected, confirmatory testing is done by inspiratory fluoroscopy (sniff test) and electromyography of the phrenic nerve. To determine if the conduction path of the phrenic nerve is intact from the cervical region to the diaphragm, the key test is fluoroscopic visualization of the diaphragm with transcutaneous stimulation of the phrenic nerve in the neck. If the diaphragm moves during stimulation then the phrenic nerve is intact, but there is a disruption of the signal pathway from the respiratory center in the brain to the phrenic nerve causing the diaphragm not to function. With the use of fluoroscopic visualization during stimulation, false-positive phrenic nerve conduction studies are virtually eliminated. However, because of difficulties in locating the phrenic nerve in the cervical region there is a significant potential for false-negative studies, especially in inexperienced hands. The most common causes of an intact phrenic nerve with diaphragm paralysis are high cervical spinal cord injury or central hypoventilation syndrome (CHS or Ondine's Curse). In almost all of these cases the diaphragm paralysis is bilateral. Unilateral paralysis of the diaphragm usually involves a nonfunctioning phrenic nerve with the causes in decreasing order of frequency: idiopathic, postsurgical (cardiac, neck, and thoracic

surgeries), and trauma. Although sniff tests and phrenic nerve conduction studies with fluoroscopic observation can identify intact phrenic nerves, the negative results of these tests do not necessarily determine the extent or location of damage. Localized damage to the myelin sheath or acute edema will result in negative results and loss of central control of the diaphragm. Remyelinization or resolution of the edema may occur over a number of days to years.[1]

Diaphragm pacing for ventilatory support has been in use for over 30 years since first reported by Glenn.[2] There are several diaphragm pacing systems available including the conventional ones in which phrenic nerve cuff electrodes are placed with staged bilateral thoracotomies. The cervical electrode placement while utilized in the past is discouraged for the following reasons: there is an accessory branch from the lower segment of the cervical spinal cord that joins the phrenic nerve trunk in the thorax so that neck stimulation may result in incomplete diaphragm activation; brachial plexus nerves are in close proximity and may be activated resulting in pain or undesirable movement; and neck movements can increase mechanical stress on the nerve/electrode system which may increase the risk of nerve injury. There have been recent reports of placing the system thoracoscopically.[3,4] Diaphragm pacing with direct phrenic nerve electrodes is underutilized because of the scope of the operation, risk of phrenic nerve injury, and theoretical concerns about using it 24h/day. There is a more recent option that involves laparoscopic implantation of intramuscular electrodes at the motor point of the diaphragm.[5] This has been implanted in 18 spinal cord patients with excellent results. This is an outpatient operation with no risk of phrenic nerve injury and allows 24-h use with the longest patient continuing to pace full-time for over 5 years. In brief, this procedure involves laparoscopic mapping of the diaphragm to identify the motor point which is the area where a electrical stimulus can cause maximal contraction of the diaphragm.[6] Two electrodes are then placed on each hemi-diaphragm with a specially designed laparoscopic implant instrument (Synapse Biomedical, Oberlin, OH) and tunneled externally to the power source.[7]

Both the phrenic nerve cuff electrode system and the laparoscopic motor point diaphragm pacing stimulation system require an intact phrenic nerve. The conduction pathway is the phrenic nerve and if that is not intact none of the systems can deliver a stimulus to the target diaphragm muscle. Almost all causes of unilateral diaphragm paralysis in non-spinal-cord-injured patients involve a phrenic nerve that is nonfunctional, at least to some extent, below the cervical region. The medical literature describes nerve transfers to the phrenic nerve and use of a diaphragm pacing system[8] as an option in patients with an injured phrenic nerve. This procedure essentially involves the coaption of a proximal foreign nerve to the distal denervated nerve to reinnervate the latter by the donated axons. Cortical plasticity appears to play an important physiological role in the functional recovery of the reinnervated muscles. An independent electrical pacing system is necessary because the nerve that is transferred has no connection to the central respiratory system so it must be stimulated to cause independent diaphragm contraction to augment respiration.

This chapter will review the extant evidence to assess whether diaphragm pacing is an option for patients with unilateral paralysis of the diaphragm when there is an intact phrenic nerve and when there is no intact nerve.

45.1. Available Evidence

The initial review will assess the evidence of diaphragm pacing when there is diaphragmatic dysfunction but an intact phrenic nerve. Over the past 30 years, electrical activation of the phrenic nerves has been used to provide artificial ventilation in patients with chronic respiratory insufficiency. Despite their clinical effectiveness, their use has been limited to a carefully selected group of patients with bilateral diaphragmatic dysfunction and intact phrenic nerves. The benefits of diaphragm pacing have been well described in large series and include: decreased barotrauma with the use of natural negative pressure ventilation with their own diaphragm; increased mobility without need for ventilator; improved speech; improved olfactory sensation; and decreased risk for pulmonary infection.[9-14] In some of the early series, diaphragm pacing was considered successful for ventilatory support in only 50% of patients.[11,15,16] These early studies are not reflective of the modern-day experience with diaphragm pacing, as the technology and patient selection methods were not well defined. There have been few reports of modern-day success rates though several papers describe the use of diaphragm pacing for over 15 years.[17,18]

Three commercial systems are in current use for trans-thoracic direct phrenic nerve stimulation: Avery Biomedical Devices (Commack, NY), Atrotech OY (Tampere, Finland), and Medimplant Biotechnisches Labor (Vienna, Austria). These systems differ primarily in the electrode design and stimulus parameters. Phrenic pacers have been implanted in over 1500 patients worldwide. Drawbacks to these systems include the risk of injury to the phrenic nerve either by surgical manipulation or by the electrode itself, system component failure, and the high cost of the systems. Although the risk of injury to the nerve has decreased, it does exist because a section of the nerve must be mobilized for electrode placement. The incidence of component failure has declined as the systems have undergone revisions. However, all three require some extracorporeal component. Unlike the cardiac pacemaker, traditional phrenic pacers require an external transmitter and antenna to transmit both the power and control signal to an implanted receiver/stimulator. Also, at present, none of the systems has any feedback or timing mechanism to make them physiologically responsive, nor are they synchronized with the upper airway. Development of such a mechanism would be an added benefit to phrenic pacers over conventional mechanical ventilators. Cost is perhaps a larger hurdle to overcome. The phrenic nerve electrode pacing systems available today cost nearly $100,000 (for the system, implant, and rehabilitation). Unlike cardiac pacemakers, because of the low number of potential candidates for these systems and the relatively low profit potential, there is little interest from major manufacturers of medical devices. This may explain the limited effort to develop improved pacing systems.

An alternative to the trans-thoracic phrenic nerve stimulation is the laparoscopic diaphragm pacing stimulation (DPS) system. There have been 22 human subjects implanted with the DPS system [18 spinal cord injury patients and 4 amyotrophic lateral sclerosis (ALS) patients]. The results of the DPS system for spinal cord patients indicated that the DPS system produced a significant mean percentage increase in tidal volume relative to the basal required tidal volume.[19] The procedure has overcome the learning curve for the operation, with the implantation standardized in an outpatient surgical procedure.[20] Overall there has been a 94% success rate for the spinal cord injured patients with the only failure being the second patient who had a false-positive inclusion criterion. The laparoscopic motor point electrode DPS system is an easy application for diaphragmatic stimulation when the phrenic nerve is intact. It overcomes many of the shortcomings of the available phrenic nerve electrode systems. The development of a totally implantable system is feasible and under way.[21] It would be a significant advancement over presently available systems.

For patients with nonfunctioning phrenic nerves, electrical activation of the intercostal muscles is one approach to treat respiratory insufficiency. Unlike the diaphragm, these muscles are innervated by a group of nerves (intercostal nerves originating from the ventral rami of T2–T12). However, by placing a single electrode in the epidural surface of the spinal cord through a dorsal laminectomy, this group of nerves/muscles can be activated which can provide up to 40% of vital capacity through the parasternal and external intercostals that are primarily inspiratory. Electrical activation of the intercostal muscles alone has been used in patients, however, the maximum duration of intercostal pacing (without mechanical ventilation or spontaneous breathing activity) remained relatively short (<3h) and is not a viable option on its own.[22] Based on this, individuals with only one intact phrenic nerve had a combined intercostal system with a conventional diaphragm pacing system placed unilaterally. This system was successful in maintaining long-term ventilatory support in the four patients but presently is not in any further trials.[23]

In those patients with a nonfunctioning phrenic nerve, diaphragm pacing is not an option unless a nerve is transferred to the phrenic nerve to re-animate the diaphragm. With advances in microsurgical techniques for neural anastomosis and a better understanding of axonal degeneration and regeneration, the repair or transfer of a nerve to the phrenic nerve and subsequent reinnervation of the diaphragm is a possibility. With a viable nerve, diaphragmatic pacing is then an option. Krieger successfully described transferring a brachial nerve to the phrenic nerve in cats in 1983.[8] After a recovery period to allow for growth of axons down the anastomosed phrenic nerve (16–32 weeks), they were able to stimulate the nerve and have adequate diaphragm contractions. Following this initial study, Krieger and colleagues investigated using an intercostals nerve in place of the brachial nerve for the anastomosis. The intercostals nerve was a good donor because of its proximity to the phrenic nerve (reducing the time for axonal regeneration), its physiological function (activation of skeletal muscle for respiration), and its size (comparable to the phrenic nerve). The initial article describes a single case and a letter to the editor describes two additional cases.[24,25] Subsequently a series of six patients was then described in 2000.[26] All of the patients had spinal cord injury with the time from injury to nerve transfer ranging from 6 months to 3 years. In this series of six patients there were a total of 10 nerve transfers. Two patients only had single nerve transfer because the other nerve on direct exploration was found to be intact. Only four patients were available for study. The fifth patient is on a progressive pacing schedule and the sixth patient was only 1 month postoperative and with accepted growth of regenerating axons of 1 mm per day the distance from the anastomosis to the diaphragm of 50 mm could not have been covered. In this series the average time for diaphragmatic response was 7 months with the shortest 6 months and the longest 13 months, so the true growth rate can be as slow at 1 mm every 8 days. Two of the patients are classified as capable of pacing but presently are not being paced because of depression in one and one died of unrelated causes. In neither of these cases were the tidal volumes or diaphragmatic movement with stimulation given. Two patients (a total of three nerve transfers) are using the system 24 h/day, but again no data are given concerning the tidal volumes or diaphragmatic excursion with stimulation. Overall, of the eight nerve transfers that could be studied, all eight showed diaphragm motion with stimulation, which is impressive given the authors' own description of the operation as difficult because of the angles and the fact the anastomosis occurs on the beating heart. There is some concern of the long-term viability of this technique in these patients, though. There was a letter to the editor by a separate physician stating that one of the patients that was reported as a success is in actuality not using the system at all.[27] To date there has been no other reports of this technique in the literature although it is mentioned often in the literature as a possibility both for spinal cord–injured patients and also patients with isolated phrenic nerve injuries.

45.2. Summary of Evidence and Current Recommendations

Overall, none of the available data concerning diaphragm pacing specifically identify its use with unilateral diaphragm paralysis. The reason for this is that unilateral paralysis usually involves an injured phrenic nerve and therefore the diaphragm cannot be paced unless the diaphragm is re-innervated with a nerve transfer. So let us first look at the evidence for diaphragm function with intercostal transfer and diaphragm pacing. The level of evidence for diaphragm pacing using an intercostal nerve transfer is level 4 because it is a case series that only measured end results with tidal volumes with stimulation and measurements of outcomes in less than 80%

of the patients. Without more centers reporting their results or this series re-analyzing their results with a long-term follow-up, the recommendation grade is C. With this scarcity of evidence patients should not be given the hope of diaphragm pacing for a unilateral paralysis of the diaphragm unless they have an intact nerve.

> Patients should not be given the hope of diaphragm pacing for a unilateral paralysis of the diaphragm unless they have an intact nerve (level of evidence level 4; recommendation grade C).

The results of diaphragm pacing when the phrenic nerve is intact are excellent. The evidence for the ability to pace the diaphragm and provide tidal volumes is level 1 because of the long history of success of pacing in multiple centers and the all or none ability to assess the results. The patient's diaphragm either provides a tidal volume for ventilation with stimulation or is nonfunctional and the patient requires a mechanical ventilator when the device is turned off. The major change in diaphragm pacing is that it can now be done more safely and as an outpatient through the laparoscopic motor point stimulation technique with a higher success rate. The recommendation grade is A for *bilateral* diaphragm pacing when both phrenic nerves are intact.

> When both phrenic nerves are intact, results of *bilateral* diaphragm pacing are excellent (level of evidence 1; recommendation grade A).
>
> For *unilateral* diaphragm paralysis pacing is not beneficial because the phrenic nerve is usually not functional (level of evidence 5; recommendation grade D).

Unfortunately, for *unilateral* diaphragm paralysis there is no evidence that pacing is done because the phrenic nerve is usually not functional. If the nerve is intact but the diaphragm is nonfunctional then the level of evidence for pacing is 5 and the recommendation grade is D because it is only based on the physiology of the system and has not been reported in the literature. Presently, the discussions of an earlier chapter in this text concerning diaphragm plication may offer the most hope for patients with unilateral dennervated diaphragms.

45.3. Future Research

Future research should involve ways to help a damaged phrenic nerve recover in unilateral paralysis. When diaphragmatic dysfunction is identified after a thoracic or cardiac procedure, instead of waiting to see if recovery occurs we should be proactive in trying to help that recovery process. Functional electrical stimulation has been shown to help recovery of injured nerves and, with the intramuscular laparoscopic diaphragm pacing technique now in clinical use, we may have a way to stimulate the diaphragm so that some afferent affects along the nerve will promote recovery. There is now some preliminary data in a disease where the phrenic nerve is dying at a set rate – amyotrophic lateral sclerosis (Lou Gehrig's disease; unpublished results). By beginning a process of conditioning the diaphragm with the DPS system, we have been able to maintain diaphragmatic function in our early patients. This is partly due to the afferent effects of electrical stimulation but also preserving and strengthening the motor units that are left. The continuous decline in forced vital capacity of these initial patients has decreased which will increase their expected lifespan. This technique of using DPS can be expanded into acutely injured phrenic nerves in the hopes of reversing or improving the affects of acute phrenic nerve injuries. This technique would not require any nerve transfers and if the nerve recovers it can be easily removed. A prospective trial of using DPS is necessary to show if this would help.

There is also a significant number of patients who were told they have a negative phrenic nerve conduction test (a nonfunctioning nerve) when, on repeat evaluation in our laboratory, we were able to show diaphragmatic movement with a nerve conduction study. Phrenic nerve studies are difficult to reproduce, especially in patients that are overweight or have thick necks. We were able to subsequently implant these patients with the laparoscopic motor point electrode system. With a simple laparoscopic mapping stimulation tool, before giving up on diaphragmatic function or prior to plication, the diaphragm should be surgically studied. If at the time of plication the diaphragm responds to intraoperative stimulation, a motor point electrode with the DPS system should be placed and diaphragm function maintained. This may be a better long-term option than plication. This hopefully will be an option in our armentarium for unilateral diaphragm function in the future.

References

1. Oo T, Watt JW, Soni BM, Sett PK. Delayed diaphragm recovery in 12 patients after high cervical spinal cord injury. A retrospective review of the diaphragm status of 107 patients ventilated after acute spinal cord injury. *Spinal Cord* 1999;37:117–122.
2. Glenn WW, Holcomb WG, Hogan J, et al. Diaphragm pacing by radiofrequency transmission in the treatment of chronic ventilatory insufficiency. Present status. *J Thorac Cardiovasc Surg* 1973;66:505–520.
3. Morgan JA, Ginsburg ME, Sonett JR, et al. Advanced thoracoscopic procedures are facilitated by computer-aided robotic technology. *Eur J Cardiothorac Surg* 2003;23:883–887; discussion 887.
4. Shaul DB, Danielson PD, McComb JG, Keens TG. Thoracoscopic placement of phrenic nerve electrodes for diaphragmatic pacing in children. *J Pediatr Surg* 2002;37:974–978; discussion 978.
5. DiMarco AF, Onders RP, Kowalski KE, Miller ME, Ferek S, Mortimer JT. Phrenic nerve pacing in a tetraplegic patient via intramuscular diaphragm electrodes. *Am J Respir Crit Care Med* 2002;166:1604–1606.
6. Onders RP, Aiyar H, Mortimer JT. Characterization of the human diaphragm muscle with respect to the phrenic nerve motor points for diaphragmatic pacing. *Am Surg* 2004;70:241–247; discussion 247.
7. Aiyar H, Stellato TA, Onders RP, Mortimer JT. Laparoscopic implant instrument for the placement of intramuscular electrodes in the diaphragm. *IEEE Trans Rehabil Eng* 1999;7:360–371.
8. Krieger AJ, Danetz I, Wu SZ, Spatola M, Sapru HN. Electrophrenic respiration following anastomosis

of phrenic with branchial nerve in the cat. *J Neurosurg* 1983;59:262–267.

9. Dobelle WH, D'Angelo MS, Goetz BF, et al. 200 cases with a new breathing pacemaker dispel myths about diaphragm pacing. *ASAIO J* 1994;40:M244–M252.

10. Elefteriades JA, Quin JA, Hogan JF, et al. Long-term follow-up of pacing of the conditioned diaphragm in quadriplegia. *Pacing Clin Electrophysiol* 2002;25:897–906.

11. Tibballs J. Diaphragmatic pacing: an alternative to long-term mechanical ventilation. *Anaesth Intensive Care* 1991;19:597–601.

12. Creasey G, Elefteriades J, DiMarco A, et al. Electrical stimulation to restore respiration. *J Rehabil Res Dev* 1996;33:123–132.

13. DiMarco A. Diaphragm pacing in patients with spinal cord injury. *Topics Spinal Cord Rehabil* 1999;5:6–20.

14. Glenn WW, Phelps ML, Elefteriades JA, Dentz B, Hogan JF. Twenty years of experience in phrenic nerve stimulation to pace the diaphragm. *Pacing Clin Electrophysiol* 1986;9:780–784.

15. Carter RE, Donovan WH, Halstead L, Wilkerson MA. Comparative study of electrophrenic nerve stimulation and mechanical ventilatory support in traumatic spinal cord injury. *Paraplegia* 1987;25:86–91.

16. Weese-Mayer DE, Silvestri JM, Kenny AS, et al. Diaphragm pacing with a quadripolar phrenic nerve electrode: an international study. *Pacing Clin Electrophysiol* 1996;19:1311–1319.

17. Elefteriades JA, Quin JA. Diaphragm pacing. *Chest Surg Clin North Am* 1998;8:331–357.

18. Elefteriades JA, Hogan JF, Handler A, Loke JS. Long-term follow-up of bilateral pacing of the diaphragm in quadriplegia. *N Engl J Med* 1992;326:1433–1434.

19. DiMarco AF, Onders RP, Ignagni A, Kowalski KE, Mortimer JT. Phrenic nerve pacing via intramuscular diaphragm electrodes in tetraplegic subjects. *Chest* 2005;127:671–678.

20. Onders RP, Dimarco AF, Ignagni AR, Mortimer JT. The Learning curve for investigational surgery: lessons learned from laparoscopic diaphragm pacing for chronic ventilator dependence. *Surg Endosc* 2005;19(5):633–637.

21. Cosendai G, de Balthasar C, Ignagni AR, et al. A preliminary feasibility study of different implantable pulse generators technologies for diaphragm pacing system. *Neuromodulation* 2005;8:203–211.

22. DiMarco AF, Supinski GS, Petro JA, Takaoka Y. Evaluation of intercostal pacing to provide artificial ventilation in quadriplegics. *Am J Respir Crit Care Med* 1994;150:934–940.

23. DiMarco AF, Takaoka Y, Kowalski KE. Combined intercostal and diaphragm pacing to provide artificial ventilation in patients with tetraplegia. *Arch Phys Med Rehabil* 2005;86:1200–1207.

24. Krieger AJ, Gropper MR, Adler RJ. Electrophrenic respiration after intercostal to phrenic nerve anastomosis in a patient with anterior spinal artery syndrome: technical case report. *Neurosurgery* 1994;35:760–763; discussion 763–764.

25. Krieger AJ. Electrophrenic respiration after intercostal to phrenic nerve anastomosis in a patient with anterior spinal artery syndrome: technical case report [letter]. *Neurosurgery* 1995;37:553.

26. Krieger LM, Krieger AJ. The intercostal to phrenic nerve transfer: an effective means of reanimating the diaphragm in patients with high cervical spine injury. *Plast Reconstr Surg* 2000;105:1255–1261.

27. Fodstad H. Electrophrenic respiration after intercostal to phrenic nerve anastomosis on a patient with anterior spinal artery syndrome: technical case report. *Neurosurgery* 1996;38:420.

46
Optimal Crural Closure Techniques for Repair of Large Hiatal Hernias

Carlos A. Galvani and Santiago Horgan

Since the advent of laparoscopic anti-reflux surgery (LARS) in 1991,[1] this approach rapidly became more acceptable not only for surgeons but also for the medical community. As a consequence the number of referrals for surgery increased considerably. Numerous reports in the literature have shown that minimally invasive surgery for reflux disease offers excellent results in 85% to 95% of patients, with short hospital stay, decreased postoperative discomfort, and early return to regular activities.[2] Over the years the increasing experience gathered with this procedure has made the technique available even for the most technically challenging operations, such as large hiatal hernias. Despite the encouraging low morbidity and mortality rates, the reported rates of anatomical failure have been from 12% to 42%.[3-6] This variation in results might represent the objective postoperative evaluation (i.e., barium esophagram) performed in some centers comparedentmeicantly related (p < 0.05) to centers that only consider symptomatic recurrences. The most frequent anatomical failure reported after laparoscopic fundoplication is the transdiaphragmatic migration of the wrap, with or without disruption.[7-9] Soper and colleagues[7] observed in multivariate analysis that postoperative vomiting, diaphragmatic stressors, and hiatal hernia size were associated with anatomical fundoplication failure. Furthermore, these investigators noted that the fundoplication was three times most likely to fail in patients with larger hiatal hernias at the time of the first intervention. Similarly, among the several technical elements implicated as possible mechanisms leading to anatomical failures; inadequate crural closure accounts for more than a half of the failures.[7,9]

Different methods have been used in an attempt to prevent hiatal hernia recurrence. The proponents of the prosthetic reinforcement of crural closure with mesh have suggested that this approach can be protective, reducing the incidence of transdiaphragmatic migration of the wrap.[10-13] For other authors, however, the use of mesh still remains controversial due to the increased risk of complications that the procedure entails.[4,14] Herein we analyze the experience reported in the literature with traditional crural approximation techniques and the use of synthetic reinforcement of the diaphragmatic closure and the associated outcomes.

46.1. Classification of Hiatal Hernias

Hiatal hernias may be classified into three types according to their anatomical characteristics:

Type I or sliding hiatal hernia: Is the most common type (95%), in which there is a migration of the gastroesophageal junction (GEJ) along with the upper portion of the stomach into the posterior mediastinum.

Type II or paraesophageal hernia: This type is the least common. A pure paraesophageal hernia exits when the fundus of the stomach herniates into the thorax alongside the esophagus, while the GEJ remains in its abdominal position.

Type III or mixed paraesophageal hernia: This type is more common than the type II. It is a combination of the type I and type II hernia; consequently they have a sliding component and a paraesophageal component. They tend to be large in size and most of the time asymptomatic.

Type IV hiatal hernia: The hernia sac contains abdominal viscera or solid organs such as the omentum, spleen, colon, and the small bowel.

46.2. Diagnostic Studies

Diagnostic studies influence how the hernia repair is performed. In patients with achalasia and paraesophageal hernia or patients with ineffective peristalsis, the fundoplication is tailored to accommodate the patients' esophageal motility disorder.

46.2.1. Barium Swallow

A barium swallow is the procedure of choice in a patient in whom a hiatal hernia is suspected; however, it should not be used to detect gastroesophageal reflux disease (GERD). Barium esophagogram findings can demonstrate and define the anatomical location of the esophagogastric junction relative to the diaphragm, and can also elucidate the location of the stomach and possible complications of reflux disease (strictures).

46.2.2. Esophagogastroduodenoscopy

This is a useful tool for evaluating the presence of strictures, Barrett's esophagus, esophagitis, and gastric ulceration. Upper endoscopy can help to differentiate between type II and type III hernias.

46.2.3. Esophageal Manometry

This should be performed during the preoperative evaluation if surgical treatment is planned. It is usually helpful in the assessment of the LES (lower esophageal sphincter) pressure, and location. Esophageal body motility should be assessed to rule out primary esophageal motility disorders (e.g., esophageal achalasia) or ineffective esopha-

geal motility (IEM), in which case the fundoplication will be tailored accordingly.

46.2.4. Twenty-Four-Hour pH Monitoring

It is helpful in identifying associated GERD. Is not a diagnostic tool for paraesophageal hernias.

46.3. Laparoscopic Repair of Large Hiatal Hernias

46.3.1. Technical Aspects

Several surgical principles should be observed when performing these repairs to minimize complications and optimize outcomes.[9]

46.3.1.1. Reduction of the Hernia and Dissection of the Sac

The first step consists of gently reduction of the herniated stomach into the abdomen avoiding tears of the serosa. If complete reduction is not possible, early division of the short gastric vessels and incision of the sac beginning at its junction with the left crus (left crura approach), facilitates bringing the gastroesophageal junction and upper fundus of the stomach into the abdomen.[15] Next, using a combination of blunt dissection and harmonic scalpel, the hernia sac is dissected off its mediastinal attachments, reduced into the abdomen, and left at the GE junction level or removed.[4,5,16] Resection of the sac is performed as much as possible always avoiding injuring the anterior vagus nerve. Leaving the sac in the chest can lead to cyst or seroma formation or hernia recurrence.

46.3.1.2. Esophageal Mobilization

Once the left crus has been exposed and the greater curvature of the stomach is completely free, the dissection is extended to the posterior mediastinum and to the right side of the esophagus. During this maneuver a lighted bougie, the endoscope, or a bougie are used for better identification of the esophagus. The bougie is usually pulled back to the esophagus during the dissection of the hiatus. The right crus is separated from the esophagus with a combination of blunt dissection and harmonic scalpel. The mobilization continues with the dissection of the posterior aspect of the esophagus and the creation of the posterior window. The posterior vagus nerve is identified at this point and preserved. A Penrose drain is used to encircle and retract the esophagus and the vagus nerve.[4,15,17]

46.3.1.3. Closure of the Crura

After the complete mobilization of the esophagus is achieved and after the GE junction is observed to be well into the abdomen, closure of the diaphragmatic defect is started. The crura closure can be performed either primarily without reinforcement or with reinforcement of the crura with prosthetic material.

1. *Primary crura closure*: This is always started at the junction of the right and left crus, and is carried out anteriorly as far as possible. Closure of the crura posterior to the esophagus is started as low as possible to decrease tension on every stitch. The bougie is pulled back into the esophagus before starting the closure. The assistant retracts the esophagus elevating it ventrally and to the left. In patients with large defects, complete closure of the defect posterior to the esophagus may result in excessive anterior angulation of the esophagus. In those patients, complete the closure of the hiatal defect by placing one or two sutures anteriorly is advisable. The closure is performed using the Endostitch (USSC) with either intracorporeal or extracorporeal knots.[14,15] Use of a 52F to 54F bougie prevents postoperative dysphagia.

2. *Synthetic crura closure*: Two different kinds of synthetic crura closure have been described:
   - *Non–tension-free techniques*: This is by far the most commonly used approach. In this technique a primary crura closure is performed with interrupted nonabsorbable sutures, furthermore, prosthesis is used to reinforce the closure of the diaphragmatic defect. A bougie is passed regularly down the esophagus during the repair to tailor the closure and to avoid postoperative dysphagia. In the majority of cases the mesh is placed posterior to the esophagus.

   Granderath and colleagues,[13,18] in addition to closing the crura primarily closure with nonabsorbable interrupted sutures, utilized a 1×3 cm polypropylene mesh. The mesh is included in one of the stitches while approximating the right and left crura. The stitches are tied extracorporeal.

   Champion and colleagues,[10] in patients with hiatal defects of 5 cm or more, performed primary crura closure around a 50F bougie. After this, a 3×5 cm polypropylene mesh is employed to cover the closure as an on-lay buttress. The mesh is secured in place with staplers along the edges of the crura.

   Frantzides and colleagues[11] advocate a cruroplasty with ePTFE (Dual Mesh Gore-Tex, W. L. Gore and Assoc., Flagstaff, AZ). In this procedure a primary closure of the crura is performed over a 50F bougie, accompanied by an oval ePTFE mesh with a 3-cm hole. The mesh is appropriately secured to the crura with staplers.

   Zilberstein[17] described a primary crura closure anterior and posterior. If this closure is considered to be under tension, a Dacron mesh U shape is placed on top of the diaphragmatic closure and fixed with marginal staplers.

   Huntington and associates[19] and later Horgan and colleagues[3] proposed a direct crura closure and a relaxing incision if excessive tension is noted. The relaxing incision is carried out over the right crus to decrease the tension of the crura repair. Additionally, a polypropylene mesh is employed to close the defect. By utilizing this approach the authors avoided the mesh to be in direct contact with the posterior wall of the esophagus.

   Oelschlager and coworkers[16] performed primary crura closure by approximating the crura with interrupted nonabsorbable sutures. In addition, a surgisis U-shaped mesh made of porcine small intestine submucosal (SIS) is used to cover the repair. The mesh is tacked to the edge of the right and left crura with staplers.

   Mattar and colleagues described another non–tension-free approach with the use of pledgets.[20] In this technique, interrupted pledgeted nonabsorbable sutures are used to approximate the crura.

- *Tension-free techniques*: In which the diaphragmatic defect is left unsutured and prosthetic materials are used to patch the defect. A bougie is not routinely used during the crura closure. This repair can be performed either anterior or posterior to the esophagus and the material may vary among authors.

Anterior mesh placement: Described by Paul and colleagues, in which a triangular piece of expanded polytetrafluoroethylene of 5 × 10cm (Gore-Tex soft tissue patch), is placed anterior to the esophagus to close the diaphragmatic defect. The mesh is fixed to the crura with intracorporeal ePTFE sutures.[21] After this, the fundus of the stomach is fixed to the right crura for intraabdominal fixation.

Posterior mesh placement: *Tension-free hiatoplasty.*[12] The hiatus is closed with a 3 × 4cm polypropylene mesh. The mesh is fixed with titanium staplers to the right and left pilar of the crus. A 360° fundoplication is interposed between the mesh and the posterior esophageal wall.

Casaccia and colleagues[22] described a hiatoplasty by using an A-shaped mesh (Bard® Composix™ mesh) composed of polypropylene-polytetrafluoroethylene (PTFE). If the diaphragmatic defect is of 3 to 4cm, a primary closure is attempted at the beginning. Whenever the defect is larger a tension-free approach is chosen. The A-shaped mesh is placed encircling the esophagus and closing the diaphragmatic defect. The mesh is sutured in place with staplers.

Anti-reflux procedure: Once the crura repair is finished, the addition of an anti-reflux procedure is performed in the majority of cases.[4,6,9–12,16,17,20] The construction of a floppy tension-free fundoplication is gauged over a bougie (50F/52F–54F/60F). If an anti-reflux procedure is not added a good number of patients will develop reflux postoperatively due to the wide dissection needed for the reduction of the hernia. Secondly, anchoring the repair underneath the diaphragm is potentially an additional protective measure to avoid anatomical failure.

46.4. Controversial Points Regarding the Use of Crural Reinforcement

Currently it is accepted that minimally invasive surgery for the treatment of large hiatal hernias has prevailed over the open approach by decreasing morbidity and mortality. Yet the reported recurrence rate with the laparoscopic approach is rather high,[4,5] resulting in substantial disagreement concerning the technical aspects of the operation. Horgan and coworkers, based on principles learned through re-operative anti-reflux surgery,[9] identified some of the reasons for postoperative failure and provided technical factors that applied during the initial procedure could decrease the recurrence rate. First, extensive mobilization of the esophagus in the posterior mediastinum is necessary to bring 3 to 4cm of esophagus below the diaphragm. Second, proper closure of the diaphragmatic defect must be achieved, followed by intrabdominal anchoring of the wrap. Analogous observations have been made by others.[5,7,8,14,20] Furthermore, Soper and Dunnegan[7] found an association between early postoperative stressors (e.g., vomiting) and the size of the hiatal hernia at the initial operation as potential reasons for anatomical fundoplication failure. Despite these observations, disruption of the crural closure and wrap migration continue to be the most common cause of anatomical postfundoplication failure.[6]

Several authors concur that in the presence of small-to-moderate hiatal hernias primary closure of the crura is indicated.[10,16,17,20,23] However, in the case of hiatal hernias with large diaphragmatic defects, primary closure of the crura creates tension and the best repair remains controversial. More than a few authors have recommended, when the size of the hiatal defect is considerable, the use of prosthetic material as a reinforcement to decrease tension on the repair and as an effective measure to prevent reherniation.[11–13,16–18]

Most of the published results available concerning laparoscopic repair of large hiatal hernias are merely observational studies of small series and not randomized, controlled trials.[12,16–21] (Table 46.1) There are only two prospective, randomized trials evaluating the results of the classic primary crura repair with a prosthetic cruro-

TABLE 46.1. Results of nonrandomized trials laparoscopic hiatal hernia repair with mesh prosthesis.

Reference	Type of procedure	N	Age (years)	Follow-up (months)	Recurrence (no. patients)
Tension-free					
Paul[21]	Cruroplasty w/PTFE	3	77	12	0
Casaccia[22]	Cruroplasty w/composite	27	60	27	1 (3.7%)
Basso[12]	Simple cruroplasty	65	47.8	48.3	9 (13.8%)
	Tension-free cruroplasty w/ polypropylene	67	47.8	22.5	0
Non–tension-free					
Zilberstein[17]	Simple cruroplasty + cruroplasty w/Dacron	7	56	16	0
Oelschlager[16]	Simple cruroplasty + cruroplasty w/SIS	9	63	8	1 (11%)
Champion[10]	Simple cruroplasty + cruroplasty w/polypropylene	52	57	25	1 (1.9%)

plasty[11-13] (Table 46.2). The first study was carried out by Frantzides and associates.[11] The authors randomly performed either primary crura closure or prosthetic reinforcement in 72 patients with hiatal defects of more than 8cm. They found that operative time was longer, and that the costs of the operation were also increased in the mesh group in contrast with the simple repair. Objective follow-up (i.e., barium swallow) after at least 12 months was available in almost every patient (average, 3.3 years). No recurrence was found in the mesh group, compared with 22% recurrence rate in the non-mesh group. Five of these patients underwent a second operation, and an onlay mesh repair was used in all of them. No mesh-related complications were seen. These investigators concluded that simple cruroplasty and mesh reinforcement, contrasting with the simple cruroplasty alone, helps to decrease the incidence of postoperative wrap herniation to nil.[11] The other prospective, randomized trial was published recently by Granderath and associates.[13] In the study, the authors randomized 100 patients for either simple cruroplasty or crura reinforcement with a polypropylene mesh. About 60% of patients in each arm had a hiatal defect greater than 5cm. The results of this study demonstrated an increased rate of postoperative dysphagia at 6-week and 3-month follow-ups in the mesh group compared to the non-mesh group (12% vs. 4%; $p < 0.05$). At 1-year follow-up, however, the incidence of postoperative dysphagia was equivalent. It is valuable to note that the authors observed that both surgical approaches were equally effective in reducing acid esophageal exposure proven by pH monitoring. As shown by postoperative X ray, anatomical postfundoplication failure was more frequent among patients who underwent a simple cruroplasty (26% vs. 8%). These excellent results are comparable with those of Frantzides,[11] and seem to encourage the routine use of mesh for reinforcement of the crura closure in patients

TABLE 46.2. Results of prospective, randomized trials comparing simple cruroplasty and cruroplasty with mesh.

Reference	Type of procedure	N	Age (years)	Operation time (min)	Morbidity	Mortality	Follow-up (years)	Recurrence (no. patients)
Frantzides[11]	Simple cruroplasty	36	63	126	Pneumothorax	0	3.3	8 (22%)
	Cruroplasty w/ PTFE	36	58	156	–	0	3.3	0
					Pneumonia Urinary retention			
Granderath[13]	Simple cruroplasty	50	48	56	na	0	12	13 (26%)
	Cruroplasty w/polypropylene	50	48	58	na	0	12	4 (8%)

Abbreviations: na, not applicable.

with large hiatal defects. Primary crural closure is appropriate for patients with small- and moderate-sized hiatal defects. Patients with large defects should have crural reinforcement at the time of repair (level of evidence 1–; recommendation grade A).

> Primary crural closure is appropriate for patients with small- and moderate-sized hiatal defects. Patients with large defects should have crural reinforcement at the time of repair (level of evidence 1–; recommendation grade A).

Additional nonrandomized reports (level of evidence 3) have also proven the efficacy of the synthetic crural closure compared with primary cruroplasty.[10,16,17,22] Although these publications represent the authors' longitudinal experience instead of being a true comparison between the two approaches, their observations remain significant. For example, Champion and colleagues switched to prosthetic reinforcement of the crura after observing a disappointing 10.6% recurrence rate with simple cruroplasty. Consequently, at the average follow-up of 25 months, they observed a decrease in the incidence of postoperative intrathoracic wrap herniation to 2% with the use of prosthetic reinforcement.[10] Similarly, Basso and associates[12] divided their experience into two chronological periods in a nonrandomized comparative study. In the first period they performed primary closure of the diaphragmatic defect. In the second part of the authors' experience, a tension-free hiatoplasty was performed in every patient. Inclusion criteria for this study included hiatal hernia or GERD. In the first period migration of the wrap into the chest was observed in 13.8% of patients, whereas no patient experienced this complication in the second period.

One of the major arguments against the utilization of mesh for the crura repair seems to be the occurrence of complications, such as esophageal erosions and strictures.[14] For this reason, another unresolved controversy is the choice of the synthetic material. It is accepted that the ideal prosthetic material should be non-reabsorbable, have a low risk of adhesions, be resistant, and be malleable to enable its use during laparoscopic

surgery.[24] Currently several types of mesh are used as a prosthetic material, among them most commonly used are polypropylene mesh,[10,12,13] PTFE mesh,[11,21] composite mesh (PTFE plus polypropylene), and Dacron mesh.[17] Recently, a new type of biomaterial derived from porcine SIS became available to repair tissue defects.[16,25]

Regardless of the type of material, mesh-related complications still take place. Carlson[26] reported esophageal erosion in one patient with a polypropylene mesh. Similar findings were reported when using a Dacron mesh by Zilberstein.[17] In Edelman's experience, one patient (20%) developed dysphagia and esophageal stenosis after tension-free repair with polypropylene mesh.[27] In order to overcome this feared complication, Casaccia and colleagues have used a composite mesh (polypropylene–PTFE).[22] However, Schauer and associates[28] described a delayed esophageal perforation, re-operation, and mesh removal in a patient in whom a PTFE mesh was used. No adhesions or erosion have been described with the use of the SIS mesh to this point.[16] The characteristics of the SIS mesh are such that after implantation the material induces ingrowth of collagen and thus the regenerated tissue is stronger than native tissue. However, long-term experience with the use of this material in the esophageal hiatus is still scant, and there is insufficient data to permit recommendations for which material to use. The tendency of most authors seems to be toward the use of softer materials that create less inflammatory response and less adhesion formation. Up to now, there are several undefined issues regarding the use of prosthetic materials for hiatal hernia repair, such as the shape, location, and the choice of material.

> There is insufficient data to permit recommendations regarding the type of material that should be used for crural reinforcement.

46.5. Conclusion

As this report has indicated, numerous techniques are available for the laparoscopic repair of large hernias. Evidence shows that synthetic reinforcement for the treatment of large hiatal hernias can be performed safely without excessive morbidity. In the presence of small-to-moderate hiatal hernias, primary cruroplasty may be employed. Reinforcement of the hiatus with prosthetic material is suggested in patients with larger crural defects. Prospective, randomized trials showed that prosthetic materials appear to significantly lengthen the stability of the anatomical repair when utilized in combination with essential technical factors, such as: (1) tension-free reduction of the stomach and esophagus with hernia sac resection; (2) crural closure; and (3) intraabdominal anchoring of the stomach with an anti-reflux procedure. Further comparative, prospective, randomized studies between different techniques will help to elucidate whether one approach is superior to the other, costs, and synthetic materials for the reconstruction of the esophageal hiatus. Longer follow-up is also necessary to evaluate anatomical failures and mesh-related complications.

References

1. Dallemagne B, Weerts JM, Jehaes C, et al. Laparoscopic Nissen fundoplication: preliminary report. *Surg Laparosc Endosc* 1991;1:138–143.
2. Horgan S, Pellegrini CA. Surgical treatment of gastroesophageal reflux disease. *Surg Clin North Am* 1997;77:1063–1082.
3. Horgan S, Eubanks TR, Jacobsen G, et al. Repair of paraesophageal hernias. *Am J Surg* 1999;177: 354–358.
4. Hashemi M, Peters JH, DeMeester TR, et al. Laparoscopic repair of large type III hiatal hernia: objective followup reveals high recurrence rate. *J Am Coll Surg* 2000;190:553–560; discussion 560–561.
5. Aly A, Munt J, Jamieson GG, et al. Laparoscopic repair of large hiatal hernias. *Br J Surg* 2005;92: 648–653.
6. Wu JS, Dunnegan DL, Soper NJ. Clinical and radiologic assessment of laparoscopic paraesophageal hernia repair. *Surg Endosc* 1999;13:497–502.
7. Soper NJ, Dunnegan D. Anatomic fundoplication failure after laparoscopic antireflux surgery. *Ann Surg* 1999;229:669–676; discussion 676–677.
8. Hunter JG, Smith CD, Branum GD, et al. Laparoscopic fundoplication failures: patterns of failure and response to fundoplication revision. *Ann Surg* 1999;230:595–604; discussion 604–606.
9. Horgan S, Pohl D, Bogetti D, et al. Failed antireflux surgery: what have we learned from reoperations? *Arch Surg* 1999;134:809–815; discussion 815–817.
10. Champion JK, Rock D. Laparoscopic mesh cruroplasty for large paraesophageal hernias. *Surg Endosc* 2003;17:551–553.
11. Frantzides CT, Richards CG, Carlson MA. Laparoscopic repair of large hiatal hernia with polytetrafluoroethylene. *Surg Endosc* 1999;13:906–908.
12. Basso N, De Leo A, Genco A, et al. 360 degrees laparoscopic fundoplication with tension-free hiatoplasty in the treatment of symptomatic gastroesophageal reflux disease. *Surg Endosc* 2000;14: 164–169.
13. Granderath FA, Schweiger UM, Kamolz T, et al. Laparoscopic Nissen fundoplication with prosthetic hiatal closure reduces postoperative intrathoracic wrap herniation: preliminary results of a prospective randomized functional and clinical study. *Arch Surg* 2005;140:40–48.
14. Gantert WA, Patti MG, Arcerito M, et al. Laparoscopic repair of paraesophageal hiatal hernias. *J Am Coll Surg* 1998;186:428–432; discussion 432–433.
15. Casabella F, Sinanan M, Horgan S, et al. Systematic use of gastric fundoplication in laparoscopic repair of paraesophageal hernias. *Am J Surg* 1996;171:485–489.
16. Oelschlager BK, Barreca M, Chang L, et al. The use of small intestine submucosa in the repair of paraesophageal hernias: initial observations of a new technique. *Am J Surg* 2003;186:4–8.
17. Zilberstein B, Eshkenazy R, Pajecki D, et al. Laparoscopic mesh repair antireflux surgery for treatment of large hiatal hernia. *Dis Esophagus* 2005;18:166–169.
18. Kamolz T, Granderath FA, Bammer T, et al. Dysphagia and quality of life after laparoscopic Nissen fundoplication in patients with and without prosthetic reinforcement of the hiatal crura. *Surg Endosc* 2002;16:572–577.
19. Huntington TR. Laparoscopic mesh repair of the esophageal hiatus. *J Am Coll Surg* 1997;184:399–400.
20. Mattar SG, Bowers SP, Galloway KD, et al. Long-term outcome of laparoscopic repair of paraesophageal hernia. *Surg Endosc* 2002;16:745–749.
21. Paul MG, DeRosa RP, Petrucci PE, et al. Laparoscopic tension-free repair of large paraesophageal hernias. *Surg Endosc* 1997;11:303–307.
22. Casaccia M, Torelli P, Panaro F, et al. Laparoscopic tension-free repair of large paraesophageal hiatal hernias with a composite A-shaped mesh: two-

year follow-up. *J Laparoendosc Adv Surg Tech A* 2005;15:279–284.

23. Leeder PC, Smith G, Dehn TC. Laparoscopic management of large paraesophageal hiatal hernia. *Surg Endosc* 2003;17:1372–1375.

24. Targarona EM, Bendahan G, Balague C, et al. Mesh in the hiatus: a controversial issue. *Arch Surg* 2004;139:1286–1296; discussion 1296.

25. Helton WS, Fisichella PM, Berger R, et al. Short-term outcomes with small intestinal submucosa for ventral abdominal hernia. *Arch Surg* 2005;140: 549–560; discussion 560–562.

26. Carlson MA, Condon RE, Ludwig KA, et al. Management of intrathoracic stomach with polypropylene mesh prosthesis reinforced transabdominal hiatus hernia repair. *J Am Coll Surg* 1998;187:227–230.

27. Edelman DS. Laparoscopic paraesophageal hernia repair with mesh. *Surg Laparosc Endosc* 1995;5:32–37.

28. Schauer PR, Ikramuddin S, McLaughlin RH, et al. Comparison of laparoscopic versus open repair of paraesophageal hernia. *Am J Surg* 1998;176:659–665.

47
Management of Acute Diaphragmatic Rupture: Thoracotomy Versus Laparotomy

Seth D. Force

Acute traumatic diaphragmatic rupture is diagnosed in 0.8% to 7% of patients following blunt trauma and in as many as 15% of patients following penetrating trauma.[1,2] However, unrecognized diaphragmatic injuries following laparotomy have also been documented; therefore the actual incidence may be higher than previously reported.[3] Whether to use an abdominal or thoracic exposure to repair the diaphragmatic injury has been debated for years with preference usually for the body cavity containing the most severely injured associated organs. This chapter will review the current literature on the various techniques to diagnose diaphragmatic injuries as well as the optimal choice of exposure for repair.

47.1. Mechanism of Injury

Stabbings and gun shot wounds are the most common mechanisms for penetrating injury to the diaphragm. Due to the significant elevation of the diaphragm during expiration, all stab wounds that enter the thoracic cavity at the fourth intercostal space or lower must be considered for possible diaphragmatic injury. Injuries from gunshot wounds vary depending on the type of ammunition used, the trajectory of the bullet, and the range from which the victim is shot. The mechanism for blunt diaphragmatic injury is unclear. Increased abdominal pressure may lead to direct rupture or herniation through weak points caused by congenital abnormalities or fractured ribs. The propensity for left-sided injuries in blunt diaphragmatic trauma has been postulated to be due to the protective nature of the liver on the right side and anatomical weak points in the left diaphragm.[4]

47.2. Mortality and Associated Injuries

Mortality tends to be high in patients diagnosed with a diaphragmatic injury as a result of the many associated injuries that are often incurred at the time of the trauma. Williams and colleagues reviewed the records of 731 patients with traumatic diaphragmatic injuries and found a 23% mortality rate. A revised trauma score (RTS) less than 5 and the number of organs injured were among the significant variables that adversely affected survival.[5]

Diaphragmatic injuries may be relatively less important in patients with other major injuries who present in shock. Rowlands and colleagues found that 75% of patients presenting to their hospital who were subsequently diagnosed with traumatic diaphragmatic injuries had other injuries. The average injury severity score in these patients was 21 and the mortality rate was 12.5%.[6] Sarna and coworkers reported on 41 patients with diaphragmatic rupture following blunt trauma and found that all of the patients had associated injuries, and 84% had injury to abdominal organs.[7] Similarly, in 65 patients diagnosed with traumatic rupture due to blunt or penetrating injury, Mihos and coworkers found associated injuries in 95% with the majority being injury to abdominal organs, most commonly liver, spleen, or intestine. This study also described an increase in mortality associated with a higher injury severity score (ISS). The mean ISS among survivors was 18 versus 41 for nonsurvivors.[8] The fact that these injuries usually occur in acutely ill patients along with other injuries makes the diagnosis of diaphragmatic trauma particularly difficult.

47.3. Diagnosis

Diagnosing traumatic diaphragmatic injuries may be difficult in the multiply injured patient. However, it is important to look for and identify diaphragmatic injuries, despite the fact that a trauma patient may have other more pressing issues at the time of presentation. Although the location of penetrating injuries or significant blunt force may heighten the clinician's suspicion, signs and symptoms of a diaphragmatic injury are nonspecific and the injury may not be recognized. Reber reported a series of 38 patients identified with traumatic diaphragmatic injuries over a 16-year period. Ten patients were found to have diaphragmatic injuries that were missed on initial evaluation. The time between the trauma and discovery of the diaphragmatic injury ranged from 20 days to 28 years and all 10 patients presented with chest or abdominal complaints. One patient died in the postoperative period and three patients developed significant complications. A retrospective blinded review by a radiologist of the patients' initial presenting chest radiographs revealed evidence for diaphragmatic injury in 4 of the 10 patients.[2] This study highlights the difficulty of accurately recognizing these injuries. Currently there are a number of diagnostic tools that the clinician may use to help identify diaphragmatic injuries.

The literature describing the various diagnostic modalities for the identification of diaphragmatic injuries consists only of cohort studies and case series. Chest radiographs have long been used to evaluate patients for diaphragmatic rupture. Findings that are suggestive of, but not specific for, diaphragmatic injury include elevated hemidiaphragm, evidence of abdominal viscera or nasogastric tube in the chest, contra-lateral mediastinal shift, and pleural effusion. However, any condition obscuring the pleural space, such as a hemothorax or a lung contusion, can mask a diaphragmatic injury. Furthermore, diaphragmatic injuries without visceral herniation may not have any specific findings on chest radiograph. Gelman and colleagues and Smithers and colleagues used chest radiographs to diagnose diaphragmatic rupture in 46% and 54%, respectively, of patients who presented with blunt trauma.[9,10] Therefore, diaphragmatic injuries will be missed in up to half of patients who present with blunt diaphragmatic injuries. Both of these studies depended heavily on the presence of viscera in the chest to diagnose the diaphragmatic injury. Importantly, the absence of herniated viscera does not rule out diaphragmatic injury.

Ultrasound has also been used to diagnose diaphragmatic injuries. Typical sonographic findings include abnormal diaphragm movement and visualization of a diaphragmatic tear or flap. The ability to perform ultrasound in the emergency room during the initial resuscitation is one of the benefits of this procedure. However, there are only a few studies that review this technique and only in patients following blunt trauma. Kim and associates performed a retrospective review of 12 patients who suffered traumatic diaphragmatic rupture and who also underwent abdominal ultrasound by a radiologist. Eight of the patients were diagnosed by ultrasound with diaphragmatic rupture, and seven of these were confirmed at the time of surgery. One patient was found to have a paper-thin diaphragm without evidence of rupture.[11] Nau and colleagues reported very different results in their review of 31 patients diagnosed with diaphragmatic rupture due to penetrating and blunt trauma. Twenty-nine of the patients were evaluated by ultrasound in the emergency room, but none was diagnosed with a diaphragmatic injury by this method.[12] The discrepancy in detection rates between the two studies may be due to operator-dependent differences. The diagnosis of diaphragmatic injury relies heavily on the skill of the sonographer, and not all hospitals have in-house sonographers who are comfortable evaluating the diaphragm. Additionally, there are no agreed upon criteria for the diagnosis of diaphragmatic rupture by ultrasound.

Computerized tomography (CT) may also aid in diagnosing diaphragmatic rupture. Because chest and abdominal CT scanning is routinely performed in trauma victims, it may provide a more convenient way to detect diaphragmatic injuries. However, most studies have not shown this to be a more sensitive test than chest radiography. Karaaslan and Trupka found, in their respective studies, that CT did not add any additional benefit to chest radiograph in diagnosing diaphragmatic rupture.[13,14] Shapiro and coworkers found CT scans and chest radiographs to be equally unreliable in diagnosing diaphragmatic injuries with approximately half of the injuries missed by either test.[15] The previously mentioned study by Nau and coworkers found that CT was only able to identify 5 patients out of 16 who had diaphragmatic injury due to blunt trauma and in none of the 11 patients who had penetrating trauma.[12] Bergin and coworkers have suggested using certain radiographic findings termed the *dependent viscera sign* to increase the accuracy of CT scanning in identifying diaphragmatic injuries. Using this technique, they found that the radiologists were able to retrospectively identify traumatic diaphragmatic injuries in 9 out 10 patients evaluated.[16] However, there are no other studies that corroborate these findings. In summary, CT does not appear to provide significant additional benefit over chest radiographs for the diagnosis of acute diaphragmatic rupture.

One final radiographic test that deserves a brief mention is magnetic resonance imaging (MRI). Shanmuganathan and colleagues found that, out of 16 patients with suspected diaphragmatic injury on chest radiograph, MRI correctly identified a diaphragmatic defect in 7 patients.[17] Although this modality may be highly accurate, it is not currently safe or feasible to bring critically ill trauma patients to the MRI scanner.

Invasive diagnostic tests may also be used to detect diaphragmatic injuries due to trauma. Prior to the advent of laparoscopy and thoracoscopy, diagnostic peritoneal lavage (DPL) was the only invasive test for identifying injuries in trauma patients who were too unstable to undergo prolonged radiographic evaluation. Freeman and colleagues retrospectively reviewed 38 patients with blunt traumatic diaphragmatic rupture who underwent peritoneal lavage. False negative lavages were found in eight patients and in all four patients who had isolated diaphragmatic injuries.[18]

More recently, thoracoscopy and laparoscopy have been used to identify traumatic diaphragmatic injuries. Spann and colleagues reported on 26 patients, following blunt trauma, who underwent diagnostic thoracoscopy and laparotomy to identify diaphragmatic injuries. Eight patients with diaphragmatic injury were identified by both techniques, and thus the authors concluded that thoracoscopy is as accurate as laparotomy for the identification of these injuries.[19] Other studies have made similar claims about laparoscopy, but this procedure is not suitable for the unstable trauma patient.[20] Thoracoscopy and laparoscopy probably do not have any benefit in the trauma patient requiring laparotomy, but these procedures may improve our ability to diagnose occult diaphragmatic injuries in clinically stable trauma patients.

47.4. Diaphragmatic Repair

The surgical considerations for repair of a ruptured diaphragm initially center on stabilizing the patient and diagnosing any associated injuries. These patients will fall into two categories: (1) isolated diaphragmatic injuries (less than 10% of all trauma patients with diaphragmatic trauma); and (2) diaphragmatic hernia associated with multiple injuries. Patients with isolated diaphragmatic injuries may be treated best with thoracoscopy or laparoscopy. Mineo and colleagues studied 36 patients who underwent thoracoscopy following isolated blunt chest trauma (level of evidence 2–). They were able to either rule out significant trauma or treat the thoracic injuries using thoracoscopy alone in 20 of these patients, including 5 who had diaphragmatic injuries.[21] These techniques can be used to diagnose and safely repair small- to moderate-sized diaphragmatic defects. Larger defects, including those with major organ herniation or large central defects, may be better repaired through a laparotomy or thoracotomy. Unfortunately, because of the rarity of this injury, there are no large studies evaluating the use of minimally invasive techniques.

Given that the majority of patients with blunt or penetrating traumatic diaphragmatic injuries have other intraabdominal injuries, it follows that laparotomy would be the exposure of choice to diagnose and treat all of these injuries. This conclusion has been supported by the thoracic and trauma literature over the past three decades. Shah and colleagues reviewed 22 papers including 980 patients with traumatic diaphragmatic injuries (level of evidence 3). Almost 90% of these patients had some combination of pelvic and/or abdominal injury. The authors remarked that since "the majority of the patients have associated intra-abdominal injuries most writers . . . recommend laparotomy as the preferable approach."[22] Niville and colleagues derived their preference for a laparotomy approach from their patient series in which 34 out of 40 patients were operated on through an abdominal incision alone (level of evidence 3). The authors stated, "when confronted by a recent diaphragmatic rupture, we almost always use an abdominal incision knowing that it can easily be extended into the chest if necessary."[23]

Despite the overwhelming support for laparotomy some authors still recommend thoracotomy for repairing traumatic diaphragmatic injuries. McCune and colleagues and Johnnson and colleagues preferred thoracotomy to repair right-sided diaphragmatic defects (level of evidence 3).[24,25] Right diaphragmatic injuries repaired in a delayed fashion may also be better approached through a right thoracotomy.

Galan and colleagues reviewed 1696 patients who suffered blunt thoracic trauma and found 40 patients with diaphragmatic injuries requiring immediate repair (level of evidence 3). Thirty-four patients underwent thoracotomy to repair the defect, including 27 left-sided injuries and 7 right-sided injuries. However, the authors do not explain their reason for choosing thoracotomy as the preferred exposure in these patients.[26] Possible explanations for a thoracotomy approach may have included other intrathoracic pathology such as pulmonary lacerations, hemothoraces, and descending aortic injures. This argument is supported by findings in a paper by Meyers and colleagues, in which 12 out of 54 patients underwent thoracotomy either alone in combination with

laparotomy (level of evidence 3). Their reasons for choosing thoracotomy included further evaluation for positive pericardial window, persistent thoracic bleeding, bleeding from dome of liver, aortic injury, and need for aortic crossclamping.[27]

Thoracotomy may be necessary for aortic injuries occurring in the presence of diaphragmatic injuries following blunt trauma. Among 69 trauma patients with diaphragmatic injuries, Rizoli and coworkers found 7 who also had a descending aortic injury (level of evidence 3). Five of these patients underwent repair of both injuries while one had repair of only the diaphragmatic injury and one died intraoperatively. All five patients who underwent repair of both injuries had laparotomies followed by thoracotomies.[28]

The type of diaphragmatic closure appears to be fairly noncontroversial. The majority of authors prefer a single layer of interrupted nonabsorbable suture, although there are no prospective or retrospective studies comparing closure techniques. The use of mesh patches is reserved for chronic diaphragmatic hernias and there are no reports of its use in acute traumatic diaphragmatic injuries.

47.5. Conclusion

In summary, acute traumatic diaphragmatic injuries are rare and usually occur in critically ill, multiply injured patients. There are no large, prospective studies evaluating the means for diagnosis and repair. The majority of papers that discuss this entity are case series or case reports (level of evidence evidence) and thus recommendations regarding diagnosis and treatment rely more on clinical opinion than on scientific results. Based on the evidence, recommendation grade D exists for laparotomy as choice for exposure in the majority of patients who have suffered a traumatic diaphragmatic injury. The exceptions include isolated right diaphragmatic injuries and diaphragmatic injuries occurring in the setting of other thoracic injuries requiring repair where thoracotomy may be more appropriate. Minimally invasive techniques appear to provide equal efficacy, compared to open techniques, for diaphragmatic repair in stable patients, but there are currently few studies evaluating these methods.

> Laparotomy is the optimal choice for exposure in the majority of patients who have suffered a traumatic diaphragmatic injury (level of evidence 3; recommendation grade D). The exceptions include isolated right diaphragmatic injuries and diaphragmatic injuries occurring in the setting of other thoracic injuries requiring repair, where thoracotomy may be more appropriate.

References

1. Rodriguez-Morales G, Rodriguez A, Shatney C. Acute rupture of the diaphragm in blunt trauma: analysis of 60 patients. *J Trauma* 1986;26:438.
2. Reber PU, Schmied B, Seiler CA, Baer HU, Patel AG, Buchler MW. Missed diaphragmatic injuries and their long-term sequelae. *J Trauma* 1998;44:183–188.
3. Feliciano DV, Cruse PA, Mattox KL, et al. Delayed diagnosis of injuries to the diaphragm after penetrating wounds. *J Trauma* 1988;28:1135.
4. Carter BN, Giuseffi J, Felson B. Traumatic diaphragmatic hernia. *AJR Am J Roentgenol* 1951;65:56–82.
5. Williams M, Carlin A, Tyburski JG, et al. Predictors of mortality in patients with traumatic diaphragmatic rupture and associated thoracic and/or abdominal injuries. *Am Surg* 2004;70:157–162.
6. Simpson J, Lobo DN, Shah AB, Rowlands BJ. Traumatic diaphragmatic rupture: associated injuries and outcome. *Ann R Coll Surg Engl* 2000;82:97–100.
7. Sarna S, Kivioja A. Blunt rupture of the diaphragm: a retrospective analysis of 41 patients. *Ann Chir Gynaec* 1995;84:261–265.
8. Mihos P, Konnstantinos P, Gakidis J, et al. Traumatic rupture of the diaphragm: experience with 65 patients. *Injury* 2003;34:169–172.
9. Gelman R, Mirvis SE, Gens D. Diaphragmatic rupture due to blunt trauma: sensitivity of plain chest radiograph. *AJR Am J Roentgenol* 1991;156:51–57.
10. Smithers BM, O'Loughlin B, Strong RW. Diagnosis of ruptured diaphragm following blunt trauma:

results from 85 cases. *Aust N Z J Surg* 1991;61:737–741.
11. Kim HH, Young RS, Kim KJ, et al. Blunt traumatic rupture of the diaphragm: sonographic diagnosis. *J Ultrasound Med* 1997;16:593–598.
12. Nau T, Seitz H, Mousavi M, Vescei V. The diagnostic dilemma of traumatic rupture of the diaphragm. *Surg Endosc* 2001;15:992–996.
13. Tugrul K, Meuli R, Androux R, et al. Traumatic chest lesions in patients with severe head trauma: a comparative study with computed tomography and conventional chest roentgenograms. *J Trauma* 1995;39:1081–1086.
14. Trupka A, Waydhas KK, Hallfeldt KKJ, et al. Value of computed tomography in the first assessment of severely injured patients with blunt chest trauma: results of a prospective study. *J Trauma* 1997;43:405–412.
15. Shapiro MJ, Heiberg E, Durham RM, Luchfefeld W, Mazuski JE. The unreliability of CT scans and initial chest radiographs in evaluating blunt trauma induced diaphragmatic rupture. *Clin Rad* 1996:51;27–30.
16. Bergin D, Ennis R, Keogh C, Fenlon HM, Murray JG. The "dependent viscera" sign in CT diagnosis of blunt traumatic diaphragmatic rupture. *AJR Am J Roentgenol* 2001;177:1137–1140.
17. Shanmuganathan K, Mirvis SE, White CS, Pomerantz SM. MR imaging evaluation of hemidiaphragms in acute blunt trauma: experience with 16 patients. *AJR Am J Roentgenol* 1996;167:397–402.
18. Freeman T, Fischer RP. The inadequacy of peritoneal lavage in diagnosing acute diaphragmatic rupture. *J Trauma* 1976;16:538–542.
19. Spann JC, Nwariaku FE, Wait M. Evaluation of video-assisted thoracoscopic surgery in the diagnosis of diaphragmatic injuries. *Am J Surg* 1995;170:628–630.
20. Matz A, Alis M, Charuzi I, Kyzer S. The role of laparoscopy in the diagnosis and treatment of missed diaphragmatic rupture. *Surg Endosc* 2000;14:537–539.
21. Mineo TC, Ambrogi V, Cristino B, Pompeo E, Pistolese C. Changing indications for thoracotomy in blunt chest trauma after the advent of videothoracoscopy. *J Trauma* 1999;47:1088–1091.
22. Shah R, Sabanathan S, Mearns AJ, Choudhury AK. Traumatic rupture of diaphragm. *Ann Thorac Surg* 1995;60:1444–1449.
23. Niville EC, Himpens JM, Bruos PL, Gruwez JA. The use of laparotomy in the treatment of recent diaphragmatic rupture due to blunt trauma. *Injury* 1983;15:153–155.

24. McCune RP, Roda CP, Eckert C. Rupture of the diaphragm caused by blunt trauma. *J Trauma* 1976;16:531.

25. Johnson CD. Blunt injuries of the diaphragm. *Br J Surg* 1988;75;226.

26. Galan G, Penalver JC, Paris F, et al. Blunt chest injuries in 1696 patients. *Eur J Cardiothorac Surg* 1992;6:284–287.

27. Meyers BF, McCabe CJ. Traumatic diaphragmatic hernia: occult marker of serious injury. *Ann Surg* 1993;218:783–790.

28. Rizoli SB, Brenneman FD, Boulander BR, Maggisano R. Blunt diaphragmatic and thoracic aortic rupture: an emerging injury complex. *Ann Thorac Surg* 1994;58:1404–1408.

Part 5
Airway

48
Stenting for Benign Airway Obstruction

Loay Kabbani and Tracey L. Weigel

Surgery has been the standard treatment for benign tracheal stenosis for decades, as it has shown durable results and low morbidity.[1] However, the low incidence of these lesions, the intrinsic technical difficulty of the surgery, and frequent patient comorbidities lead to significant postoperative complications including anastomotic dehiscence and re-stenoses, make stenting an attractive alternative. Most of the experience with stents comes from the palliation of malignant airway strictures, with an estimated 20% to 30 % of patients with lung cancer developing some degree of airway obstruction during the course of their disease.[2] The incidence of benign airway stenoses is unknown.

There are no large randomized trials to assess the best treatment strategy for patients with benign airway obstructions with good justification. It would be difficult to select a uniform cohort, it is unethical to randomize patients who are symptomatic to the noninterventional arm, and it would not be possible to randomize patients into double-blind studies. Therefore the literature is full of individual case reports and case series with few to no case controlled studies. Despite the lack of prospective, randomized data, the new stent technology is quickly being embraced due to its ready availability and ease of deployment. So the question is no longer, "Is stent therapy helpful?"; rather it is rapidly becoming, "Is stenting or surgery best for a particular patient?"[3]

In this chapter, we present the main controversies of stent therapy for benign tracheobroncheal strictures, including endobronchial stent place-
ment, type, and duration of stent therapy. Medline was searched for keywords "benign airway stenoses" and "stents". The search was limited to the English language. The titles were reviewed and the relevant abstracts were read. The pertinent articles were reviewed along with all their significant references. We did not review single case reports. No trials were found in the Cochrane Central Register of Controlled Trials or the Cochrane Database of Systematic Reviews.

48.1. Controversies and How Published Data Impacts Our Clinical Practice

48.1.1. Common Clinical Indications for Stents

48.1.1.1. Postintubation Stenosis/ Post-tracheostomy Stenosis

Historically, the gold standard for the management for a tracheobronchial stricture has been tracheal sleeve resection followed by end-to-end anastomosis (see Table 48.1). Grillo's group[1,4] reported good results in 95% of their 901 patients with 4% of their patients requiring tracheostomies or T tubes. Similar results were reported by others[5,6]. Gaissert[7] advised against stenting surgically favorable patients in his case series of 15 patients with stent complications.

Surgical resection, however, may be associated with increased risk in patients with insufficient tracheobronchial length for an end-to-end,

TABLE 48.1. Potential indications for stent placement in benign tracheobronchial disease.

Tracheal stenosis
  Congenital
    Endotracheal tube injury (PIS)
    Post-tracheotomy related (PTS)
  Secondary to systemic disease
    Wegener's syndrome
    Relapsing polychrondritis
    Amyloidosis
Bronchial stenosis
  Post–lung transplantation
  Relapsing polychondritis
  Postinfectious (tuberculosis)
Tracheomalacia
  Congenital
  Idiopathic
  Tracheobronchomegaly (Mounier–Kuhn syndrome)
  Relapsing polychondritis
  Tracheotomy related
  Post–lung transplant
  Radiation therapy related
Tracheobroncheal compression
  Compression by vascular abnormalities and malformation
  Fibrosing mediastinitis
  Kyphoscoliosis
Tracheal perforation

tension-free anastomosis, in patients who are in poor health, or in those who develop recurrent strictures.[8] Cooper[9] described his experience with Montgomery T tubes in 47 patients (36 with benign lesions) (Table 48.2). However, this required a tracheostomy for stabilization and secretion management.

This paved the way for Dumon's silicone tube, introduced in 1990, which was met with widespread use due to its ease of insertion with a rigid bronchoscope and avoidance of a tracheostomy. In his original series,[10] which included 66 patients (28 with benign strictures) and a mean follow-up of 3 months, he gave a preliminary outcome describing the feasibility and safety of this stent. In his follow-up study[11] of four institutions and 1058 patients, 263 of them had benign stenosis. In the benign group, complications included migration in 18%, obstruction in 5.7%, and granulation tissue formation in 17.2%. Removal of the stent without subsequent recurrence of the stenosis was achieved in 24% of patients.

In a retrospective study by Martinez-Ballarin[12] comprising 63 patients with benign tracheal stenoses (82% with postintubation stenosis (PIS)/post-tracheostomy stenosis (PTS)), 48 patients had silicone stents placed with curative intent and 15 patients had the stents placed for palliative reasons. After 18 months, 27 patients had their stents removed (6 for migration), 4 patients needed stent replacement, and 17 patients were cured. Sixteen patients were still being followed up at the time the article was printed, and six patients

TABLE 48.2. Stenting for benign tracheal stenosis.

Reference	Duration of follow-up	No. patients	Population	Level of evidence	Stent used	Conclusions
Cooper[9] 1989	na	36	Mixed	3	Montgomery	Montgomery T tube can be used as palliation, adjunct to surgery, or as a destination therapy.
Dumon[10] 1990	3 months	28	Mixed	3	Dumon	Dumon stents are safe to use in both benign and malignant tracheobroncheal stenosis.
Martinez-Ballarin[12] 1996	8 months	64	Postintubation	3	Dumon	Highly effective in relieving symptoms; good patient tolerance; 1 patient dies secondary to occlusion of the stent with secretions.
Brichet[13] 1999	28 months	32	PIS/PTS	3	Dumon	Interventional bronchoscopy was curative in 1/3 of patients
Sesterhenn[15] 2004	16 months	11	Postintubation	3	National	National stents should be considered for treatment of benign stenosis.
Noppen[16] 2005	2 months	39	Postintubation	3	Ultraflex	25% of patients required stent removal; national stent removal was safe and feasible.
Puma[20] 2000	10 months	45	PIS/PTS	3	Silicone	3 lesion types: (1) circumferential lesions, stents good as bridge to surgery; (2) inflammatory, also stents good as a bridge until inflammation dies down; (3) extensive subglotic damage where surgery will have poor results, stents are good long-term palliation.

Abbreviations: na, not available; PIS/PTS, postintubation stenosis/post-tracheostomy stenosis.

needed another intervention including surgical resection of stenoses, T-tube placement, or tracheostomy. Brichet[13] presented a multidisciplinary approach to the management of postintubation stenoses, which included laser resection of isolated webs in 15 patients (10 were cured) and stent placement using Dumon silicone stents for the more complex strictures (17 patients). Only 3 of the 17 stented patients were cured, 4 underwent surgery, and 9 had permanent palliative stent placement. His protocol called for stent removal in 6 months. Brichet noted that most patients with tracheal stenoses are acutely ill and stenting may be a way to bridge them into a healthier state. In his series, three patients died shortly after stenting from other, non–stent-related causes.

Puma[14] reported on 71 patients with PIS/PTS; 26 were treated by immediate surgery and 45 patients underwent stenting first. In nine patients stenting was used as a bridge to surgery; these patients usually had severe inflammatory lesions and the stent was used until healing stabilized. In 37 patients, stenting was considered the definitive treatment. In 14 of these patients the stent was removed with no recurrence of symptoms in 10 patients. Dumon stents were used for most lesions, Montgomery stents were used for patients who required frequent suctioning, and dynamic Y stents were used for those with distal lesions. He concluded that some stenoses can be treated by stents only, and cure may be achieved after up to 2 years of stenting. A normal airway is never seen after stent placement, but the lumen is large enough to allow normal breathing. Epithilization, airway diameter, and chondromalacia were important determinants of whether stents could be removed.

Sesterhenn[15] presented his data on PIS using uncovered nitinol stents. All patients were relieved of their symptoms and no stents were removed. Noppen used nitinol stents to treat 39 patients with benign tracheobroncheal disorders. Fifteen patients had PIS. Stents were removed in 25% of patients due to complications, and cure was achieved in only two patients.

48.1.1.1.1. Duration of Stent Implantation and Stent Removal

Dumon had initially recommended a period of 6 to 12 months[10] before attempting removal of his stent. In Brichet's study,[13] they were left in for 6 months with a 16% rate of successful removal. Martinez-Ballarin[12] set an arbitrary interval of 18 months before stent removal; 35% of his group were cured with stents alone with 16 patients still waiting until the end of the 18-month period. Noppen[16] removed 10 covered Nitinol stents from his series of 35 adult patients (8 for complications and 2 after healing of the tracheal lesion). Removal was successful without any major complications. Significant bleeding occurred in two patients who were treated successfully using conservative measures.

48.1.1.1.2. Recommendations

While resection offers the best therapy and long-term results for benign tracheal stenosis, stents may be palliative or provide a bridge to surgery for patients who are considered unfit for surgery. A trial of stenting for cure may be attempted, as some success has been reported with stenting and close supervision. Most data support using silicone stents for this disease, however, data on the use of the covered Ulraflex stents are increasing. Up to 18 months of stenting may be required for PTS/PIS; clinical judgment is important in determining the timing of safe stent removal. In the case of metallic stents, removal should be performed in the operating room where extracorpoveal membrane oxygenation (ECMO) back up is available in case of acute airway obstruction or hemorrhage. These data consist of case series and case reports, therefore the grade of our recommendation for treatment of PIS/PTS is C.

> Resection offers the best therapy and long-term results for benign tracheal stenosis. Stents may be palliative or provide a bridge to surgery for patients who are considered unfit for surgery (level of evidence 4; recommendation grade C).

48.1.1.2. Idiopathic Tracheobroncheomalacia

In children the goal of stenting is to support the airway till it gains its structural integrity with growth. Silicone stents compromise the lumen due to their unfavorable wall-to-lumen ratio, significantly reducing the cross-sectional diameter; they repeatedly become obstructed with

TABLE 48.3. Stenting for idiopathic tracheomalacia.

Reference	Duration of follow-up	No. patients	Level of evidence	Stent used	Conclusions
Filler[17]	16 months	16	3	Palmaz	Stents may be used effectively in tracheobroncheomalacia; removal may be required for complications.
Furman[43]	6 month	6	3	Palmaz	BEMS work well for tracheobroncheomalacia not responsive to conventional therapy.
Geller[18,44]	na	9	3	Palmaz	4 patients died secondary to bronchial hemorrhage; stent suitable as final resort; high complication rate.
Nicolai[19]	32 months	9	3	Nitinol	Nitinol stents offer a therapeutic option for inoperable central airway malacia or stenosis in children with minimal morbidity.

Abbreviations: BEMS, balloon-expanded metal stents; na, not available.

secretions and have a high migration rate of up to 30%. Metal stents have a thin wall and are easily deployed in infants with tracheobroncho-malacia. The Palmaz stent is frequently used in children because of the availability of small stents.

Filler[17] reported his experience with the Palmaz stents in critically ill children. Sixteen patients with a median age of 9 months received 30 stents. Safe removal of stents was reported at an average age of 14 months. One patient died during stent removal from tracheal hemorrhage. In Geller's case series[18] of nine patients using Palmaz stents, three patients died from tracheal hemorrhage and one died from recurrent pneumonia. He recommended that stents be used only as a last resort and after careful consideration. Nicolai[19] deployed Ultraflex stents in five infants: 2 tracheal and 11 bronchial stents. Four stents required removal and replacement for suboptimal position with forceps/rotation technique endoscopically without incident. The longest follow-up was 6 years (see Table 48.3).

48.1.1.2.1. Removal and Duration of Stent

Filler[17] recommended stent removal at 1 year, yet Puma[20] believed that at least 2 years are necessary before attempting stent removal in severe circumferential stenoses with associated tracheal malacia.

48.1.1.2.2. Recommendation

Idiopathic tracheobronchomalacia is a difficult disease to treat. Stents do improve the short-term results; what will happen as the child reaches adulthood is speculative at present. The longest follow-up is only 7 years. Palmaz stents are the most commonly used stents in children. However, good results can be obtained with Ultraflex stents. The timing of stent removal is controversial and we advocate removing metallic stents in the operating room (OR) with ECMO backup in case there is loss of the airway or hemorrhage. The data are based on case series and case reports; therefore our recommendation grade for treatment of tracheomalacia is C.

Idiopathic tracheobronchomalacia is a difficult disease to treat. Stents improve the short-term clinical results (level of evidence 4; recommendation grade C). What will happen as the child reaches adulthood is speculative at present.

48.1.1.3. Anastomotic Strictures (Lung Transplantation/Sleeve Resection)

Stents are used to treat anastomotic strictures, bronchiomalacia, and anastomotic dehiscences (Table 48.4). Both silicone[9] and metallic stents[21,22] have been used with good results. Mild stenoses are treated with simple balloon dilation; however, severe and persistent stenoses, tracheomalacia, and dehiscences often require stenting. In Chhajed's study, 13% of all lung transplants had a bronchial complication. They recommended dilation first, as 20% of patients responded to dilation alone. All tracheomalacia patients did well with stents. The stents did not relieve the air leak in the dehiscence group. Mughal[23] looked at nitinol stents in seven patients with bronchial

TABLE 48.4. Stenting for bronchial strictures or anastomotic complications.

Reference	Duration of follow-up	No. patients	Patient population	Level of evidence	Stent used	Conclusions
Mughal[23]	13 months	7	Lung transplant	3	Ultraflex	In uncovered stents granulation tissue helps healing of dehiscence; difficulty of stent removal not mentioned.
Saad[50]	20.1 months	12	Mixed	3	SEMS	Stents are effective in this sick and high-risk population with acceptable complications.
Chhajed[21]	na	33	Lung transplant	3	Mixed	Balloon dilation of airway obstruction in lung transplant patients is not very successful; tracheobroncheal stents are clearly useful.
Herrera[57]	25 months	18	Lung transplant	3	Gianturco	Stent therapy is effective treatment for lung transplant airway obstruction.

Abbreviation: na, not available.

anastomotic dehiscences. He was able to remove the stents within 21 to 57 days in all five patients, two of whom required repeat stenting for broncheomalacia. He did not use covered metal stents due to their high incidence of bacterial colonization,[24] and advocates the use of uncovered stents for dehiscence on the basis that this promotes granulation tissue and healing.

48.1.1.3.1. Recommendation

Most authors recommend metal stents in broncheomalacia, as silicone stents migrate.[25] Strictures can be treated with balloon dilation, and stenting should be observed for recalcitrant strictures. Covered stents should be removed after 6 to 8 weeks, as their long-term complications have not been all elucidated. For bronchial or anastomotic dehiscence, covered metallic stents are preferred. The data consists entirely of case series and case reports, therefore our recommendation

grade for treatment of anastomotic, post–lung transplant strictures is C.

> Metallic stents are useful for treatment of bronchial strictures after sleeve lobectomy or lung transplantation (level of evidence 4; recommendation grade C).

48.1.1.4. Tuberculous Strictures

Lee reported stenting for tuberculous strictures in his series of 59 patients[26] (Table 48.5). Stents were inserted into 5 out of the 59 patients who were refractory to repeated balloon dilations. In another study from Korea,[27] 19 patients underwent dilation and placement of 5 Z stents. One stent fractured and another had severe ingrowth of granulation tissue.

Wan[28] reported his series of seven patients, all of whom did well with significant improvement of

TABLE 48.5. Stenting for tuberculous strictures.

Reference	Duration of follow-up	No. patients	Patient population	Level of evidence	Stent used	Conclusions
Lee[26]	32 months	33	TB	3	Metallic	Nitinol stents can be used successfully in patients who fail balloon dilation.
Lee[27]	na	19	TB	3	Metallic Z stents	Balloon dilation as initial therapy had good results; metallic Z stents has a high complication rate.
Wan[28]	na	7	TB	3	Dumon	Dumon stents can be used along with balloon dilation in airway obstruction secondary to TB.
Kim[29]	5–52 months	9	TB	3	Metallic	Nitinol retrievable strents good option for TB strictures; stent removal after 6 months has a low incidence of relapse.

Abbreviations: na, not available; TB tuberculosis.

their symptoms. Kim[29] reported a series of nine patients with tuberculosis strictures and used nitinol stents for an average of 4 to 6 months. None of the four patients who had a stent in for 6 months had recurrence, whereas 3/5 patients who had the stent in for only 2 months had recurrence.

48.1.1.4.1. Recommendation

Balloon dilation is first-line therapy for tracheo-broncheal stenosis secondary to tuberculosis. Stents have a role in intractable stenosis. Both nitinol and silicone stents can be used. Removal of the stents seems reasonable after 6 months. The data is based on case series and case reports, therefore our recommendation grade for treatment of tuberculosis strictures is D.

> Balloon dilation is first-line therapy for tracheobroncheal stenosis secondary to tuberculosis. Stents have a role in managing intractable stenosis (level of evidence 4 to 5; recommendation grade D).

48.1.2. Choice of Stent

48.1.2.1. Silicone Stents

48.1.2.1.1. Dumon Stents (Nova Tech, Abayone)

Introduced by Dumon in 1990, this stent is considered the standard by many physicians (Table 48.6). The main advantage includes the ability to be repositioned at a latter time. The disadvantages include migration, mucus plugging, and granuloma formation, albeit with less ferocity than is evident with metal stents. The need for rigid bronchoscopy for insertion is another disadvantage, as fewer than 10% of pulmonologists can perform rigid bronchoscopy.[30]

Dumon[31] reported results from 1574 stents placed in 1058 patients. Benign disease accounted for 360 patients. In this group stent migration occurred in 15%, stent obstruction by secretion in 8%, and granulation tissue formation occurred in 18%. There have been some fatalities reported from acute obstruction with secretions and failure of immediate referral.[31] Two studies address the issue of silicone stent migration with new designs. The first, by Vergnon,[32] had no stent migration in his series of 13 patients using a new stent with variable diameters. The second, by Noppen,[33] looked at a screw thread stent compared to the Dumon stent. Stent migration occurred in more patients who received Dumon stents (24% vs. 5%), although the difference was not statistically significant.

Several stents, such as the Polyflex stents,[34] which incorporate both silicone and metal in their design, attempt to remedy some of the drawbacks of pure silicone or metal devices. Hybrid stents consist of expandable metal struts, which resist compression, covered by a silicone membrane. In Bolliger's[34] study, 25 patients with terminal cancer had the Polyflex placed with a migration rate of only 3.7%; no other complications were noted.

48.1.2.2. Metallic Stents

The stents used in airways include the balloon-expanded metal stents (BEMS), most commonly the Palmaz stent, and the self-expanding metal stents (SEMS), most commonly, the nitinol/Ultraflex. The Wallstent and the Gianturco stent are rarely used today.

48.1.2.2.1. Gianturco Stent (William Cook, Denmark)

Today, placing Gianturco stents in the airways is considered obsolete by all experts, in spite of their

TABLE 48.6. Silicone stents.

Reference	Duration of follow-up	No. patients	Level of evidence	Stent used	Conclusions
Dumon[10,11]	na	690	3	Dumon	Dumon stents are effective in treating benign tracheal stenosis with a cure rate of around 24%.
Noppen[33]	Up to 6 years	23	3	Silicone (Dumon vs. Screw-thread)	New stent had less migration than Dumon stent.
Vergnon[32]	19 months	13	3	Silicone (Tracheobronxane ST stent)	New silicone stent had no migration and less granulation tissue formation.

Abbreviation: na, not available.

seemingly easy insertion.[35,36] This is because of the high rate of complications, which include stent fracture,[37] fistula formation,[38,39] and rapid re-occlusion of the airway with granulation tissue.[39] In an animal study from Italy,[40] three types of stents were compared in 12 sheep: (1) bare self-expandable metallic stents (Gianturco); (2) silicone stents (Dumon); and (3) covered self-expandable synthetic stents (Polyflex). They found the Gianturco stent proved unsafe in the long term, owing to the risk of severe airway wall damage and perforation. The Polyflex stent was well tolerated but presented a high migration rate. The silicone stent showed several limitations but appear to be well tolerated by the host mucosa.

48.1.2.2.2. Palmaz Stent (Johnson and Johnson, Warren, NJ)

This is a balloon expandable stainless-steel mesh stent. Availability in small diameters made it attractive for the pediatric population, especially for tracheobroncheomalacia (Table 48.7). It has plastic behavior and therefore does not re-expand after being deformed. Filler and colleagues[41] reported results in 16 patients, most of whom had tracheomalacia. The stents were removable, and granulation tissue was seen in approximately 20% of the group. Perini and coworkers[42] treated eight patients with benign tracheobronchial disorders with 24 stents. Stent migration occurred in two patients (25%) and stent deformation in three patients (38%). Furman and associates[43] reported their series of six patients. He had to remove one stent due to severe granulation tissue formation; two patients died from sepsis. Geller and coworkers[44] reported their experience in nine children with benign stenosis. Four patients died, three due to tracheal hemorrhage and one due to recurrent pneumonias. Sommer and Forte[45] believe use of this stent is the preferred management for significant tracheobronchomalacia in children. Susanto and colleagues[46] used 11 Palmaz stents in seven patients with either bronchial stenosis or malacia after lung transplantation. Complications after stent placement included partial dehiscence of the stent from the bronchial wall in two patients, stent migration in three patients, partial obstruction of a segmental bronchial orifice by a stent in the main bronchus, and longitudinal stent collapse.

48.1.2.2.3. Wallstent (Boston Scientific Co., Watertown, MA)

This is a self-expanding metal stent made from a cobalt alloy. It is rarely used today. The utility of the device remains compromised by difficulty in repositioning and removing it.[47] Nitinol stents have better characteristics and have replaced Wallstents.

48.1.2.2.4. Ultraflex Stent (Boston Scientific Co., Watertown, MA)

Nitinol is a nickel–titanium alloy that exhibits a shape memory phenomenon known as the Marmen effect. The Ultraflex is a self-expanding

TABLE 48.7. Palmaz stents in the pediatric population.

Reference	No. patients	Patient population	Level of evidence	Stent used	Conclusions
Perini[42]	8	Lung transplant	3	Palmaz	Palmaz stents are subject to deformity and migration from repeated external stress.
Furman[43]	6	Neonatal	3	Palmaz	BEMS work well for tracheobronchomalacia not responsive to conventional therapy.
Geller[18,44]	9	Tracheomalacia	3	Palmaz	4 patients dies secondary to bronchial hemorrhage; stent suitable as final resort; high complication rate.
Filler[17]	16	Benign	3	Palmaz	Stents may be used effectively in tracheobronchomalacia; removal may be required for complications.
Susanto[46]	7	Lung transplant	3	Palmaz	Easy insertion and removal; this stent has significant complications.

Abbreviations: BEMS, balloon-expanded metal stents; na, not available.

TABLE 48.8. Ultraflex stents vs. Wallstents.

Reference	Duration of follow-up	No. patients	Level of evidence	Stent used	Conclusions
Noppen[16]	16.2 months	39	3	Wallstent	25% of patients required stent removal; nitinol stent is safe and feasible.
Sesterhenn[58]	16 months	11	3	Nitinol	Nitinol stents should be considered for treatment of benign stenosis.
Madden[49]	41 months	10	3	Ultraflex	Good long-term results; complications include halitosis and granulation formation.
Mughal[23]	13 months	7	3	Ultraflex	In uncovered stents, granulation tissue hels healing of dehiscence; difficulty of stent removal not mentioned.
Saad[50]	20.1 months	12	3	Wallstent	Stents are effective in this sick and high-risk polulation with acceptable complications.

device made of nitinol. It has a cylindrical open knitted loop design made from a single strand of nitinol wire and available in 8 to 20mm diameters. It does not fully expand to its austenitic state immediately after release, allowing time to readjust the position. The flexibility also allows it to fit to complex stenotic shapes. It can be easily removed before complete epithelization.

Jantz[48] reported their series of 34 patients, 16 of whom had benign disorders (Table 48.8). The average follow-up was 19.5 months. No patient had excessive granuloma formation or secretions. One patient had his stent removed without difficulty.

Noppen[16] reported his series of 34 patients who underwent stent placement for benign disease. Twenty-five percent of these required removal (five patients with granuloma formation, one patient with stent failure and restenosis). There were two cases of stent fracture, and two patients were considered to have had successful treatment. All the implanted stents were covered. His conclusions were that even though stents are regarded as permanent, removal was safe and with out major sequelae.

Sesterhenn and colleagues[15] reported their experience with nitinol stents in 11 patients with benign diseases. In their follow-up (mean, 67 weeks), one patient developed granuloma that required laser resection and one patient developed a dislocation of the stent requiring restinting. All his patients were nonoperable candidates. None of the stents were removed because all the patients tolerated it well. Madden[49] treated nine patients with benign diseases with 11 covered nitinol stents. All patients improved significantly. There was one patient who devel-

oped granulation tissue distal to the stent, sputum retention occurred in one patient, and two patients developed halitosis.

As mentioned previously, Mughal[23] described his experience with nitinol stents in seven lung-transplant patients. He recommended uncovered stents to prevent bacterial colonization and enhance granulation formation in dehiscence. He was able to remove the stents in five patients without complications. Saad[50] described the Cleveland Clinic experience using self-expanding stents in 82 patients using both Wallstents and Ultraflex stents. Fifty patients had cancer, 11 patients had undergone a lung transplants, and 21 had other miscellaneous benign disorders. Clinical infection occurred in 15.9%, obstructive granulomas in 14.6%, and migration in 4.7%. The complication rate was not related to the type of stent (Wallstents vs. Ultraflex), or the version (covered vs. uncovered). There was no difference in complication rates among the three groups.

48.1.2.3. Recommendations

The Dumon stent is safe. Disadvantages include the need for rigid bronchoscope, difficulty in conforming to irregular airways, interference with mucociliary clearance, and a relatively high rate of migration.

We do not recommend the use of the Gianturco stents due to their potential complications.

The Palmaz stent is not suited for adults secondary to its mechanical properties and reported complications. It may be useful in the pediatric population due to its size availability. Nitinol stents are being used with increased frequency in its place.

The Ultraflex stent is probably the stent of choice. The elasticity of this alloy biodynamically closely resembles that of the tracheobronchial tree, in contrary to stainless steel.[2] The austenitic characteristic is very important, because after expansion, the nitinol stent does not increase its pressure on the airway wall. This contrasts with the expandable metallic stent, in which there is constant elastic pressure on the airway.[2] The risk of airway perforation is theoretically lower with nitinol stents because they do not change length once expanded and are flexible enough to change shape with a cough, yet have radial strength during constant compression by tumor or stenosis. However, there is no evidence to prove this. Migration seems to be less than with other stents, and the covered stents seem safe, in terms of removal. It is probably as good as silicone stents in tracheal lesions and we prefer them over silicone stents in bronchial lesions.[36]

> The Dumon stent is safe, but its disadvantages include the need for rigid bronchoscope, difficulty in conforming to irregular airways, interference with mucociliary clearance, and a relatively high rate of migration.
>
> The Palmaz stent is not suited for adults secondary to its mechanical properties and reported complications. It may be useful in the pediatric population due to its size availability.
>
> The Ultraflex stent is a probably the stent of choice (level of evidence 3 to 4; recommendation grade C).

48.2. Future Studies and Trends

Poly-L-lactic acid and polyglycolic acid (PLPG) resorbable external stents may offer a potential solution to the problem of tracheomalacia.[51] These have been placed externally in animal models with good results when compared to the internal Palmaz stent[52] and silicone stents.[53] Advantages of this material include its strength, its versatile shaping characteristics, and its resorbability, which would obviate the need for surgical removal and allow for infant airway growth. Dexamethasone (DXM)-eluting, covered, self-expanding metallic stents have been evaluated in the canine bronchus[54] and were compared to a covered metallic stent. There were less epithelial erosions and less granulation tissue associated with the DXM-eluting covered stent. A completely absorbable stent made of polyglactin 910 (Vicryl) filaments in a homogenous polydioxanone (PDS) melt has been studied in an animal model. The stent, however, was completely absorbed within 4 weeks. The stent did show complete biodegradability and sufficient suspensor properties.[55] Future stents will combine the advantages of the metal and silicone varieties, and the indications for placing pure metal stents will likely decline.

48.3. Personal Views and Conclusion

There are no randomized studies directly comparing long-term outcomes after stenting versus resection for benign airway stenoses. We do need to continue to collect data on the different stents being used. This is difficult in single institutions due to the comparatively low number of patients. I would suggest that a database be set up by the stent companies, biased as they may be, to further study the long-term results and gain further insights.

Most physicians placing stents are pulmonologists with little rigid bronchoscopic experience.[30] Therefore, we will continue to see the advancement of stents that can be inserted through flexible bronchoscopes. The most comprehensive assessment and therapy are generally provided by centers with multidisciplinary airway teams specializing in compromised airways. Brichet[13] developed an algorithm for the management of tracheal stenoses. The algorithm was designed by thoracic surgeons, otorhinolaryngologists, anesthesiologists, and pulmonologists. Their approach primarily relied on rigid bronchoscopy with laser therapy and stent placement, followed by surgery, in appropriate candidates who developed disease recurrence. This multidisciplinary approach was also suggested by Jones.[56] This multidisciplinary approach to the care of patients ensures that patients will receive the most appropriate intervention, and hopefully will generate answers to the increasing number of questions concerning the diagnosis and management of this group of patients.

References

1. Grillo HC, Mathisen DJ, Waen JC, et al. Laryngotracheal resection and reconstruction for subglottic stenosis. *Ann Thorac Surg* 1992;53:54–63.
2. Ginsberg RJ, Vokes EE, Ruben A. Non-small cell lung cancer. In: DeVita VT, Hellman S, Rosenberg SA, eds. *Cancer: Principles and Practice of Oncology*. 5th ed. Philidelphia: Lippincott-Raven; 1997: 858–911.
3. Ernst A, Feller-Kopman D, Becker HD, Mehta AC. Central airway obstruction. *Am J Respir Crit Care Med* 2004;169:1278–1297.
4. Wright CD, Grillo HC, Wain J, et al. Anastomotic complications after tracheal resection: prognostic factors and management. *J Thorac Cardiovasc Surg* 2004;128:731–739.
5. Couraud L, Jougon JB, Velly JF. Surgical treatment of nontumoral stenoses of the upper airway. *Ann Thorac Surg* 1995;60:250–259; discussion 259–260.
6. Rea F, Callegaro D, Loy M, et al. Benign tracheal and laryngotracheal stenosis: surgical treatment and results. *Eur J Cardiothorac Surg* 2002;22:352–356.
7. Gaissert HA, Grillo HC, Wright CD, et al. Complication of benign tracheobronchial strictures by self-expanding metalstents. *J Thorac Cardiovasc Surg* 2003;126:744–747.
8. Donahue DM, Grillo HC, Wain JC, et al. Reoperative tracheal resection and reconstruction for unsuccessful repair of postintubation stenosis. *J Thorac Cardiovasc Surg* 1997;114:934–938.
9. Cooper JD, Pearson FG, Patterson GA, et al. Use of silicone stents in the management of airway problems. *Ann Thorac Surg* 1989;47:371–378.
10. Dumon JF. A dedicated tracheobronchial stent. *Chest* 1990;97:328–332.
11. Dumon JF, Cavaliere S, Diaz-Jimenez JP, et al. Seven year experience with the Dumon prosthesis. *J Bronchol* 1996;3:6–10.
12. Martinez-Ballarin JI, Diaz-Jimenez JP, Castro MJ, et al. Silicone stents in the management of tracheobronchial stenoses. *Chest* 1996;109:626–629.
13. Brichet A, Verkindre C, Dupont J, et al. Multidisciplinary approach to management of postintubation tracheal stenosis. *Eur Respir J* 1999;13:888–893.
14. Puma F, Ragusa M, Nicola A, et al. The role of silicone stents in the treatment of criatricial tracheal stenosis. *J Thorac Cardiovasc Surg* 2002;120:1064–1069.
15. Sesterhenn AM, Wagner H, Alfke H. Treatment of benign tracheal stenosis utilizing self-expanding nitinol stents. *Cardiovasc Intervent Radiol* 2004; 27:355–360.
16. Noppen M, Stratakos G, D'Haese J, et al. Removal of covered self-expandable metallic airway stents in benign disorders: indications, technique, and outcomes. *Chest* 2005;127:482–487.
17. Filler RM, Forte V, Chait P. Tracheobronchial stenting for the treatment of airway obstruction. *J Pediatr Surg* 1998;33:304–311.
18. Geller KA, Wells WJ, Koempel JA, et al. Use of the Palmaz stent in the treatment of severe tracheomalacia. *Ann Otol Rhinol Laryngol* 2004;113:641–647.
19. Nicolai T, Huber RM, Reiter K, Merkenschlager A, Hautmann H, Mantel K. Metal airway stent implantation in children: follow up of seven children. *Pediatr Pulmonol* 2001;31:289–296.
20. Puma F, Ragusa M, Avenia N. The role of silicone stents in the treatment of cicatricial tracheal stenoses. *J Thorac Cardiovasc Surg* 2000;120:1064–1069.
21. Chhajed PN, Malouf MA, Tamm M. Ultraflex stents for the management of airway complications in lung transplant recipients. *Respirology* 2003;8:59–64.
22. Orons P, Amesur N, Dauber J, et al Balloon dilation and endobronchial stent placement for bronchial strictures after lung transplantation. J Vasc Intervent Radiol 2000;11:89–99.
23. Mughal M, Gildea T, Murthy S, et al. Short term deployment of self-expanding metallic stents facilitates healing of bronchial dehiscence. *Am J Respir Crit Care Med* 2005;172:768–771.
24. Noppen M, Pierard D, Meysman M. Bacterial colonization of central airways after stenting. *Am J Respir Crit Care Med* 1999;160:672–677.
25. Mulligan M. Edoscopic management of airway complications after lung transplantation. *Therap Bronchosc* 2001;11:907–915.
26. Lee KH, Ko GY, Song HY. Benign tracheobronchial stenoses: long-term clinical experience with balloon dilation. J Vasc Intervent Radiol 2002;13: 909–914.
27. Lee KW, Im JG, Han JK, et al. Tuberculous stenosis of the left mail bronchus: results of treatment with balloons and metallic stents. *J Vasc Intervent Radiol* 1999;10:352–358.
28. Wan IYP, Lee TW, Lam HCK, et al. Tracheobronchial stenting for tuberculosis airway stenosis. *Surg Laprosc Endsc Perc Tech* 2000;10:41–43.
29. Kim JH, Shin JH, Shim TS, et al. Results of temporary placement of covered retrievable expandable nitinol stents for tuberculous bronchial strictures. J Vasc Intervent Radiol 2004;15:1003–1008.
30. Colt HG, Prakash UB, Offord KP. Bronchoscopy in North America: survey by the American Assiciation for Bronchology. *J Bronchol* 2000;7:8–25.

31. Dumon JF, Cavalier S, Diaz-Jimenez JP, et al. Seven year experience with the Dumon prostehesis. *J Bronchol* 1996;3:6–10.

32. Vergnon JM, Costes F, Polio JC. Efficacy and tolerance of a new silicone stent for the treatment of benign tracheal stenosis: preliminary results. *Chest* 2000;118:422–426.

33. Noppen M, Meysman M, Claes I, et al. Screwthread vs Dumon endoprothesis in the management of tracheal stenosis. *Chest* 1999;115:532–535.

34. Bolliger CT, Breitenbuecher A, Brutsche M, et al. Use of studded Polyflex stents in patients with neoplastic obstructions of the central airways. *Respiration* 2004;71:83–87.

35. Noppen M, Van Renterghem D, Vanderstraeten P. The wrong stent at the wrong time: a cautionary tale. *Respiration* 2003;70:313–316.

36. Jantz MA, Silvestri GA. Silicone stents versus metal stents for management of benign tracheobronchial disease. Pro: Metal stents. *J Bronchol* 2000;7:177–183.

37. Hermeic JE, Haasler GB. Tracheal wire stent complications in malacia: implications of position and design. *Ann Thorac Surg* 1997;63:209–212.

38. Bolot G, Poupart M, Pignat JC, et al. Self-expanding mstal stents for the management of bronchial stenosis and bronchomalacia after lung transplantation. *Larygoscope* 1998;108:1230–1233.

39. Nashef SAM, Dromer C, Velly JC, et al. Expanding wire stents for tracheobronchial disease: indications and complications. *Ann Thorac Surg* 1992;54:937–940.

40. Puma F, Farabi R, Urbani M, et al. Long-term safety and tolerance of silicone and self-expandable metal stents: an experimental study. *Ann Thorac Surg* 2000;69:1030–1034.

41. Fraga JC, Filler RM, Forte V, et al. Experimental trial of balloon-expandable, metallic Palmaz stent in the trachea. *Arch Otolaryngol Head Neck Surg* 1997;123:522–528.

42. Perini S, Gordon RL, Golden JA, et al. Deformation and migration of Palmaz stents after placement in the tracheobronchial tree. *J Vasc Interv Radiol* 1999;10:209–215.

43. Furman RH, Backer CL, Dunham ME, et al. The use of balloon-expandable stents in the treatment of pediatric tracheomalacia and bronchomalacia. *Arch Otolaryngol Head Neck Surg* 1999;125:203–207.

44. Geller KA, Wells WJ, Koempel JA, et al. Use of the palmaz stent in the treatment of sever tracheomalacia. *Ann Otol Rhinol Laryngol* 2004;113:641–647.

45. Sommer D, Forte V. Advances in the management of major airway collapse: the use of airway stents. *Otolaryngol Clin North Am* 2000;33:163–177.

46. Susanto I, Peters JI, Levine SM, et al. Use of balloon-expandable metallic stents in the management of bronchial stenosis and bronchomalacia after lung transplantation. *Chest* 1998:114:1330–1335.

47. Bolliger CT, Arnoux A, Oeggerli MV, et al. Covered Wallstent insertion in a patient with conical tracheobronchial stenosis. *J Bronchol* 1995;2:215.

48. Jantz MA, Silvestri GA. Silicone stents versus metal stents for the management of benign tracheobronchial disease. Pro: metal stents. *J Bronchol* 2000;7:177–183.

49. Madden BP, Park JE, Abhijat S. Medium-term follow-up after deployment of Ultraflex expandable metallic stents to manage endobronchial pathology. *Ann Thorac Surg* 2004;78:1898–1902.

50. Saad CP, Sudish M, Krizmanich G. Self-expanding metallic airway stents and flexible bronchoscopy. *Chest* 2003;124:1993–1999.

51. Nalwa SS, Hartig GK, Warner T, Connor NP, Thielman MJ. Evaluation of poly-L-lactic acid and polyglycolic acid resorbable stents for repair of tracheomalacia in a porcine model. *Ann Otol Rhinol Laryngol* 2001;110:993–999.

52. Sewall GK, Warner T, Connor NP, Hartig GK. Comparison of resorbable poly-L-lactic acid-polyglycolic acid and internal Palmaz stents for the surgical correction of severe tracheomalacia. *Ann Otol Rhinol Laryngol* 2003;112:515–521.

53. Saito Y, Minami K, Kobayashi M. New tubular bioabsorbable knitted airway stent: biocompatibility and mechanical strength. *J Thorac Cardiovasc Surg* 2002;123:161–167.

54. Shin JH, Song HY, Seo TS, et al. Influence of a dexamethasone-eluting covered stent on tissue reaction: an experimental study in a canine bronchial model. *Eur Radiol* 2005;15:1241–1249.

55. Lochbihler H, Hoelzl J, Dietz HG. Tissue compatibility and biodegradation of new absorbable stents for tracheal stabilization: an experimental study. *J Pediatr Surg* 1997;32:717–720.

56. Jones LM, Mair EA, Fitzpatrick TM. Multidisciplinary airway stent team: a comprehensive approach and protocol for tracheobronchial stent treatment. *Ann Otol Rhinol Laryngol* 2000;109:889–898.

57. Herrera JM, McNeil KD, Higgins RS, et al. Airway complications after lung transplantation: treatment and long-term outcome. *Ann Thorac Surg* 2001;71:989–993.

58. Sesterhenn AM, Wagner HJ, Alfke H, Werner JA, Lippert BM. Treatment of benign tracheal stenosis utilizing self-expanding nitinol stents. *Cardiovasc Intervent Radiol* 2004;27(4):355–360.

49
Tracheal Resection for Thyroid or Esophageal Cancer

Todd S. Weiser and Douglas J. Mathisen

The goals of major resection of the trachea or carina for malignant invasion by thyroid or esophageal carcinomas should be the opportunity for cure or for the palliation of symptoms related to these secondary tracheal neoplasms. Due to the differences in the natural history of these two distinct malignant processes, airway resection and reconstruction should usually only be considered for tracheal invasion by adjacent thyroid carcinomas. Major airway resection for locally invasive carcinomas of the esophagus is almost never indicated.

In general, patients with noninvasive thyroid malignancies achieve meaningful long-term survival after surgical resection.[1] Tracheal invasion by differentiated thyroid carcinoma at primary presentation occurs infrequently, with an estimated occurrence rate of between 1% and 6.5%.[2] Patients may present with hoarseness, hemoptysis, or dyspnea. The goal in treating these patients should be similar to that for patients with noninvasive thyroid cancers: the extirpation of all locoregional disease. The thyroid surgeon usually discovers airway involvement during elective thyroid resection and often attempts to shave off the neoplasm from the wall of the trachea. Despite adjuvant therapies, this approach unfortunately often leads to tumor recurrence with potentially profound morbidity and mortality from subsequent hemorrhage and suffocation.[3] To avoid airway obstruction and hemoptysis, tracheal resection and reconstruction can be performed. Grillo was the first to report a case of tracheal resection and reconstruction for airway involvement by thyroid carcinoma in 1965.[4] Even patients with incurable thyroid carcinoma with slow-growing distant metastatic disease can benefit from palliative resection of the thyroid cancer and involved trachea.

Techniques have been developed for simple sleeve resection of the trachea. Thyroid cancers that invade part of the cricoid cartilage can be resected and reconstructed by removing the involved airway and preserving one half of the cricoid cartilage and opposite recurrent laryngeal nerve. The distal airway is shaped to fit the resulting defect in a jigsaw fashion (Figure 49.1). Although demanding technically, this can be safely done with preservation of voice and airway. Alternative palliative options include rigid bronchoscopy with coring out the invading malignancy, laser ablative approaches, or external beam radiotherapy. These options incompletely address the oncological process and are best reserved for patients with limited life expectancies.

Carcinoma of the esophagus can potentially invade the tracheal wall. Radiographic evaluation of the patient with esophageal carcinoma, especially when combined with bronchoscopy and esophageal ultrasound, can help identify those patients at high risk for airway involvement.[5] Subsequent tracheoesophageal fistulae (TEF) can occur as the result of direct erosion and necrosis of the esophageal carcinoma or due to the effects of therapy resulting in necrosis of the tumor and tracheal wall. Unfortunately, patients with malignant esophagorespiratory fistulae have a dismal prognosis and esophagectomy with airway resection and reconstruction is almost never warranted. Most patients with

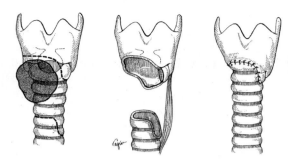

FIGURE 49.1. A complex type of resection in a patient with a recurrent thyroid carcinoma, presenting 2 years after thyroidectomy. [Reprinted with permission from Grillo HC, Zannini P. Resectional management of airway invasion by thyroid carcinoma. *Ann Thorac Surg* 1986;42:287–298, with permission from Society of Thoracic Surgeons.]

malignant TEF are diagnosed after the appearance of the fistula, but there are cases in which an impending fistula is discovered. In these latter cases, airway involvement is typically noted on bronchoscopic evaluation. Airway resection and reconstruction combined with esophagectomy interrupts the tracheal blood supply, greatly increasing the risk of airway anastomotic complications.

49.1. Published Data

Since Grillo's initial description of tracheal resection and reconstruction for locally invasive thyroid carcinoma, the techniques for airway resection have been refined and standardized. This has led to a significant improvement in morbidity and mortality associated with tracheal surgery. Accordingly, several centers, mainly in the United States and Japan, have pursued aggres-

sive surgical treatment of well-differentiated thyroid carcinoma with airway invasion. Major series are listed in Table 49.1. Due to the relative infrequency of this clinical situation, all reports are uncontrolled case series with a level of evidence of 4 based on the criteria established by the Oxford Centre for Evidenced-Based Medicine.

49.1.1. Thyroid Cancer Invading the Trachea

There is no consensus in the literature on the optimal surgical management of patients with thyroid carcinoma invading the trachea. Fujimoto and associates[6] published the first large experience in 1986. They treated 20 patients with locally invasive papillary thyroid cancer involving the airway. Six patients underwent tracheal sleeve resection and reconstruction, shave procedures were performed in 7 patients, 3 underwent window resection of the trachea, and a laryngotracheoesophagectomy was carried out in 1 patient. Resection was not possible in three patients due to very advanced local disease. One perioperative death occurred among the 17 patients who underwent resection. One local recurrence was reported and this occurred in one patient undergoing a shave procedure. No information was given on relief of symptoms. In follow-up, thyroid carcinoma resulted in death in three patients: one patient with a local recurrence after a shave procedure and in two patients in which resection could not be performed due to extensive local disease.

Ishihara and colleagues[7] reported results of airway resection for locally advanced thyroid cancers. This series was the first in the literature in which the patients were treated with circumferential airway resection and reconstruction. Of

TABLE 49.1. Major reports of surgical management of thyroid carcinoma with tracheal invasion.

Author	Year	Survival data						Level of evidence
		Shave resection			Radical resection			
		N	5-year (%)	10-year (%)	N	5-year (%)	10-year (%)	
Ishihara[7]	1991	–	–	–	50	66.6	60.2	4
Czaja[9]	1997	75	90	86	34	93	90	4
McCarty[11]	1997	35	90	85	5	66.6	nr	4
Grillo[13]	1992	–	–	–	27	59	50	4

Abbreviation: nr, not reported.

60 patients, laryngotracheal reconstruction was performed in 41 patients, while the remaining 19 had a tracheal resection and reconstruction. The malignancy in two thirds of these patients represented recurrent disease. Thirty-four patients underwent complete resections with 5- and 10-year survivals of 78% and 78%, while the 5- and 10-year survivals of those undergoing incomplete resection were 43.7% and 24.3%, respectively. Among the 26 patients in whom resection was incomplete, adequate resection of involved airway was not possible in 18 patients. No mention of symptom palliation was noted in this study. The authors demonstrated that complete resection enables improved overall survival, but notably, long-term survival can be achieved in those patients with incomplete resections.

To determine the effects of the extent of tracheal resection in patients with invasive thyroid carcinoma, Ozaki and colleagues[8] histologically examined specimens from 21 circumferential sleeve resections of involved trachea. Five specimens in cross-sectional analysis had more extensive mucosal than adventitial involvement. In these five cases, once the tracheal rings were invaded and tumor reached the submucosal space, growth continued circumferentially beyond what was appreciated from the adventitial surface. Therefore, residual tumor may be left behind when performing partial wedge resections of the airway based on involvement of the tracheal adventitia. No patients developed a local recurrence during long-term follow-up. The authors propose that when technically feasible, circumferential tracheal sleeve resections should be performed for thyroid cancers with airway involvement.

In 1997, Czaja and McCaffrey retrospectively reviewed their experience with 124 patients surgically managed on the basis of depth of malignant invasion of the airway.[9] Comparison of survival rates was made between patients who underwent either complete tumor removal ($n = 34$), shave excision ($n = 75$), or incomplete resection with tracheotomy to relieve airway obstruction ($n = 15$). The complete tumor removal group included a wide array of surgical procedures: total or partial laryngectomy, tracheal resection with primary anastomosis, or tracheal window resection. Shave excision included thyroid resections where (1) the

tumor was firmly attached to a wall of the areodigestive tract, (2) a portion of the tracheal wall was resected, with no gross residual disease remaining, and (3) microscopic margins were presumed positive. Adjuvant therapy, although not explicitly described, was administered to these patients postoperatively. In this series, survival rates of patients who underwent shave excision were not statistically different from those who underwent complete resection. When patients who underwent complete excision and shave excision were compared with those who underwent incomplete excision, there was a significant decrease in survival seen in the incomplete resection group. The authors therefore concluded that shaving the tumor off of the trachea is a viable option to treat tumors with minimal invasion.

Nishida and associates[10] reviewed their results treating 117 patients with differentiated thyroid carcinoma invading adjacent structures. Airway involvement was present in 69 patients who were managed based on the extent of laryngotracheal involvement. Deep invasion was defined as that existing through the cartilaginous layer. Fifty-four patients presented with deep tracheal invasion and 15 had superficial involvement. Patients with deep tracheal invasion were offered concomitant airway resection at the time of thyroidectomy. Forty patients consented to airway resection, while 14 did not. These latter 14 patients underwent thyroidectomy with no airway resection, leaving macroscopic tumor in the trachea. The mean overall survival was 8.7 ± 1.1 years for the concomitant airway resection group versus 1.5 ± 0.4 years for the thyroidectomy-only group. Thirteen of 15 patients whose tumors were firmly adherent to or abutting the external perichondrium of the trachea were treated with shave procedures. The patients in this group had similar local, regional, and distant recurrences when compared to a group of patients with no airway involvement, but who had tumors that invaded other local structures ($n = 48$). The mean overall survival was 12.9 ± 2.2 years versus 11.9 ± 1.1 years, respectively, between these two groups. Only two patients with superficial invasion were treated with airway resection. Conclusions reached by the authors in this work were that patients with deep tracheal invasion should be treated by resection of the invaded trachea, while those with limited invasion can be treated successfully without concomitant tracheal resection.

In another report, McCarty and colleagues[11] treated 40 patients with thyroid carcinoma and laryngotracheal involvement. Thirty-five of these patients were deemed to have had superficial invasion and were treated with cartilage shave procedures and adjuvant external beam radiotherapy. The remaining five patients had full-thickness tracheal wall involvement and were treated with airway resection, including tracheal sleeve resection ($n = 3$) and total laryngectomy ($n = 2$). Of the cartilage shave group, 25 patients were alive and without evidence of recurrence at a mean follow-up of 82 months. Five patients developed local recurrences and were managed with total laryngectomy ($n = 1$), tracheal resection ($n = 1$), or repeat radiotherapy ($n = 3$). The 10-year disease-free and overall survival rates for all patients were 47.9% and 83.9%, respectively. These authors concluded that a conservative surgical approach to minimally invasive thyroid carcinomas with cartilage shave procedures and adjuvant radiotherapy is a reasonable treatment option.

Grillo and colleagues[12,13] in 1986, with an update in 1992, reported our experience at the Massachusetts General Hospital with 52 patients with this disease entity. Resection was not performed in 18 of these patients, mainly because of extensive disease. Of the remaining 34 patients undergoing surgical management, 27 patients were reconstructed and 7 patients underwent cervicomediastinal exenteration. Early in the experience, 1 of the 27 reconstructed patients had a wedge resection of the trachea; the remaining 26 received cylindrical resections. Ten of the 27 reconstructions involved laryngotracheal anastomoses. The average length of airway resected was 3.5cm (range, 1.5–7cm). No patient in this series required laryngeal release.

In Grillo's series, 2 of the 27 patients who had airway reconstruction died in the postoperative period. One death was due to local necrosis of the anastomosis in a patient who had received 48Gy of irradiation 6 years previously. This patient was operated on in the time prior to the use of omental transfer for vascular augmentation of irradiated airways. The second patient expired from com-

plications surrounding a respiratory arrest. The morbidity was quite minimal in this series: one patient developed anastomotic granulation tissue, another had a mild air leak that resolved with nonoperative therapy, and one patient had a postoperative, unilateral, vocal cord paralysis.

The best results in this series were obtained when airway resection and reconstruction were performed at the time of thyroidectomy. Patients referred promptly for tracheal resection after the thyroid carcinoma was shaved off of the trachea also achieved prolonged survival, although not as long as those resected primarily. Airway recurrence developed in only 2 of the 25 survivors undergoing airway resection with construction. It should also be noted that resection was also performed in some patients for palliation or prevention of airway symptoms in the presence of slowly growing pulmonary metastases. The average survival for the seven patients with known pulmonary metastases was 4.2 years, with the longest surviving 10.5 years.

Gaissert[14] has further updated our experience with the surgical treatment of thyroid carcinomas with tracheal invasion. This series now reports on segmental airway resections in 82 of 110 patients who presented to the Massachusetts General Hospital over a 40-year period of time. Of note, 33 patients (40.2%) had prior tracheal shave excision. To date, 69 patients have undergone resection and reconstruction, with 29 tracheal and 40 laryngotracheal resections performed. No additional mortalities have occurred since Grillo's report in 1992. Mean follow-up is now 5.9 years, with 15-year follow-up complete in 67% of the patients. In those undergoing airway reconstructions, mean survival was 9.5 years and 10-year survival was 41.7%. Thirteen patients received salvage operations: laryngectomy ($n = 5$) or cervical exenteration ($n = 8$). The mean survival for this group was 5.8 years with 10-year survival being 16.9%. In 37 patients with well-differentiated carcinomas and complete resection, mean survival was 13.8 years and 10-year survival was 61.8% (Table 49.2). Disease-free survival was also significantly higher in patients with complete resection.

Gaissert also compared outcomes according to time of presentation for airway resection. Twenty-eight patients presented with recurrent,

TABLE 49.2. Overall and disease-free survival (DFS) in patients undergoing airway resection for invasive, well-differentiated thyroid carcinoma.

	Overall (n = 62)	Reconstruction (n = 56)	Salvage (n = 6)	Complete resection	
				Yes (n = 37)	No (n = 25)
Mean survival (years)	10.2	10.6	6.1	13.8	5.3
5-year survival (%)	60	63	33	74	39
10-year survival (%)	42	45	17	61	17
15-year survival (%)	25	26	17	44	0
Mean DFS (years)	6.5	7.0	1.7	8.5	2.9
5-year DFS (%)	37	41	0	50	18
10-year DFS (%)	22	25	0	28	14
15-year DFS (%)	19	22	0	28	7

Source: Data from Gaissert et al.[14]

loco-regional disease late after prior thyroidectomy (delayed presentation), while 11 patients were either referred for tracheal resection directly after thyroidectomy (n = 8) or underwent airway resection (n = 3) at the time of thyroidectomy (early presentation). Overall and disease-free survivals were significantly longer in the early presentation group (Table 49.3). Table 49.4 compares outcomes in patients with differentiated carcinoma who underwent concomitant shave procedure and subsequent airway resection for recurrence (delayed airway resection) to patients who underwent airway resection either at the time of thyroidectomy or shortly thereafter (early airway resection). The mean overall survival was 13.1 and 17.9 years in the delayed and early resection groups, respectively. The disease-free survival was also significantly higher in the early resection group when compared to delayed resection, 14.6 versus 5.1 years, respectively.

49.1.2. Esophageal Cancer Invading the Trachea

The first description of combined major airway resection in association with esophagectomy for esophageal carcinoma was performed by Thompson[15] in 1973. Review of the literature for evidence of successful tracheal resection for patients with esophageal malignancies since that time yields only sparse, small series and case reports. Martins[16] described four patients (3 cervical esophageal carcinomas, 1 postcricoid carcinoma) who underwent posterior tracheal wall resection with en bloc total pharyngolaryngoesophagectomy and gastric transposition. The tracheal defect was subsequently reconstructed utilizing the serosa of the transposed stomach. Two patients suffered from early postoperative death unrelated to the gastrotracheal anastomosis and

TABLE 49.3. Overall and disease-free survival (DFS) according to time of presentation.

	Delayed presentation (n = 28)	Early presentation (n = 11)
Mean survival (years)	7.5	17.6
5-year survival (%)	50	89
10-year survival (%)	32	89
15-year survival (%)	26	59
Mean DFS (years)	4.7	14.2
5-year DFS (%)	31	67
10-year DFS (%)	11	67
15-year DFS (%)	11	50

Source: Data from Gaissert et al.[14]

TABLE 49.4. Overall and disease-free survival (DFS) in patients with differentiated thyroid carcinoma who underwent thyroidectomy with shave procedure and later airway resection for recurrence compared to patients whose airway resection was performed with thyroidectomy or shortly thereafter.

	Delayed airway resection (n = 15)	Early airway resection (n = 11)
Mean time to airway resection (months[a])	67	3
Mean survival (years[a])	13.1	17.6
20-year[a] survival (%)	24	59
Mean DFS (years[a])	5.1	14.2
20-year[a] DFS (%)	0	50

[a]From the date of thyroidectomy.
Source: Data from Gaissert et al.[14]

the remaining two patients received palliation for 9 and 18 months. No gastrotracheal fistulae developed in this small series. Another potential mode of airway reconstruction in this clinical scenario involves the use of a free radial forearm flap to recreate the posterior tracheal wall.[17]

The largest series of noncylindrical resections of the major airways was presented by Matsubara and colleagues,[18] who reviewed their experience with 55 patients whose squamous cell carcinomas of the thoracic esophagus involved the trachea or main bronchi. This group performed varying degrees of partial tracheal wall resections with concurrent esophagectomy for the invading malignancy. The group of patients that underwent thick-wall resection had their partial tracheal wall defects repaired with either a latissimus dorsi or intercostal muscle flap. The overall in-hospital mortality was significant, with 10 deaths in these 55 patients (18%). The 1- and 2-year survival after esophagectomy was 44% and 25%, respectively. Improved survival was observed in those not having viable carcinoma at the surgical margin after preoperative therapy.

In patients with esophageal malignancies, the appearance of an esophagorespiratory fistula is a serious complication with a dismal prognosis. If left untreated, these fistulae will lead to continued airway contamination, which frequently result in pulmonary sepsis and death. To address this problem, several palliative treatment modalities have been utilized to minimize tracheobronchial soilage. These techniques include esophageal and airway stenting, esophageal exclusion or bypass, and fistula resection, to name a few. Burt and colleagues[19] found a median survival of 5 weeks in 207 patients with esophagorespiratory fistulae receiving all modes of treatment. As would be expected with this bleak prognosis, no patients in this series were treated with combined esophageal and airway resection and reconstruction.

49.2. Clinical Practice Based on Published Data

It is worth noting that the authors of each of the studies described all have a relatively strong bias towards one approach. For example, some insti-

tutions performed segmental resections of the airway for locally invasive thyroid carcinomas, whereas others feel less invasive techniques can adequately address this problem. Institutional experience in these procedures will therefore influence outcomes in the surgical treatment of these processes. We, for example, have developed a strong interest in disease processes of the airway. Hence, airway resection and reconstruction is an endeavor we feel fairly comfortable with and our morbidity and mortality with this procedure remains relatively low. Accordingly, we treat well-differentiated thyroid carcinomas that invade the airway with segmental resections of the larynx and trachea.

It is therefore quite difficult to compare clinical series addressing the most effective surgical treatment for locally invasive thyroid malignancies and arrive at a consensus opinion. The literature to date evaluating tracheal resection to address invasion by thyroid carcinoma consists entirely of uncontrolled case reports and case series. The relative infrequency of these clinical situations plays a major role in the paucity of studies available to analyze and make subsequent treatment recommendations. An argument can be made to approach these lesions with partial airway wall resections, as proposed by some experts; an equally effective treatment strategy is to perform cylindrical airway resections with reconstruction (level of evidence 4; recommendation grade C). Regardless of the actual surgical technique employed, one certain conclusion is that this clinical scenario is best remedied by a surgical approach.

> Thyroid carcinoma invading the trachea may be approached with partial airway wall resection or by cylindrical airway resection with reconstruction; the outcomes of these approaches are similar (level of evidence 4; recommendation grade C).

It is even more difficult to arrive at a consensus statement with regards to the optimal surgical treatment strategy for addressing airway invasion by esophageal carcinomas due to the significant lack of data available in the world's literature. Due to the considerable mortality associated with even partial wall airway resection and concurrent esophagectomy in Matsubara's experience,[18] there is insufficient evidence to make a specific treatment recommendation for this dismal clinical dilemma.

> There is considerable mortality associated with even partial wall airway resection and concurrent esophagectomy; there is insufficient evidence to make a specific treatment recommendation for this dismal clinical dilemma.

49.3. Personal View of the Data

We believe that the well-described series by Grillo[13] and Ishihara[7] have adequately demonstrated that airway resection and reconstruction for differentiated thyroid cancer is safe, has an associated low incidence of morbidity and mortality, and offers the potential for cure. This approach also provides prolonged palliation and can prevent death by asphyxiation or hemorrhage. We do not feel shaving techniques adhere to standard oncological principles. We have in fact seen an increasing amount of patients referred to us with local recurrences after this approach.[14] The surgical motivation behind shaving these tumors off of the airway is based on the false premise that segmental resection and reconstruction is associated with high risk.

The ideal method to settle this controversy is to perform a randomized study of the two techniques. Again, due to the rarity of this condition and the institutional experiences that are inherent in our practices, this question may never be adequately answered. We will continue to support a policy of complete resection of all known tumors at the time of initial operation. Preoperative evaluation may identify those at risk for airway invasion and these should be evaluated with bronchoscopy prior to thyroidectomy. If unsuspected airway invasion is encountered at initial surgical intervention, then expeditious referral to a center well versed in these problems should be performed.

In contradistinction, segmental resection and reconstruction of the trachea is not advised for esophageal carcinomas with direct airway invasion. Generally, the extent of airway involvement is often of significant length to prohibit reconstructive techniques. Also, the airway anastomosis is at great risk for ischemia and necrosis because the blood supply to the trachea is significantly affected by adjacent esophagectomy. Segmental tracheal vascular branches are often disrupted by esophagectomy. Matsubara[18] attempted to circumvent this high risk of anastomotic complications by performing partial tracheal wall resections with muscle flap repair. This is one option to this difficult anatomical dilemma, but the limited prognosis for these patients does not warrant aggressive surgical therapy in most cases. The dismal life expectancy in patients with esophagorespiratory fistulae also impacts the techniques employed to provide palliation. We feel that fistula resection with concomitant airway reconstruction is rarely warranted in these patients. More appropriate palliative techniques include esophageal and airway stents whose description is beyond the scope of this chapter.

References

1. Beahrs OH, Kiernan PD, Hubert JP Jr. Cancer of the thyroid gland. In: Suen JY, Myers EN, eds. *Cancer of the Head and Neck*. New York: Churchhill Livingston; 1981:599–632.
2. Lawson W, Som MP, Biler HF. Papillary carcinoma of the thyroid invading the upper air passages. *Ann Otol Rhinol Laryngol* 1997;86:751–755.
3. Silliphant WM, Klinck GH, Levitin MS. Thyroid carcinoma and death: a clinicopathlgical study of 193 autopsies. *Cancer* 1964;17:513–525.
4. Grillo HC. Circumferential resection and reconstruction of the mediastinal and cervical trachea. *Ann Surg* 1965;162:374–388.
5. Riedel M, Hauck RW, Stein HJ, et al. Preoperative bronchoscopic assessment of airway invasion by esophageal cancer: a prospective study. *Chest* 1998;113:687–695.
6. Fujimoto Y, Obara T, Ito Y, et al. Aggressive surgical approaches for locally invasive papillary carcinoma of the thyroid in patients over forty-five years of age. *Surgery* 1986;100:1098–1107.
7. Ishihara T, Kobayaski K, Kikuchi K, et al. Surgical treatment of advanced thyroid carcinoma invading the airway. *J Thorac Cardiovasc Surg* 1991; 102:717–720.

8. Ozaki O, Sugino K, Mimura T, et al. Surgery for patients with thyroid carcinoma invading the trachea: circumferential sleeve resection followed by end-to-end anastomosis. *Surgery* 1995;117:268–271.

9. Czaja JM, McCaffrey TV. The surgical management of laryngotracheal invasion by well-differentiated papillary thyroid carcinoma. *Arch Otolarygol Head Neck Surg* 1997;123:484–490.

10. Nishida T, Nakao K, Hamaji M. Differentiated thyroid carcinoma with airway invasion: indication for tracheal resection based on the extent of cancer invasion. *J Thorac Cardiovasc Surg* 1997;114:84–92.

11. McCarty TM, Kuhn JA, Williams WL Jr, et al. Surgical management of thyroid carcinoma invading the airway. *Ann Surg Oncol* 1997;4:403–408.

12. Grillo HC, Zanninni P. Resectional management of airway invasion by thyroid carcinoma. *Ann Thorac Surg* 1986;24:866–870.

13. Grillo HC, Suen HC, Mathisen DJ, et al. Resectional management of thyroid carcinoma invading the airway. *Ann Thorac Surg* 1992;54:3–9.

14. Gaissert H, Honnings J, Grillo HC, et al. Segmental laryngotracheal and tracheal resection for invasive thyroid carcinoma. *Ann Thorac Surg* 2006;82(1):268–272.

15. Thompson DT. Lower tracheal and carinal resection associated with subtotal oesophagectomy for carcinoma of the oesophagus involving trachea. *Thorax* 1972;28:257–260.

16. Martins AS. Total posterior tracheal wall resection and reconstruction with pharyngolaryngo-esophagectomy. *Surgery* 1999;125:357–362.

17. Nakatsuka T, Kato H, Ebihara S, et al. Free forearm flap reconstruction of the posterior tracheal wall invaded by esophageal carcinoma. *J Reconstr Microsurg* 1998;14:305–308.

18. Matsubara T, Ueda M, Nakajima T, et al. Can esophagectomy cure cancer of the thoracic esophagus involving the major airways? *Ann Thorac Surg* 1995;59:173–177.

19. Burt M, Diehl W, Martini N, et al. Malignant esophagorespiratory fistula: management options and survival. *Ann Thorac Surg* 1991;52:1222–1229.

Part 6
Pleura and Pleural Space

50
Pleural Sclerosis for Malignant Pleural Effusion: Optimal Sclerosing Agent

Zane T. Hammoud and Kenneth A. Kesler

Malignant pleural effusions are frequent sequelae of metastatic cancer. Approximately half of all patients with metastatic cancer will develop a pleural effusion, with lung and breast cancer accounting for 75% of cases.[1] The development of a malignant pleural effusion often leads to symptoms, such as dyspnea and cough, which significantly reduce the quality of life. Unfortunately, most malignant effusions do not respond to systemic therapy, thereby necessitating other forms of treatment when symptomatic. Currently the main options for the palliative treatment of symptomatic malignant pleural effusion include repeated thoracenteses, placement of indwelling pleural catheters, and pleurodesis. Repeated thoracenteses and indwelling pleural catheters are reasonable options for patients with very short life expectancies. Over time, repeated thoracenteses are inconvenient and the patient must tolerate recurrent symptoms as the fluid reaccumulates. Indwelling pleural catheters minimize the recurrence of symptoms but can be burdensome to patients.

Pleurodesis is a treatment with the goal of producing fibrosis between the visceral and parietal pleura, thereby obliterating the pleural space. If successful, pleurodesis prevents the reaccumulation of the effusion with permanent relief of symptoms. A variety of techniques have been used to achieve pleurodesis. Most commonly, a chemical sclerosant is instilled into the pleural space during thoracoscopy or through an indwelling tube thoracostomy. A number of prospective and retrospective clinical studies have been undertaken to determine the optimal strat-

egy to achieve pleurodesis. If there is evidence to support the superiority of one strategy over other strategies, then it may be possible to achieve standardization of the treatment of symptomatic malignant pleural effusions. The aim of this chapter is to determine the optimal sclerosing agent as well as to determine the optimal technique to achieve successful pleurodesis in the palliative treatment of symptomatic malignant pleural effusions based on current evidence.

50.1. Sclerosing Agents

50.1.1. Talc

Talc is considered to be one of the most successful sclerosing agents that achieves pleurodesis. A recent survey of pulmonologists from five English-speaking countries found talc to be the sclerosing agent of choice in 68% of respondents.[2] Talc is a soft anhydrous compound mainly composed of magnesium silicate and contains particles of varying size. Talc can be aerosolized into the pleural space as a powder or instilled as a slurry. While the precise mechanism by which talc induces pleural sclerosis is unclear, there is evidence to suggest that basic fibroblast growth factor plays an important role in this process.[3]

50.1.2. Bleomycin

Bleomycin is an anti-neoplastic antibiotic used to treat head and neck, cervical, and germ cell malignancies. As an anti-neoplastic agent, bleomycin has well-known pulmonary and cutaneous toxicities, which limits total intravenous dosage. Bleomycin has been successfully utilized as a pleural sclerosing agent for many years.

50.1.3. Tetracycline (Doxycycline)

Tetracycline is a broad spectrum antibiotic derived from *Streptomyces*. The parenteral form of the drug is no longer commercially available in United States, thereby precluding its use as a sclerosing agent. Doxycycline, a close pharmacological relative, has been used as an alternative agent with similar efficacy.

50.1.4. Other Agents

Silver nitrate was one of the first agents described for pleural sclerosis, abandoned for unclear reasons. There are recent reports of silver nitrate being reintroduced as a sclerosing agent.[4] Paschoalini and colleagues, in a prospective, randomized trial, found 0.5% silver nitrate to be at least equally efficacious to talc slurry for producing a pleurodesis.[5] OK-432 is a preparation of *Streptococcus pyogenes* that is widely used for pleural sclerosis in Japan, where talc is not commercially available.[6] Mitoxantrone is a synthetic anti-neoplastic drug that has been used for pleural sclerosis in patients with malignant effusion secondary to ovarian cancer.[7] Other rarely employed agents include interferon α and quinacrine.[4,8]

50.2. Choice of Sclerosing Agent

Chemical sclerosing agents have been the subject of many reports. The agents most frequently studied have been talc, either in powder or slurry form, bleomycin, and tetracycline or tetracycline derivatives. In a prospective, randomized trial involving 29 patients, Zimmer and colleagues[9] reported no statistically significant difference in the control of malignant effusions between talc slurry and bleomycin. At a mean follow-up of 1.7 months, control of effusion, defined as no evidence of fluid re-accumulation by routine chest radiograph, was achieved in 79% of patients receiving bleomycin and in 90% of those receiving talc. These authors concluded that talc, in

slurry form, is the agent of choice, due only to a significant cost advantage over bleomycin. Diacon and colleagues[10] reported the results of a prospective, randomized trial comparing talc aerosolized under thoracoscopic guidance versus bleomycin instillation. In this study involving 31 patients, talc was superior with respect to reducing the recurrent effusion rates. After 180 days, 65% of patients who underwent pleurodesis with bleomycin recurred compared to only 13% of patients who received talc. After a preliminary interval of 30 days the two agents had similar efficacy however. Haddad and coworkers[11] found no significant difference in success rate between talc slurry and bleomycin instilled through an indwelling chest catheter in a prospective, randomized trial of 71 patients after a median follow-up of 2.5 months. These authors also however recommend the use of talc slurry on the basis of lower costs.

Tetracycline, and its derivative doxycycline, has been compared to other sclerosing agents. Martinez-Moragon and colleagues[12] reported no difference in successful pleurodesis between tetracycline and bleomycin in a randomized, controlled trial of 62 patients with malignant pleural effusion. In a prospective, randomized trial of bleomycin versus doxycycline for pleurodesis, Patz and coworkers[13] found no significant difference in efficacy between the two agents in a total of 58 evaluable patients after 30 days of follow-up. Hartman and associates[14] reported their results of aerosolized talc under thoracoscopic guidance compared with historical controls treated with either tetracycline or bleomycin. These authors found talc to be superior to the other two agents for control of malignant pleural effusions.

A recently published Cochrane Database review attempted to establish the optimal sclerosing agent as well as the optimal technique to accomplish pleurodesis in the treatment of malignant pleural effusion.[15] This review encompased a total of 36 randomized, controlled trials, which enrolled 1499 patients. In 10 trials, comprising 308 patients, talc was compared to other agents. Overall, talc was found to be the more effective sclerosing agent, with a relative risk to achieve successful pleurodesis of 1.34 [95% confidence interval (95% CI), 1.16–1.55]. Five of these 10 trials compared talc to bleomycin, with a relative risk of 1.23 (95% CI, 1.00–1.50) favoring talc. Three of the trials studied talc and tetracycline or doxycycline, which again favored talc at a relative risk for success of 1.32 (95% CI, 1.01–1.72). Bleomycin was evaluated against other sclerosing agents in a total of 18 trials comprising 718 patients. There was no overall benefit of utilizing bleomycin compared to any other agent. Specifically, bleomycin was compared to tetracycline or doxycycline in eight trials, with the relative risk for successful pleurodesis of 1.03 (95% CI, 0.89–1.20). Tetracycline or doxycycline was compared to several other agents in 18 trials. The relative risk of successful pleurodesis was 0.98 (95% CI, 0.88–1.09), suggesting that tetracycline or its derivative were also not superior to any other agents studied.

Although talc has been shown to be an effective sclerosing agent, concern has been raised regarding safety. Reports of respiratory failure secondary to adult respiratory distress syndrome after talc administration have led some authors to voice caution.[16-18] The exact incidence of this complication is unknown but appears to be uncommon, with most reports citing rates below 3%. There is also evidence to suggest that the risk of pulmonary complications is dose related (>5g) and related to smaller talc particles (<15µm).[19] Long-term side effects[20] are not relevant to the vast majority of patients with malignant pleural effusion and limited life expectancy.

50.3. Technique of Pleurodesis

The Cochrane Database review also attempted to determine the optimal technique of achieving pleurodesis by analyzing studies that compared delivery of a sclerosing agent during operative thoracoscopy to bedside instillation through an indwelling thoracostomy tube. Overall, a total of five studies were included. The relative risk of successful pleurodesis favored thoracoscopic delivery, with a ratio of 1.68 (95% CI, 1.35–2.10). Of these five studies, two, with a total of 112 patients, used talc in both arms. The pooled estimate of these two studies favored talc aerosolized under thoracoscopic guidance with a success ratio of 1.19 (95% CI, 1.04–1.36). Moreover, there was no difference in mortality or morbidity between thoracoscopic and bedside talc pleurodesis.

A multi-institutional cooperative trial led by the Cancer and Leukemia Group B (CALGB) randomized 501 patients with malignant pleural effusion to receive talc aerosolized under thoracoscopic guidance or talc slurry instilled at bedside through a thoracostomy tube.[16] In this large trial, there was no statistical difference in the rate of successful pleurodesis between the two treatment approaches at 30 days. In subset analysis however, the thoracoscopic approach was significantly favored in the group of patients who demonstrated >90% lung re-expansion as well as patients with effusions secondary to breast or lung cancer. Among patients who were available for 30-day follow-up and who had >90% lung re-expansion, the thoracoscopic approach achieved successful pleurodesis in 82% while talc slurry achieved successful pleurodesis in only 67% ($p = 0.02$). A report by Yim and colleagues[21] randomized 57 patients with good performance status and symptomatic malignant pleural effusions to thoracoscopic talc insufflation versus talc slurry instilled through tube thoracostomy. This study found no statistical difference in the rate of recurrent effusion at a mean follow-up of 10 months, with recurrence in 1 of 28 patients after thoracoscopy and in 3 of 29 patients after talc slurry.

Viallat and coworkers[22] reported on their experience with thoracoscopic talc insufflation in a review of 360 cases. Of the 327 patients who could be assessed at 1 month, 90.2% had successful pleurodesis. Furthermore, 265 of these patients were followed up to 12 months. In this group of patients with longer follow-up 82.1% continued to demonstrate no evidence of recurrent effusion. Although no other agent or technique was studied, these authors recommended thoracoscopic insufflation over talc slurry on the basis of the excellent long-term results achieved in their series. In another large single-institution series of patients undergoing thoracoscopic talc instillation, Cardillo and colleagues[23] reported successful pleurodesis in 92.7% of patients available for long-term follow-up. The total number of patients in this study was 690, 611 of whom had a malignant effusion. These authors also recommended the thoracoscopic approach due to

TABLE 50.1. Selected reports with level of evidence 1.

Author	Comparison	Level of evidence
Shaw[15]	Various agents	1a
Martinez-Moragon[12]	Tetracycline vs. bleomycin	1b
Haddad[11]	Talc vs. bleomycin	1b
Diacon[10]	Talc vs. bleomycin	1b
Zimmer[9]	Talc vs. bleomycin	1b
Patz[13]	Bleomycin vs. doxycycline	1b
Yim[21]	VATS vs. talc slurry	1b
Dresler[16]	VATS vs. talc slurry	1b
Paschoalini[5]	Silver nitrate vs. talc	1b

Source: Oxford Centre for Evidence-based Medicine Levels of Evidence (May 2001).

TABLE 50.2. Selected reports with other levels of evidence.

Author	Subject	Level of evidence	Recommendation grade
Hartmann[14]	VATS talc vs. tetracycline/ bleomycin	4	C
Brega-Massone[24]	Chemical pleurodesis	4	C
Viallat[22]	VATS talc	4	C
Dikensoy[4]	Pleurodesis agents	2a	B

Source: Oxford Centre for Evidence-based Medicine Levels of Evidence (May 2001).

efficacy and safety. Level of evidence 1 studies for pleurodesis strategy in the treatment of malignant pleural effusions are given in Table 50.1. Table 50.2 lists studies with other levels of evidence.

50.4. Conclusions

Based on current evidence, talc is the sclerosing agent of choice for the treatment of symptomatic malignant pleural effusion (level of evidence 1; recommendation grade A). Talc is widely available, inexpensive, and highly effective. There have, however, been pulmonary complications reported including deaths secondary to respiratory failure. Such toxicity appears uncommon and possibly can be avoided by using talc doses under 5 g and talc preparations with large particle size.

> Talc is the sclerosing agent of choice for the treatment of symptomatic malignant pleural effusion (level of evidence 1; recommendation grade A).

The optimal method of talc delivery is somewhat more controversial. There appears to be sufficient evidence to favor thoracoscopic-guided insufflation over bedside instillation through indwelling chest catheters. The use of thoracoscopy facilitates fluid evacuation, including loculated fluid, and allows lysis of pleural space

adhesions, resulting in maximal lung re-expansion. Under thoracoscopic guidance, talc can be evenly distributed over the entire visceral and parietal pleural surfaces. These features of thoracoscopy can only serve to increase the chance of successful pleurodesis and are difficult if not impossible to duplicate by other methods. Therefore, a patient with the diagnosis of a malignant pleural effusion who is deemed a candidate for pleurodesis should be offered thoracoscopic insufflation of talc to optimize the likelihood of achieving durable symptomatic relief (level of evidence 1; recommendation grade A).

> A patient with a malignant pleural effusion who is deemed a candidate for pleurodesis should be offered thoracoscopic insufflation of talc to optimize the likelihood of achieving durable symptomatic relief (level of evidence 1; recommendation grade A).

References

1. American Thoracic Society. Management of malignant pleural effusions. *Am J Respir Crit Care Med* 2000;162:1987–2001.
2. Lee YCG, Baumann MH, Maskell NA, et al. Pleurodesis practice for malignant pleural effusions in five English-speaking countries. *Chest* 2003;124:2229–2238.
3. Antony VB, Nasreen N, Mohammed KA, et al. Talc pleurodesis: basic fibroblast growth factor mediates pleural fibrosis. *Chest* 2004;126:1522–1528.
4. Dikensoy O, Light RW. Alternative widely available, inexpensive agents for pleurodesis. *Curr Opin Pulm Med* 2005;11:340–344.

5. Paschoalini M, Vargas FS, Marchi E, et al. Prospective randomized trial of silver nitrate vs talc slurry in pleurodesis for symptomatic malignant pleural effusions. *Chest* 2005;128:684–689.

6. Kishi K, Homma S, Sakamoto S, et al. Efficacious pleurodesis with OK-432 and doxorubicin against malignant pleural effusions. *Eur Respir J* 2004;24: 263–266.

7. Barbetakis N, Vassiliadis M, Kaplanis K, Valeri R, Tsilikas C. Mitoxantrone pleurodesis to palliate malignant pleural effusion secondary to ovarian cancer. *BMC Palliative Care* 2004;3:4.

8. Sartori S, Tssinari D, Ceccoti P, et al. Prospective randomized trial of intrapleural bleomycin versus interferon alfa-2b via ultrasound-guided small-bore chest tube in the palliative treatment of malignant pleural effusions. *J Clin Oncol* 2004;22: 1228–1233.

9. Zimmer PW, Hill M, Casey K, Harvey E, Low DE. Prospective randomized trial of talc slurry vs bleomycin in pleurodesis for symptomatic malignant pleural effusions. *Chest* 1997;112:430–434.

10. Diacon AH, Wyser C, Bolliger CT, et al. Prospective randomized comparison of thoracoscopic talc poudrage under local anesthesia versus bleomycin instillation for pleurodesis in malignant pleural effusions. *Am J Respir Crit Care Med* 2000;162: 1445–1449.

11. Haddad FJ, Younes RN, Gross JL, Deheinzelin D. Pleurodesis in patients with malignant pleural effusions: talc slurry or bleomycin? Results of a prospective randomized trial. *World J Surg* 2004; 28:749–754.

12. Martinez-Moragon E, Aparicio J, Rogado MC, Sanchis J, Sanchis F, Gil-Wuay V. Pleurodesis in malignant pleural effusions: a randomized study of tetracycline versus bleomycin. *Eur Respir J* 1997;10:2380–2383.

13. Patz EF, McAdams HP, Erasmus JJ, et al. Sclerotherapy for malignant pleural effusions: a prospective randomized trial of bleomycin vs doxycycline with small-bore catheter drainage. *Chest* 1998;113:1305–1311.

14. Hartman DL, Gaither JM, Kesler KA, Mylet DM, Brown J, Mathur PN. Comparison of insufflated talc under thoracoscopic guidance with standard tetracycline and bleomycin pleurodesis for control of malignant pleural effusions. *J Thorac Cardiovasc Surg* 1993;105:743–748.

15. Shaw P, Agarwal R. Pleurodesis for malignant pleural effusions. *The Cochrane Library* 2005;2.

16. Dresler CM, Olak J, Herndon JE, et al. Phase III intergroup study of talc poudrage vs talc slurry sclerosis for malignant pleural effusions. *Chest* 2005;127:909–915.

17. Light RW. Talc should not be used for pleurodesis. *Am J Respir Crit Care Med* 2000;162:2024–2026.

18. Rehse DH, Aye RW, Florence MG. Respiratory failure following talc pleurodesis. *Am J Surg* 1999;177:437–440.

19. Maskell NA, Lee YCG, Gleeson FV, Hedley EL, Pengelly G, Davies RJO. Randomized trials describing lung inflammation after pleurodesis with talc of varying particle size. *Am J Respir Crit Care Med* 2004;170:377–382.

20. Lange PJ, Mortensen J, Groth S. Lung function 22–35 years after treatment of idiopathic spontaneous pneumothorax with talc poudrage or simple drainage. *Thorax* 1988;43:753–758.

21. Yim APC, Chan ATC, Lee TW, Wan IYP, Ho JKS. Thoracoscopic talc insufflation versus talc slurry for symptomatic malignant pleural effusion. *Ann Thorac Surg* 1996;62:1655–1658.

22. Viallat JR, Rey F, Astoul P, Boutin C. Thoracoscopic talc poudrage pleurodesis for malignant effusions: a review of 360 cases. *Chest* 1996;110: 1387–1393.

23. Cardillo G, Facciolo F, Carbone L, et al. Long-term follow-up of video-assisted talc pleurodesis in malignant recurrent pleural effusions. *Eur J Cardiothorac Surg* 2002;21:302–306.

24. Brega-Massone PB, Lequaglie C, Magnani B, Ferro F, Cataldo I. Chemical pleurodesis to improve patients' quality of life in the management of malignant pleural effusions: the 15 year experience of the national cancer institute of Milan. *Surg Laparosc Endosc Percutan Tech* 2004;14:73–79.

51
Management of Malignant Pleural Effusion: Sclerosis or Chronic Tube Drainage

Joe B. Putnam, Jr.

Numerous benign, infectious, and malignant diseases lead to recurrent pleural effusions.[1,2] Patients with cancer often develop current malignant pleural effusions secondary to their underlying disease. These malignant pleural effusions (MPE) frequently cause dyspnea and functional impairment. After other causes of dyspnea have been excluded, drainage of the MPE by simple thoracentesis can improve dyspnea and assist in improving ambulation and general activities. Malignant pleural effusion often recurs, challenging the physician, the patient, and the patient's family in balancing the benefits of symptomatic improvement with the risk and inconvenience of therapy. In addition, most patients with MPE will have a median life expectance of 90 days (range, 3–9 months) depending upon the histological subtype of the primary tumor.[3-5]

Treatment for patients with initial or recurrent MPE should focus on relief of symptoms of dyspnea and restoration of normal activity.[6,7] Traditionally, pleurodesis (e.g., visceral and parietal pleural symphysis with obliteration of the pleural space) has been achieved by in-hospital drainage of the effusion by tube thoracostomy (chest tube) or thoracoscopy followed by sclerosis with talc or other agents. Pleurodesis is necessary prior to removal of the chest tube and discharge home. Once hospitalized for treatment of MPE, other interventions may occur that could affect quality of life. A significant portion of anticipated future survival time could be spent inside the hospital. If pleurodesis cannot be achieved or if the fluid recurs, the treatment was then desig-

nated as having failed; the patient was then treated with the best available remaining therapy.

An alternative paradigm is a patient-centered treatment that focuses on relief of the patient's symptoms of dyspnea and restoration of more normal function. Relief of dyspnea by repeated drainage using a chronic indwelling catheter could accomplish these goals on an outpatient basis, thereby eliminating hospitalization. This chronic indwelling pleural catheter would relieve dyspnea by consistently achieving fluid removal and allowing the underlying subclinical pleural inflammation to achieve pleurodesis. Once the catheter ceases to drain fluid, it may be removed.

The optimal choice of therapy can sometimes be identified by grading current evidence on the topic and using this evidence to provide objective support for recommendations.[8] Using these techniques, guidelines for the management of pleural diseases have been established by professional organizations.[6,7]

51.1. Therapeutic Overview

Treatment options for MPE are varied and often tailored to the clinician's specialty and expertise, the patient's physical performance status, hospitalization status, and individual desires. Treatment options include thoracentesis or repeat thoracentesis; tube thoracostomy with drainage and sclerosis with talc, bleomycin, or other material; or thoracoscopy with drainage and talc insufflation.[9] Alternatives to pleurodesis include chronic dwelling pleural catheter (Pleurx®, Denver Biomedical, Inc., Golden, CO)[5] and pleuro-peritoneal shunt.[10,11]

All treatment options include one or more of the following items:

- Drainage of the pleural space.
- Apposition of the visceral and pleural surfaces with complete expansion of the lung (usually).
- Dispersion of a sclerosing agent throughout the pleural space.
- Maintenance of the pleural apposition until chemical or inflammatory pleuritis occurs.
- Obliteration of the pleural surface, for example, pleurodesis.

51.2. Diagnostic/Therapeutic Thoracentesis

Complete drainage of the effusion (to dryness) should be performed to assess the degree in which the MPE is causing the dyspnea, and the completeness of lung expansion, and for diagnosis. This process will provide physical relief and a determination of whether the pleural fluid was the mechanical cause of the patient's dyspnea, or other symptoms. In a small percentage of patients, the symptoms may be related to underlying pleural disease and not to the effusion (e.g., mesothelioma or other chronic pleural disease).

Complications of thoracentesis or pleural biopsy include pneumothorax, bleeding, hypotension (vasovagal related), re-expansion pulmonary edema, or infection. Symptoms related to thoracentesis include paroxysmal cough (from rapid expansion of alveoli in the previously deflated lung), and pain at the visceral and parietal membranes make initial contact. The pain may commonly occur in the shoulder or upper back. This technique may provide relief for several weeks before recurrence.

Outpatient serial thoracentesis may be considered although the inconsistent application and drainage may result in loculations and further physical embarrassment to the patient. The pleural effusions can re-accumulate rapidly. After diagnostic and therapeutic thoracentesis,

the patient should have follow-up for recurrent symptoms develop. If the pleural effusion recurs, the patient may be treated in a more definitive manner.

51.3. Drainage Volume

The amount of fluid drained during thoracentesis should be sufficient to obtain a diagnosis, relieve symptoms of dyspnea, and to avoid re-expansion pulmonary edema or pneumothorax. General guidelines have suggested that no more than 1500 mL be removed from one hemithorax during a single procedure. However, this arbitrary number does not consider the individual patient's height and weight. As a general rule, the surgeon may consider it appropriate to drain up to 20 mL pleural fluid per kilogram body weight as an initial volume.

51.4. Small Bore Catheters and Sclerosis

Various temporary and semi-permanent catheters have been used to palliate symptoms of dyspnea (level of evidence 3).[12-14] Simple small-bore drainage catheters (10F–14F) have been used effectively. Gravity drainage of the pleural fluid can be accomplished and pleurodesis achieved with several agents. In one study, small-bore catheters yielded outcomes equivalent to patients receiving chest tube after diagnostic thoracoscopy, and in addition were more comfortable (level of evidence 1b).[15] Additional small studies have been performed with early success using bleomycin or talc sclerotherapy.[16-19]

Small-bore catheters with drainage can allow for more rapid pleurodesis using oxytetracycline or bleomycin compared to a more traditional drainage and subsequent sclerosis[20] (level of evidence 2a). A shorter hospital stay results, and the response at 1 to 6 months after pleurodesis was equivalent between the two groups (level of evidence 2a).[21] An earlier randomized trial also noted that pleurodesis following rapid drainage (median chest tube duration, 2 days) was equivalent to pleurodesis performed after drainage was less than 150 mL/day (median chest tube duration, 7 days). The recommended approach would be the one which would minimize hospitalization.[22] In summary, drainage of MPE using small bore catheter drainage and rapid pleurodesis achieves results similar to prolonged drainage prior to pleurodesis (level of evidence 1b to 3; recommendation grade B).

> Drainage of MPE using small bore catheter drainage and rapid pleurodesis achieves results similar to prolonged drainage prior to pleurodesis (level of evidence 1b to 3; recommendation grade B).

51.5. Pleurodesis/Sclerosis

Pleurodesis: [pleuro + Greek desis, binding together (from dein, to bind).]

Pleurodesis is generally considered standard treatment for recurrent MPE. Many agents have been used with variable success. Additional factors that impact on the success of pleurodesis include initial drainage time, chest drain diameter, management of the chest drain (suction, no suction), etc. Pleurodesis is performed to inflame the visceral and parietal pleura, and to fuse the pleura together obliterating the potential pleural space. A sclerosing agent instilled within the ipsilateral thorax induces an inflammatory reaction. With pleurodesis, the pleural fluid cannot accumulate, or compress the functioning lung or (at the extreme) the mediastinum.[23]

51.5.1. Sclerosing Agents

Almost all sclerosing agents can produce fever, tachycardia, chest pain, and nausea.[24] As sclerosing agents may cause pain (talc, doxycycline, tetracycline, etc.), the patient should be premedicated with pain medication (usually narcotics) prior to instillation of the sclerosing agent.

Talc is a common, inexpensive, and effective sclerosing agent.[25] With complete expansion of the lung and apposition of the visceral and parietal pleura, pleural symphysis can occur. Talc

may cause adverse reactions such as microemboli and granulomatous tissue reactions.[26] Although many agents have been evaluated for pleurodesis, talc is the most common agent used today. It is generally considered the most effective agent for pleurodesis. A systematic review through 1992[27] and another organized review[28] confirmed the clinical and cost effectiveness of talc (level of evidence 1a; recommendation grade A). Talc has been studied in comparison with tetracycline and bleomycin. Tetracycline is no longer on the market and has been replaced with doxycycline. Talc has been found to be the better agent whenever compared with an alternative sclerosing agent and is much cheaper (level of evidence level 1b).[29-31]

More recent studies suggest that both thoracoscopic pleurodesis (in the operating room) and bedside instillation of talc slurry were equivalent in effectiveness (level of evidence level 1b; recommendation grade A).[32] Bedside drainage and talc slurry installation provide good resolution of symptoms, and are a cost-effective solution to the expensive alternatives of general anesthesia, thoracoscopy or thoracotomy, and inpatient hospitalization (level of evidence level 3).[16]

> Talc is the agent of choice for pleurodesis (level of evidence 1a to 1b; recommendation grade A).
>
> Bedside instillations of talc slurry and thoracoscopic talc insufflation in the operating room have similar effectiveness (level of evidence 1b; recommendation grade A).

51.5.2. Talc Instillation

Various techniques are used to instill talc within the pleural cavity. Three randomized, controlled trials have evaluated video-assisted thoracic surgery (VATS) with talc insufflation and bedside chest tube with installation of talc slurry, and the results suggested that either method was effective.[32-34] Talc slurry is commonly used following placement of a chest tube at the bedside. One study suggested fewer recurrences in patients with talc insufflation[33] following talc insufflation, but no such difference was noted in the other two studies in which bedside application of talc slurry appeared to be more effective. An additional benefit of thoracoscopy is that tissue diagnosis, pleural biopsy, printable biopsy, breakdown of adhesions, etc., can be achieved. If a tissue diagnosis has been obtained, bedside drainage and instillation of talc slurry appears to be a clinically effective and cost-effective method of achieving pleurodesis.

Although the bedside application of talc slurry can be easily done, the distribution of this talc slurry may not be completely uniform. Two randomized, controlled studies identified that physical maneuvers of turning the patient for various periods of time in various positions (typically lateral decubitus, prone, opposite lateral decubitus, supine) do not enhance distribution of agents.[35,36] These two radiographic studies used a -labeled suspension and demonstrated no improvement in distribution or outcome with rotation (level of evidence 1b; recommendation grade A).

> Rotation of the patient's body to enhance dispersal of the sclerosing agent it not recommended (level of evidence 1b; recommendation grade B).

51.5.3. Talc Dose

Talc administered as slurry through a chest tube or pleural catheter may be as effective as direct insufflation of talc via thoracoscopy.[37,38] Typically, a slurry of 5g in a solution of 50 to 100mL saline (with or without lidocaine) is instilled.[39] Single institutional studies suggest that either 5g or 2g of talc can be used with similar results. There may be relationship between the size of talc particles or specific contaminants and complications of talc use. In addition, a higher incidence of respiratory failure in may be related to the use of 10g of talc. Complications of talc sclerosis for MPE must be considered. In one study, respira-

tory failure was noted in 4% of patients undergoing bedside instillation of talc slurry compared to 8% in patients undergoing thoracoscopic talc insufflation.[32] Respiratory problems have been noted in a small fraction of patients in other studies.[39]

51.5.4. Alternatives to Talc

Tetracycline has been commonly used in the past in association with tube thoracostomy.[40] Instillation of the tetracycline solution provides a faster pleurodesis and pleural symphysis than chest tube drainage alone; however, it may cause significant pain. Doxycycline is an available alternative to tetracycline and is felt to have roughly equal effectiveness.[4,41,42] Bleomycin (60 units) has been shown useful and may be of equivalent effectiveness to tetracycline; however, it is expensive and can have systemic toxicity.[43,44] Talc was shown to be much cheaper than bleomycin in one study: $12 for talc compared to almost $1000 for bleomycin.[38] Talc was recommended as the first choice in two small randomized studies evaluating alternatives to talc including silver nitrate[45] and quinaquin.[30]

51.6. Thoracoscopy and Sclerosis

Thoracoscopy may also be considered as a means for obtaining pleural sclerosis in the management of MPE. After drainage and biopsy, the sclerosing agent is placed under direct visualization onto the pleural surface. Complications with this procedure include requirements for intubation and general anesthesia, and a small risk for bleeding and infection. A pneumothorax is uniformly present and requires a chest tube for a short time after the procedure. Proponents of this procedure believe the sclerosing agent can be more efficiently applied to the pleura. However, there are no studies showing one method to be superior to the other. Several agents can be used for pleurodesis, including talc, bleomycin, and doxycycline.[46,47]

Surgical techniques, such as thoracoscopy, drainage, and talc poudrage, may not carry any objective advantages over simple drainage and instillation of talc slurry. Mechanical abrasion of the parietal pleura using gauze, or other techniques (such as laser or argon beam coagulator) can be applied by thoracoscopic or open techniques. One single-institution study noted that mechanical pleurodesis (abrasion of the parietal pleura under thoracoscopic guidance) appeared to be more effective (less complications, shorter hospitalization) than talc pleurodesis.[48] Pleurectomy carries excessive risk of mortality and cannot be generally recommended. Unintended benefits of a thoracoscopic approach include inspection of the pleura, lysis/division of adhesions, and obliteration of loculations. Directed or random pleural biopsy should also be considered. Thoracoscopy has high accuracy in diagnosis of pleural disease, greater than 90%.[49]

In patients in whom a diagnosis must be obtained for treatment considerations, drainage, multiple pleural biopsies, and treatment may all be performed under a single anesthetic. Surgical exploration or thoracoscopy in most patients carries risk of anesthesia and thoracic manipulation. Thoracoscopy or open exploration is warranted only in highly selected patients. The value of this technique to the end-stage patient may be very limited and more simple strategies may be considered.

51.7. Tube Drainage and Sclerosis Versus Thoracoscopy and Sclerosis

A recent prospective, randomized trial was performed by cancer and leukemia group B (CALGB) to evaluate the efficacy, safety, and instillation technique for talc for pleurodesis for treatment of MPE.[32] The trial evaluated 501 patients who were randomized to thoracoscopy with talc insufflation talc poudrage (TTI, $n = 242$) or thoracostomy and talc slurry (TS, $n = 240$). The primary end point was 30-day freedom from radiographic MPE recurrence among surviving patients whose lungs initially re-expanded more than 90%. Morbidity, mortality, and quality of life were also assessed.

Patient demographics and primary malignancies were similar between study arms. A significant portion of patients died within 30 days (13% TS; 9.4% TTI). In evaluable patients who survived at least 30 days, the freedom from recurrence was 70% (TS) and 79% (TTI), somewhat lower than the expected 90% to 100% effectiveness anticipated. Overall, there was no difference between patients with successful 30-day outcomes based upon the instillation technique (TTI, 78%; TS, 71%). Subgroup analysis suggested that patients with primary lung or breast cancer had better success with TTI than with TS (82% vs. 67%). Treatment-related mortality occurred in nine TTI patients and seven TS patients. Common morbidity included fever, dyspnea, and pain. Respiratory complications were more common following TTI than TS (14% vs. 6%) including respiratory failure (TS = 4%; TTI = 8%), and toxic deaths (TS = 5; TTI = 6). The authors suggested that the etiology and incidence of respiratory complications from talc need further exploration.

Based on this single study, outcomes of chest tube placement and sclerosis and thoracoscopy with talc insufflation for management of MPE are similar (level of evidence 1b; recommendation grade B). There may be an advantage to performing a thoracoscopy approach in patients with MPE related to lung cancer or breast cancer.

> Outcomes of chest tube placement and sclerosis and thoracoscopy with talc insufflation for management of MPE are similar (level of evidence 1b; recommendation grade B).
>
> There may be an advantage to performing a thoracoscopy approach in patients with MPE related to lung cancer or breast cancer.

51.8. Chronic Indwelling Pleural Catheter

The Pleurx® catheter (Denver Biomedical Inc.) is a chronic indwelling Silastic catheter communicating within the pleural space. The patient or caregiver connects the catheter to a disposable vacuum bottle every other day to drain the pleural fluid, provide relief of dyspnea, and potentially achieve spontaneous pleurodesis.[5,50] The technique of insertion of a chronic indwelling pleural catheter has been described elsewhere.[5,9]

Between 1994 and 1999, a prospective, multicenter, randomized clinical trial was conducted to compare the effectiveness and safety of an indwelling pleural catheter with the effectiveness and safety of a chest tube and doxycycline sclerosis for treatment of cancer patients with symptomatic recurrent MPE.[5] The anticipated benefits of catheter-based treatment were outpatient management, improved quality of life, reduced medical costs, and improved function.

A total of 144 patients were randomly assigned to either an indwelling pleural catheter or a chest tube and doxycycline sclerosis (talc was not available at all centers at the time of the study.) Chest tubes were placed in a standard fashion. A modified Borg scale, the dyspnea component of the Guyatt chronic respiratory questionnaire, and Karnofsky performance status score were assessed and used for making comparisons between groups. Outcomes measured included control of pleural effusion, length of hospitalization, morbidity, and survival.

There was no difference between the two groups in initial (pretreatment) performance status or initial dyspnea scores. Median survival was 90 days in both the chest tube and pleural catheter groups. Patients with lung or breast cancer had a 90-day survival rate of approximately 70%; patients with other cancer types (as a group) had a 90-day survival rate of less than 40%. After treatment, both the chest tube and pleural catheter groups showed similar significant improvements in the Guyatt chronic respiratory questionnaire scores and had similar morbidity rates. There were no treatment-related deaths.

Initial treatment success rates (pleurodesis achieved in the chest tube group; drainage of effusion and relief of dyspnea in the pleural catheter group) were 64% in the patients treated with a chest tube and sclerosis, compared to 92% of those treated with a chronic indwelling catheter. Seventy percent of patients treated with a pleural

catheter experienced spontaneous pleurodesis. Seventy-one percent of patients with a chest tube had pleurodesis, although 28% of these patients developed a recurrence of their pleural effusion after treatment. The hospitalization was shorter in the pleural catheter patients: 1 day versus 6.5 days. An overnight hospitalization stay was standard protocol treatment for the patients receiving a pleural catheter. On the basis of initial treatment outcomes, both chest tube and sclerosis and chronic pleural drainage have similar success rates (level of evidence 1b; recommendation grade B). Whether there is a significantly higher rate of recurrent pleural effusion long term after using the chest tube/sclerosis technique remains to be seen.

On the basis of the successful multi-institutional experience with indwelling pleural catheters, an analysis of the results of outpatient management of patients with MPE and an indwelling pleural catheter was conducted.[51] Hospitalization and early charges between patients treated with pleural catheters were compared to those treated with chest tube drainage and sclerosis. One hundred consecutive patients treated with the pleural catheter (40 inpatients, 60 outpatients) and 68 consecutive patients treated with chest tube drainage and sclerosis (all inpatients) were analyzed. Outcomes evaluated were control of pleural effusion, length of hospitalization, morbidity, and survival.

There were no pretreatment or post-treatment differences in physical performance status or symptoms between the two groups. Mean hospitalization time was 8 days for inpatients whether they were treated with a chest tube or a pleural catheter. Overall survival was 50% at 90 days. Survival did not differ by treatment among the groups. In patients treated with pleural catheters, there were no catheter-related deaths, no emergency operations, and no major bleeding. Eighty-one percent of patients treated with pleural catheters experienced no side effects. The economic impact of pleural catheters was significant. For patients treated in hospital, mean charges ranged from $7000 to $11,000. Patients treated as outpatients (60 pleural catheter patients) had mean charges of $3400. Outpatient pleural catheter drainage was safe, cost efficient, and successful, and was associated with minimal morbidity.

No hospitalization was required for patients initially evaluated as outpatients. Outpatient management of MPE can be considered a standard of care (level of evidence 3; recommendation grade C).

> Chest tube/sclerosis and chronic pleural drainage have similar success rates (level of evidence 1b; recommendation grade B).
>
> Outpatient management of MPE can be considered a standard of care for patients undergoing chronic pleural drainage (level of evidence 3; recommendation grade C).

51.9. Special Circumstances: Trapped Lung

Patients with a trapped lung represent another difficult clinical challenge.[52] After drainage of a pleural effusion, the underlying lung may remain collapsed from adhesions or pleural carcinomatosis. To the inexperienced physician, this may mimic a pneumothorax. A chest tube may be placed, but the trapped lung will not expand. Long-term use of the chest tube in an attempt to re-expand the lung may increase the risk of pleural empyema. Standard techniques of thoracotomy and decortication may be considered to remove the pleural peel. Decortication is usually performed in patients with benign diseases in whom the pleural peel restricts ventilation with progressive and refractory dyspnea. Expansion of the normal underlying lung can improve symptoms of dyspnea. However, this intervention is sometimes drastic and may be contraindicated in patients with extensive malignancy.

The Pleurx® catheter and the pleuro-peritoneal shunt (Denver Biomedical, Inc.) have been used in selected patients with a trapped lung. The pleuro-peritoneal shunt has two fenestrated limbs that are placed into the pleural cavity and into the peritoneum, respectively. A one-way valve within a subcutaneous or external pumping chamber allows the patient or caregiver to pump and drain the fluid (from the pleural cavity to the peritoneal cavity) on a daily basis.

The Pleurx® catheter may be used to drain fluid from a trapped lung if symptoms of dyspnea occur. Use of the catheter allows the patient and/or his or her caregiver to relieve the dyspnea while draining the pleural fluid at home. In this manner the patient and caregiver can intervene directly against symptoms of dyspnea that the patient experiences as a result of the recurring pleural effusion. Drainage is typically performed every other day. Patients tolerate this well and are able to maintain an independent and functional life outside hospital.

51.10. Conclusions

The management of recurrent MPE requires selection among treatment options based on a careful assessment of the benefits of the therapy and the associated risks. Patients with MPE have limited life expectancy. Therefore, efforts to palliate or eliminate dyspnea help to optimize function, eliminate hospitalization, and reduce excessive end-of-life medical care costs, and may be achieved with both pleurodesis and an indwelling pleural catheter. Pleurodesis is an effective means of treating patients with MPE. The approach consisting of tube thoracostomy, drainage, and sclerosis with talc slurry is more cost effective than thoracoscopy with drainage and talc poudrage. Completeness of drainage appears to be advantageous for patients with MPE. Most patients currently have a large chest tube placed rather than a small-bore 12F to16F pigtail catheter, although the small-bore catheter appears to be equally effective and more comfortable. Further prospective studies are necessary to clarify this potential advantage for the small-bore catheters. Careful decisions by the clinician in coordination with the patient and his/her family are necessary to select the optimal therapy for the patient (Figure 51.1). Various effective solutions exist that can be individually tailored to the patient with malignant pleural effusion.

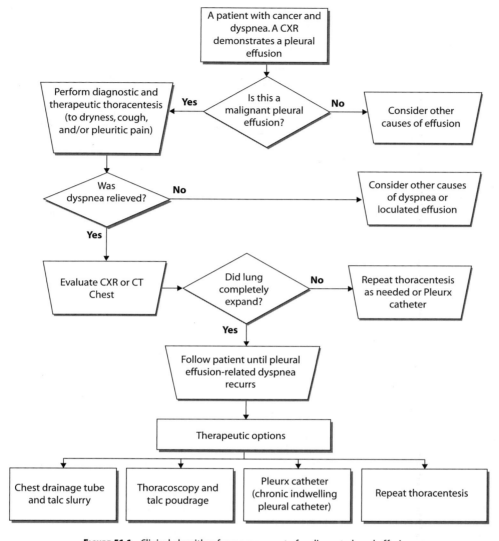

FIGURE 51.1. Clinical algorithm for management of malignant pleural effusion.

References

1. Light RW. Management of pleural effusions. *J Formosan Med Assoc* 2000;99:523–531.
2. Light RW. Useful tests on the pleural fluid in the management of patients with pleural effusions [editorial]. *Curr Opin Pulm Med* 1999;5:245–249.
3. Sanchez-Armengol A, Rodriguez-Panadero F. Survival and talc pleurodesis in metastatic pleural carcinoma, revisited. Report of 125 cases. *Chest* 1993;104:1482–1485.
4. Patz EF, Jr. Malignant pleural effusions: recent advances and ambulatory sclerotherapy. *Chest* 1998;113(suppl 1):74S–77S.
5. Putnam JB Jr, Light RW, Rodriguez RM, et al. A randomized comparison of indwelling pleural catheter and doxycycline pleurodesis in the management of malignant pleural effusions. *Cancer* 1999;86:1992–1999.
6. American Thoracic Society. Management of malignant pleural effusions. *Am J Respir Crit Care Med* 2000;162:1987–2001.

7. Antunes G, Neville E, Duffy J, Ali N, and the Pleural Diseases Group SoCCBTS. BTS guidelines for the management of malignant pleural effusions. *Thorax* 2003;58(suppl):38.

8. National Institute for Clinical Excellence. *Information for National Collaborating Centres and Guideline Development Groups*. London: National Institute for Clinical Excellence; 2001.

9. Putnam JB Jr. Malignant pleural effusions. *Surg Clin North Am* 2002;82:867–883.

10. Ponn RB, Blancaflor J, D'Agostino RS, Kiernan ME, Toole AL, Stern H. Pleuroperitoneal shunting for intractable pleural effusions. *Ann Thorac Surg* 1991;51:605–609.

11. Lee KA, Harvey JC, Reich H, Beattie EJ. Management of malignant pleural effusions with pleuroperitoneal shunting. *J Am Coll Surg* 1994; 178:586–588.

12. Sahin U, Unlu M, Akkaya A, Ornek Z. The value of small-bore catheter thoracostomy in the treatment of malignant pleural effusions. *Respiration* 2001;68:501–505.

13. Saffran L, Ost DE, Fein AM, Schiff MJ. Outpatient pleurodesis of malignant pleural effusions using a small-bore pigtail catheter. *Chest* 2000;118:417–421.

14. Smart JM, Tung KT. Initial experiences with a long-term indwelling tunnelled pleural catheter for the management of malignant pleural effusion. *Clin Radiol* 2000;55:882–884.

15. Clementsen P, Evald T, Grode G, Hansen M, Krag JG, Faurschou P. Treatment of malignant pleural effusion: pleurodesis using a small percutaneous catheter. A prospective randomized study. *Respir Med* 1998;92:593–596.

16. Belani CP, Pajeau TS, Bennett CL. Treating malignant pleural effusions cost consciously. *Chest* 1998;113(suppl 1):78S–85S.

17. Marom EM, Patz EF Jr, Erasmus JJ, McAdams HP, Goodman PC, Herndon JE. Malignant pleural effusions: treatment with small-bore-catheter thoracostomy and talc pleurodesis. *Radiology* 1999;210:277–281.

18. Bloom AI, Wilson MW, Kerlan RK Jr, Gordon RL, LaBerge JM. Talc pleurodesis through small-bore percutaneous tubes. *Cardiovasc Intervent Radiol* 1999;22:433–436.

19. Parulekar W, Di Primio G, Matzinger F, Dennie C, Bociek G. Use of small-bore vs large-bore chest tubes for treatment of malignant pleural effusions. *Chest* 2001;120:19–25.

20. Sartori S, Tombesi P, Tassinari D, et al. Sonographically guided small-bore chest tubes and sonographic monitoring for rapid sclerotherapy of recurrent malignant pleural effusions. *J Ultrasound Med* 2004;23:1171–1176.

21. Yildirim E, Dural K, Yazkan R, et al. Rapid pleurodesis in symptomatic malignant pleural effusion. *Eur J Cardiothorac Surg* 2005;27:19–22.

22. Villanueva AG, Gray AWJ, Shahian DM, Williamson WA, Beamis JF Jr. Efficacy of short term versus long term tube thoracostomy drainage before tetracycline pleurodesis in the treatment of malignant pleural effusions. *Thorax* 1994;49:23–25.

23. Rodriguez-Panadero F, Antony VB. Therapeutic local procedures: pleurodesis. *Eur Respir Mon* 2002;22:311–326.

24. Schafers SJ, Dresler CM. Update on talc, bleomycin, and the tetracyclines in the treatment of malignant pleural effusions. *Pharmacotherapy* 1995;15:228–235.

25. Antony VB. Pathogenesis of malignant pleural effusions and talc pleurodesis. *Pneumologie* 1999; 53:493–498.

26. Kennedy L, Rusch VW, Strange C, Ginsberg RJ, Sahn SA. Pleurodesis using talc slurry. *Chest* 1994;106:342–346.

27. Eccles M, Mason J. How to develop cost-conscious guidelines. *Health Technol Assess* 2001;5:2001.

28. Shaw PAR. Pleurodesis for malignant pleural effusions. *Cochrane Database Systematic Rev* 2004;1: CD002916.

29. Tan C. Pleurodesis for malignant effusion. In: Treasure T, Keogh B, Pagano D, Hunt I, eds. *The Evidence for Cardiothoracic Surgery*. Malta: Gutenberg Press Ltd.; 2005:119–129.

30. Haddad FJ, Younes RN, Gross JL, Deheinzelin D. Pleurodesis in patients with malignant pleural effusions: talc slurry or bleomycin? Results of a prospective randomized trial. *World J Surg* 2004;28:749–753.

31. Diacon AH, Wyser C, Bolliger CT, et al. Prospective randomized comparison of thoracoscopic talc poudrage under local anesthesia versus bleomycin instillation for pleurodesis in malignant pleural effusions. *Am J Respir Crit Care Med* 2000;162: t-9.

32. Dresler CM, Olak J, Herndon JE, et al. Phase III intergroup study of talc poudrage vs talc slurry sclerosis for malignant pleural effusion. *Chest* 2005;127:909–915.

33. Manes N, Rodriguez-Panadero F, Bravo JL, Hernandez H, Alix A. Talc pleurodesis. Prospective and randomized study. Clinical follow-up. *Chest* 2000;118:131S.

34. Yim AP, Chan AT, Lee TW, Wan IY, Ho JK. Thoracoscopic talc insufflation versus talc slurry for

symptomatic malignant pleural effusion [see comment]. *Ann Thorac Surg* 1996;62:1655–1658.

35. Dryzer SR, Allen ML, Strange C, Sahn SA. A comparison of rotation and nonrotation in tetracycline pleurodesis. *Chest* 1993;104:1763–1766.

36. Mager HJ, Maesen B, Verzijlbergen F, Schramel F. Distribution of talc suspension during treatment of malignant pleural effusion with talc pleurodesis. *Lung Cancer* 2002;36:77–81.

37. Hartman DL, Gaither JM, Kesler KA, Mylet DM, Brown JW, Mathur PN. Comparison of insufflated talc under thoracoscopic guidance with standard tetracycline and bleomycin pleurodesis for control of malignant pleural effusions. *J Thorac Cardiovasc Surg* 1993;105:743–747.

38. Zimmer PW, Hill M, Casey K, Harvey E, Low DE. Prospective randomized trial of talc slurry vs bleomycin in pleurodesis for symptomatic malignant pleural effusions. *Chest* 1997;112:430–434.

39. Janssen JP. Is thoracoscopic talc pleurodesis really safe? [review]. *Monaldi Arch Chest Dis* 2004;61:35–38.

40. Martinez Moragon E, Aparicio Urtasun J, Sanchis Aldas J, et al. Tetracycline pleurodesis for treatment of malignant pleural effusions. Retrospective study of 91 cases. *Med Clin* 1993;101:201–204.

41. Prevost A, Nazeyrollas P, Milosevic D, Fernandez-Valoni A. Malignant pleural effusions treated with high dose intrapleural doxycycline: clinical efficacy and tolerance. *Oncol Rep* 1998;5:363–366.

42. Herrington JD, Gora-Harper ML, Salley RK. Chemical pleurodesis with doxycycline 1g. *Pharmacotherapy* 1996;16:280–285.

43. Ong KC, Indumathi V, Raghuram J, Ong YY. A comparative study of pleurodesis using talc slurry and bleomycin in the management of malignant pleural effusions. *Respirology* 2000;5:99–103.

44. Noppen M, Degreve J, Mignolet M, Vincken W. A prospective, randomised study comparing the efficacy of talc slurry and bleomycin in the treatment of malignant pleural effusions. *Acta Clinica Belgica* 1997;52:258–262.

45. Paschoalini MS, Vargas FS, Marchi E, et al. Prospective randomized trial of silver nitrate vs talc slurry in pleurodesis for symptomatic malignant pleural effusions. *Chest* 2005;128:684–689.

46. de Campos JR, Vargas FS, de Campos WE, et al. Thoracoscopy talc poudrage: a 15-year experience. *Chest* 2001;119:801–806.

47. Schulze M, Boehle AS, Kurdow R, Dohrmann P, Henne-Bruns D. Effective treatment of malignant pleural effusion by minimal invasive thoracic surgery: thoracoscopic talc pleurodesis and pleuroperitoneal shunts in 101 patients. *Ann Thorac Surg* 2001;71:1809–1812.

48. Crnjac A, Sok M, Kamenik M. Impact of pleural effusion pH on the efficacy of thoracoscopic mechanical pleurodesis in patients with breast carcinoma. *Eur J Cardiothorac Surg* 2004;26:432–436.

49. Petrakis I, Katsamouris A, Drossitis I, Bouros D, Chalkiadakis G. Usefulness of thoracoscopic surgery in the diagnosis and management of thoracic diseases. *J Cardiovasc Surg* 2000;41:767–771.

50. Pollak JS, Burdge CM, Rosenblatt M, Houston JP, Hwu WJ, Murren J. Treatment of malignant pleural effusions with tunneled long-term drainage catheters. *J Vasc Intervent Radiol* 2001;12:201–208.

51. Putnam JB Jr, Walsh GL, Swisher SG, et al. Outpatient management of malignant pleural effusion by a chronic indwelling pleural catheter. *Ann Thorac Surg* 2000;69:369–375.

52. Pien GW, Gant MJ, Washam CL, Sterman DH. Use of an implantable pleural catheter for trapped lung syndrome in patients with malignant pleural effusion. *Chest* 2001;119:1641–1646.

52
Initial Spontaneous Pneumothorax: Role of Thoracoscopic Therapy

Faiz Y. Bhora and Joseph B. Shrager

The management of spontaneous pneumothorax (SP) is complicated by the many clinical settings in which it occurs and the lack of accepted guidelines for management. Primary spontaneous pneumothorax (PSP) occurs in persons without obvious underlying lung disease with a reported incidence of 7.4 to 18/100,000 per year for men and 1.2 to 6/100,000 per year for women.[1] Secondary spontaneous pneumothorax (SSP) complicates an underlying lung disease, most often chronic obstructive pulmonary disease (COPD), with a reported incidence similar to that of PSP. Because of the additional presence of the patient's underlying lung disease, SSP is considered a potentially life-threatening event, while PSP is rarely life threatening.[2,3] In this chapter, we will focus on the possible role of video-assisted thoracic surgery (VATS) as first-line therapy for patients presenting with their first episode of PSP, in contrast to the traditional approach of initial nonoperative management with surgical therapy reserved only for recurrent PSP. We will also briefly discuss the limited role of VATS as initial therapy for patients presenting with their first episode of SSP.

52.1. Initial Decision: Observation Versus Intervention

The initial questions to be answered when faced with a patient with SP are: When is simple observation sufficient, and, on the other hand, when is intervention necessary? Size of pneumothorax is one criteria by which to choose between observations and intervention strategies. Although it is difficult to accurately assess the size of a pneumothorax from a two-dimensional chest radiograph, the volume of a pneumothorax approximates the ratio of the cube of the lung diameter to the hemithorax diameter, and as a result the size is often underestimated. For example, a 1-cm pneumothorax on the posterior-anterior (PA) chest radiograph occupies about 27% of the hemithorax volume if the lung diameter is 9cm and the hemithorax is 10cm [$(10^3 - 9^3)/10^3 = 27\%$]. By the same principle, a 2-cm radiographic pneumothorax occupies 49% of the hemithorax. The British Thoracic Society (BTS) recommends intervention for any PSP greater than 2cm regardless of symptoms, quantifying these as large pneumothoraces.[4] If more precise size estimates are required, computed tomography (CT) scanning is the most accurate approach.[5] However, CT scan is only required initially in cases where it is difficult to differentiate a pneumothorax from suspected bullae in cases of complex cystic lung disease.[6]

Hence, at least one guideline recommends observation alone for small (<2cm) minimally symptomatic PSP[7-9] and this is one reasonable approach. The mean rate of resolution/reabsorption of pneumothoraces without an ongoing air leak is 1.8% per day and full re-expansion of a 15% pneumothorax occurs in 8 to 12 days.[9] Patients with these small PSPs do not require hospital admission, but all would agree that they should be observed in the emergency room for 4 to 6h with a repeat chest radiograph showing no enlargement of the pneumothorax. They can then be discharged with clear advice to return in the event of worsening breathlessness, and they should be seen in the outpatient clinic 1 to 2 weeks later to assure continued resolution. Observation alone is inappropriate in more than minimally symptomatic patients regardless of the size of the pneumothorax on a chest radiograph.

Unlike PSP, all patients with SSP require either inpatient observation or intervention. For SSP less than 1 cm with minimal symptoms, inpatient observation with serial films is recommended by the BTS. All other cases should receive active intervention, most often in the form of intercostal tube drainage. It is our advice, on the basis of the lung volume reduction surgery experience, that no suction should be placed upon the chest tubes of patients with SSP unless the lung fails to expand initially, after which time the minimal amount of suction allowing near-complete re-expansion should be applied.

52.2. Which Intervention?

52.2.1. Simple Aspiration Versus Tube Thoracostomy

Once it has been determined that intervention is needed for PSP, there are three main options: simple aspiration; intercostal tube drainage with or without chemical pleurodesis; and surgical strategies. Both the BTS and an American College of Chest Physicians Delphi Consensus Statement[10] recommend simple aspiration as first-line treatment for all PSP and most SSP needing intervention. This recommendation is based on the fact that successful initial re-expansion of the lung occurs in 59% to 83% of cases of PSP and 33% to 67% in SSP[11-13] and the fact that intercostal drainage with a tube can always be performed as second-line treatment should simple aspiration fail. Successful aspiration in these series depended on age (under 50 years, 70%–81% success; over 50 years, 19%–31% success); the presence of chronic lung disease (27%–67% success); and the size of the pneumothorax (<3 L aspirated, 89% success; >3 L aspirated, no success; >50% pneumothorax on chest film, 62% success; <50% pneumothorax on chest film, 77% success).

Several prospective, randomized trials have shown no difference in initial success rates of lung re-expansion (59% vs. 63%) or recurrence of pneumothorax at 3 months (20% vs. 28%) between simple aspiration and chest tube thoracostomy[13,14] Touted advantages of needle or small-catheter–based simple aspiration are a reduction in total pain scores during hospitalization and shorter hospital stays in some series.[15] Although there may be some advantages of simple aspiration stemming from less invasiveness and perhaps lower cost compared to tube thoracostomy, small-bore chest tubes can be placed with minimal morbidity and provide greater versatility in cases of initial nonexpansion of the lung in the form of application of suction and if needed, pleurodesis. It is certainly reasonable, and in our opinion optimal, therefore, to move directly to small-bore chest tube placement in most patients with SP who fall into the intervention subset, especially those with larger pneumothoraces, the elderly, and those with underlying lung disease (SSP). It is our opinion that most SSP larger than 1 cm and all SSP larger than 2 cm should be treated by intercostal tube drainage. If simple aspiration is performed in patients with SSP, prompt progression to intercostal tube drainage should be performed at the first sign of incomplete drainage. Although some have even recommended that consideration be given to a second attempt at aspiration for SP,[11] this would seem unwise to us after an unsuccessful first attempt under any circumstances.

There is no published evidence to suggest that larger tubes (20F–24F) are any better than small tubes (10F–14F),[16] although the authors' personal experience favors using at least a 20F tube in these circumstances, as this size tube is far less likely to become kinked or clogged with blood or tissue, thereby causing ineffective evacuation of the pleural space. Furthermore, if one opts to perform talc pleurodesis through the tube (as may be done for some cases of SSP), this can be difficult to perform through a very small tube.

Whether or not to place suction upon an intercostal tube after tube insertion is controversial. We believe that for PSP, a brief period (1–2 h) of −20 cm suction should be applied after tube insertion to promote initial re-expansion, but that the tube should subsequently be placed to water seal regardless of the presence of air leak. For SSP, where underlying bullous disease may be torn by even low levels of suction, we believe suction should not be applied even initially. A low level (−10cm) of suction can be added after 24 to 48h if there is failure of the lung to expand. It should be mentioned that here is no evidence to support the routine initial use of suction applied to chest tubes placed for the treatment of SP[17,18]; on the contrary, there is accumulating evidence that suction in many situations may only serve to prolong air leaks.[19,20] The addition of suction immediately after insertion of a chest tube in cases where a pneumothorax is large and may have been present for several days additionally risks precipitating re-expansion pulmonary edema.

52.2.2. Role of Video-Assisted Thorascopic Procedures

The role of video-assisted thorascopic surgery (VATS) in the first-line treatment of SP is continuing to evolve. Until fairly recently, the widely accepted gold standard for initial management of a first episode of PSP was observation for a small pneumothorax and simple aspiration versus tube thoracostomy for larger or symptomatic pneumothoraces. Before the advent of VATS in 1991, the gold standard procedure when surgical intervention was felt to be indicated was bleb excision and apical parietal pleurectomy via standard posterior–lateral thoracotomy or axillary thoracotomy.[21,22] This was virtually always reserved for recurrent ipsilateral pneumothorax, first contralateral pneumothorax, first episode of tension pneumothorax, bilateral pneumothorax, and first episode of pneumothorax in patients unable to receive prompt medical care or in high-risk professions such as airline pilots and scuba divers. Because recurrence rates of pneumothorax with conservative therapy (observation, simple aspiration, and tube thoracostomy) in most studies exceeds 40%,[14,15,23] other less invasive first-line modalities such as medical pleurodesis with teracycline and talc had been investigated but with disappointing results.[24]

As surgeons' experience with the VATS procedure has matured over the last decade, VATS blebectomy with pleurodesis/pleurectomy has come to be accepted as the new gold standard operative procedure for PSP. It has been demon-strated to have similar recurrence rates and likely lower morbidity as compared to thoracotomy.[25,26] The following question is therefore increasingly being asked: Is a VATS procedure appropriate not only after recurrent PSP and in special situations, but also as a routine in the first episode of PSP?

The first paper to look at this question was published in 1996 and reported that VATS was more effective in treating patients with first time *and* recurrent spontaneous pneumothorax, with less morbidity and potentially decreased total costs compared to conservative therapy.[27] This study retrospectively looked at two groups of patients, comparing 112 patients in group I (conservative therapy, 1985–1989) to 97 patients in group II (VATS, 1991–1994). In group II, 70/97 patients were cases of first-time SP. The groups were fairly well matched. For group I, tube thoracostomy was only performed if the pneumothorax was over 15% or progressed during observation. Of the 112 patients in group I, 97 underwent tube thoracostomy. Follow-up was obtained in 78 patients in group I. The 2-year recurrence rate was 22%. In group II, the 2-year recurrence rate was 4% ($p < 0.02$). Total tube drainage time and hospitalization time was also significantly lower in group II. This Dutch study did not report a significant difference in cost, but extrapolated that costs would have been lower for group II if the 4-day waiting period before operation could be shortened and if the costs of treatment of the recurrent cases were factored in.

The next series to look specifically at the role of VATS for first-time PSP was published in 1998 and retrospectively looked at the results in 61 patients who presented with the first episode of PSP between 1995 and 1997 and were treated with VATS.[28] There was no control group. If the patient was clinically stable and the size of the pnemothorax was less than 20%, the patient was observed. Otherwise, a chest tube was inserted without the application of suction. All 61 patients underwent high resolution CT (HRCT) and 48 had visible blebs. Surgery was recommended to these 48 patients and 45 consented. The operative procedure consisted of three- port thoracopy, apical blebectomy, and mechanical pleurodesis with a piece of electrocautery tip cleaner. Median operating time was 42min. The mean duration of chest tube drainage after surgery was 3.2 ± 1.9 days and the mean hospitalization after operation was 4.5 ± 1.9 days. Two cases had prolonged air leak more than 7 days and were treated by talc pleurodesis. Follow-up duration was 6 months. One recurrence was detected. The authors' conclusion that their protocol "decreases recurrence, shortens the time needed before the decision for operative intervention, decreases the time a chest tube is needed, and shortens the hospital stay" is not entirely supported by the evidence presented. Further, there is conflicting evidence as to whether the presence or absence of apical blebs has a significant impact on the natural history of PSP, and thus whether there is any justification for using HRCT results as an indication for surgery. The data on CT in predicting a recurrence is conflicting[29,30] and further, several studies show that blebs found on CT are not always the site of the air leak[31] and have no predictive value for recurrence in PSP.[32] However, this paper does validate the low morbidity and recurrence rate of pnemothorax following primary VATS over a short follow-up period.

The next series to address this question had a longer follow-up period of 53.2 months.[33] Between 1991 and 1997, 109 patients underwent VATS for SP. Fifty-three patients had first-episode PSP and 9 patients had first-episode SSP. Seventy-two patients had leaks or blebs identified at operation. Video-assisted thorascopic surgery was performed within 24h of hospital admission. No invasive procedure was performed if the size of pneumothorax did not exceed 20%. All others received a chest tube prior to VATS. If no blebs or air leaks were identified, only apical pleurodesis was performed. This was done in a variety of ways: electrocautery, partial or total pleurectomy, or talc pleurodesis. Mean operating time was 57 ± 2 min. Three patients (2.7%) had prolonged air leak more than 48h and underwent re-operation. The median postoperative stay in the PSP group was 4 days and in the SSP group 8 days. The long-term recurrence was 4.6% and was seen in patients who had not received a pleural procedure at the time of treatment by VATS. Because they calculated that almost 50% of patients with first-time SP will require operation either because of persistent air leak or subsequent recurrence, the authors argue in favor of extending the indica-

tion for immediate VATS to patients presenting with their first episode of SP.

A larger series of 156 patients presenting with initial PSP and treated with semi-elective VATS on presentation was presented in 2003 with some interesting results.[34] All patients presenting to the emergency room between 1992 and 2001 with PSP were initially managed with admission without chest tube placement. Within 12 hours, all patients underwent VATS, bleb resection, mechanical pleurodesis with an electrocautery cleaning pad *and* talc pleurodesis. Mean hospital stay was 2.4 ± 0.5 days. Surprisingly, blebs were found in all cases, there were no reported air leaks at 24h, and there were no recurrences with a median follow-up of 62 months (attributed to the use of both mechanical and talc pleurodesis in all cases). Certainly, placing a patient with a pneumothorax on positive-pressure ventilation prior to a VATS procedure without a chest tube in place, as was done in this series, must be done only under very careful observation, with urgent chest decompression as needed.

The only study to compare conservative treatment, open thoracotomy, and VATS was recently published in 2005 and is a retrospective study carried out between 1989 and 2001 in 281 patients with PSP.[35] Mean follow-up duration was 78 months. Before 1993, first-episode SP was treated conservatively if no blebs were seen on CT, and by thoracotomy if blebs were identified. After 1993, operative intervention was by VATS, replacing thoracotomy. When looking at first episode only, 181 patients received conservative therapy, 13 patients underwent thoracotomy, and 87 patients underwent VATS. Recurrence rates for each group were: 54.7% conservative group ($p < 0.05$), 7.7% thoracotomy, and 10.3% VATS (no statistical difference). Hospital stay was significantly shorter in the VATS group compared to open thoracotomy (4.1 vs. 11.5 days). The authors concluded that the "outcome of VATS was very good compared to conservative treatment and equal to that of thoracotomy in the first episode of spontaneous pneumothorax."

All of the above studies were merely suggestive of a role for VATS in first-episode SP by virtue of their retrospective design. The only prospective (but still nonrandomized) study to evaluate chest tube drainage versus VATS was published in 2000.[36] This Italian paper divided 70 patients presenting with first SP into two groups of 35 patients between 1996 and 1999. The first group underwent pleural drainage by chest tube and the second underwent VATS. The operative procedure consisted of blebectomy of visible blebs (80%) or apical wedge resection and pleurectomy if a bleb or air leak was not identified. The average operative time was a swift 18min. Prolonged air leaks more than 6 days were seen in 11.4% of patients who underwent pleural drainage versus 5.7% in the VATS group. Mean hospital time was shorter in the VATS group (6 days vs. 12 days) and recurrence at 12 months was 2.8% with VATS and 22.8% with pleural drainage. Total extrapolated direct hospital costs were lower in the VATS group (however, the cost-analysis assumptions used in this Italian study are not applicable to the U.S. model of health care, where lengths of stay are markedly lower). The authors conclude that, "The use of VATS at first spontaneous pneumothorax is justified in the interest of both patients and healthcare administrators as demonstrated by decreased recurrences and economy savings resulting from the use of VATS."

Although both the American College of Chest Physicians Delphi Consensus Statement (2001) and The British Thoracic Society (2003) guidelines continue to recommend simple aspiration as the first therapy for initial PSP, it would appear that the paradigm has begun to shift as increasing evidence accumulates that VATS as primary therapy for the initial episode of PSP may be appropriate. On the basis of nonrandomized data, it appears likely that this approach leads not only to significantly lower rates of recurrence, but also to improved patient quality-of-life indices and lower costs.[37] A prospective, randomized study looking at simple aspiration versus chest tube drainage versus VATS for first-episode PSP, with a carefully performed cost–benefit analysis would be needed to answer this question conclusively. Certainly, VATS blebectomy and pleurodesis or pleurectomy is the procedure of choice for recurrent PSP. The decision making involved in when to operate versus choosing conservative therapy for a patient with first-episode or recurrent SSP is more complicated and varies according to the overall condition of these often ill patients. A detailed discussion of these issues is beyond the space limits of this chapter.

52.3. Suggested Algorithm for Initial Management of First Episode of Spontaneous Pneumothorax

Based on the literature and our large personal experience with this problem, we feel that the following approach is the optimal overall algorithm for patients presenting with the first episode of PSP (Figure 52.1). As a routine, we do not obtain a chest CT scan. For a small pneumothorax (<20%; approximately 1-cm rim) and minimal symptoms, simple observation with repeat chest radiograph in the emergency room in 4 to 6h is appropriate. If the pneumothorax is stable, the patient can be discharged with careful instructions about seeking attention for increased pain or shortness of breath and a plan for a repeat radiograph at about 2 weeks to ensure near or complete resolution (recommendation grade B).

> For a small initial primary spontaneous pneumothorax and minimal symptoms, simple observation is appropriate; if the pneumothorax is stable, the patient can be observed on an outpatient basis (level of evidence 2 to 3; recommendation grade B).
>
> All patients with initial secondary spontaneous pneumothoraces should be admitted to a medical facility; for those with small pneumothoraces, initial observation is sufficient (level of evidence 2 to 3; recommendation grade B).

All SSP patients should be admitted to a medical facility for observation and/or intervention. For small SSP less than 1cm, initial careful observation is sufficient (recommendation grade B). For larger, progressive, or symptomatic SSP, chest-tube intervention is recommended as first-line therapy (recommendation grade B), and we believe that at least a 20F tube should be placed (large enough to remain patent and allow possible subsequent talc pleurodesis) (recommendation grade D). Computed tomography scan is generally useful in SSP patients as it will help delineate the severity and distribution of emphysematous changes, which may be useful in

FIGURE 52.1. Algorithm for initial management of first-episode primary spontaneous pneumothorax.

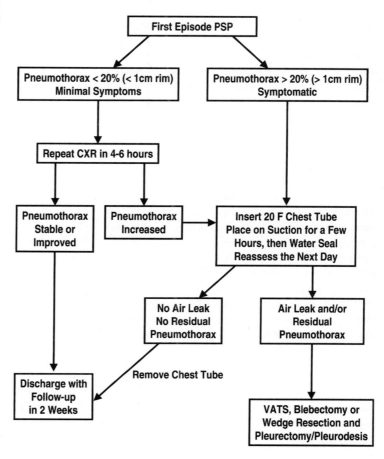

guiding the therapeutic approach. In some cases it is important to obtain an urgent CT even before chest tube placement, as a giant bulla can easily be mistaken for a pneumothorax. Pleurodesis via the chest tube or surgical intervention, preferably by VATS, can then be planned on a case-by-case basis.

In a first episode of PSP, if the pneumothorax is greater than 20% and/or the patient has significant shortness of breath or pain, intervention is indicated. We believe that the current literature does not clearly delineate which is best among the choices of simple aspiration, intercostal tube drainage alone, or primary VATS. In this setting of inconclusive data (Table 52.1), the approach which we have adopted and believe is most appropriate is as follows. First, despite the literature that demonstrates some effectiveness of simple aspiration and small-bore, soft drainage cathe-

ters at centers that use these routinely, it is our personal belief that these are to be avoided. It is our experience that both of these procedures tend to be performed by physicians or staff who are less experienced and not specialists in pulmonary medicine or surgery: thus, a needle used to drain the pleural space will not infrequently result in torn visceral pleura, leading to a greater

TABLE 52.1. Level of evidence of studies reporting results of VATS procedure in first-episode PSP.

Study	Reference	Study period	Level of evidence
Schramel, 1996	27	1985–1994	2+
Kim, 1998	28	1995–1997	3
Hatz, 2000	33	1991–1997	3
Torresini, 2000	36	1996–1999	2+
Margolis, 2003	34	1992–2001	3
Sawada, 2005	35	1989–2001	2+

problem than would otherwise be present. We have found further that the small drainage catheters often kink or otherwise become obstructed, failing to drain the pleural space adequately, leading to recurrent pneumothorax requiring additional therapy. We therefore favor placement of a 20F standard thoracostomy tube as initial therapy in first-episode PSP patients who are deemed to require intervention (recommendation grade D).

> In an initial primary spontaneous pneumothorax, if it is greater than 20% and/or the patient has significant shortness of breath or pain, intervention is indicated. There is insufficient data to make a recommendation as to whether simple aspiration, intercostal tube drainage, or VATS is the best initial intervention. For larger, progressive, or symptomatic secondary spontaneous pneumothoraces, chest-tube intervention is recommended as first-line therapy (level of evidence 2 to 3; recommendation grade B).

Once this chest tube has been inserted, the tube is placed to water seal after a brief period of suction and chest radiograph showing complete re-expansion. If on the following day there is no air leak and no significant pneumothorax, we remove the tube and discharge the patient. If on that day the patient has an air leak or a recurrent pneumothorax, we take that patient to the operating room for VATS as soon as possible (recommendation grade C). This approach is based upon two main concepts: First, we feel that a patient should not be subjected to general anesthesia and a surgical procedure when up to 60% of such patients do not require the procedure because they would not have suffered a recurrent pneumothorax without the procedure. The VATS procedure, though fairly straightforward, is not completely without morbidity. Second, in those publications that have found a cost–benefit to VATS in first episodes PSP, this conclusion rests largely upon (1) a protocol by which the procedure is done early after presentation (thus reducing hospital stay), and (2) those patients not undergoing VATS having a prolonged hospital stay. Our approach both allows a nonsurgical

approach to patients who will require only a one-night hospital stay, and it assures that those patients who might otherwise have a prolonged stay with chest tube drainage have their leaks repaired early. VATS blebectomy and pleurodesis or pleurectomy is preferable to thoracotomy for blebectomy and pleurectomy or pleurodesis whenever a decision to operate has been made in PSP (recommendation grade B).

> In patients treated with a chest tube in whom a chest radiograph shows complete lung re-expansion, if there is no pneumothorax or air leak on the day following chest tube placement, the tube is removed and the patient is discharged. If on that day the patient has an air leak or a recurrent pneumothorax, VATS intervention is recommended (level of evidence 3 to 4; recommendation grade C).

Our personal technique of VATS includes resection of all sites of air leak and blebs with endostapling devices, and total parietal pleurectomy. If there are no visible blebs, we perform an apical wedge excision to be sure microscopic blebs have not been missed and to allow diagnosis of any rare underlying lung disease that may be present. In women, we routinely examine the diaphragm for the fenestrations or endometrial implants that have been associated with catamenial pneumothorax. We favor pleurectomy over pleurodesis because the original procedure done via thoracotomy that became the gold standard for this condition included pleurectomy, and pleurectomy is quite easily performed via VATS (the slightly higher recurrence rates generally reported for VATS vs. thoracotomy may in fact be due to the typical use of pleurodesis as opposed to pleurectomy at VATS). We keep a single chest tube to suction for 48h following the operation to allow adhesions to begin to form, and if there is no leak at that time, the tube is removed and the patients are discharged. We do not feel that chemical pleurodesis via any tube for first-episode PSP is appropriate, as it is clearly less effective than VATS, and it may make a subsequent VATS procedure for a recurrence impossible and necessitate a thoracotomy at that time.

References

1. Melton LJ, Hepper NCG, Offord KP. Incidence of spontaneous pneumothorax in Olmsted County, Minnesota: 1950–1974. *Am Rev Respir Dis* 1979;29: 1379–1382.

2. Noppen M, Baumann MH. Pathogenesis and treatment of primary spontaneous pneumothorax: an overview. *Respiration* 2003;70:431–439.

3. Noppen M, Schramel F. Pneumothorax. *Eur Respir Monogr* 2002;7:279–296.

4. Henry M, Arnold T, Harvey J. BTS guidelines for the management of spontaneous pneumothorax. *Thorax* 2003;58:ii, 39.

5. Engdahl O, Toft T, Boe J. Chest radiograph: a poor method for determining the size of a pneumothorax. *Chest* 1993;103:26–29.

6. Philips GD, Trotman-Dickenson B, Hodson ME, et al. Role of CT in the management of pneumothorax in patients with complex cystic lung disease. *Chest* 1997;112:275–278.

7. Selby CD, Sudlow MF. Deficiencies in the management of spontaneous pneumothoraces. *Scot Med J* 1994;39:75–76.

8. Serementis MG. The management of spontaneous pneumothorax. *Chest* 1970;57:65–68.

9. Flint K, Al-Hillawi AH, Johnson NM. Conservative management of spontaneous pneumothorax. *Lancet* 1984;ii:687–688.

10. Baumann MH, Strange C, Heffner JE, et al. Management of spontaneous pneumothorax. *Chest* 2001;119:590–602.

11. Archer GJ, Hamilton AAD, Upadhyag R, et al. Results of simple aspiration of pneumothoraces. *Br J Dis Chest* 1985;79:177–182.

12. Ng AWK, Chan KW, Lee SK. Simple aspiration of pneumothorax. *Singapore Med J* 1994;35:50–52.

13. Noppen M, Alexander P, Driesen P, et al. Manual aspiration versus chest tube drainage in first episode of primary spontaneous pneumothorax. *Am J Respir Crit Care Med* 2002;165:1240–1244.

14. Andrivert P, Djedaim K, Teboul J-L, et al. Spontaneous pneumothorax: comparison of thoracic drainage vs. immediate or delayed needle aspiration. *Chest* 1995;108:335–340.

15. Harvey J, Prescott RJ. Simple aspiration versus intercostal tube drainage for spontaneous pneumothorax in normal lungs. *BMJ* 1994;309:1338–1339.

16. Tattersal DJ, Traill ZC, Gleeson FV. Chest drains: Does size matter? *Clin Radiol* 2000;55:415–421.

17. So SY, Yu DY. Catheter drainage of spontaneous pneumothorax: suction or no suction, early or late removal? *Thorax* 1982;37:46–48.

18. Sharma TN, Agrihotri SP, Jain NK, et al. Intercostal tube thoracostomy in pneumothorax: factors influencing re-expansion of lung. *Ind J Chest Dis Allied Sci* 1988;30:32–35.

19. Marshall MB, Deeb ME, Bleir JI, et al. Suction vs water seal after pulmonary resection: a randomized, prospective study. *Chest* 2002;121: 831–835.

20. Cerfoloi RJ, Bryant AS, Singh S, et al. The management of chest tubes in patients with a pneumothorax and an air leak after pulmonary resection. *Chest* 2005;128:816–820.

21. O'Rourke JP, Yee ES. Civilian spontaneous pneumothorax. *BMJ* 1971;4:86–88.

22. Weedon D, Smith GH. Surgical experience in the management of spontaneous pneumothorax, 1972–1982. *Thorax* 1983;38:737–743.

23. Light RW. Pneumothorax. In: Light RW, ed. *Pleural Diseases*. 3rd ed. Baltimore: Wilkins and Wilkins; 1995:242–277.

24. Massard G, Thomas P, Wihlm JM. Minimally invasive management for first and recurrent pneumothorax. *Ann Thorac Surg* 1998;66:592–599.

25. Freixinet JL, Canalis E, Julia G, et al. Axillary thoracotomy versus videothoracoscopy for the treatment of primary spontaneous pneumothorax. *Ann Thorac Surg* 2004;78:417–420.

26. Samtambrogio L, Nosotti M, Bellaviti N, et al. Videothoracoscopy versus thoracotomy for the diagnosis of the indeterminate solitary pulmonary nodule. *Ann Thorac Surg* 1995;59:868–870.

27. Schramel FMNH, Sutedja TG, Barber JCE, et al. Cost-effectiveness of video-assisted thoracoscopic surgery versus conservative treatment for first time or recurrent spontaneous pneumothorax. *Eur Respir J* 1996;9:1821–1825.

28. Kim J, Kim K, Shim YM, et al. Video-assisted thoracic surgery as a primary therapy for primary spontaneous pneumothorax. *Surg Endosc* 1998;12: 1290–1293.

29. Warner BE, Bailey WW, Shipley RT. Value of CT of the lung in the management of bullae in patients with primary spontaneous pneumothorax. *Am J Surg* 1991;162:39–42.

30. Mitlehner W, Friedrich M, Dissmann W. Value of CT in the detection of bullae in patients with primary spontaneous pneumothorax. *Respiration* 1992;59:221–227.

31. Noppen M. Do blebs cause primary spontaneous pneumothorax? Con: blebs do not cause primary spontaneous pneumothorax. *J Bronchol* 2002;9:319–323.

32. Schramel FMNH, Zanen P. Blebs and/or bullae are of no importance and have no predictive value for

recurrences in patients with primary spontaneous pneumothorax. *Chest* 1976;119:1976–1977.

33. Hatz RA, Kaps MF, Meimarakis G, et al. Long-term results after video-assisted thoracoscopic surgery for first-time and recurrent spontaneous pneumothorax. *Ann Thorac Surg* 2000;70:253–257.

34. Margolis M, Gharagozloo F, Tempesta B, et al. Video-assisted thoracic surgical treatment of initial spontaneous pneumothorax in young patients. *Ann Thorac Surg* 2003;5:1661–1664.

35. Sawada S, Watanabe Y, Shigeharu. Video-assisted thoracoscopic surgery for primary spontaneous pneumothorax: evaluation of indications and long-term outcome compared with conservative treatment and open thoracotomy. *Chest* 2005;126: 2226–2230.

36. Torresini G, Vaccarili M, Divisi D, et al. Is video-assisted thoracic surgery justified at first spontaneous pneumothorax? *Eur J Cardiothorac Surg* 2002;20:42–45.

37. Ng CSH, Wan S, Yim APC. Letter to the editor. Paradigm shift in surgical approaches to spontaneous pneumothorax: VATS. *Thorax* 2004;59: 357.

53
Intrapleural Fibrinolytics

Jay T. Heidecker and Steven A. Sahn

Pleural space infection (complicated parapneumonic effusion and empyema) is common and causes significant morbidity and mortality of up to 10%. The incidence of community-acquired pneumonia in the United States is estimated at 3.5 to 4 million cases per year with about 20% of patients requiring hospitalization.[1] A parapneumonic effusion develops in approximately half of hospitalized patients with pneumonia,[2] translating into 300,000 to 350,000 parapneumonic effusion annually. Most are small and resolve with antibiotics alone without pleural space sequelae. However, the effusion can progress to a complicated parapneumonic effusion (CPE) or empyema. Management ranges from observation to thoracotomy with decortication. The use intrapleural fibrinolytics, such as streptokinase, urokinase, and tissue plasminogen activator (tPA) to augment chest-tube drainage of a CPE and empyema is widespread; however, case series, cohort studies, and small randomized, controlled trials have conflicting conclusions. Recently, a large, multicenter, randomized clinical trial [First Multicenter Intrapleural Sepsis Trial (MIST-1)] found no benefit of intrapleural streptokinase for CPE and empyema[3]; therefore, the use of intrapleural fibrinolytics must be selective and needs further study.

The classification of pleural space infection can be confusing. For simplicity, an uncomplicated parapneumonic effusion is a pleural effusion that occurs as a result of pneumonia that resolves with antibiotic therapy alone. A CPE (pleural fluid pH <7.20 and/or positive gram stain or culture) is a pleural effusion associated with pneumonia that requires drainage for the resolution of pleural sepsis. An empyema thoracis is pus in the pleural space[2] and represents the final stage of a parapneumonic effusion that always requires pleural space drainage.

53.1. Pathophysiology of Parapneumonic Effusions and Empyema

Parapneumonic effusions are prototypical exudative effusions that occur as a result of altered microvascular permeability.[4] The natural history of a parapneumonic effusion evolves over three stages: exudative, fibrinopurulent, and organizing. The exudative stage begins shortly after the onset of the pneumonic process. Neutrophils bind to cell wall components on bacteria in the distal alveoli and secrete interleukin-1(IL-1), IL-6, IL-8, tissue necrosis factor α (TNF-α), and platelet activating factor (PAF).[5] IL-8 and PAF recruit neutrophils, which secrete additional cytokines that recruit more neutrophils and increase vascular permeability of both pulmonary and adjacent parietal pleural microvessels. A neutrophil-predominant, protein-rich fluid with an elevated lactate dehydrogenase (LDH) is formed in the pleural space.[6] Prompt and appropriate antibiotic therapy in this stage controls the inflammatory process, obviating the need for pleural space drainage with or without fibrinolytics.

The fibrinopurulent stage is characterized by continued exudation of plasma proteins, including coagulation factors, as well as dysregulation of fibrinolysis, resulting in altered fibrin turnover, septation, and loculation within the pleural space. During the development of a parapneumonic effusion, the mesothelial cell is stimulated by TNF-α, IL-1, lipopolysaccharide, and interferon γ (INF-γ).[7] In parapneumonic effusion and empyema, levels of plasminogen activator inhibitors 1 and 2 (PAI-1 and PAI-2) are significantly elevated,[8-10] inhibiting fibrinolysis and promoting fibrin formation.[10,11] Fibrin strands form, causing loculation. Extensive loculation can lead to lung entrapment.[12] Because the central pathology appears to be disordered fibrin turnover, it has been postulated that intrapleural fibrinolytics would be effective in the drainage of pleural fluid in the early fibrinopurulent stage, preventing progression to an empyema. The conflicting data regarding the effectiveness of intrapleural fibrinolytics may reflect the presence of collagen formation along this fibrin skeleton and crosslinking of fibrin strands rendering fibrinolytics ineffective during the late fibrinoproliferative and organizing phase.

The third stage of a parapneumonic effusion is the organizing stage, which results in an empyema. Progression to this stage typically occurs over 2 to 4 weeks in the absence of adequate treatment. The empyema fluid (pus) becomes viscous because of fibrin, cellular debris, and coagulation proteins which often contain viable bacteria.[13] Fibroblasts enter the pleural space and promote collagen deposition on the fibrin neomatrix and along the pleural surface. The result is an inelastic visceral pleural peel that limits lung expansion. Due to collagen deposition and the maturity of the visceral pleural peel, a fibrinolytic agent would not be expected to be useful in a mature empyema.

53.2. Management of Complicated Parapneumonic Effusions

Most CPEs require pleural space drainage, in addition to antibiotic therapy. Success rates of image-guided, small-bore catheters and standard chest tubes for CPEs are similar.[14,15] Ultrasonographic and computed tomography (CT)[16]-directed, small-bore chest tubes can be placed

into small loculations that may be difficult to reach with blind insertion, such as apical loculations, loculations abutting the mediastinum, and loculations with underlying lung consolidation. Each loculus should be drained, if possible. Small-bore chest tubes should be flushed regularly via a three-way valve[17]; intrapleural fibrinolytics can easily be administered through a side port of most small-bore chest tubes.

53.2.1. Management of Empyema

For the patient with empyema, initial therapy should include drainage of the pleural space and intravenous antibiotics. The optimal mode of drainage is controversial. Although success with small-gauge, image-guided pigtail catheters is reported,[14] a large-bore (28F–32F) chest tube is the preferred initial drainage modality of non-loculated empyema.[18] However, in pooled data from 21 case series reporting treatment of CPE and empyema, patients treated with tube thoracostomy as the primary intervention required a second intervention 40% of the time.[19] Wait and colleagues[20] found that early treatment of loculated empyema with video-assisted thoracoscopic surgery (VATS) resulted in a significantly decreased hospital stay compared to streptokinase in a small series of patients; however, the methodology was biased toward the VATS arm. A Cochrane review of all trials comparing medical and surgical therapy for empyema excluded most series for methodological reasons[21-23] and, therefore, could not reach definitive conclusions.[24] The most important aspect of management of empyema is the prompt initiation of effective drainage of the pleural space. Delays in completing drainage, regardless of the initial approach selected, contribute to increased morbidity.[25]

53.2.2. Evaluation of Chest-tube Drainage

When tube thoracostomy is the initial management choice for CPE and empyema, chest-tube output should be monitored accurately. When drainage approaches 50cc/day or the patient's symptoms have not improved, a posterior-anterior (PA) and lateral chest radiograph or CT scan should be performed to assess adequacy of drainage and tube position. If there is residual fluid, the tube should be flushed with sterile saline to ensure patency.[17] If kinked, it can be withdrawn slightly to relieve the obstruction. There are commercial dressings available that secure a small-bore chest tube to the chest wall without kinking. Computed tomography is able to demonstrate whether the chest tube is correctly positioned in the fluid collection and whether there are additional loculations that are not in communication with the tube. In some instances, however, tube thoracostomy alone is inadequate.

The options available to manage inadequate drainage include additional chest tubes, intrapleural fibrinolytics, VATS, limited thoracotomy, standard thoracotomy with decortication, and open surgical drainage. The choice of an additional drainage modality depends upon the presence of ongoing pleural sepsis, maturity of the empyema, degree of restriction of lung function from a mature pleural peel, familiarity with the treatment modalities, and debility of the patient.

53.2.3. Intrapleural Fibrinolytics

Intrapleural fibrinolytics have been used when there is occlusion of the chest tube with thick, viscous material or when there are multiple pleural loculations that fail to drain.[13] The three primary fibrinolytics that have been used are streptokinase, urokinase, and tissue plasminogen activator (tPA). Streptokinase is dosed by adding 250,000 units to 20 to 100mL of normal saline. If urokinase is chosen, 100,000 units are used; however, it is not currently available in the United States.[26] In children, 4mg tPA in 50mL saline has been used.[27] The fibrinolytic is instilled into the pleural space, and the chest tube is clamped for 2 to 4h.[28,29] The chest tube is then unclamped and returned to suction. Daily or up to three times per day instillations have been employed. We favor three instillations daily so we can assess a patient's response relatively rapidly and avoid an unnecessarily delay of surgery if there is an inadequate response to the fibrinolytic. Mechanistically, administration of intrapleural fibrinolytics would appear to be an effective approach in disrupting pleural loculations if given when fibrin stranding predominates prior to fibrin strand crosslinking and collagen deposition.

The literature regarding the effectiveness of intrapleural fibrinolytics is conflicting. Many case series have suggested improvement in clinical and radiographic outcomes with intrapleural streptokinase or urokinase.[29-39] Small randomized, controlled trials report improvement in the volume of fluid drained,[26,28,40-42] radiographic appearance of the pleural space,[26,28,38] decreased hospital stay,[26,41] and decreased need for surgery[26,40,41] in patients receiving intrapleural fibrinolytics (streptokinase or urokinase). The patients in these studies were heterogenous. In some studies, only patients with empyema were studied; in others, a mixed population of empyemas and CPE were represented. A summary of the case series and randomized studies involving intrapleural fibrinolytics is shown in Tables 53.1 and 2.

While there have been numerous studies documenting apparent efficacy of intrapleural fibrinolytics, the majority of the reports are small retrospective case series. A Cochrane review of three randomized, controlled trials of good methodological quality[26,28,41] found that intrapleural fibrinolytics appeared to decrease hospital stay, need for surgery, and time to defervesence, and showed improvement in the chest radiograph. However, these findings were not uniform and the number of patients was small. Therefore, the Cochrane review did not recommend use of intrapleural fibrinolytics for the management of CPE and empyema.[43]

A double-blind, randomized clinical trial in the United Kingdom of 454 patients (MIST-1) examined the utility of intrapleural streptokinase in patients with empyema (pus) or CPE (pH of <7.20 or positive gram stain with signs of infection, such as fever, elevated white-cell count, or elevated C-reactive protein). Results in 427 patients enrolled did not show a difference in mortality rates, need for surgery, or hospital stay.[3] However, 83% of the patients had empyema, corresponding to the organizational stage of a parapneumonic effusion. The median time from initial symptoms of pneumonia to randomization of 14 days reflects an advanced pathophysiological stage of the parapneumonic effusion. Therefore, it would not be anticipated that these patients would have a positive response from intrapleural fibrinolytic therapy. We believe that the results from the MIST-1 trial should not be applied to all

TABLE 53.1. Studies with at least 10 patients involving fibrinolytics in adults.

Reference	Level of evidence	Design	Agent	N (type)	Comments
Bergh (1977)[30]	4	Retrospective case series	Streptokinase 250,000 U/day	12 empyemas	83% increased drainage or CXR improvement
Henke (1992)[31]	4	Retrospective case series	Streptokinase 250,000 U/day	12 CPE	67% increased drainage or CXR improvement
Taylor (1994)[32]	4	Retrospective case series	Streptokinase 250,000 U/day	11 empyemas	73% increased drainage or clinical, CXR, US improvement
Laisaar (1996)[33]	4	Retrospective case series	Streptokinase 250,000 U/day	1 CPE 21 empyemas	68% increased drainage clinical or CXR improvement
Roupie (1996)[34]	4	Retrospective case series	Streptokinase 250,000 U/day	16 empyemas	88% increased drainage or CT imiprovement
Moulton (1989)[35]	4	Retrospective case series	Urokinase 80–150,000 U several times/day	11 empyemas	91% clinical improvement
Park (1996)[36]	4	Retrospective case series	Urokinase 80,000 U t.i.d.	10 empyemas	60% improved lung expansion on CXR
Bouros (1994)[37]	4	Prospective case series	Streptokinase 250,000 U/day	15 CPE 5 empyemas	95% clinical or CXR improvement
Jerjes-Sanches (1996)[38]	4	Prospective multicenter series	Streptokinase 250,000 U/day	30 empyemas	93% increased drainage, CXR or pft improvement
Bouros (1996)[39]	4	Prospective case series	Urokinase 50,000 U/day	13 CPE 7 empyemas	95% increased drainage or improved CXR or US
Lim (1999)[21]	3b	Prospective sequential cohort	Streptokinase 250,000 U/day vs. SK + surgery vs. no treatment	19 CPE 63 empyemas	Decreased mortality 3% vs. 24% with SK + surgery vs. nothing; trend toward mortality benefit in SK vs. nothing but not significant
Chin (1997)[29]	2b	Case control	Chest tube alone or streptokinase 250,000 U/day	12 CPE 40 empyemas	Increased drainage but no improvement in fever, need for surgery, hospital stay, or mortality
Davies (1997)[28]	2b	Randomized, controlled trial	Streptokinase 250,000 U/day vs. NS	11 CPE 13 empyemas	Increased drainage and CXR improvement in streptokinase group
Wait (1997)[20]	1b	Randomized series	Streptokinase 250,000 U/day vs. VATS	20 CPE or empyemas	VATS decrease hospital days and increase success of drainage
Bouros (1999)[26]	1b	Randomized, controlled trial	Urokinase 100,000 U/day × 3 days vs. NS	21 CPE 10 empyemas	Urokinase decrease hospital days, increase success 87% vs. 25%, decrease VATS need 14% vs. 38%
Tuncozgur (2001)[41]	1b	Randomized, controlled trial	Urokinase 100,000 U/day × 5 days vs. placebo	49 CPE or empyemas	Urokinase decrease hospital stay 14 vs. 21 days and need for surgery 29% vs. 60%
Diacon (2004)[40]	1b	Randomized, controlled trial	Streptokinase 250,000 U/day vs. NS	7 CPE 37 empyemas	Streptokinase increase success and decrease need for surgery 14% vs. 32%; all patients got rinse of NS or SK
Bouros (1997)[42]	1b	Randomized, double-blind trial	Streptokinase 250,000 U/day vs. urokinase 100,000 U/day	39 CPE 11 empyemas	Both improve drainage, no difference in amount of drainage or need for surgery
Maskell (2005)[3]	1b	Randomized, double-blind trial	Streptokinase 250,000 U bid × 3 days vs. placebo	355 empyemas 75 CPE	No difference in need for surgery, mortality, hospital stay, residual pleural thickening; study population skewed with high percentage mature empyema
Cameron (2004)[43] (Cochrane review)	1a	High-quality meta-analysis	Evaluated the RCTs available at time	144 patients with CPE or empyema	Fibrinolytics appear to decrease need for surgery and length of stay; unable to give firm recommendations due to low number of patients

Abbreviations: CPE, complicated parapneumonic effusion; CXR, chest radiograph; NS, normal saline; pft, author, please supply definition; RCT, randomized, controlled trial; tPA, tissue plasminogen activator; US, ultrasound.

TABLE 53.2. Studies with at least 10 patients involving fibrinolytics in children.

Reference	Level of evidence	Design	Agent	N (type)	Comments
Hawkins (2004)[60]	4	Retrospective case series	tPA	58 empyemas in children	93% successful without need for additional treatment
Weinstein (2004)[27]	3a	Retrospective cohort	Early, late, or no tPA 4 mg	8 empyemas 45 CPE; all in children	Decreased chest-tube time in patients with early tPA, no operations required; sequential no tPA, then after 1999 all early or late tPA
Yao (2004)[57]	3a	Prospective & retrospective cohort	Streptokinase 12,000 U/kg/day	19 CPE 23 empyemas in children	Streptokinase increase drainage, decrease fever days 5.3 vs. 7.9 days, decrease surgery 10% vs. 41%
Singh (2004)[59]	1b	Randomized, controlled trial	Streptokinase 15,000 U/kg/day × 3 days vs. NS	40 empyemas in children	No difference in clinical or sonographic outcome
Thomson (2002)[56]	1b	Randomized, multicenter, double-blind, controlled trial	Urokinase 40,000 U bid × 3 days vs. placebo	60 CPE or empyemas in children	Urokinase decrease hospital stay 7.2 vs. 9.4 days; only 5 VATS needed 3 in placebo 2 in urokinase

Abbreviations: CPE, complicated parapneumonic effusion; CXR, chest radiograph; NS, normal saline; tPA, tissue plasminogen activator; US, ultrasound.

patients with CPEs because the group that potentially would be responsive (those in the early fibrinopurulent stage) was under-represented in this trial. The message from MIST-1 is that there is no role for intrapleural fibrinolytics in the late fibrinopurulent or organizational stage of a parapneumonic effusion. The value of intrapleural fibrinolytics can only be judged when given earlier in the pathophysiological process. Further studies assessing the efficacy of intrapleural fibrinolytics must recognize that parapneumonic effusion and empyema represent a heterogeneous spectrum of disorders. Trials should not enroll patients with mature empyema as these patients bias the results toward a negative treatment effect.

The use of intrapleural fibrinolytics is not without adverse effects. There are case reports of localized pleural and systemic bleeding[44,45] and acute respiratory distress syndrome after intrapleural instillation of streptokinase and urokinase.[46] Streptokinase is a bacterial protein and, therefore, can induce neutralizing antibodies. These antibodies could theoretically interfere with its efficacy and cause an anaphylactic reaction if streptokinase is given in subsequent hospitalizations. Patients who have received streptokinase should receive a card indicating their exposure and should receive urokinase or tPA for future thrombolysis.

Other agents may be better suited to disrupt pleural loculations. Single-chain urokinase appears to work only on plasminogen that is bound to fibrin strands[47]; and therefore, it is not active against free-floating plasminogen within the pleural space. This selective binding may offer two distinct benefits. First, by being active only on bound plasminogen, it activates plasminogen that can cleave fibrin strands, causing loculations instead of being utilized on free-floating fibrinogen. Second, binding to plasminogen on fibrin strands may shield it from plasminogen activator inhibition and prolong its effects.[47,48] Further study is needed to clarify the apparent advantage of single-chain urokinase compared to streptokinase and other urokinase preparations. Tissue plasminogen activator may be more effective in disrupting loculations than urokinase or streptokinase preparations, as it does not require binding to plasminogen to be active. Retrospective cohorts of children with empyema and CPE suggest that tPA may increase drainage without significant bleeding risk.[27,49] However, there is a paucity of literature in adults reporting its use.[50] Given its increased cost, widespread use of tPA for CPE and empyema cannot currently be advocated. There may be a role for fibrinolytics in combination with deoxyribonuclease (DNase) or collagenases. The initial use of intrapleural streptokinase was from bacterial cultures that contained both streptokinase as well as streptococcal DNase.[51] In comparison to streptokinase alone, the addition of DNase caused marked reduction in the viscosity of the pus in vitro[52] and has been successfully used in humans.[53] Mechanistically, these two agents used together would lyse fibrin strands and decrease viscosity of the pus, promoting better drainage. However, before widespread use of these combinations can be advocated, randomized studies or large, well-designed cohort trials would be required.

In the absence of high-grade evidence from adequately performed trials, we limit the use of fibrinolytic therapy to patients with late exudative or early fibrinopurulent parapneumonic effusions who do not drain rapidly and completely following chest-tube insertion. Parapneumonic effusions in these early stages are more likely to be amenable to fibrinolytic therapy compared with effusions in the organized stage (empyema). Once we have verified that the chest tube remains within a loculation by CT scan, we dose streptokinase three times per day, clamping the tube for 2h. If we do not achieve radiographic improvement with three doses, we either insert an additional chest tube under ultrasound or CT guidance or consider surgical drainage. If an additional chest tube(s) does not result in adequate drainage, surgery should be performed without delay if there are no absolute contraindications.

52.2.4. Conclusion

Based on the evidence available, the authors recommend that intrapleural fibrinolytics should not be used for mature empyema (level of evidence 1a to 1b; recommendation grade A), may be considered for early fibrinopurulent complicated parapneumonic effusion (level of evidence 1b to 2b; recommendation grade B), but their use should not delay surgical intervention where appropriate.

> Intrapleural fibrinolytics should not be used for management of mature empyema (level of evidence 1a to 1b; recommendation grade A).
>
> Intrapleural fibrinolytics may be considered for management of early fibrinopurulent complicated parapneumonic effusion (level of evidence 1b to 2b; recommendation grade B), but their use should not delay surgical intervention where appropriate.

52.2.5. Empyema in Children

Management of empyema in children is similar to adults with some notable exceptions. First, the epidemiology of empyema differs in children and adults. Most children with empyema are healthy. They have less altered mental status, airway protection issues, and aspiration, and are, in general, not at risk for anaerobic pathogens. The majority of children present with cough, dyspnea, respiratory distress, and fever; poor feeding is a rare presentation.[54] In the western world, children virtually never die from empyema; the difference in mortality between adults and children with empyema is related to the comorbidities in adults. It is unclear whether immediate drainage is necessary in pediatric patients who have complicated (by pleural fluid analysis, ultrasound, or CT scan appearance) parapneumonic effusions. Pediatric patients with exudative parapneumonic effusions have been treated successfully with antibiotics alone[54] or with serial thoracentesis as opposed to chest-tube drainage.[55] Small-bore chest tubes appear effective in draining pediatric empyema and resulted in a significant decrease in hospital stay in one study.[56] Intrapleural fibrinolytics, including tPA,[27,49] appear to decrease febrile days, the need for surgical intervention,[57] and hospital stay.[56] Fibrinolytics also appear to be safe in children.[58] As death is rare in pediatric empyema in the western world, assessment of this end point is problematic (Table 53.2).

53.2.6. Conclusion

Based on the paucity of studies and conflicting conclusions of the two randomized, controlled trials,[56,59] there is insufficient evidence to provide a recommendation on the use of fibrinolytics in children; however, the use of intrapleural fibrinolytics appears to be safe.

> There is insufficient evidence to provide a recommendation on the use of fibrinolytics for management of empyema in children.

References

1. Bernstein JM. Treatment of community-acquired pneumonia – IDSA guidelines. Infectious Diseases Society of America. *Chest* 1999;115:9S–13S.

2. Strange C, Sahn SA. The definitions and epidemiology of pleural space infection. *Semin Respir Infect* 1999;14:3–8.

3. Maskell NA, Davies CW, Nunn AJ, et al. U.K. controlled trial of intrapleural streptokinase for pleural infection. *N Engl J Med* 2005;352:865–874.

4. Sahn SA. The pathophysiology of pleural effusions. *Annu Rev Med* 1990;41:7–13.

5. Kroegel C, Antony VB. Immunobiology of pleural inflammation: potential implications for pathogenesis, diagnosis and therapy. *Eur Respir J* 1997; 10:2411–2418.

6. Light RW, Girard WM, Jenkinson SG, et al. Parapneumonic effusions. *Am J Med* 1980;69: 507–512.

7. Antony VB, Hott JW, Kunkel SL, et al. Pleural mesothelial cell expression of C-C (monocyte chemotactic peptide) and C-X-C (interleukin 8) chemokines. *Am J Respir Cell Mol Biol* 1995;12: 581–588.

8. Philip-Joet F, Alessi MC, Philip-Joet C, et al. Fibrinolytic and inflammatory processes in pleural effusions. *Eur Respir J* 1995;8:1352–1356.

9. Idell S, Girard W, Koenig KB, et al. Abnormalities of pathways of fibrin turnover in the human pleural space. *Am Rev Respir Dis* 1991;144: 187–194.

10. Idell S, Zwieb C, Boggaram J, et al. Mechanisms of fibrin formation and lysis by human lung fibroblasts: influence of TGF-beta and TNF-alpha. *Am J Physiol* 1992;263:L487–L494.

11. Idell S, Zwieb C, Kumar A, et al. Pathways of fibrin turnover of human pleural mesothelial cells in vitro. *Am J Respir Cell Mol Biol* 1992;7:414–426.

12. Strange C, Tomlinson JR, Wilson C, et al. The histology of experimental pleural injury with tetracycline, empyema, and carrageenan. *Exp Mol Pathol* 1989;51:205–219.

13. Sahn SA. Management of complicated parapneumonic effusions. *Am Rev Respir Dis* 1993;148: 813–817.

14. Silverman SG, Mueller PR, Saini S, et al. Thoracic empyema: management with image-guided catheter drainage. *Radiology* 1988;169:5–9.

15. vanSonnenberg E, Nakamoto SK, Mueller PR, et al. CT- and ultrasound-guided catheter drainage of empyemas after chest-tube failure. *Radiology* 1984;151:349–353.

16. Klein JS, Schultz S, Heffner JE. Interventional radiology of the chest: image-guided percutaneous drainage of pleural effusions, lung abscess, and pneumothorax. *AJR Am J Roentgenol* 1995;164: 581–588.

17. Davies CW, Gleeson FV, Davies RJ. BTS guidelines for the management of pleural infection. *Thorax* 2003;58(suppl 2):ii18–ii28.

18. Light R. Parapneumonic effusions and empyema: current management strategies. *J Crit Illness* 1995;10:832–839.

19. Colice GL, Curtis A, Deslauriers J, et al. Medical and surgical treatment of parapneumonic effusions: an evidence-based guideline. *Chest* 2000;118: 1158–1171.

20. Wait MA, Sharma S, Hohn J, et al. A randomized trial of empyema therapy. *Chest* 1997;111:1548–1551.

21. Lim TK, Chin NK. Empirical treatment with fibrinolysis and early surgery reduces the duration of hospitalization in pleural sepsis. *Eur Respir J* 1999;13:514–518.

22. Sasse S, Nguyen TK, Mulligan M, et al. The effects of early chest tube placement on empyema resolution. *Chest* 1997;111:1679–1683.

23. Lee SH LS, Lee SY, Park SM, et al. A comparative study of three therapeutic modalities in loculated tuberculous pleural effusions. *Tuberculosis Respir Dis* 1996;43:683–692.

24. Coote N. Surgical versus non-surgical management of pleural empyema. *Cochrane Database Syst Rev* 2002:CD001956.

25. Ashbaugh DG. Empyema thoracis. Factors influencing morbidity and mortality. *Chest* 1991;99:1162–1165.

26. Bouros D, Schiza S, Tzanakis N, et al. Intrapleural urokinase versus normal saline in the treatment of complicated parapneumonic effusions and empyema. A randomized, double-blind study. *Am J Respir Crit Care Med* 1999;159:37–42.

27. Weinstein M, Restrepo R, Chait PG, et al. Effectiveness and safety of tissue plasminogen activator in the management of complicated parapneumonic effusions. *Pediatrics* 2004;113: e182–e185.

28. Davies RJ, Traill ZC, Gleeson FV. Randomised controlled trial of intrapleural streptokinase in community acquired pleural infection. *Thorax* 1997;52:416–421.

29. Chin NK, Lim TK. Controlled trial of intrapleural streptokinase in the treatment of pleural empyema and complicated parapneumonic effusions. *Chest* 1997;111:275–279.

30. Bergh NP, Ekroth R, Larsson S, et al. Intrapleural streptokinase in the treatment of haemothorax and empyema. *Scand J Thorac Cardiovasc Surg* 1977;11:265–268.

31. Henke CA, Leatherman JW. Intrapleurally administered streptokinase in the treatment of acute

loculated nonpurulent parapneumonic effusions. *Am Rev Respir Dis* 1992;145:680–684.

32. Taylor RF, Rubens MB, Pearson MC, et al. Intrapleural streptokinase in the management of empyema. *Thorax* 1994;49:856–859.

33. Laisaar T, Puttsepp E, Laisaar V. Early administration of intrapleural streptokinase in the treatment of multiloculated pleural effusions and pleural empyemas. *Thorac Cardiovasc Surg* 1996; 44:252–256.

34. Roupie E, Bouabdallah K, Delclaux C, et al. Intrapleural administration of streptokinase in complicated purulent pleural effusion: a CT-guided strategy. *Intensive Care Med* 1996;22: 1351–1353.

35. Moulton JS, Moore PT, Mencini RA. Treatment of loculated pleural effusions with transcatheter intracavitary urokinase. *AJR Am J Roentgenol* 1989;153:941–945.

36. Park CS, Chung WM, Lim MK, et al. Transcatheter instillation of urokinase into loculated pleural effusion: analysis of treatment effect. *AJR Am J Roentgenol* 1996;167:649–652.

37. Bouros D, Schiza S, Panagou P, et al. Role of streptokinase in the treatment of acute loculated parapneumonic pleural effusions and empyema. *Thorax* 1994;49:852–855.

38. Jerjes-Sanchez C, Ramirez-Rivera A, Elizalde JJ, et al. Intrapleural fibrinolysis with streptokinase as an adjunctive treatment in hemothorax and empyema: a multicenter trial. *Chest* 1996;109:1514–1519.

39. Bouros D, Schiza S, Tzanakis N, et al. Intrapleural urokinase in the treatment of complicated parapneumonic pleural effusions and empyema. *Eur Respir J* 1996;9:1656–1659.

40. Diacon AH, Theron J, Schuurmans MM, et al. Intrapleural streptokinase for empyema and complicated parapneumonic effusions. *Am J Respir Crit Care Med* 2004;170:49–53.

41. Tuncozgur B, Ustunsoy H, Sivrikoz MC, et al. Intrapleural urokinase in the management of parapneumonic empyema: a randomised controlled trial. *Int J Clin Pract* 2001;55:658–660.

42. Bouros D, Schiza S, Patsourakis G, et al. Intrapleural streptokinase versus urokinase in the treatment of complicated parapneumonic effusions: a prospective, double-blind study. *Am J Respir Crit Care Med* 1997;155:291–295.

43. Cameron R, Davies HR. Intra-pleural fibrinolytic therapy versus conservative management in the treatment of parapneumonic effusions and empyema. *Cochrane Database Syst Rev* 2004: CD002312.

44. Porter J, Banning AP. Intrapleural streptokinase. *Thorax* 1998;53:720.

45. Temes RT, Follis F, Kessler RM, et al. Intrapleural fibrinolytics in management of empyema thoracis. *Chest* 1996;110:102–106.

46. Frye MD, Jarratt M, Sahn SA. Acute hypoxemic respiratory failure following intrapleural thrombolytic therapy for hemothorax. *Chest* 1994;105: 1595–1596.

47. Idell S, Mazar A, Cines D, et al. Single-chain urokinase alone or complexed to its receptor in tetracycline-induced pleuritis in rabbits. *Am J Respir Crit Care Med* 2002;166:920–926.

48. Antony VB. Fibrinolysis in the pleural space: breaking the bonds that bind. *Am J Respir Crit Care Med* 2002;166:909–910.

49. Ray TL, Berkenbosch JW, Russo P, et al. Tissue plasminogen activator as an adjuvant therapy for pleural empyema in pediatric patients. *J Intensive Care Med* 2004;19:44–50.

50. Walker CA, Shirk MB, Tschampel MM, et al. Intrapleural alteplase in a patient with complicated pleural effusion. *Ann Pharmacother* 2003;37:376–379.

51. Tillett W, Sherry S. The effect in patients of streptococcal fibrinolysin (streptokinsae) and streptococcal deoxyribonuclease on fibrinous, purulent, and sanguinous pleural exudations. *J Clin Invest* 1949;28:173–190.

52. Simpson G, Roomes D, Heron M. Effects of streptokinase and deoxyribonuclease on viscosity of human surgical and empyema pus. *Chest* 2000;117:1728–1733.

53. Simpson G, Roomes D, Reeves B. Successful treatment of empyema thoracis with human recombinant deoxyribonuclease. *Thorax* 2003;58:365–366.

54. Chan W, Keyser-Gauvin E, Davis GM, et al. Empyema thoracis in children: a 26-year review of the Montreal Children's Hospital experience. *J Pediatr Surg* 1997;32:870–872.

55. Shoseyov D, Bibi H, Shatzberg G, et al. Short-term course and outcome of treatments of pleural empyema in pediatric patients: repeated ultrasound-guided needle thoracocentesis vs chest tube drainage. *Chest* 2002;121:836–840.

56. Thomson AH, Hull J, Kumar MR, et al. Randomised trial of intrapleural urokinase in the treatment of childhood empyema. *Thorax* 2002; 57:343–347.

57. Yao CT, Wu JM, Liu CC, et al. Treatment of complicated parapneumonic pleural effusion with intrapleural streptokinase in children. *Chest* 2004; 125:566–571.

58. Kilic N, Celebi S, Gurpinar A, et al. Management of thoracic empyema in children. *Pediatr Surg Int* 2002;18:21–23.

59. Singh M, Mathew JL, Chandra S, et al. Randomized controlled trial of intrapleural streptokinase in empyema thoracis in children. *Acta Paediatr* 2004;93:1443–1445.

60. Hawkins JA, Scaife ES, Hillman ND, et al. Current treatment of pediatric empyema. *Semin Thorac Cardiovasc Surg* 2004;16:196–200.

54
Diffuse Malignant Pleural Mesothelioma: The Role of Pleurectomy

Jasleen Kukreja and David M. Jablons

Diffuse malignant pleural mesothelioma (MPM) is an aggressive tumor with dismal prognosis that has largely been associated with exposure to asbestos. As a disease of industrialized nations predominantly, it is expected to have its peak incidence around year 2020. In the United States alone, 2500 to 3000 new cases of MPM are diagnosed annually and its incidence is increasing.[1-4] Based on a 20- to 50-year latency period between exposure and disease manifestation, there might still be another surge in incidence in the mid 21st century associated with asbestos exposure from the unfortunate events of September 11, 2001, at the World Trade Center in New York City. Despite important advances in our understanding of this disease, long-term survivors are rare due to delay in diagnosis and rapid disease progression. Malignant pleural mesothelioma poses a significant healthcare problem not only for patients and their caregivers, but also for industry and government in terms of the enormous cost of compensation.

Median survival for untreated patients is reported to be between 4 to 18 months from the time of diagnosis. Unlike other thoracic malignancies, patients usually succumb to locoregional disease with invasion of vital structures such as lungs, heart, great vessels, and esophagus, rather than metastases. Hence, early diagnosis is critical in the treatment of MPM.[5,6] With the advent of aggressive local control such as extrapleural penumonectomy and radical pleurectomy/decortication with systemic multimodality therapies, patients are living longer but presenting with more systemic failures and metastases.

Brain metastases, for example, while once exceedingly rare in MPM, are now seen commonly.

Computed tomography (CT) is the primary modality of choice for evaluating MPM. Computed tomography findings can be used to preclude surgery in patients with obviously unresectable tumors (e.g., diffuse extension of tumor into the chest wall, mediastinum, vital organs, peritoneum, or distant metastasis).[7] Magnetic resonance imaging (MRI) has been recommended occasionally as an adjunct to more accurately define invasion of the diaphragm and endothoracic fascia.[7-9] Recently, flourodeoxyglucose–positron emission tomography (PET-FDG) has emerged as a new imaging modality in the evaluation of MPM with reportedly a better sensitivity, specificity, and accuracy (97%, 80%, and 94%, respectively) for detecting all histological types of MPM lesions when compared with CT (83%, 80%, and 82%, respectively).[10] Positron emission tomography may also help ascertain the biological aggressiveness of the tumor and hence determine the prognosis in patients with MPM. In a recent study, those with higher FDG uptake had a significantly shorter survival time.[11] Based on these criteria, a decision can be made whether to pursue an aggressive approach or not. More recently, fusion PET-CT scanning has replaced PET scans for a better correlation of anatomical detail with metabolic activity. Currently, however, FDG-PET based scanning is not widely used for MPM staging in the United States.

Despite the imaging modalities mentioned above, some patients still require surgical staging/confirmation of N2 status. Video-assisted thoracoscopic surgery (VATS) has become the current gold standard for establishing a histological diagnosis,[12] as well as for staging patients. In addition to stage, age, performance status, and epithelial histology have a significant impact on survival in MPM.[13] The presence of chest pain, weight loss, high platelet counts (>400K), low hemoglobin, high white-blood-cell count, and high lactate dehydrogenase (>500 IU/L) impact negatively on patient survival.[14] No clear consensus exists as to a specific biomarker or set of biomarkers that are either prognostic or can clearly direct therapy. Yet progress in understanding the molecular pathogenesis of MPM does hold promise for being able to identify in the future a specific set of genes and/or biomarkers that can predict biological aggressiveness, the chance of metastasis, and the likelihood that aggressive combined modality interventions will confer a long-term survival advantage. The science, however, is not here yet.

54.1. Therapy

There is no universally accepted standard therapy for MPM. Treatment options include chemotherapy, radiation therapy, surgery, or some combination of these modalities. Single-modality therapy has had limited success in the treatment of this disease. The median survival for patients receiving supportive care alone has been reported to be as low as 6 months.[15,16] As in most orphan and understudied diseases, however, the interpretation of any data is fraught with significant bias and hampered by underpowered, nonrandomized, nonprospective studies. In addition, because of the nonstandardized staging system for MPM, many observations cannot be extrapolated across institutions or countries. Given that most data (with a few exceptions noted below) are from retrospective, small single-institution trials that spanned years if not decades to accrue patients with evolving staging techniques and modalities, it is difficult to draw firm conclusions regarding best treatment option(s).

54.1.1. Single-Modality Therapy

54.1.1.1. Chemotherapy

Up until recently, the median survival time of patients treated with chemotherapy alone, either as single agent or some combination, was no better than 7 months.[14] However, newer agents, in particular gemcitabine and pemetrexed in combination with platinum analogs, have recently been shown to improve response rates and quality of life. In a phase II study, Byrne and colleagues achieved a partial response rate of 47% in patients with advanced-stage pleural mesothelioma treated with combination of cisplatin and gemcitabine.[17]

Pemetrexed, a novel multitargeted anti-folate that inhibits DNA synthesis, in combination with platinum analogs in two phase I studies, achieved a partial response (PR) rates of 32% and 45%, respectively.[18–20] Based on the encouraging results of the aforementioned trials, Vogelzang and coworkers[21] conducted a phase III trial to determine whether combination pemetrexed/cisplatin conferred a survival advantage in patients with MPM compared with cisplatin alone.

In this multicenter, international, randomized study, 456 patients with unresectable MPM were randomized to receive either a combination of pemetrexed and cisplatin or cisplatin alone. Combination pemetrexed/cisplatin significantly improved time to relapse (5.7 months vs. 3.9 months; $p = 0.001$) and, most importantly, survival (12.1 months vs. 9.3 months; $p = 0.02$). The 2.8-month survival benefit in the combination chemotherapy group translated into an improved hazard ratio of 0.77 or, conversely, a meaningful relative risk of death reduction of 23%. Therefore, combination pemetrexed/cisplatin is now routinely used for advanced-stage biopsy proven MPM (level of evidence 1a).

54.1.1.2. Radiation

The role of radiation as single-modality therapy is difficult to evaluate due to the fact that radiation has generally been used as part of either bimodality or multimodality therapy in conjunction with chemotherapy, surgery, or both. Effectiveness of radiation therapy alone is limited by the comparatively radio-resistant nature of the disease, the high doses, and/or the extensive target areas required. Radiation, however, has been used to palliate areas of symptomatic tumor invasion.[22] Radiotherapy has also been used effectively to prevent biopsy tract site malignant seeding. In a recent randomized study comparing those receiving daily sessions of local radiotherapy to the invasive/diagnostic entry site with those receiving no radiation, none of the patients treated with radiation developed entry tract metastasis as opposed to 40% of the untreated that did.[23] This study supports the use of early local radiotherapy in preventing malignant seeding at the biopsy site or chest-tube site (level of evidence 1b).

54.1.2. Surgery

Similar to chemotherapy and radiation, surgery as a single-modality therapy has not been overly successful in the treatment of MPM. Furthermore, only 20% to 30% of patients at the time of presentation are amenable to resection. Of those, 20% are unresectable at the time of operation. Because MPM is predominantly a loco-regional disease, surgical strategies have focused on loco-regional control. Current surgical therapy for patients with MPM includes radical surgery (extrapleural penumonectomy), debulking surgery (pleurectomy/decortication), and palliation (drainage effusion and pleurodesis). Surgery in MPM, like any operation for cancer, has the most benefit when an R0 or nearly R0 resection can be achieved. R0 status after resection has been shown by a few groups to confer a survival advantage compared to those that received lesser degree of resection. This philosophy has significant import in approaching patients with MPM for surgical treatment. While palliative decortications alone can make patients less dyspneic and offer better quality of life in the short term, no real evidence exists to suggest that it confers any survival advantage. Radical pleurectomy (visceral and parietal) with skeltonization of hilar and mediastinal pericardial and diaphragmatic pleura, however, can lead to a meaningful cytoreduction and chance of increased survival if R0 status can be achieved. The evidence of data, however, is limited.

Historically, extrapleural pneumonectomy (EPP) entailing en bloc resection of the pleura, lung, ipsilateral hemidiaphragm, and pericardium has been limited by high operative mortality (30%).[24] As a result, pleurectomy/decortication (P/D) that only removes all gross pleural disease

without removing the underlying lung, pericardium, or diaphragm has been preferred over EPP by some surgeons due to lower associated morbidity and mortality (1.5% to 5%).[25] However, the last couple of decades have seen improvements in the operative technique, anesthesia, perioperative care, and patient selection, resulting in a significant reduction in operative mortality rate to less than 4% for EPP in centers with significant experience.[26]

Despite the theoretical advantage, radical surgery, however, failed to confer a survival advantage over debulking surgery in a multicentered Lung Cancer Study Group (LCSG) prospective trial. Between 1985 and 1988, the LCSG enrolled patients with biopsy proven MPM. Of the 83 patients accrued, only 20 were eligible for EPP. The remaining patients either underwent P/D or were treated nonsurgically. The postoperative mortality was 15% in the EPP group. While the recurrence-free survival was significantly longer for those who underwent EPP, there was no difference in overall survival among these three groups (level of evidence 2b). Furthermore, the authors did acknowledge that the observed difference in recurrence-free survival among the three groups might not be entirely attributable to the surgical approach because it was not adjusted for other prognostic indicators.[27]

54.1.3. Multimodality Therapy

Due to disappointing results with single-modality therapy, the consensus among experienced groups is that surgery is best combined with adjuvant chemotherapy, radiation, or a combination of these. Of all treatment approaches attempted, EPP, in combination with chemoradiation, has been most consistently associated with long-term disease-free survival and has provided for the greatest amount of cytoreduction.

54.1.3.1. Evidence for Extrapleural Pneumonectomy and Adjuvant Therapy

The largest experience to date supporting EPP followed by adjuvant therapy came from Brigham and Women's Hospital and Dana Farber Cancer Institute (BWH/DFCI). In this retrospective review of 183 patients, Sugarbaker and colleagues reported an overall median survival of 19 months, with 2-year and 5-year survivals of 38% and 15%, respectively, with an impressive operative mortality of 3.8%. A highly selected subset of 31 patients (roughly 15% of the series) with epithelial type, negative surgical margins, and negative lymph nodes demonstrated an impressive median survival of 51 months, with 2- and 5-year survivals of 68% and 46%, respectively. Survival correlated significantly with the stage of the disease.[28]

Similarly, in a phase II single-institution (Memorial Sloan-Kettering Cancer Center; MSKCC) study of EPP (62 patients) versus P/D (5 patients) followed by hemithoracic radiation (54 Gy), the median survival in the EPP group was noted to be 17 months with an overall survival at 3 years of 27%.[29] In contrast to the 51 months median survival in early stage in Sugarbaker's study, early-stage disease (stage I and II) "good" prognosis patients in this study had a median survival of 33.8 months only. A number of factors could account for the observed differences, namely trimodality therapy in Sugarbaker and colleagues study as opposed to bimodality therapy in Rusch and colleagues study; different staging criteria; etc. Due to the extremely small patient numbers, the survival was not assessed in the P/D group.

While both studies seem to support the aggressive surgical approach entailing EPP followed by some form of adjuvant therapy in early-stage MPM (level of evidence 2b), the efficacy of EPP over P/D has not been studied in a controlled clinical trial setting, making it difficult to draw any firm conclusions. In support of the above, Maziak and associates, in their systematic review of the surgical management of MPM, found only one prospective study by Pass and colleagues showing a significant difference in survival between the EPP (9.4 months) and P/D (14.5 months) treatment arms ($p = 0.012$). But patients were generally preselected for a specific surgical treatment in this series.[30,31] None of the retrospective studies that included some form of adjuvant treatment reported a significant or consistent difference or advantage in median survival for EPP when compared to P/D. Unfortunately, interpretation of these trials is difficult, leaving the practitioner unsure as to which approach may offer the greatest benefit or least harm to the patient. Despite the relative lack of data and clarity some consensus and trends in patient management are emerging across centers of excellence for MPM treatment (discussed below).

54.1.3.2. Evidence for Pleurectomy/Decortication with Adjuvant Therapy

As most patients succumb to local tumor invasion rather than metastases, reducing the volume of tumor may be an important determinant of postoperative survival and can improve quality of life (QOL). Debulking surgery, whilst not curative, has the potential to obtain effective local control due to the protracted time before a significant amount of tumor re-accumulates to provoke symptoms. The choice of operation, EPP versus P/D, is dictated by several factors. The difference in the operative mortality between the two operations plays a major role in determining the suitability of one surgical approach over the other. The amount of disease and vital organs involvement further governs which operation is most suitable for a given patient. Patient factors such as inadequate cardiopulmonary reserve or comorbidities may preclude the more aggressive EPP approach. For this subgroup of patients, P/D offers a better therapeutic option. Yet, the real question as to whether P/D compared to nonoperative treatment prolongs survival has not been addressed in carefully controlled, prospective, randomized trials.

While retrospective studies have typically shown a survival advantage for patients undergoing surgery of any kind (P/D or EPP) versus nonoperated upon patients, these studies suffer from similar selection bias flaws in that the surgery arms of the studies all selected for better performance status low tumor burden patients, etc. As a debulking procedure, P/D inherently has a high local failure rate. Similar to the EPP experience, most institutions use combined modality therapy to reduce regional recurrences in P/D. The role of adjuvant chemotherapy, administered both locally and systemically, following P/D has also been investigated. The rationale for local intrapleural instillation of chemotherapy relies on the proclivity of MPM to remain localized even when advanced.

A significant amount of work has been performed by investigators at MSKCC in New York using intrapleural chemotherapy following P/D in the treatment of MPM. In a phase II trial of P/D, Rusch and colleagues reported their experience with 27 patients with biopsy-proven MPM who underwent P/D followed immediately in the postoperative period with intrapleural instillation of cisplatin and mitomycin via chest tubes and subsequently systemic administration of the two agents 3 to 5 weeks later. The median progression-free survival was 13.6 months with an overall survival at 2 years of 40% (with the median overall survival of 18.3 months). While the overall survival in this phase II trial was better than supportive care alone and comparable to other combined modality regimens, local relapse remained a major problem. Similar to the EPP experience, the investigators found that epithelial histology conferred significantly better survival than nonepithelial histology.[32] One can cautiously conclude from this trial (feasibility nonrandomized trial) that in a select cohort with epithelial histology and an R0 resection with P/D, that P/D offers a viable option in an adjuvant setting (level of evidence 2b). However, once again, trials such as these emphasize the need for multi-institutional and multidisciplinary approach to this rare disease entity in a phase III setting.

Memorial Sloan-Kettering Cancer Center investigators in their continual effort to better understand this disease to improve outcome reported their largest experience to date with P/D followed by radiation. In this retrospective review, 123 patients between 1974 and 2003 underwent P/D. Postoperatively, the entire hemithorax was irradiated externally to a median dose of 42.5Gy with a mixed photon electron beam technique to reduce damage to the underlying lung. Fifty-four patients also received intraoperative brachytherapy to any residual gross disease following P/D. In this series, the median survival and 2-year overall survival were 13.5 months and 23%, respectively. Nonepithelial histology, left-sided disease, radiation dose less than 40Gy, and the use of implants were all noted to be negative predictors of overall survival in multivariate analysis. Despite this intensive treatment, 67% had local relapse. While this low-dose mixed photon–electron beam likely spared the underlying lung, it failed to produce long-term survivors or effective local control. The authors,

therefore, concluded that adjuvant radiation is not an effective treatment option for eradicating residual disease following P/D and that a more aggressive, that is, greater cytoreductive surgical approach was necessary[33] (level of evidence 2b). Several other authors have reported a median survival ranging from 10 to 18 months with P/D followed by radiation again in small series with inherent biases.

We at University of California, San Francisco, have similarly performed a retrospective review of radical pleurectomy/decortication and intraoperative radiotherapy (IORT) followed by external beam radiation therapy with or without chemotherapy for diffuse malignant pleural mesothelioma. Of the 32 patients that were initially evaluated between 1995 and 2000, 26 that underwent successful radical P/D were entered into analysis. Twenty-four patients received IORT for a median dose of 15Gy. The same number of patients also received postoperative either three-dimensional (3D) conformal RT (14 patients) or IMRT (10 patients). The median dose of external beam radiation was 41.4Gy. Some, but not all, patients were given platinum-based chemotherapy. A median overall survival of 18.1 months and an overall 2-year survival of 32% were demonstrated. Radical pleurectomy/decortication with aggressive radiotherapy with or without chemotherapy might offer an alternative treatment option to those who cannot tolerate extrapleural pneumonectomy.[34] Yet, IORT is challenging to administer to sufficient tissue planes at risk (interlobar fissures, diaphragm, and pericardial/mediastinal pleura) and is not universally available. Whether the combined IORT radical P/D offered enhanced local control was not clear. Also, newer effective chemotherapy regimens with a pemetrexed backbone may achieve more for residual disease post P/D than IORT could offer. Finally, in these patients, although they benefited initially from improved pulmonary function, their pulmonary function gradually deteriorated with time (especially in the long-term survivors) such that the pneumonectomy-sparing value of radical P/D was diminished. In essence, they developed a slow-motion autopneumonectomy due to postoperative changes, injury or sacrifice of the phrenic nerve, and long-term radiation sequelae. Additionally, as shown in other series, higher dose external beam radiation especially when not 3D conformal and/or IMRT, has been associated with significantly higher toxicity.

The role of P/D with intraoperative photodynamic therapy has also been investigated. Pass and colleagues in a phase III study randomized 63 patients to intraoperative PDT or not followed by postoperative immunochemotherapy. Forty-eight patients met the preoperative criteria for randomization. Twenty-three patients underwent P/D and the remaining EPP. The median survival for this cohort was 14.4 months, compared with 7.7 months for those who were not debulked. Although pilot studies on the use of intraoperative photodynamic therapy as adjuvant therapy were promising, this phase III trial showed no apparent benefit for either progression-free (8.5 vs. 7.7 months) or overall survival (14.4 vs. 14.1 months) for intraoperative PDT. A trend, however, for longer survival was noted for those undergoing P/D as opposed to EPP (22 months vs. 11 months; $p = 0.07$) regardless of intraoperative PDT (level of evidence 2b).[35,36] Unfortunately, the study was not powered to detect the superiority of one surgical approach over the other.

54.1.3.3. Evidence for Extrapleural Pneumonectomy and Neoadjuvant Therapy

Neoadjuvant therapy is standard although somewhat controversial in certain locally advanced cancers such as stage IIIA (N2) non-small cell lung cancer. Recent advances in chemotherapy for MPM have led some groups to investigate the feasibility of induction chemotherapy prior to EPP in MPM patients as well. In a phase II trial, the MSKCC group enrolled patients with advanced disease to first undergo induction therapy with gemcitabine and cisplatin followed in 3 to 5 weeks by EPP and adjuvant 54 Gy radiation 4 to 6 weeks, postoperatively. The patients not only tolerated this regimen but their resectability rate was better (88%) when compared with the historical resectability rate of 75% to 80%. Despite the original concern that chemotherapy induced fibrosis might make the dissection more difficult, no operative mortality was noted.[37]

Similarly, a Swiss group reported no perioperative mortality and a median survival of 23 months in their series of 20 patients following induction chemotherapy with gemcitabine and cisplatin followed by EPP with or without adjuvant radiation. Interestingly, this was far superior to their own experience of EPP with adjuvant chemoradiation (a median survival of 13 months).[38] A recently opened multicentered, prospective, randomized, phase III trial is underway in the United Kingdom comparing induction chemotherapy (pemetrexed–platinum doublet) alone to induction chemotherapy (same drugs) followed by EPP. While we await the results of this trial, the preliminary results appear promising and may translate into prolonged survival. Regardless, it does not appear that induction chemotherapy, especially regimens with pemetrexed, which is exceptionally well tolerated, increased surgical morbidity or mortality and is well tolerated even in the setting of EPP.

54.2. The Debate

In experienced centers, the surgical mortality associated with EPP is in the range of 3.8% to 5%, comparable to 1.5% to 5% for P/D, which is a remarkable achievement given the frequent extent of disease encountered and the magnitude of the procedure being performed. Amazingly, in some centers the operative mortality with EPP is significantly less than the operative mortality for routine pneumonectomy for lung cancer (5%–8%). Therefore, operative mortality by itself should not preclude the more radical EPP approach. While EPP provides a more complete removal of gross disease, in patients with early disease both procedures allow for complete removal of gross disease. Extrapleural pneumonectomy may be more appropriate for those with advanced disease infiltrating the fissures and encasing the lung in whom P/D may not get rid of all gross disease. Furthermore, EPP facilitates the feasibility of adjuvant radiotherapy. Pneumonectomy allows the entire hemithorax to be irradiated at a higher more effective dose (approx 50–60 Gy) as opposed to P/D, where the underlying lung is at risk of radiation fibrosis, thus limiting the field and radiation dose. Extraplueral pneumonectomy, has better relapse-free survival. Unfortunately, despite these stated advantages, the evidence to date in support of EPP has failed to establish definitively a significant overall survival advantage over P/D. Of course, the real trial comparing the two approaches head to head prospectively has not been done. Yet, there is movement among MPM centers to consider such a trial. Now that there are multiple centers with teams of thoracic surgeons, medical and radiation oncologists who are experts in MPM, sufficient numbers of patients could be accrued both in the United States and Europe to answer the question.

Recent advances in chemotherapy in MPM have been encouraging. As mentioned previously, the combination of pemetrexed/cisplatin in unresectable disease has shown decent response. Currently, clinical trials are underway where this regimen is being studied in a neoadjuvant setting for those with resectable disease by EPP. There is a high likelihood that bulky disease may be reduced and render a patient a candidate for the lesser of the two aggressive procedures, that is, P/D, but still delivering a R0 resection. Our single-institution preliminary experience in a relatively small number of patients supports this hypothesis. We also have had anecdotal success in rendering those who were initially unresectable that after chemotherapy became amenable to resection.

In the final analysis, the optimal treatment of MPM remains to be determined by continued carefully planned and performed clinical trials. It is for this reason that patients with MPM should be referred to centers with established programs that are participating in multi-institutional efforts to allow the right questions to be asked and hopefully answered. For now, in the absence of irrefutable solid trial data, it is common practice for patients to be treated based on individual institutional biases and dependent on the multiple determinants, comorbidities, and performance status of the patient (Figure 54.1). The best evidence to date suggests that a subset of patients with favorable criteria such as epithelial histology, limited bulk of disease, and who are mediastinal (N2) node negative (i.e., early stage I or II) will benefit from enhanced local control and possible chance of cure with EPP and combined systemic chemotherapy and adjuvant radiation. The advent of molecular assessment of tumors and gene profiling should allow determination of the innate biological aggressiveness of an individual patient's tumor (perhaps regardless of other classic staging parameters such as T or N status) and this may help guide resection choice. Patients in whom long-term survival is less likely would benefit from non-pneumonectomy approaches that are still being developed. In the interim,

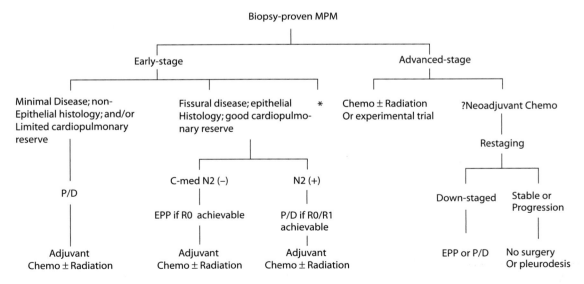

FIGURE 54.1. Algorithm for managing MPM. C-med, cervical mediastinoscopy; EPP, extrapleural pneumonectomy; N2, ipsilateral lymph node station; P/D, pleurectomy/decortication; *, neoadjuvant chemotherapy followed by EPP or P/D.

current practice guidelines suggest that there is a role for radical P/D with intra-operative mediastinal node sampling as part of a combined modality approach in patients who cannot tolerate EPP and in whom an R0 or R1 resection can be delivered (Figure 54.1). Palliative (>R1) P/D, on the other hand, probably has a limited role.

> There is a role for radical P/D with intra-operative mediastinal node sampling as part of a combined modality approach in patients who cannot tolerate EPP and in whom an R0 or R1 resection can be delivered (level of evidence 2b; recommendation grade B).
> Palliative (>R1) P/D has a limited role in the management of MPM.

References

1. Enterline PE and VL Henderson. Geographic patterns for pleural mesothelioma deaths in the United States, 1968–81. *J Natl Cancer Inst* 1987;79:31–37.
2. Connelly RR, Spirtas R, Myers MH, et al. Demographic patterns for mesothelioma in the United States. *J Natl Cancer Inst* 1987;78:1053–1060.
3. Spirtas R, Beebe GW, Connelly RR, et al. Recent trends in mesothelioma incidence in the United States. *Am J Ind Med* 1986;9:397–407.
4. Devesa SS, Blot WJ, Stone BJ, et al. Recent cancer trends in the United States. *J Natl Cancer Inst* 1995;87:175–182.
5. Marom EM, Erasmus JJ, Pass HI, et al. The role of imaging in malignant pleural mesothelioma. *Semin Oncol* 2002;29:26–35.
6. Steele JPC. Prognostic factors in mesothelioma. *Semin Oncol* 2002;29:36–40.
7. Wang ZJ, Reddy GP, Gotway MB, et al. Malignant pleural mesothelioma: evaluation with CT, MR imaging, and PET. *Radiographics* 2004;24:105–119.
8. Heelan RT, Rusch VW, Begg CB, et al. Staging of malignant pleural mesothelioma: comparison of CT and MR imaging. *Am J Roentgenol* 1999;172:1039–1047.
9. Patz EF, Shaffer K, Piwnica-Worms DR, et al. Malignant pleural mesothelioma: value of CT and MR imaging in predicting resectability. *AJR Am J Roentgenol* 1992;159:961–966.
10. Gerbaudo VH, Sugarbaker DJ, Britz-Cunningham S, et al. Assessment of malignant pleural mesothelioma with (18)F-FDG dual-head gamma-camera coincidence imaging: comparison with histopathology. *J Nucl Med* 2002;43:1144–1149.
11. Benard F, Sterman D, Smith RJ, et al. Pro-gnostic value of FDG PET imaging in malignant pleural mesothelioma. *J Nucl Med* 2000;41:1443–1444.
12. Boutin C, Rey F. Thoracoscopy in the pleural malignant mesothelioma: a prospective study of 188 consecutive patients. Part I: diagnosis. *Cancer* 1993;72:389–393.
13. Baas P. Predictive and prognostic factors in malignant pleural mesothelioma. *Curr Opin Oncol* 2003;15:127–130.
14. Herndon J, Green M, Chahinian AP, et al. Factors predictive of survival among 337 patients with mesothelioma treated between 1984 and 1994 by the Cancer and Leukemia Group B. *Chest* 1998;113:723–731.
15. Ruffie PA. Pleural mesothelioma. *Curr Opin Oncol* 1991;3:328–334.
16. DePangher-Manzini V, Brollo A, Franceschi S, et al. Prognostic factors of malignant mesothelioma of the pleura. *Cancer* 1993;72:410–417.
17. Byrne MJ, Davidson JA, Musk AW, et al. Cisplatin and gemcitabine treatment for malignant mesothelioma: a phase II study. *J Clin Oncol* 1999;17:25–30.
18. Taylor EC. Design and synthesis of inhibitors of folate-dependent enzymes as antitumor agents. *Adv Exp Med Biol* 1993;338:387–408.
19. Thodtmann R, Depenbrock H, Dumez H, et al. Clinical and pharmacokinetic phase I study of multitargeted antifolate (LY231514) in combination with cisplatin. *J Clin Oncol* 1999;17:3009–3016.
20. Calvert AH, Hughes AN, Calvert PM, et al. ALIMTA in combination with carboplatin demonstrates clinical activity against malignant mesothelioma in a phase I trial. *Lung Cancer* 2000;29:73–74.
21. Vogelzang NJ, Rusthoven JJ, Symanowski J, et al. Phase III study of pemetrexed in combination with cisplatin versus cisplatin alone in patients with malignant pleural mesothelioma. J Clin Oncol 2003;21:2636–2644.
22. Baldini EH. External beam radiation therapy for the treatment of pleural mesothelioma. *Thorac Surg Clin* 2004;14:543–548.
23. Boutin C, Rey F, Viallat JR. Prevention of malignant seeding after invasive diagnostic procedures in patients with pleural mesothelioma: a randomized trial of local radiotherapy. *Chest* 1995;108:754–758.
24. Butchart EG, Ashcroft T, Barnsley WC, et al. Pleuropneumonectomy in the management of diffuse

diffuse malignant mesothelioma of the pleura. Experience with 29 patients. *Thorax* 1976;31:15–24.

25. Rusch VW. Pleurectomy/decortication in the setting of multimodality treatment of diffuse malignant pleural mesothelioma. *Semin Thorac Cardiovasc Surg* 1997;9:367–372.

26. Sugarbaker DJ, Jaklitsch MT, Bueno R, et al. Prevention, early detection, and management of complications after 328 consecutive extrapleural pneumonectomies. *J Thorac Cardiovasc Surg* 2004;128:138–146.

27. Rusch VW, Piantadosi S, Holmes EC, et al. The role extrapleural pneumonectomy in malignant pleural mesothelioma. A lung cancer study group trial. *J Thorac Cardiovasc Surg* 1991;102:1–9.

28. Sugarbaker DJ, Flores RM, Jaklitsch M, et al. Resection margins, extrapleural nodal status, and cell type determine postoperative long-term survival in trimodality therapy of malignant pleural mesothelioma: results in 183 patients. *J Thorac Cardiovasc Surg* 1999;117:54–65.

29. Rusch VW, Rosenzweig K, Venkatraman E, et al. A phase II trial of surgical resection and adjuvant high dose hemithoracic radiation for malignant pleural mesothelioma. *J Thorac Cardiovasc Surg* 2001;122:788–795.

30. Pass HI, Kranda K, Temeck BK, et al. Surgically debulked malignant pleural mesothelioma: results and prognostic factors. *Ann Surg Oncol* 1997;4:215–222.

31. Maziak DE, Gagliardi A, Haynes AE, et al. Sugical management of malignant pleural mesothelioma: a systematic review and evidence summary. *Lung Cancer* 2005;48:157–169.

32. Rusch VW, Saltz L, Venkatraman E, et al. A phase II trial of pleurectomy/decortication followed by intrapleural and systemic chemotherapy for malignant pleural mesothelioma. *J Clin Oncol* 1994;12:1156–1163.

33. Gupta V, Mychalczak B, Krug L, et al. Hemithoracic radiation therapy after pleurectomy/decortication for malignant pleural mesothelioma. *Int J Radiat Oncol Biol Phys* 2005;63:1045–1052.

34. Lee TT, Everett DL, Shu HG, et al. Radical pleurectomy/decortication and intraoperative radiotherapy followed by conformal radiation with or without chemotherapy for malignant pleural mesothelioma. *J Thorac Cardiovasc Surg* 2002;124:1183–1189.

35. Friedberg JS, Mick R, Stevenson J, et al. A phase I study of Foscan-mediated photodynamic therapy and surgery in patients with mesothelioma. *Ann Thorac Surg* 2003;75:952–959.

36. Pass HI, Temeck BK, Kranda K, et al. Phase III randomized trial of surgery with or without intraoperative photodynamic therapy and postoperative immunochemotherapy for malignant pleural mesothelioma. *Ann Surg Oncol* 1997;4:628–633.

37. Flores RM. Induction chemotherapy, extrapleural pneumonectomy, and radiotherapy in the treatment of malignant pleural mesothelioma: the Memorial Sloan-Kettering experience. *Lung Cancer* 2005;49:S71–S74.

38. Weder W, Kestenholz P, Taverna C et al. Neoadjuvant chemotherapy followed by extrapleural pneumonectomy in malignant pleural mesothelioma. *J Clin Oncol* 2004;22:3451–3457.

55

Treatment of Malignant Pleural Mesothelioma: Is There a Benefit to Pleuropneumonectomy?

Stacey Su, Michael T. Jaklitsch, and David J. Sugarbaker

Malignant pleural mesothelioma (MPM) is a rare but highly aggressive tumor of the pleura that has defied standard approaches to treatment. Left untreated, the disease carries a grave prognosis, with median survival ranging from 4 to 12 months. Surgery serves as the mainstay of treatment: the strategy with resectable tumors is to widely remove all gross disease and apply adjunctive treatments for maximal local and systemic control. This approach is necessarily aggressive, with the goal of prolonging survival and the hope of cure for patients who are treated early in the course of the disease. Extrapleural pneumonectomy (EPP), the en bloc resection of the lung, visceral and parietal pleura, pericardium, and ipsilateral diaphragm, represents the most radical surgical approach to eradicate all macroscopic tumor burden. Other surgical options, such as pleurectomy and decortication, serve to debulk tumors but inevitably leave gross residual disease within the hemithorax. Against the background of a dismal disease, the combination of EPP with different adjuvant regimens has yielded promising outcomes. Furthermore, studies of these multimodal treatments have led to a revised staging system that may more appropriately stratify the biological variants of this disease.

To date, there are no evidence-based consensus guidelines on the management of MPM. Given the rarity of MPM, there are no randomized, controlled trials that compare different surgical approaches with one another or compare surgery to alternative treatments. The cumulative evidence in the literature lies in retrospective case series reports and prospective, noncontrolled studies, further confounded by the changing classification and staging of MPM over the years. This chapter critically evaluates the evidence that supports the role of EPP, in combination with adjuvant therapies, in prolonging survival of patients with MPM.

55.1. Published Data

55.1.1. Single-modality Treatment

The failure of EPP to extend survival in the context of a single-modality regimen is well established (Table 55.1).[1-4] Butchart's series quoted an operative mortality of 31%, a 5-year survival of 3%, and a median survival of 10 months. Although it provided a brief period of local control, EPP alone did not improve the natural history of the disease. Poor response rates to chemotherapy and limitations in the maximum radiation dose allowable by surrounding intrathoracic viscera led caregivers to recommend supportive care alone.

55.1.2. Multimodality Treatment

A seminal article by Antman and colleagues in 1980 at the Sidney Farber Cancer Institute (renamed the Dana–Farber Cancer Institute in 1983) advocated a multimodality approach to MPM after a retrospective review suggested an advantage to aggressive intervention.[5] Thereafter, a prospective multimodality protocol was issued, including EPP followed by adjuvant chemotherapy (cyclophosphamide/doxorubicin/

TABLE 55.1. Reported mortality of extrapleural pneumonectomy with and without adjuvant therapy.

Reference	Number Epp	Adjuvant Therapy	Epithelial Histology	Operative Mortality(%)	% Survival				
					1-yr	2-yr	3-yr	5-yr	Median (mos)
Worn, 1974[1]	62	None	–	ns		37		10	
Butchart, 1976[2]	29	None	11	31		10		3	
DaValle, 1986[3]	33	C[d]	20	9.1		24	14		
Ruffie, 1991[4]	23	–	–	13		17		–	9
Allen, 1994[5]	40	C or RT	26	7.5		22.5		10	
Rusch, 1991[6]	20	None		15		33			10
Pass, 1997[14]	39	PDT							9.4
Rusch, 1999	115	C or RT, CRT	–	3.5					*
Sugarbaker, 1993[7]	52	CAP + RT[a]	50	5.8[b]		50		–	
Sugarbaker, 1999[8]	183	CAP + RT[a]	103	3.8		37		14	
Maggi, 2001[39]	23	CP + RT[a]		6.3					77%[c]
Rusch, 2001[17]	62	RT[a]	60	11			27		17
Aziz, 2002[40]	64	CE	35	9.1	84		48	18	35
Sugarbaker, 2004[18]	328	C + RT		3.4					
Stewart, 2004[15]	53	None[e]		7.5					17

Abbreviations: C, adjuvant chemotherapy; CAP, cyclophosphamide (600 mg/m^2) + doxorubicin (60 mg/m^2) + cisplatin (70 mg/m^2), 4 to 6 cycles; CE, carboplatin + epirubicin and postoperative systemic chemotherapy; CP, carboplatin (at an area under the curve of 6) + paclitaxel (200 mg/m^2), 4 cycles; RT, adjuvant radiotherapy.
[a]RT up to 55 Gy.
[b]All cell types combined ($n = 52$).
[c]21/27 (77%) alive at median follow-up of 12.5 months.
[d]Doxorubicin or RT or both in 52% of patients.
[e]Essentially EPP only, a few patients had adjuvant chemotherapy, but most in United Kingdom are advised to wait until disease recurs.
*Median survival: stage I, 29 months; stage II, 19 months; stage III, 10 months; stage IV, 8 months.

cisplatin, or CAP) and radiation therapy (RT). In 1991, Sugarbaker and colleagues published their first case series of 31 patients who underwent EPP in a trimodality setting, demonstrating a low rate of mortality (6%).[6] This study identified trends toward improved survival in the subset of patients with negative histological margins.

Coincident with the 1991 Sugarbaker study, several other centers produced case series reporting improved rates of operative mortality with EPP.[3,7] A prospective trial by Rusch and coworkers in 1991 noted a longer progression-free survival with EPP but showed no difference in survival when compared to patients who underwent less radical procedures or nonsurgical treatment.[4] Allen and associates published a retrospective case series of patients who underwent both EPP and pleurectomy/decortication (P/D) with postoperative adjuvant therapy of either computed tomography (CT) or RT; there was a trend toward higher median survival in those who underwent EPP, although it was not statistically significant.[8]

Over the next several years, Sugarbaker and colleagues worked to refine their surgical technique and improve patient selection. A 1992 update (44 patients) described a substantial reduction in mortality (4.6%).[9] In 1993, the Brigham and Women's Hospital (BWH) and Dana–Farber Cancer Institute (DFCI) combined cancer treatment program identified a subset of patients with epithelial histology and node-negative status that exhibited improved survival.[10] Dissatisfied with the ability of current staging systems to stratify patients according to survival, they proposed a revised staging system (Table 55.2). The next update in this series (120 patients) reported a median survival of 21 months.[11] The previously published staging criteria were validated, with survival stratifying according to the BWH pathological stage: stage I median survival, 22 months; stage II median survival, 17 months; stage III median survival, 11 months ($p = 0.04$). Although there was no surgical control group, this study suggested a survival

TABLE 55.2. Staging systems of malignant pleural mesothelioma.

Brigham and Women's Hospital (BWH) Revised Staging System

I.   Disease confined to the capsule of the parietal pleura: ipsilateral pleura, lung, pericardium, diaphragm, or chest-wall disease limited to previous biopsy types.
II. All stage I with positive intrathoracic (N0, N1) lymph nodes.
III. Local extension of disease into chest wall or mediastinum, heart, or through diaphragm, peritoneum, with or without extrathoracic or contralateral (N2, N3) lymph node involvement.
IV. Distant metastatic disease.

International Mesothelioma Interest Group (IMIG) Staging System

T.   Primary tumor and extent
T1. a. Tumor limited to ipsilateral parietal pleura, including mediastinal and diaphragmatic pleura: no involvement of the visceral pleura.
     b. Tumor involving the ipsilateral parietal pleura, including mediastinal and diaphragmatic pleura; scattered foci or tumor also involving the visceral pleura.
T2. Tumor involving each of the ipsilateral pleural surfaces (parietal, mediastinal, diaphragmatic pleura; scattered foci or tumor also involving the visceral pleura.)
     • Involvement of diaphragmatic muscle.
     • Confluent visceral pleura (including the fissures) or extension of tumor from visceral pleura into the underlying pulmonary parenchyma/
T3. Describes locally advanced but potentially resectable tumor; tumor involving all of the ipsilateral pleural surfaces (parietal, mediastinal, diaphragmatic, and visceral pleura) with at least one of the following features.
     • Involvement of the endothoracic fascia.
     • Extension into mediastinal fat.
     • Solitary, complete resectable focus or tumor extending into the soft tissues of the chest wall.
     • Nontransmural involvement of the pericardium.
T4. Describes locally advanced technically nonresectable tumor; tumor involving all of the ipsilateral pleural surfaces (parietal, mediastinal, diaphragmatic, and visceral pleura) with at least one of the following features.
     • Diffuse extension or multifocal mass of tumor in the chest wall, with or without associated rib destruction.
     • Direct transdiaphragmatic extension of the tumor to the peritoneum.
     • Direct extension of tumor to the contralateral pleura.
     • Direct extension of tumor to one or more mediastinal organs.
     • Direct extension of tumor into the spine.
     • Tumor extending through the internal surface of the pericardium without or without a pericardial effusion or tumor involving the myocardium.

N.   Lymph nodes
Nx. Regional lymph nodes cannot be assessed.
N0. No regional lymph node metastases.
N1. Metastases in ipsilateral bronchopulmonary or hilar lymph nodes.
N2. Metastases in the subcarinal or the ipsilateral mediastinal lymph nodes, including the ipsilateral internal mammary nodes.
N3. Metastases in contralateral mediastinal, contralateral internal mammary, ipsilateral, or contralateral supraclavicular scalene lymph nodes.

M.   Metastases
Mx. Presence of distant metastases cannot be assessed.
M0. No (known) metastasis.
M1. Distant metastasis present.

Stage grouping

I.   a. T1aN0M0
     b. T1bN0M0
II. T2N0M0
III. Any T3M0, any N1M0, any N2M0
IV. Any T4, any N3, any M1

benefit for patients with epithelial histology and negative nodes.

While Sugarbaker and colleagues confirmed the validity of their revised staging system with the results from their updated data set, a consortium led by Rusch called the International Mesothelioma Interest Group (IMIG) developed another staging system.[12] The International TNM staging was based on emerging data about the impact of T (tumor) and N (node) status on survival. The T descriptor provided the precise anatomical definition of the extent of the primary tumor, while the N descriptor referred to the same nodal sets used in the International Lung Cancer Staging System. However, the validity of the International TNM staging system was called into question with the subsequent update on 183 patients published by Sugarbaker and colleagues in 1999.[13] Multivariate analysis of this data set showed that the most important predictor of poor outcome after undergoing EPP in a trimodal setting was histological subtype (mixed or sarcomatoid), followed by N2 nodal disease and positive resection margins. The identification of these three prognostic factors led the authors to modify the BWH staging system, incorporating positive margins and extrapleural nodes into the classification. N2 nodes were reclassified as defining stage III (instead of stage II) disease beyond the pleural envelope. The revised BWH staging system improved the survival stratification of the cohort of 183 patients ($p = 0.0011$) as compared to the stratification yielded by the previously published BWH staging system. However, the International TNM staging system failed to stratify survival when applied to the Sugarbaker data set. The TNM staging designated the majority of the patients as stage III, coalescing patients with different tumor characteristics and obscuring survival benefits associated with such prognostic markers. Furthermore, the T descriptor was not a statistically significant predictor of survival on log rank testing, reflecting the failure of the TNM staging system to represent the biological behavior of MPM in this largest patient series to date.

Nonetheless, the TNM staging continues to be the more widely used staging system. Rusch and coworkers published a prospective, noncontrolled study of a cohort of MPM patients treated with either EPP or P/D followed by adjuvant treatment. Tumor stage had a significant impact on overall survival when considered across all four stage groups: stage I ($n = 21$) had a median survival of 30 months, stage II ($n = 40$) 19 months, stage III ($n = 102$) 10 months, and stage IV ($n = 68$) 8 months. It should be noted that stage I comprises T1N0 tumors of strikingly minimal disease and is the least common stage at which patients present. This study showed that the data also

stratified by the number of positive nodes (0–3 nodes positive vs. ≥4 nodes positive) and adjuvant therapy. The study overall encouraged treatment of early disease with surgical resection and adjuvant therapy. Although there was no significant difference in survival based on the type of surgical resection (EPP vs. P/D), it should be noted that P/D was performed in patients with minimal visceral pleural tumor while those with more locally advanced tumor underwent EPP. The bias in operative planning undermines Rusch's conclusion that the type of surgical resection does not have an impact on survival. A similar bias is present in the study from the National Cancer Institute (NCI) by Pass and associates, who reported a retrospective review of 95 patients, divided between EPP and P/D followed by intraoperative photodynamic therapy (PDT) and immunochemotherapy.[14] The median survival for EPP was 9.4 months compared to 14.5 months for P/D; however, the study acknowledged that patients with lesser volume of tumor burden underwent P/D. Additionally, the technique of EPP was less than radical, with a dissection that spared a portion or all of the diaphragm.

There remains much controversy as to the importance of the type of surgical resection between EPP and P/D. This is likely to remain unresolved in the absence of randomized, controlled trials comparing the two approaches. Improvements in operative technique and patient selection have reduced the mortality risk of EPP to 4% in the Sugarbaker series, matching the quoted risk of P/D (1%–5%). Thus the argument against EPP due to high operative mortality does not apply to select high-volume centers. Unless patients fail the eligibility criteria for EPP (Table 55.3), the evidence strongly suggests that resectable MPM should be treated with radical resection via EPP followed by adjuvant chemoradiotherapy. This trimodal approach offers the best chance for long-term survival in select patient subgroups. A recent case series by Stewart and colleagues supports the benefit of EPP over P/D, showing a longer progression-free survival and longer time to local disease progression with EPP.[15] The identification of negative microscopic margins as a prognostic marker of survival in patients, as elucidated by Sugarbaker and col-

TABLE 55.3. Eligibility criteria for extrapleural pneumonectomy.

Karnofsky performance > 70
Renal function: Creatinine < 2
Liver function: AST < 80 IU/L, total bilirubin < 1.9 mg/dL, PT < 15 s
Pulmonary function: Postoperative FEV$_1$ > 0.8 L as per PFTs and
   quantitative V/Q scans
Cardiac function: Normal EKG and echocardiogram (EF > 45%)
Extent of disease: limited to ipsilateral hemithorax, with no transdia-
   phragmatic, transpericardial, or extensive chest wall involvement

Abbreviations: AST, aspartate aminotransferase; EF, ejection fraction;
EKG, electrocardiogram; FEV$_1$, forced expiratory volume in 1 s; PFT, pul-
monary function tests;
PT, prothrombin time; V/Q, lung ventilation/perfusion quotient.

leagues, provides an additional argument in favor of EPP because P/D inevitably leaves gross residual disease.

Studies of patterns of failure have pointed to loco-regional recurrence as the most common site of treatment failure. A study by Baldini revealed the ipsilateral hemithorax to be the most common site of relapse after trimodality therapy (35%), followed by abdomen (26%) and contralateral thorax (17%).[16] Distant recurrence was rare (8%). This study highlights the locally aggressive nature of MPM and strongly argues for strategies to achieve maximal local tumor control. Different means have been studied to eradicate microscopic foci of tumor burden: intrapleural chemotherapy, intraoperative RT and PDT, postoperative RT, IMRT, and brachytherapy. On the other hand, Rusch and coworkers published a phase II trial of patients who underwent EPP followed by high-dose hemithoracic radiation.[17] This trial reported a higher proportion of distant metastases (30%) as the first site of relapse, rather than loco-regional recurrence (2%). This finding highlights the need for adjuvant chemotherapy to target systemic spread of the disease. It should be noted that the Rusch study defined distant metastases to include those that occurred in the abdomen and contralateral thorax. Other groups consider these sites to possibly represent contiguous spread or tumor seeding from the primary disease process; instead, distant metastases are specified as those in the brain, bone, or other areas more likely to represent hematogenous or lymphatic spread of the primary disease.

55.2. Impact of Published Data on Clinical Practice

The evidence presented herein consists of a cumulative experience gained from retrospective case series and prospective, noncontrolled phase I/II trials. There are no prospective, randomized, controlled trials comparing surgical resection to alternative modalities, nor comparing different surgical approaches (EPP vs. P/D) against one another. These shortcomings are inherent in the evaluation of a rare disease such as MPM. Additionally, it can be argued that randomized, controlled trials may not be an appropriate standard of evidence by which to evaluate most surgical treatments, which necessarily rely on observational studies to show that standards of practice are safe and beneficial. Thus, the above heterogeneity of evidence must be critically evaluated with full awareness of the biases intrinsic to the study design.

The data highlight MPM as an insidious, locally aggressive disease whose biological behavior can be assessed based on a limited number of known prognostic markers. Better prognosis is associated with epithelial histology, negative nodes, and negative microscopic margins. Extrapleural pneumonectomy has been shown to be a surgical procedure with acceptable risk of mortality and morbidity in high-volume centers, one that trades its aggressive approach and attendant risks for the hope of achieving maximal local tumor control and long-term survival under the aegis of a multimodality strategy. Extrapleural pneumonectomy in a trimodality setting of adjuvant chemoradiation has been the best studied in the largest retrospective case series by Sugarbaker and coworkers.[18] In this series, a patient subset has been identified by prognostic markers to have a 5-year survival of nearly 50% after undergoing EPP and adjuvant chemoradiation.

One of the challenges in the treatment of MPM lies in incorporating pathological, genetic, or other tumor markers into the staging system so as to optimally stratify patients according to prognosis. Accurate staging leads to better patient selection for appropriate treatments. To improve patient selection, the use of preresectional nodal testing via mediastinoscopy, thoracoscopy, or laparoscopy will likely improve the sensitivity and specificity of our current radiologic tools to detect extrapleural extension of disease. The key lies in finding the multimodality regimen that offers the maximal benefit of local and systemic control with minimal toxicity and risk. New modalities will be instituted as the armamentarium of chemomodulatory drugs and adjuvant delivery systems expands. However, consensus guidelines on how to standardize treatment will not be available in the absence of prospective, randomized controlled trials. On the basis of published data, EPP is an essential element of multimodality therapy for MPM in the setting of adequate cardiorespiratory reserve, careful pre-resectional surgical and radiographic staging, and epithelial subtype. This is based on a 2++ level of evidence and is given a B recommendation grade. Extrapleural pneumonectomy is likely not useful in the setting of poor functional status, sarcomatoid or mixed histology, mediastinal nodal involvement, and spread of disease beyond the pleural envelope. This is based on a 2++ level of evidence and granted with a B recommendation grade.

> Extrapleural pneumonectomy is an essential element of multimodality therapy for malignant pleural mesothelioma in the setting of adequate cardiorespiratory reserve, careful pre-resectional surgical and radiographic staging, and epithelial subtype (level of evidence 2++; recommendation grade B).
>
> Extrapleural pneumonectomy is likely not useful in the setting of poor functional status, sarcomatoid or mixed histology, mediastinal nodal involvement, and spread of disease beyond the pleural envelope (level of evidence 2++; recommendation grade B).

55.3. Personal View of the Data

The primary role of extrapleural pneumonectomy in multimodality therapy for malignant pleural mesothelioma is to enable a macroscopic complete resection (MCR). Adjuvant therapy with local and systemic modalities is intended to eliminate micrometastatic disease that remains at local margins or as a consequence of hematog-

enous or lymphangitic spread. Current local and systemic modalities are inadequate to effect a cure, and hence, the secondary goal of surgery is to improve the quality and duration of life. Extrapleural pneumonectomy offers the eligible patient the best chance for overall and disease-free survival. Treating a patient with P/D leaves a substantial residual tumor burden that lessens the efficacy of adjuvant therapies. Because the time interval between treatment and death is proportional to the number of viable tumor cells remaining at the completion of therapy, the ability to achieve maximal cytoreduction is thought to be integral to the ability to extend survival. A host of innovative adjuvant therapies are currently being investigated and may hold the key to long-term survival or cure for victims of this horrible disease, but it is unlikely that a single solution will work for all patients. Each of these modalities has specific advantages in select subsets of patients. Ongoing clinical trials comparing the effectiveness of surgical cytoreduction in conjunction with adjuvant treatment regimens are key to extending survival.

55.4. Present and Future Investigations

55.4.1. Hyperthermic Intracavitary Intraoperative Chemotherapeutic Lavage

The culprits of recurrent disease are thought to be (1) residual tumor cells from positive resection margins, (2) free intrathoracic cancer cells that have penetrated the pleura prior to resection, and (3) spillage of tumor at the time of resection.[19-21] In the 1990s, several groups began investigating the benefits of heated and unheated intracavitary or intraperitoneal chemotherapeutic lavage immediately after surgical debulking as a means of completing the cytoreductive process at micrometastatic levels. The role of intracavitary chemotherapy has been studied in a variety of malignancies and the results have been favorably reported in the literature.

In 1992, Markman and Kelson[22] of Memorial Sloan-Kettering Cancer Center applied the concept of intraperitoneal lavage in patients with malignant peritoneal mesothelioma. Cisplatin and mitomycin were infused through a peritoneal catheter after surgical debulking. Cisplatin ($100 mg/m^2$) was given every 28 days and mitomycin (5–10 mg) was given 7 days after each intraperitoneal cisplatin dose. No patient was able to tolerate more than five courses because of disease progression or catheter failure. Although the median survival was only 19 months, there were a few long-term survivors. Four patients (21%) lived for more than 3 years and two were clinically disease-free more than 5 years from the start of the intraperitoneal treatment.

In 1996, Alberts and colleagues presented a retrospective, randomized trial in which intraperitoneal cisplatin was administered to patients with stage III ovarian cancer after cytoreductive surgery.[23] Estimated median survival was significantly longer in the group receiving intraperitoneal cisplatin (49 months) compared with the group receiving intravenous cisplatin (41 months). The Memorial Sloan-Kettering Cancer Center in New York has completed two studies of intrapleural chemotherapy following radical pleurectomy for MPM.[24–26] The intrapleural chemotherapeutic regimen was cisplatin ($100 mg/m^2$) and mitomycin ($8 mg/m^2$). This treatment was well tolerated, but the most common site of recurrent disease remained the ipsilateral hemithorax.

Tumor cells have a higher sensitivity to heat compared with normal cells.[27] Hyperthermia increases cell permeability, alters the cellular metabolism, and increases the transport of drugs across cell membranes. Stehlin[28] used hyperthermic melphalan to perfuse the limbs of patients with melanoma of the extremities. Five-year survival of 30 patients treated with hyperthermic melphalan was superior to the normothermic group (80% vs. 20%). These findings have been confirmed by Santinami and coworkers of the National Cancer Institute of Milan, Italy.[29]

Van Ruth and coworkers have used doxorubicin and cisplatin in intraoperative heated chemotherapy for malignant mesothelioma.[30] Doxorubicin was able to penetrate into the intercostal muscle specimen. They determined that it was safe and had limited systemic side effects. Paul Sugarbaker of the Washington Cancer Institute investigated heated intraperitoneal chemotherapy for peritoneal carcinomatosis of gastrointestinal malignancies.[31]

These studies and the work of Roberts,[32] Rusch,[26] and others influenced the BWH/DFCI team to offer radical pleurectomy to patients unable to tolerate EPP in the context of a series of phase I and II trials designed to examine the efficacy of surgical cytoreduction followed by intracavitary hyperthermic cisplatin lavage. A paper reporting the efficacy of P/D with intracavitary heated chemotherapy was recently published.[33] The EPP study is close to accrual.

55.4.2. Antifolate Antagonists

The molecular basis of MPM is not well understood, but the key to finding therapies that will halt the progression of MPM lies at the molecular interface. The Thoracic Surgery Oncology Laboratory at BWH has been using bioinformatics tools to analyze how gene expression is modified in MPM tumors compared with normal lung and pleura. In one study, Bueno and colleagues identified the human α-folate receptor as being highly expressed in 44 of 61 MPM tissues.[34] Other investigators have noted that methotrexate, which blocks folate metabolism, has a significant response in MPM.[35] Two anti-folate–based chemotherapy combinations emerged in 2000: pemetrexed/cisplatin and raltitrexed/cisplatin. A phase I trial of pemetrexed/cisplatin showed objective responses in 5 of 11 patients (45%), while a phase I trial of pemetrexed/carboplatin showed responses in 9 of 29 patients (31%).[35] A phase III multinational trial that randomized 456 patients with MPM to cisplatin with or without pemetrexed showed response rates in 41% in the double-agent arm versus 17% in the cisplatin arm alone ($p < 0.0001$).[36] Median survival was prolonged when pemetrexed was added (12 months vs. 9 months; $p = 0.02$). This evidence holds promise for a multimodality treatment protocol that may eventually incorporate the use of pemetrexed in an adjuvant setting.[36]

55.4.3. Gene Ratios

Oligonucleotide and cDNA microarrays can be used to identify cancer-related genes in tumor tissues such as MPM; the expression profiles of these genes can be correlated with clinical parameters, including diagnosis and outcome.

Microarray data can often be difficult to interpret because of the complex statistical analysis involved, the number of samples needed to draw statistically significant conclusions, and the quantity of RNA required. In 2002, Gordon and colleagues discovered gene expression ratios incorporating specific genes that could be useful in distinguishing between diagnosis of MPM and adenocarcinoma of the lung.[37] These investigators used a training set of 32 discarded MPM and lung adenocarcinoma samples ($n = 16$ each) to identify five and three highly expressed genes with reciprocal average expression levels in MPM and lung adenocarcinoma tissue, respectively. Expression data for these eight genes were used to calculate all 15 possible gene pair ratios by placing a MPM overexpressed gene in the numerator and an adenocarcinoma overexpressed gene in the denominator. A diagnosis was then predicted by comparing each ratio value to a threshold of 1. Ratios greater than 1 predicted MPM and ratios less than 1 predicted adenocarcinoma. These 15 pairs each proved to be between 91% and 98% accurate at predicting the correct diagnosis of an additional 149 MPM and adenocarcinoma tumors. Accuracy was increased to 95% to 99% by combining multiple gene pair ratios.

Gordon and colleagues have also used gene ratios to predict survival in MPM patients receiving standard BWH trimodality therapy. A four-gene prognostic expression ratio test accurately predicted treatment-related patient outcome in MPM independent of histology.[38] A recent study by the same group validated the concept of gene ratio–based prognostic tests in a cohort of 39 tumor specimens obtained from patients receiving EPP and heated intraoperative intracavitary chemotherapy. New treatment-specific prognostic genes and gene ratio–based prognostic tests identified in this study were also highly accurate and statistically significant when examined in an independent set of 52 tumors from patients undergoing similar treatment.[38] In the future, the use of gene ratios could eventually elaborate the staging system so as to help stratify patients into treatment groups and optimize treatment strategies. This novel test could also elucidate a mechanistic pathway that predisposes tumors toward treatment failure, thereby pointing the way to new (neo)adjuvant therapies.

References

1. Worn H. [Chances and results of surgery of malignant mesothelioma of the pleura]. *Thoraxchir Vask Chir* 1974;22:391–395.
2. Butchart EG, Ashcroft T, Barnsley WC, et al. Pleuropneumonectomy in the management of diffuse malignant mesothelioma of the pleura. Experience with 29 patients. *Thorax* 1976;31:15–24.
3. DaValle MJ, Faber LP, Kittle CF, et al. Extrapleural pneumonectomy for diffuse, malignant mesothelioma. *Ann Thorac Surg* 1986;42:612–618.
4. Rusch VW, Piantadosi S, Holmes EC. The role of extrapleural pneumonectomy in malignant pleural mesothelioma. A Lung Cancer Study Group trial. *J Thorac Cardiovasc Surg* 1991;102:1–9.
5. Antman KH, Blum RH, Greenberger JS, et al. Multimodality therapy for malignant mesothelioma based on a study of natural history. *Am J Med* 1980;68:356–362.
6. Sugarbaker DJ, Heher EC, Lee TH, et al. Extrapleural pneumonectomy, chemotherapy, and radiotherapy in the treatment of diffuse malignant pleural mesothelioma. *J Thorac Cardiovasc Surg* 1991;102:10–15.
7. Ruffie P, Feld R, Minkin S, et al. Diffuse malignant mesothelioma of the pleura in Ontario and Quebec: a retrospective study of 332 patients. *J Clin Oncol* 1989;7:1157–1168.
8. Allen KB, Faber LP, Warren WH. Malignant pleural mesothelioma. Extrapleural pneumonectomy and pleurectomy. *Chest Surg Clin North Am* 1994;4:113–126.
9. Sugarbaker DJ, Mentzer SJ, Strauss G. Extrapleural pneumonectomy in the treatment of malignant pleural mesothelioma. *Ann Thorac Surg* 1992;54:941–946.
10. Sugarbaker DJ, Strauss GM, Lynch TJ, et al. Node status has prognostic significance in the multimodality therapy of diffuse, malignant mesothelioma. *J Clin Oncol* 1993;11:1172–1178.
11. Sugarbaker DJ, Garcia JP, Richards WG, et al. Extrapleural pneumonectomy in the multimodality therapy of malignant pleural mesothelioma. Results in 120 consecutive patients. *Ann Surg* 1996;224:288–294.
12. Rusch VW. A proposed new international TNM staging system for malignant pleural mesotheli-

oma. From the International Mesothelioma Interest Group. *Chest* 1995;108:1122–1128.

13. Sugarbaker DJ, Flores RM, Jaklitsch MT, et al. Resection margins, extrapleural nodal status, and cell type determine postoperative long-term survival in trimodality therapy of malignant pleural mesothelioma: results in 183 patients. *J Thorac Cardiovasc Surg* 1999;117:54–65.

14. Pass HI, Temeck BK, Kranda K, et al. Phase III randomized trial of surgery with or without intraoperative photodynamic therapy and postoperative immunochemotherapy for malignant pleural mesothelioma. *Ann Surg Oncol* 1997;4: 628–633.

15. Stewart DJ, Martin-Ucar A, Pilling JE, et al. The effect of extent of local resection on patterns of disease progression in malignant pleural mesothelioma. *Ann Thorac Surg* 2004;78:245–252.

16. Baldini EH, Recht A, Strauss GM, et al. Patterns of failure after trimodality therapy for malignant pleural mesothelioma. *Ann Thorac Surg* 1997; 63:334–338.

17. Rusch VW, Rosenzweig K, Venkatraman E, et al. A phase II trial of surgical resection and adjuvant high-dose hemithoracic radiation for malignant pleural mesothelioma. *J Thorac Cardiovasc Surg* 2001;122:788–795.

18. Sugarbaker DJ, Jaklitsch MT, Bueno R, et al. Prevention, early detection, and management of complications after 328 consecutive extrapleural pneumonectomies. *J Thorac Cardiovasc Surg* 2004;128:138–146.

19. Koga S, Kaibara N, Iitsuka Y, et al. Prognostic significance of intraperitoneal free cancer cells in gastric cancer patients. *J Cancer Res Clin Oncol* 1984;108:236–238.

20. Hansen E, Wolff N, Knuechel R, et al. Tumor cells in blood shed from the surgical field. *Arch Surg* 1995;130:387–393.

21. Tanida O, Kaneshima S, Iitsuka Y, et al. Viability of intraperitoneal free cancer cells in patients with gastric cancer. *Acta Cytol* 1982;26:681–687.

22. Markman M, Kelsen D. Efficacy of cisplatin-based intraperitoneal chemotherapy as treatment of malignant peritoneal mesothelioma. *J Cancer Res Clin Oncol* 1992;118:547–550.

23. Alberts DS, Liu PY, Hannigan EV, et al. Intraperitoneal cisplatin plus intravenous cyclophosphamide versus intravenous cisplatin plus intravenous cyclophosphamide for stage III ovarian cancer. *N Engl J Med* 1996;335:1950–1955.

24. Bains MS, Ginsberg RJ, Jones WG 2nd, et al. The clamshell incision: an improved approach to bilat-

eral pulmonary and mediastinal tumor. *Ann Thorac Surg* 1994;58:30–33.

25. Rusch V, Saltz L, Venkatraman E, et al. A phase II trial of pleurectomy/decortication followed by intrapleural and systemic chemotherapy for malignant pleural mesothelioma. *J Clin Oncol* 1994;12:1156–1163.

26. Rusch VW, Niedzwiecki D, Tao Y, et al. Intrapleural cisplatin and mitomycin for malignant mesothelioma following pleurectomy: pharmacokinetic studies. *J Clin Oncol* 1992;10:1001–1006.

27. Strom R, Crifo C, Rossi-Fanelli A, et al. Biochemical aspects of heat sensitivity of tumour cells. *Recent Results Cancer Res* 1977;7–35.

28. Stehlin JS Jr, Giovanella BC, Gutierrez AE, et al. 15 years' experience with hyperthermic perfusion for treatment of soft tissue sarcoma and malignant melanoma of the extremities. *Front Radiat Ther Oncol* 1984;18:177–182.

29. Santinami M, Belli F, Cascinelli N, et al. Seven years experience with hyperthermic perfusions in extracorporeal circulation for melanoma of the extremities. *J Surg Oncol* 1989;42:201–208.

30. van Ruth S, Baas P, Haas RL, et al. Cytoreductive surgery combined with intraoperative hyperthermic intrathoracic chemotherapy for stage I malignant pleural mesothelioma. *Ann Surg Oncol* 2003;10:176–182.

31. Sugarbaker PH. Observations concerning cancer spread within the peritoneal cavity and concepts supporting an ordered pathophysiology. *Cancer Treat Res* 1996;82:79–100.

32. Roberts JR. Surgical treatment of mesothelioma: pleurectomy. *Chest* 1999;116:446S–449S.

33. Sugarbaker DJ. Macroscopic complete resection: the goal of primary surgery in multimodality therapy for pleural mesothelioma. *J Thorac Oncol* 2006;1(2):175–176.

34. Bueno R, Appasani K, Mercer H, et al. The alpha folate receptor is highly activated in malignant pleural mesothelioma. *J Thorac Cardiovasc Surg* 2001;121:225–233.

35. Fizazi K, John WJ, Vogelzang NJ. The emerging role of antifolates in the treatment of malignant pleural mesothelioma. *Semin Oncol* 2002;29:77–81.

36. Vogelzang NJ, Rusthoven JJ, Symanowski J, et al. Phase III study of pemetrexed in combination with cisplatin versus cisplatin alone in patients with malignant pleural mesothelioma. *J Clin Oncol* 2003;21:2636–2644.

37. Gordon GJ, Jensen RV, Hsiao LL, et al. Translation of microarray data into clinically relevant cancer

diagnostic tests using gene expression ratios in lung cancer and mesothelioma. *Cancer Res* 2002; 62:4963–4967.

38. Gordon GJ, Jensen RV, Hsiao LL, et al. Using gene expression ratios to predict outcome among patients with mesothelioma. *J Natl Cancer Inst* 2003;95:598–605.

39. Maggi G, Casadio C, Cianci R, Rena O, Ruffini E. Trimodality management of malignant pleural mesothelioma. *Eur J Cardiothorac Surg* 2001;19:346–350.

40. Aziz T, Jilaihawi A, Prakash D. The management of malignant pleural mesothelioma; single centre experience in 10 years. *Eur J Cardiothorac Surg* 2002;22:298–305.

41. Rusch VW, Veukatraman ES. Important prognostic factors in patients with malignant pleural mesotheliomia, managed surgically. *Ann Thorac Surg* 1999;68:1799–1804.

Part 7
Mediastinum

56
Management of Myasthenia Gravis: Does Thymectomy Provide Benefit over Medical Therapy Alone?

Vera Bril and Shaf Keshavjee

Myasthenia gravis (MG) is a disorder caused by abnormal neuromuscular transmission and can be either congenital or acquired. Acquired MG is an autoimmune disease mediated by acetylcholine receptor antibodies (AChrab) or antibodies to muscle-specific tyrosine kinase (anti-MusSK antibodies) directed against the acetylcholine receptor region of the postsynaptic membrane. Blocking and accelerated degradation of acetylcholine receptors lead to impaired neuromuscular transmission. When the safety factor for normal neuromuscular transmission is exceeded, then clinical weakness is apparent.[1,2] Myasthenia gravis has a predilection for the ocular and bulbar muscles, but generalized somatic muscle weakness, particularly of proximal groups, is also common. Fatigable weakness is the hallmark of MG and the disorder is diagnosed by the clinical presentation, abnormal electrodiagnostic findings on single-fiber electromyography and repetitive nerve stimulation tests, and elevated AChrab or anti-Musk antibodies in the patients' sera.[3]

Abnormalities of the thymus gland are commonly found in patients with MG; thymoma is present in about 10% to 15% of patients[4] and lymphoid follicular hyperplasia in about 70%.[2] In older patients, normal involution of the thymus gland produces thymic atrophy. In addition to the thymic pathology present in many patients with MG, there exists substantial data from animal models supporting the immunopathological role of the thymus in the development of autoimmune MG.[5]

56.1. Thymectomy: Background

Blalock introduced thymectomy as a therapeutic intervention for patients with MG prior to the days of controlled, randomized trials – first in patients with thymoma, and then in those without this finding.[6,7] Further clinical reports of the benefits of thymectomy led to the acceptance of this procedure for patients with generalized MG as a standard of practice. Nonetheless, controversies surrounding thymectomy abound in the literature.[8] Randomized, controlled trials, including a sham surgery arm, have not been done and as a result, some authorities question the benefits of thymectomy. Furthermore, the timing of thymectomy, whether thymectomy should be done in young children,[9] and the surgical approach for thymectomy[8] are all matters of debate.

The benefits of thymectomy are inferred partly from the natural history of MG in prethymectomy times. Up to one third of patients died during myasthenic crises prior to modern management of MG.[10] This clinical course improved after thymectomy became widely applied. However, simultaneous changes in intensive care unit (ICU) care, ventilatory support, and the introduction of immunosuppressive therapy may have also contributed to the improved outcomes in MG, regardless of thymectomy. Thus, the evidence for thymectomy is not grade A, but rather indirect and possibly misleading. Retrospective studies in children and adults suggest that patients undergoing thymectomy have higher remission rates than those who are managed medically.[11–13] Remission rates in children during a 3-year follow-up were 40% for the thymectomy group compared to 15% for the medically managed group.[13] In adults followed for about 20 years, the rates were 35% of those who had thymectomy compared to 7.5% who did not.[12] In this study, computer matching was used to find 80 nonoperated control subjects in order to compare the outcome of medical management with 104 patients who had thymectomy.

56.2. Thymectomy for Generalized Myasthenia Gravis

Despite current management that advocates the use of thymectomy for generalized MG with and without thymoma, the use of thymectomy in nonthymomatous MG remains controversial. In an effort to further examine the evidence for thymectomy, Gronseth and Barohn reviewed 21 retrospective thymectomy studies with 8490 patients from 1953 to 1998.[14] Patients having thymectomy were two times more likely to experience improvement than those who did not have this intervention (level of evidence 1). Improvement was defined as medication-free remission, asymptomatic on medications, or improved on medications. The median rates of each category of improvement were remission 25%, asymptomatic 39%, or clinically improved 70%. This meta-analysis highlighted the finding that most patients do not experience remission or achieve a completely asymptomatic state. Another study reported a multivariate analysis of prognostic factors in 756 patients with MG,[15] and found that thymectomy was significantly associated with remission, but the odds ratio was 1.6 (level of evidence 2++). Furthermore, the observation that the benefits of thymectomy are delayed with 25% achieving remission in the first year, 40% by the end of the second year, and 55% in the third year[16] suggests that other factors in addition to surgery may contribute significantly to the improvement observed after thymectomy. Currently, an international, randomized, multicenter study of whether trans-sternal thymectomy reduces corticosteroid requirements in patients with AChrab-positive, generalized MG[17] has been funded by

the National Institutes of Health (NIH) and will start enrolling patients this year. The results of this study may answer the question of whether trans-sternal thymectomy reduces the requirement for immunosuppressive medication in patients with MG, that is, indicates reduced disease activity. The exclusion of AchRab-negative patients in the study design may not be necessary[18] and will limit the generalizability of the results. In an optimal study design, a sham surgery arm would be included to avoid bias in patient reporting or perceptions. Obviously, this will not likely be carried out as the sham surgery arm provides an ethical challenge due to the risks of anesthesia and surgery without benefit to the patient, but this would provide the ultimate convincing evidence of the benefits of thymectomy in patients with MG. Still, the balance of evidence currently favors thymectomy for generalized, nonthymomatous MG (recommendation grade B).

> The balance of evidence currently favors thymectomy for generalized, nonthymomatous MG (level of evidence 2; recommendation grade B).

56.3. Thymectomy: Special Considerations

Although the current consensus is to use thymectomy for patients with nonthymomatous generalized MG, thymectomy in other patient groups, such as those with purely ocular MG, is much more controversial.[19] Based on the immunopathophysiology demonstrated in human and animal studies,[20] there is a role for thymectomy in younger patients with ocular MG, but many clinicians would hesitate to recommend surgery for this cohort[21] (level of evidence 3; recommendation grade D). Another area of debate is the upper age limit for thymectomy. Because older individuals have thymic atrophy rather than hyperplasia, the use of surgery in this group does not appear to have the same theoretical basis as in younger patients. In addition, complications of thymectomy are likely to be greater in older patients. However, there are retrospective studies reporting that thymectomy is safe in patients over age 60,[22,23] and that 16% of those over age 60 have thymic hyperplasia.[22] Despite the reported safety of thymectomy in older subjects, in this series[22] 1 patient out of the elderly cohort of 25 died compared to no deaths in the younger age group. Other retrospective series have shown that age does predict outcome in thymectomy for MG[24] with lower response rates in older subjects. In the absence of thymoma, our current practice is generally not to recommend thymectomy for patients over age 60, similar to practice in other centers[21] (level of evidence 3; recommendation grade D). At the other end of the age spectrum, thymectomy also is not recommended in very young children.[13]

56.4. Thymectomy: Surgical Approach

A final area of controversy in thymectomy for MG is the preferred surgical approach. Some centers recommend maximal thymectomy (trans-sternal + transcervical)[25] to eliminate the gland and possible extra-anatomical thymic tissue as well, whereas other centers recommend trans-sternal thymectomy or the minimally invasive transcervical thymectomy.[26,27] A more recent surgical innovation is the modification of this procedure with the introduction of video-assisted transcervical thymectomy.[28] The types of thymectomy have not been compared directly in any randomized study, but there is a school of thought that suggests that maximal thymectomy is preferred over more conservative approaches due to more complete resection of thymic tissue.[8] The meta analysis of 21 retrospective studies showing a positive benefit of thymectomy in patients with MG included all types of thymectomy approaches[14] (level of evidence 1−). Furthermore, relatively large case series have shown comparable remission and improvement rates in MG patients with different types of thymectomy[27,28] (level of evidence 3), thus it is not clear that the more extensive thymectomy procedures are more effective (recommendation grade D). Statistical reshuffling of crude data from different study reports may show different outcomes for different surgical interventions,[8] but this type of reanalysis in

itself may provide flawed results and does not provide definitive evidence of the benefits of one surgical approach over another. Ideally, a randomized trial of the different approaches would need to be done to address the issue of the most effective route for thymectomy. Such a study might be done in multiple centers with different centers undertaking their different preferred surgical approaches, if the study patients could travel to whatever center the study randomization allocated them. Currently, no such study is planned and there is no consensus on the optimal surgical approach.

> The optimal thymectomy approach is still unknown; outcomes are comparable between aggressive and conservative minimally invasive surgical approaches (level of evidence 3; recommendation grade D).

56.5. Outcome Measures in Myasthenia Gravis Studies

The outcome measures in MG have varied in different clinical trials. Most recently, efforts to standardize the assessment of MG have included the Quantitative Myasthenia Gravis Score (QMGS; Table 56.1).[29,30] This scale of 39 points quantitates the various clinical deficits observed in MG patients. Patients with milder degrees of MG have a score less than 10. A change of 3.5 units, or about 10% of the total scale, is considered to represent a clinically meaningful change on the QMGS.[29] Taking into account the variability of the QMGS on repeat testing as well as the magnitude of change considered clinically meaningful, power analysis indicates that 44 patients are necessary in a two-arm study to detect a treatment difference.[29] The relatively small number of MG patients required when using this clinical scale makes clinical trials feasible. Many studies have used the modified Osserman score that has the advantage of being simple, readily understood and has meaningful degrees of clinical change between categories[26] (Table 56.2). The clinical relevance of small changes in the QMGS is not as readily apparent as the relevance of changes in grade on the Osserman scale, but the QMGS score

TABLE 56.1. Quantitative myasthenia gravis score.[a]

Test item	None 0	Mild 1	Moderate 2	Severe 3	Score
Double vision on lateral gaze right or left (circle one), in seconds	61	11–60	1–10	Spontaneous	
Ptosis (upward gaze) in seconds	61	11–60	1–10	Spontaneous	
Facial muscles	Normal lid closure	Complete, weak	Complete	Incomplete	
Swallowing 4-oz. water (1/2 cup)	Normal	Minimal, coughing or throat clearing	Severe, coughing, choking or nasal regurgitation	Cannot swallow (test not attempted)	
Speech after counting aloud from 1 to 50 (onset of dysarthria	None at 50	Dysarthria at 30–49	Dysarthria at 10–29	Dysarthria at 9	
Right arm outstretched (90° sitting), in seconds	240	90–239	10–89	0–9	
Left arm outstretched (90° sitting) in seconds	240	90–239	10–89	0–9	
Vital capacity (# predicted)	≥80	65–79	50–64	<50	
Right hand grip (kgW)					
Men	≥45	15–44	5–14	0–4	
Women	≥30	10–29	5–9	0–4	
Left hand grip (kgW)					
Men	≥35	15–34	5–14	0–4	
Women	≥25	10–24	5–9	0–4	
Head lifted (45° supine) in seconds	120	30–119	1–29	0	
Right leg outstretched (45° supine) in seconds	100	31–99	1–30	0	
Left leg outstretched (45° supine), in seconds	100	31–99	1–30	0	
Total QMG score (range 0–39)					

[a]The QMG Score modified by Barohn et al.[29]

is valid, and detects changes of smaller magnitude than the Osserman scale, and thus may contribute to a better understanding of MG.[30] The use of a standardized, reliable method to assess MG in clinical trials allows an accurate comparison of results across studies. Although the QMGS is reflective of smaller degrees of clinical change, the concept of remission rate remains attractive as it is easy to understand and compare. One

drawback to comparison of remission rates is in the fact that many authors define remission differently using, for example, complete remission, remission, and partial remission. This heterogeneity and the lack of a standardized statistical Kaplan–Meier analysis of remission rates prevent easy comparison of results from different studies.

56.6. Patient Population in Myasthenia Gravis Studies

The population of MG patients to be included in clinical trials is also a matter of debate. In general, homogeneity of the patient population enrolled in clinical trials is desirable to maximize chances of a favorable result, but this may be at the cost of generalizability of the results to the MG popu-

TABLE 56.2. Modified Osserman classification.

Score	Details
0	Asymptomatic
1	Ocular signs and symptoms only
2	Mild generalized weakness
3	Moderate generalized weakness, or bulbar dysfunction, or both
4	Severe generalized weakness or respiratory dysfunction, or both

lation, and perhaps not necessary depending on the particular question under study. For example, the presence of AChrab may help to confirm the diagnosis of MG, but elimination of patients with seronegative MG from clinical trials begs the question of whether this group would respond to the treatment in question. Furthermore, patients with seronegative MG respond to immunomodulation and thymectomy supporting the immunopathogenic nature of their disorder.[18,21] These patients are thought to have similar underlying immunopathophysiology, but that the immune attack is directed at different epitopes of the neuromuscular junctional complex. Thus, standard immunoassays for AChrab may not detect the pathogenic antibodies in such patients. Indeed, some AChrab seronegative patients have been demonstrated subsequently to have other antibodies such as antiMusK[31,32] and these patients also respond to immunotherapy.[32] There is thus insufficient evidence to consider that this group of patients would be unresponsive to thymectomy.[33,34] Possibly other antibodies causing MG will be discovered in the future further complicating study design or generalizability.

56.7. Conclusions

In summary, MG is an autoimmune disorder mediated by thymic immunopathology. Thymectomy is a reasonable intervention given our current state of knowledge (evidence level 2+; recommendation grade B), but definitive randomized clinical trials need to be done to demonstrate the efficacy of thymectomy in MG. The optimal thymectomy approach is still debatable, but outcomes appear to be comparable between aggressive and conservative minimally invasive surgical approaches[27,28] (evidence level 3; recommendation grade D). Given the lack of definitive randomized trials comparing the different types of thymectomy, the choice of surgical approach is dictated by that method having the lesser morbidity, mortality, and cost.

References

1. Drachman DB. Myasthenia gravis. *N Engl J Med* 1994;330:1797–1810.
2. Hohlfeld R, Wekerle H. The immunopathogenesis of myasthenia gravis. In: Engel AG, ed. *Myasthenia Gravis and Myasthenic Disorders.* New York: Oxford University Press; 1999:87–104.
3. Keesey JC. Clinical evaluation and management of myasthenia gravis. *Muscle Nerve* 2004;29:484–505.
4. Morgenthaler TI, Brown LR, Colby TV, et al. Thymoma. *Mayo Clin Proc* 1993;68:1110–1123.
5. Lindstrom JM. Experimental autoimmune myasthenia gravis: induction and treatment. In: Engel AG, ed. *Myasthenia Gravis and Myasthenic Disorders.* New York: Oxford University Press; 1999: 87–104.
6. Blalock A, Mason MF, Morgan HJ, et al. Myasthenia gravis and tumors of the thymic region: report of a case in which the tumor was removed. *Ann Surg* 1939;110:544–561.
7. Blalock A, Harvey AM, Ford FR, et al. The treatment of myasthenia gravis by removal of the thymus gland: preliminary report. *JAMA* 1941;117:1529–1533.
8. Jaretzki A, Steinglass KM, Sonett JR. Thymectomy in the management of myasthenia gravis. *Semin Neurol* 2004;24:49–62.
9. Szobor A, Mattyus A, Molnar J. Myasthenia gravis in childhood and adolescence. Report on 209 patients and review of the literature. *Acta Paediatr Hung* 1988;29:299–312.
10. Oosterhuis HJ. Observations of the natural history of myasthenia gravis and the effect of thymectomy. *Ann N Y Acad Sci* 1981;377:678–690.
11. Seybold ME, Howard FM Jr, Duane DD, et al. Thymectomy in juvenile myasthenia gravis. *Arch Neurol* 1971;25:385–392.
12. Buckingham JM, Howard FM Jr, Bernatz PE, et al. The value of thymectomy in myasthenia gravis: a computer-assisted matched study. *Ann Surg* 1976;184:453–458.
13. Rodriguez M, Gomez MR, Howard FM Jr, et al. Myasthenia gravis in children: long-term follow-up. *Ann Neurol* 1983;13:504–510.
14. Gronseth GS, Barohn RJ. Practice parameter: thymectomy for autoimmune myasthenia gravis (an evidence-based review): report of the Quality Standards Subcommittee of the American Academy of Neurology. *Neurology* 2000;55:7–15.
15. Mantegazza R, Baggi F, Antozzi C, et al. Myasthenia gravis (MG): epidemiological data and prognostic factors. *Ann N Y Acad Sci* 2003;998:413–423.
16. Perlo VP, Arnason B, Poskanzer D, et al. The role of thymectomy in the treatment of myasthenia gravis. *Ann N Y Acad Sci* 1971;183:308–315.

17. Wolfe GI, Kaminski HJ, Jaretzki A 3rd, et al. Development of a thymectomy trial in nonthymomatous myasthenia gravis patients receiving immunosuppressive therapy. *Ann N Y Acad Sci* 2003;998:473–480.

18. Shahrizaila N, Pacheco OA, Vidal DG, et al . Thymectomy in myasthenia gravis: comparison of outcome in Santiago, Cuba and Nottingham, UK. *J Neurol* 2005;252:1262–1266.

19. Schumm F, Wietholter H, Fateh-Moghadam A, et al. Thymectomy in myasthenia with pure ocular symptoms. *J Neurol Neurosurg Psychiatry* 1985;48: 332–337.

20. Engel AG. *Myasthenia Gravis and Myasthenic Disorders*. New York: Oxford University Press; 1999.

21. Saperstein DS, Barohn RJ. Management of myasthenia gravis. *Semin Neurol* 2004;24:41–48.

22. Tsuchida M, Yamato Y, Souma T, et al. Efficacy and safety of extended thymectomy for elderly patients with myasthenia gravis. *Ann Thorac Surg* 1999;67:1563–1567.

23. Dohi-Iijima N, Sekijima Y, Nakamura A, et al. Retrospective analyses of clinical features and therapeutic outcomes in thymectomized patients with myasthenia gravis at Shinshu University. *Intern Med* 2004;43:189–193.

24. Budde JM, Morris CD, Gal AA, et al. Predictors of outcome in thymectomy for myasthenia gravis. *Ann Thorac Surg* 2001;72:197–202.

25. Jaretzki A 3rd, Wolff M. "Maximal" thymectomy for myasthenia gravis. Surgical anatomy and operative technique. *J Thorac Cardiovasc Surg* 1988;96:711–716.

26. Cooper JD, Al-Jilaihawa AN, Pearson FG, et al. An improved technique to facilitate transcervical thymectomy for myasthenia gravis. *Ann Thorac Surg* 1988;45:242–247.

27. Bril V, Kojic J, Ilse WK, et al. Long-term clinical outcome after transcervical thymectomy for myasthenia gravis. *Ann Thorac Surg* 1998;65:1520–1522.

28. de Perrot M, Bril V, McRae K, et al. Impact of minimally invasive trans-cervical thymectomy on outcome in patients with myasthenia gravis. *Eur J Cardiothorac Surg* 2003;24:677–683.

29. Barohn RJ, McIntire D, Herbelin L, et al. Reliability testing of the quantitative myasthenia gravis score. *Ann N Y Acad Sci* 1998;841:769–772.

30. Bedlack RS, Simel DL, Bosworth H, et al. Quantitative myasthenia gravis score: assessment of responsiveness and longitudinal validity. *Neurology* 2005;64:1968–1670.

31. Hoch W, McConville J, Helms S, et al. Autoantibodies to the receptor tyrosine kinase MuSK in patients with myasthenia gravis without acetylcholine receptor antibodies. *Nat Med* 2001;7:365–368.

32. Sanders DB, Tucker-Lipscomb B, Massey JM. A simple manual muscle test for myasthenia gravis: validation and comparison with the QMG score. *Ann N Y Acad Sci* 2003;998:440–444.

33. Leite MI, Strobel P, Jones M, et al. Fewer thymic changes in MuSK antibody-positive than in MuSK antibody-negative MG. *Ann Neurol* 2005;57:444–448.

34. Lavrnic D, Losen M, Vujic A, et al. The features of myasthenia gravis with autoantibodies to MuSK. *J Neurol Neurosurg Psychiatry* 2005;76:1099–1102.

57
Thymectomy for Myasthenia Gravis: Optimal Approach

Joshua R. Sonett

Perhaps one of the longest unresolved issues in thoracic surgery is the role of thymectomy in the treatment of myasthenia gravis (MG). Persistent questions and issues involve not only the surgical approach to thymectomy, but even the role of thymectomy itself in the treatment of myasthenia gravis. Many of these issues remain unclear because there is no level 1 evidence, and even level 2 evidence available to compare and analyze comparable study populations is limited. Results of many studies are as well not reported using appropriate Kaplan–Meier methodology, making analysis of the results even more challenging or ineffective.[1] Additionally, myasthenia gravis is an entity in itself with varying degrees of severity, time courses, and self-remissions. Alfred Blalock, who pioneered and helped introduce thymectomy for myasthenia gravis beginning in 1939,[2] was even noted in a comment in 1947 to show his doubts about the usefulness of thymectomy: "I thought we had an answer to the thymus in MG, but such does not appear to be the case"[3]; unfortunately this prophetic statement is still relevant.

57.1. Published Data

57.1.1. Thymectomy Versus Medical Treatment

To help analyze the published literature on the role of thymectomy in MG, Gronseth performed an evidence-based review of thymectomy in non-thymomatous MG between 1953 and 1998. In 310 articles discussing MG and thymectomy, 28 articles, involving 8490 patients, were found to be consistent with level 2 evidence studies.[4] Results indicated an overall benefit for patients undergoing thymectomy versus medical treatment, with the following median relative rates associated with thymectomy: medication-free remission 2.1, asymptomatic 1.6, and improvement 1.7. Overall crude uncorrected results of patients undergoing thymectomy resulted in a median rate of remission of 25%, an asymptomatic state of 39%, and an overall improvement rate of 70%. However, significant confounding differences in baseline characteristics of prognostic importance existed between thymectomy and nonthymectomy patient groups. The final conclusion, based on the level of available evidence, was that the benefit of thymectomy in nonthymomatous autoimmune MG has not been established conclusively, and that thymectomy is recommended as an option to increase the probability of improvement (level of evidence 2).

> The benefit of thymectomy in nonthymomatous autoimmune myasthenia gravis has not been established conclusively; thymectomy is recommended as an option to increase the probability of symptomatic improvement (level of evidence 2; recommendation grade B).

Thus, as we in the surgical community debate and analyze the actual different methods and techniques of thymectomy, the debate must be viewed in the context that conclusive evidence of the efficacy of thymectomy is itself still lacking many years after it was introduced as a therapeutic modality. To help define conclusively the role of thymectomy in nonthymomatous MG, a prospective multi-institutional international trial, approved for funding by the National Institutes of Health (NIH), is planned to randomize patients to thymectomy versus medical treatment beginning in 2006.[5]

57.1.2. Surgical Approaches to Thymectomy

The surgical approaches to thymectomy are varied and reflect the desire to perform a complete resection weighed against the magnitude and morbidity of the procedure. All approaches enable complete resection of the capsular thymus; what differentiates the approaches are the extent of peri-thymic mediastinal and cervical tissue that are excised. To help understand the different approaches to thymectomy and categorize the extent of resections the Myasthenia Gravis Foundation of America (MGFA) has broadly classified varying techniques of resection based on the operative approach and extent of surgical resection (Table 57.1).[6,7] In the ever dynamic surgical field, robotic approaches (T-2 a) as well as bilateral thoracoscopic approaches (T-2 b) are evolving. Overall individual case series have reported data that support the validity and success of all the approaches; however, the lack of prospective, case controlled studies do not provide a significant level of evidence that one thymectomy technique is superior.[4]

> There is insufficient evidence to determine which thymectomy technique is superior in the management of myasthenia gravis.

TABLE 57.1. Myasthenia Gravis Foundation of America (MGFA) thymectomy classification.[6,7]

T-1. Transcervical thymectomy
    a. Basic
    b. Extended
T-2. Videoscopic thymectomy
    a. VATS
    b. VATET
T-3. Trans-sternal thymectomy
    a. Standard
    b. Extended
T-4. Transcervical and trans-sternal thymectomy

Given the lack of definitive case controlled and prospective studies, this evidence-based review will highlight selective studies that are reported by established centers in the long-term treatment of MG. All data presented represents level 2 evidence. Additional literature review will examine the failure of thymectomy procedures, morbidity, and results of anatomical studies of the thymic resection. Simple comparison of reported remissions rates and partial remission rates or improvement can be and are misleading when evaluating treatment results. Many patients with MG will improve with time, thus any true reflection of surgical results should include time after thymectomy. Unfortunately, the majority of the literature does not accommodate for time and are reported as simple crude calculations of remissions (improvement divided by the number of thymic resections). The best method for comparing and understanding results of the literature would be with life table analysis using the Kaplan–Meier method.[8–10]

57.1.1.1. Extended Trans-sternal Thymectomy

Akira Masaoka[11] of Nagoya University in Japan and Alfred Jaretzki[12] of Columbia University in New York have been amongst the most articulate and persistent leaders in regards to the role extended or complete thymectomy in myasthenia gravis. In 1996, Masaoka and colleagues reported a 20-year review of their experience with extended thymectomy for MG.[11] This procedure involves en bloc resection of the anterior mediastinal fat tissue form phrenic to phrenic laterally and the diaphragm and the thyroid gland caudally and cephalad. All adipose tissues in this region is meticulously resected, including around the brachiocephalic veins, thymus, and pericardium. Cervical neck dissection is performed via the sternotomy incision, but aggressive dissection near the recurrent nerves is avoided. In a cohort of 286 patients, remission rates in nonthymomatous MG were 45.8% (5 years), 55.7% (10 years), and 67.2% at 15 years. Similar results have been consistently documented in other series of extended thymectomy. Analysis of multiple publications utilizing extended thymectomy consistently find pathological evidence of thymic tissue within the mediastinal fat out side the capsule of the primary thymus (Table 57.2).[11–16]

TABLE 57.2. Extent of thymic tissue recovered in peri-thymic mediastinal fat tissue.

Reference	Surgical approach	Extracapsular thymic tissue
Jaretzki[11]	Maximal	50 patients (98%)
Masaoka[12]	Extended	18 patients (72%)
Zielinski[13]	Extended	58 patients (56.0%)
Ashour[14]	Extended	38 patients (39.5%)
Scelsci[15]	VATET	27 patients (37%)
Mineo[16]	VATS	31 patients (32%)

Abbreviations: VATET, video-assisted thoracoscopic extended thymectomy; VATS, video-assisted thorascopic surgery.

57.1.1.2. Transcervical Thymectomy

Basic transcervical thymectomy (T-1a) as an alternative to trans-sternal thymectomy was introduced on a large scale by Kirschner and colleagues in the late 1960s.[17] However, widespread acceptance of the procedure only followed the introduction of a more extended and facilitated technique as presented by Cooper: "I do not like to get up and present a paper and look like a blithering idiot by telling people you can take out something through the neck when it is obvious to everybody that it is much easier to take it out through the chest."[18] Utilizing a sternal retractor to improve visualization and dissection of the thymus as well as perithymic fat, a series of 65 patients were presented with a 52% crude complete remission rate. These remission results have been consistently repeated by other groups, including Defilippi [50% relative risk (RR)],[19] and Calhoun (44% RR),[20] combined with reports of minimal morbidity and an median length of hospital stay of less than 1.5 days.[21]

57.1.1.3. Video-Assisted Thorascopic Surgery Thymectomy, Extended Video-Assisted Thorascopic Surgery Procedures Video-Assisted Thorascopic Extended Thymectomy

More recently, the evolution of videoscopic techniques has enabled excellent visualization and minimally invasive techniques for thymic resection. Early results were initially presented by a consortium of minimally invasive centers, describing the technique and safe encouraging initial results. Mack and colleagues[22] described 33 thymectomies (either left or right VATS) performed at three institutions with an 18.6% RR at 23 months follow-up. Yim and colleagues recently presented the most comprehensive experience with VATS thymectomy in 38 patients at a single institution. In this limited study, a crude RR (CRR) of 22% was achieved and a 75% CRR was found as measured by Kaplan–Meier survival curve.[23] In an effort to mimic the approach of the maximal thymectomy as described by Jaretzki, Novellino has described the VATET approach[24]: video-assisted thorascopic extended thymectomy, utilizing a small cervical incision and then bilateral thorascopic approach. In a very well-controlled level 2a series presented by Mantegazza, 159 patients underwent VATET, and at 6 years the CSR by life table analysis was 50.6%.[25]

57.1.1.4. Morbidity and Failures

Results of the evidence-based review by Gorsenth indicate a remarkably low mortality rate for any of the currently used procedures.[4] Peri-operative mortality rates were found to be higher prior to1970, but after that time reported rates were found to consistently less than 1%. Additionally, with present day techniques of extended trans-sternal thymectomy, particularly with special attention to avoidance of injury to the recurrent nerves, morbidity rates for the methods are not significantly different. What is clear is that patients undergoing transcervical and thoracoscopic thymectomy procedures can be discharged earlier and have earlier return to daily activities and function. Importantly, limited but important data document the failure of initial thymectomy secondary to retained thymic tissue missed at initial exploration (Table 57.3).[26–29]

TABLE 57.3 Surgical resection of persistent thymic tissue after initial thymectomy.

Reference	No. patients	Original procedure	Pathological thymus found at resection	Myasthenias improvement
Henze[26]	20	Transcervical	20/20	19/20
Masaoka[27]	6	Transcervical	6/6	3/6
Miller[28]	6	Transcervical (3) Basic trans-sternal (3)	5/6	5/6
Rosenberg[29]	13	Transcervical	11/13	6/13
Zielinski[13]	21	Transcervical (19) Trans-sternal (2)	17/21	Not reported

57.2. Summary of Published Data

Unfortunately, it is clear that many answers and approaches to the treatment of MG remain undefined based on a critical analysis of the data. Although there is no level 1 evidence supporting the role of thymectomy in MG, a preponderance of level 2 evidence supports the role of thymectomy in the treatment paradigm of MG. However, recent NIH support for a randomized trial of medical therapy versus thymectomy in the treatment of MG highlights the uncertainty of the evidence to date. In terms of the different surgical approaches to thymectomy, the literature does not definitively support any one particular surgical procedure. This must be interpreted in the context of the preponderance of data being reported as crude data in generally small single-center experiences. These equivocal results must be weighed against clear pathological evidence of extracapsular thymic tissue in the majority of patients and limited but defined reports of retained thymic tissue being the cause of some initial surgical failures. Thus some form of complete thymectomy should be the goal of any surgical approach, and this has been shown to be feasible by all the approaches described.

57.3. Personal View and Clinical Practice

I strongly believe that the evidence to date supports the role of thymectomy in the treatment of MG. This recommendation and practice is bolstered by the modern day ability to perform the procedure with a very low morbidity and mortality, thus fulfilling the basic surgical tenant of risk versus benefit. Given that recommendation and practice, I clearly understand the limits of the data to date, and would support the randomized trial of thymectomy versus medical therapy. But, as with any trial, I would have to bow to some of my biases, and would be reluctant to enter patients into the trial who present with significant respiratory failure. In terms of surgical approach, my bias is toward some type of maximal or extended thymectomy. I believe this can be accomplished best by sternotomy or by bilateral VATS with possible cervical exploration. However, this practice

paradigm must be viewed with the understanding that the published results to date do not clearly support any one particular approach and transcervical and unilateral VATS resection are used by many accomplished thoracic surgeons.

In the final analysis, the onus is on the thoracic surgical community to investigate the potential surgical benefit of thymectomy in MG. This benefit, if proven, will allow us to proceed with further studies to best define the appropriate and perhaps best approaches to resection as well as refine indications in terms of symptoms and timing of surgery. I thus would encourage and support the impending trial of thymectomy versus medical therapy in the treatment of MG.

References

1. Jaretzki A, Steinglass KM, Sonett JR. Thymectomy in the management of myasthenia gravis. *Semin Neurol* 2004;24:49–62.
2. Blacock A, Mason MF, Morgan HJ, Riven SS. Myathenias gravis and tumors of the thymic region: report of a case in which the tumor was removed. *Ann Surg* 1939;110:544–561.
3. Clagett OT, Eaton LM. Surgical treatment of myathenias gravis. *J Thorac Surg* 1947;16:62–80.
4. Gronseth SG, Barohn RJ. Practice parameter: thymectomy for autoimmune myasthenia gravis (an evidence-based review). *Neurology* 2000:55:7–15.
5. Wolfe GI, Kaminski HJ, Jaretzki A III, Swan A, Newsom-Davis J. Development of a thymecotmy trial in nonthymomatous myasthenia gravis patients receiving immunosuppressve therapy. *Ann N Y Acad Sci* 2003;998:473–480.
6. Jartzki A III, Barohn RJ, Ernstoff RN, et al. Myasthenia gravis: recommendations for clinical research standards. *Neurology* 2000;55:16–23.
7. MG Task Force. *Recommendations for Clinical Research Standards.* 2002. Available from: http://www.myasthenia.org/clinical/research/Clinical_Research_Standards.htm
8. Masaoka A, Extended trans-sternal thymectomy for myasthenia gravis. *Chest Silla Clin Na Am* 2001;11:369–387.
9. Jaretzki A III. Thymectomy for myasthenia gravis: an analysis of the controversies regarding technique and results. *Neurology* 1997;48(suppl 5):S52–S63.
10. Kaplan EL, Meier P. Nonparametric estimation from incomplete observations. *J Am Stat Assoc* 1958;53:457–481.

11. Masaoka A, Nagaoka Y, Kotake Y. Distribution of thymic tissue at the anterior mediastinum. Current procedures in thymectomy. *J Thorac Cardiovasc Surg* 1975;70:747–754.
12. Jaretzki III, Wolff M. "Maximal" thymectomy for myasthenia gravis. Surgical anatomy and operative technique. *J Thorac Cardiovasc Surg* 1988;96: 711–716.
13. Zielinski M, Kusdsal J, Szlubowski A, Soja J. Comparison of late results of basic transsternal and extended thymectomies in the treatment of myasthenia gravis. *Ann Thorac Surg* 2004;78: 253–258.
14. Ashour M. Prevalance of ectopic thymic tissue in myasthenia gravis and its clinical significance. *J Thorac Cardiovasc Surg* 1995;109:632–635.
15. Scelsi R, Ferro T, Novellino L, et al. Detection and morphology of thymic remnants after video-assisted thorcoscopic extended thymectomy (VATET) in patients with myasthenia gravis. *Int Surg* 1996;81:14–17.
16. Mineo CT, Pompeo E, Lerut T, Bernardi G, Coosemans W, Nofroni I. Thoracoscopic thymectomy in autoimmune mystheni: results of left-sided approach. *Ann Thorac Surg* 2000;69:1537–1541.
17. Krischner PA, Osserman KE, Kark AE. Studies in myasthenias gravis. *JAMA* 1969;209:906–991.
18. Cooper JD, Al-Jilaihawa AN, Pearson FG, Humphrey JG, Humphrey HE. An improved technique to facilitate transcervical thymectomy for myathenia gravis. *Ann Thorac Surg* 1988:45:242–247.
19. DeFilippi VJ, Richman DP, Ferguson MK. Transcervical thymectomy for myasthenia gravis. *Ann Thorac Surg* 1994:57:194–197.
20. Calhoun RF, Ritter JH, Guthrie TJ, et al. Results of transcervical thymectomy for myasthenia gravis in 100 consecutive patients. *Ann Surg* 1999; 230:555.
21. Ferguson MF. Transcervical thymectomy. *Semin Thorac Cardiovasc Surg* 1999;11:59–64.
22. Mack MJ, Landreneau RJ, Yim AP, Hazelrigg SR, Scruggs GR. Results of video-assisted thymectomy in patients with myasthenia gravis. *J Thorac Cardiovasc Surg* 1996;112:1352–1360.
23. Manalulu A, Lee TW, Wan I, Law CY, Chang C, Garzon JC, Yim AP. Video-assisted thoracic surgery thymectomy for nonthymomatous myasthenia gravis. *Chest* 2005;128:3454–3460.
24. Novellino L, Longoni M, Spinelli L, Andretta M, Cozzi M, Faillace G. Extended thymectomy without sternotomy performed by cervicotomy and thoracoscopic technique in the treatment of myasthenia gravis. *Int Surg* 1994;79:1378–1381.
25. Mantegazza R, Fulvio B, Bernasconi P, et al. Video-assisted thoracoscopic extended thymectomy and extended transsternal thymectomy (T-3b) in nonthymomatous myasthenia gravis patients: remission after 6 years of follow-up. *J Neurol Sci* 2003; 212:31–36.
26. Henze A, Biderfeld P, Chrisensson B, Matell G, Pirsanen R. Failing transcervical thymectomy in myasthenis gravis. An evaluation of transternal re-exploration. *Scand J Thorac Cardiovasc Surg* 1984;18:235–238.
27. Masaoka A, Monden Y, Seike Y, Tanioka T, Kagotani K. Reoperation after transcervical thymectomy for myasthenias gravis. *Neurology* 1982;32: 83–85.
28. Miller RG, Filler-Katz A, Kiprov D, Roan R. Repeat thymectomy in chronic refractory myasthenia gravis. *Neurology* 1991;41:923–924.
29. Rosenberg M, Jauregui WO, De Vewga M, Herrera MR, Roncoroni AJ. Recurrence of thymic hyperplasia after thymectomy in myasthenia gravis. Its importance as a cause of failure of surgical treatment. *Am J Med* 1983;74:78–82.

58
Management of Residual Disease after Therapy for Mediastinal Germ Cell Tumor and Normal Serum Markers

Luis J. Herrera and Garrett L. Walsh

Primary mediastinal nonseminomatous germ cell tumors (PMNGCT) are rare, representing less than 6% of all germ cell tumors (GCT) and 10% to 20% of all anterior mediastinal masses.[1,2] These tumors can be biologically aggressive, with regional involvement of adjacent structures and a high metastatic potential. The biology of extragonadal GCT is often different than their gonadal counterparts, despite having similar histological features (Table 58.1).[3,4]

Due to the aggressive behavior of these tumors, a multimodality approach is the most effective treatment strategy. Controversy still exists regarding the optimal chemotherapy regimen and the timing and indications for surgical intervention. One complex feature of PMNSGCT is the unpredictability of tumor response to induction treatment when based solely on radiographic evaluation and serum tumor marker analysis. In resected specimens after chemotherapy, tumors may exhibit extensive necrosis, teratoma, persistent malignant cells, or malignant transformation, regardless of the serum tumor marker status and the radiographic tumor response in imaging studies.[5-8]

Significant advances have occurred in the treatment of germ cell tumors over the past 30 years using multimodality therapy, with high chemotherapy response rates and dramatic improvement in long-term survivors. In most cases, surgical resection of residual disease still plays an important role in the overall management of these patients. The decision to resect residual disease after chemotherapy can be diffi-

cult, and the indication and timing for surgery is tailored to the individual patient and tumor biology. Given the rarity of this disease, the literature consists of retrospective series accumulated over several decades in selected high-volume centers. Due to the lack of controlled trials, definitive recommendations for the management of mediastinal germ cell tumors are based on these small case series only. Furthermore, patient diversity in terms of the extent of disease makes cohort studies or controlled trials difficult.

This chapter focuses on the management of PMNSGCT, with a focus on the role of surgery for the treatment of residual disease after chemotherapy with normalization of serum tumor markers, based on the best available evidence to date. Other histological types of germ cell tumors often occur in the mediastinum, including teratoma, seminoma, and metastatic gonadal germ cell tumor. This chapter primarily focuses on the management of the primary tumors of the mediastinum of nonseminomatous histology.

58.1. Clinical Evidence: Surgical Management of Primary Mediastinal Nonseminomatous Germ Cell Tumors

Primary mediastinal nonseminomatous germ cell tumors are the most malignant subgroup of germ cell tumors, with poor prognosis despite aggressive therapy. PMNSGCT are classified as

TABLE 58.1. Pathological classification of primary mediastinal germ cell tumors.

Teratomatous tumors
Benign
  Mature teratomas (well differentiated, mature elements; benign)
  Immature teratomas (immature mesenchymal or neuroepithelial tissue)
Malignant
  Teratoma with additional malignant components (germ cell elements, epithelial cancer, sarcoma)

Nonteratomatous tumors
  Seminomas
  Nonseminomatous
    Yolk sac tumors
    Embryonal carcinomas
    Choriocarcinomas
  Mixed nonseminomatous and seminomatous tumor

Source: Modified from Moran et al.[4]

poor prognosis germ cell tumors by the International Germ Cell Cancer Collaborative Group consensus classification based solely on the mediastinal location and regardless of any other variable.[9]

After confirmation of the diagnosis with serum tumor markers and, if possible with tumor biopsy, chemotherapy is the first-line treatment modality for these malignancies. Initial surgical resection or debulking of anterior mediastinal NSGCT are not indicted because it rarely achieves complete resection due to the infiltrative nature of these tumors. This will also have the negative consequence of delaying the initiation of chemotherapy. Cisplatin-based chemotherapy is standard induction therapy. First-line therapy usually consists of a combination of cisplatin with etoposide and bleomycin (BEP).[2] The response rates after chemotherapy for PMNSGCT are much lower than for the testicular malignant germ cell tumors. Serum tumor markers (STM) consist of α fetoprotein (AFP), β-human chorionic gonadotropin (β-HCG), and lactate dehydrogenase (LDH). They are elevated in up to 90% of patients with PMNSGCT.[10] Normalization of STM after chemotherapy occurs in approximately 45% to 90% of patients, with other patients demonstrating persistently elevated tumor markers and persistent disease in the mediastinum.[6,11] Normalization of STM is not necessarily associated with a complete radiographic resolution of the mediastinal mass because persistent viable tumor, residual teratoma, or necrosis can still be present in the mediastinum after induction therapy with marker stabilization or normalization.[8]

After chemotherapy, the stage of the disease is reassessed with repeat imaging and STM. Patients may either have: (1) complete radiologic and serologic response; (2) complete serologic response but with a residual mediastinal tumor; (3) growth of the tumor with normalization of STM; or (4) growth of tumor with persistently elevated markers. Surgery is felt to play an important role in groups 2 and 3, but perhaps is less warranted in groups 1 and 4. Surgery can be an adjunct to chemotherapy to achieve a complete response and it can also evaluate the nature and viability of residual masses in order to guide further therapy. In addition, the resection of residual teratomatous elements halts tumor growth and minimizes possible future complications related to growing teratoma syndrome with tumor compression or invasion of vital structures.

Because of the rarity of these tumors, no controlled or randomized clinical trials are available and perhaps will never be performed. The literature regarding PMNSGCT consists of case series reviewed retrospectively over decades (Table 58.2). Nevertheless, important points can be gathered from the available literature in order to base clinical decisions. Based on the reported literature, the ideal candidate with PMNSGCT for surgical resection has normalization of STM after first-line chemotherapy, has a residual and resectable mediastinal mass on imaging, has no evidence of extramediastinal metastatic disease, and has good performance and physiologic status (Figure 58.1). Nevertheless, many patients evaluated for surgery after first-line chemotherapy do not fulfill these criteria but may still benefit from surgical resection. Several factors must be considered prior to surgery after the completion of first-line chemotherapy: (1) the radiographic response to chemotherapy; (2) the level of serum tumor markers; (3) the presence of extramediastinal metastatic disease; (4) the extent and resectability of the residual tumor; and (5) the physiological reserve of the patient and estimated morbidity of the planned operation.

TABLE 58.2. Summary of published series of PMNSGCT treated with chemotherapy followed by surgery of residual disease.

References	PMNSGCT (n)	Year	Patients resected n (%)	Preoperative NL STM	Overall survival	Level of evidence
Schneider[15]	47	1987–2002	47 (100%)	21 (45%)	3 year, 30%	4
Takeda[19]	8	1986–2000	7 (87%)	7 (100%)	5 year, 43%	4
Bokemeyer[11]	287	1975–1996	145 (49%)	124 (45%)	5 year, 45%	4
Vuky[7]	49	1979–1999	32 (65%)	19 (59%)	2 year, 40%	4
Ganjoo[5]	75	1983–1997	62 (82%)	44 (70%)	5 year, 48%	4
Walsh[6]	20	1993–1998	11 (55%)	10 (91%)	2 year, 68%	4
Kesler[8]	92	1981–1998	79 (86%)	50 (63%)	5 year, 56%	4
Bacha[21]	14	1979–1995	6 (43%)	8 (57%)	5 year, 48%	4
Hidalgo[20]	27	1978–1995	6 (22%)	na	5 year, 31%	4
Lemarie[22]	64	1983–1990	22 (49%)	na	2 year, 53%	4
Gerl[16]	12	1981–1994	12 (100%)	na	5 year, 56%	4
Wright[10]	28	1976–1988	16 (57%)	22 (78%)	5 year, 57%	4

Abbreviations: na, not available; NL STM, normalization of serum tumor markers; PMNSGCT, primary mediastinal nonseminomatous germ cell tumor; Rec, level of recommendation.

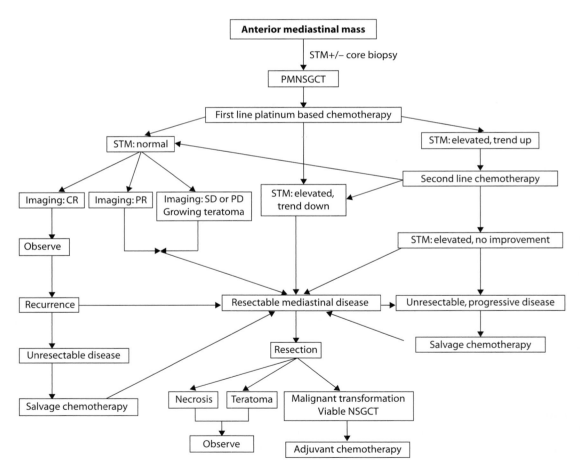

FIGURE 58.1. Algorithm for management of PMNSGCT.

58.1.1. Radiographic Response to Chemotherapy

After completion of chemotherapy, repeat imaging is obtained to reassess the extent of residual disease. In radiographic complete response with no residual tumor, observation alone is indicated. Patients with a partial response and residual resectable tumor can then be considered for surgery, particularly if STM have normalized. For patients with stable disease or disease progression that does not appear to be completely resectable, consideration to further chemotherapy is warranted.

58.1.2. Level of Serum Tumor Markers

The impact of STM levels at the time of surgical intervention for patients with PMNSGCT who have had first-line induction chemotherapy has not been well studied, but several case series have illustrated important points in the management of this disease.

Vuky and colleagues from Memorial Sloan-Kettering Cancer Center published a retrospective study of 32 patients with PMNSGCT who underwent surgical resection over a 20-year period.[7] After induction chemotherapy, normalization of STM occurred in 19 of the 32 patients (59%), but having an elevated STM level at the time of surgery did not exclude patients for resection. Patients with normal STM had less residual viable tumor (56% vs. 77%). However, in patients with persistently elevated STM, a complete surgical resection was achieved in 10 patients (77%). There was a trend towards decreased survival in patients with increasing STM at the time of surgery compared with patients with STM normalization ($p = 0.09$). Similarly, in our study at M.D. Anderson Cancer Center, all patients resected postchemotherapy had normalization of STM, and the one patient with persistent elevation had rapid progression of disease postoperatively.[6,7]

In another study, Kesler and colleagues reported a retrospective review of 92 patients with PMNSGCT, 79 of whom underwent surgery after platinum-based chemotherapy over a 16-year period.[8] Levels of STM normalized in 50 of the 79 patients (63%), with those patients who had normal levels at the time of resection having decreased incidence of viable NSGCT in the resected specimen when compared with patients with elevated STM (18% vs. 52%). On multivariate analysis, a significantly elevated AFP level (>1000 ng/mL) after first-line chemotherapy showed an associated relative risk of death of 6.5 [95% confidence interval (95% CI), 1.3–33.2; $p = 0.03$), however, AFP levels less than 1000 ng/mL had no apparent significant impact on survival.

It is unclear from the reviewed literature what is the optimal timing and role of surgery in a patient who has persistent elevation of STM after first-line chemotherapy. Several factors must be considered: (1) the absolute level and trend of STM elevation; (2) the resectability of the residual tumor; (3) the radiographic response; and (4) the feasibility of further chemotherapy cycles or alternate agents. It is important to consider that the outcome of patients treated with salvage chemotherapy due to residual disease after first-line therapy is poor, with long-term survival attainable in less than 7% of patients.[12] Such dismal results would favor surgical resection of residual tumor in selected patients, despite persistently elevated STM.

58.1.2. Impact of Extramediastinal Metastatic Disease

Patients with PMNSGCT often present with metastatic disease outside the mediastinum. As many as 15% to 65% of patients can have distant disease in the liver, bone, spine, brain, and lungs.[6,7,13,14] Intuitively, it would seem that patients with metastatic disease would fare much worse than patients with isolated mediastinal masses, but this has been varably described. In a study by Ganjoo and colleagues, of the 75 patients with PMNSGCT, 19 (25%) had visceral metastasis at the time of presentation.[5] Five-year disease-free survival was 37% for patients with metastatic disease versus 55% for patients without metastases ($p = 0.042$). Trends towards decreased survival in patients with metastatic disease has been reported in other studies, but statistically significant differences have not been consistently found.[6–8,10,15]

Patients with elevated STM after induction therapy who also present with extramediastinal disease present a particular challenge for surgeons. If the mediastinal disease is the most feasible site to resect or if it is causing local compression symptoms, it is reasonable to proceed with resection of the mediastinal tumor to assess tumor viability and guide further therapy for the other extramediastinal lesions. All disease that is amenable to resection, including lung metastases, should be resected subsequently or concomitantly. In cases of widespread metastatic disease, surgery is at times indicated as a means for tissue procurement to establish the histology of residual disease in order to guide further therapy. The most accessible or the most symptomatic site of disease is surgically resected. If possible, an aggressive approach with resection of metastatic sites is performed if the estimated morbidity is acceptable.

58.1.4. Resectability and Extent of Resection

Surgical resection of mediastinal germ cell tumors can be challenging. These tumors tend to develop an intense desmoplastic reaction, obscuring all tissue planes, and making safe dissection around vascular structures, lung, and cardiac chambers difficult. If the disease is completely resectable, en bloc resection of the mass and any invaded structures is performed, including resection of vascular structures, a phrenic nerve, lung, partial cardiac chambers, and chest wall. At times, en bloc resection of these tumors is not feasible due to encircling of both phrenic nerves, or involvement of multiple mediastinal structures. In some cases, bisecting the tumor allows safer access to the thoracic great vessels for better vascular control and delineation of the anatomy. Some authors recommend four quadrant epicenter biopsies with frozen section evaluation, and if no viable tumor is present, near total endolesional resection with preservation of lung, phrenic nerves, and vascular structures is performed.[8] If at all possible, every effort should be made to preserve lung parenchyma because many

of these patients have limited pulmonary reserve secondary to bleomycin toxicity.

58.1.5. Physiological Reserve and Estimated Morbidity

A careful physiological evaluation is performed in these patients, who, although young, can have significant compromise in their respiratory function due to chemotherapy-related toxicity. Complete pulmonary function testing including ventilation/perfusion scans and evaluation of diffusion capacity (DLCO) is necessary. The risk of the planned operation is assessed based on the patient's performance status, comorbidities, and functional reserve. These patients often develop a persistent postoperative sinus tachycardia that is not related to their volume status, hemoglobin, or pain level which may take several days to resolve.

58.1.6. Prognosis and Impact of Postresection Tumor Histology

One of the most interesting aspects of the biology of PMNSGCT is the diversity of histological features and the capacity for cellular transformation after chemotherapy. It has been shown that the histology of the residual mediastinal mass is an important predictor of survival and disease recurrence. The histology in the pathology of the resected masses may reveal necrosis (24%–27%), residual teratoma only (35%–45%), viable NSGCT (10%–26%), or malignant transformation to carcinoma or sarcoma (5%–10%).[5,6,8] Patients with necrosis have an excellent survival (mean, 139 months), compared to an intermediate survival of patients with teratoma (mean, 111 months), and the decreased but still acceptable survival of patients with residual malignant NSGCT (mean, 52 months). Malignant transformation into sarcoma has the worst prognosis with few patients alive past 57 months (Figure 58.2).[8] Current recommendations support the addition of adjuvant chemotherapy for patients with residual viable tumor in the resected specimen consisting of at least two cycles of chemotherapy. The finding of malignant transformation to an epithelial histology or to a sarcoma warrants a change in chemotherapy regimens.

FIGURE 58.2. Kaplan–Meier survival curve based on postoperative pathological category. Numbers represent the patients at risk for death. (Reprinted from Kesler KA, Rieger KM, Ganjoo KN, et al. Primary mediastinal nonseminomatous germ cell tumors: the influence of postchemotherapy pathology on long-term survival after surgery. *J Thorac Cardiovasc Surg* 1999;118:692–700, with permission from Elsevier.)

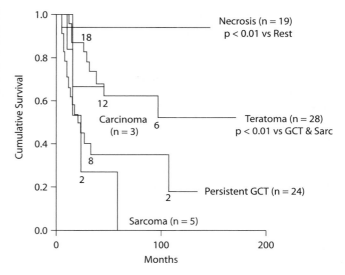

58.2. Current Evidence-Based Management of Primary Mediastinal Nonseminomatous Germ Cell Tumors

Overall, PMSCGCT have a poor prognosis when compared with testicular NSGCT; however, important advances have been made in the management of these aggressive malignancies. Due to the rarity of these tumors, few centers have accumulated significant experience with this disease, and prospective trials are not available to generate clear recommendations for treatment. With multimodality therapy, including resection of residual masses after chemotherapy, 5-year survival rates of 30% to 57% can be achieved (Table 58.2).[5–8,11,15–23]

Definite improvements have been made over the last two decades with the addition of cisplatin-based chemotherapy and surgical resection of residual disease, with much higher rates of long-term survivors. Due to limited number of cases, the basis for current practice is derived from small case series reported to date (Figure 58.1).

58.2.1. Surgical Resection of Residual Tumor after Completion of Initial Chemotherapy

Once initial chemotherapy is completed, evaluation of response is performed. There is enough literature available to support the role of surgical resection of residual mediastinal disease after induction therapy; however, the level of evidence is low due to retrospective studies of small number of patients in several series accumulated over many years. Normalization of STM is indicative of a good response and it seems clear that if the disease is resectable, surgery should be performed in physiologically fit patients with isolated mediastinal tumors (level of evidence 4; recommendation grade C). Patients with STM levels that decrease, but remain elevated, after initial chemotherapy display a trend of decreased survival after resection but some authors still recommend resection due to the low specificity of STM elevation and the poor results of salvage or second line chemotherapy (level of evidence 4 to 5; insufficient data to make a recommendation).[7,8]

> Normalization of serum tumor markers is indicative of a good response to systemic therapy; if the residual disease is resectable, surgery should be performed in physiologically fit patients with isolated mediastinal tumors (level of evidence 4; recommendation grade C).
>
> Patients with serum tumor marker levels that remain elevated after initial chemotherapy display a trend of decreased survival after resection; resection may be appropriate due to the poor results of salvage or second-line chemotherapy (level of evidence 4 to 5; insufficient data to make a recommendation).

The resectability of disease is important, and a complete resection of the disease is the goal and may require en bloc resections of vascular structures, phrenic nerve, adjacent lung, and chest wall, but this must be balanced against the morbidity associated with extensive resections. Extended resections including pneumonectomies, bilateral phrenic nerves, recurrent laryngeal nerves, or multiple vascular structures should not be performed, particularly if only teratoma or necrosis is found on tumor intraoperative biopsy, as advocated by Kesler and colleagues.[8] Patients who have other sites of metastatic disease, including lung, brain, spine, and liver, should also be considered for resection or further chemotherapy, especially if the mediastinal mass has evidence of viable tumor.

58.3. Clinical Evidence Versus Practice: Current Standard of Care and Clinical Trends in the Management of Primary Mediastinal Nonseminomatous Germ Cell Tumors

The patient with an anterior mediastinal mass and suspected germ cell tumor requires confirmation of the diagnosis in most cases. In an emergent situation, initiation of therapy based on STM elevation alone is adequate, but whenever feasible, core biopsy of the tumor has a high yield for histological confirmation. Baseline pulmonary function tests and laboratories and a search for metastatic disease are performed. The initial management of PMNSGCT consists of induction chemotherapy, disease restaging with STM, and repeat imaging and surgical resection of residual mediastinal masses. However, there is significant variability between patients and extent of disease, making standardized patient selection for surgery difficult. Clinical judgment and discussion in a multidisciplinary conference helps define which patients would benefit from resection. The decision of when to proceed with surgical resection will depend on the overall status of the patient and the availability of further chemotherapy at individual institutions.

The surgical approach is most commonly via a sternotomy, sternotomy with ipsilateral thoracotomy (hemi-clamshell), or bilateral anterior thoracosternotomy (clamshell), depending on tumor features and location. If the tumor cannot be completely resected en bloc, intraoperative biopsies with near complete resections is acceptable for nonmalignant tumors. Judicious use of intravenous fluids and low oxygen concentrations can help minimize pulmonary complications in these patients.

Significant improvements have occurred in the management of this disease, but the outcomes of patients with progression or recurrence of disease is poor. Several unanswered questions remain. Multi-institutional trials may be needed in order to developed a more standardized staging system and better define the role and timing of surgery, in particular for those patients with metastatic disease and persistently elevated STM. Improvement in salvage chemotherapy regimens would likely have a significant impact in the overall outcome of these patients. Subsequent development of hematogenous malignancies, in particular acute megakaryocytic leukemia, also limits long-term survival in some of these patients after they have overcome their initial malignancy, and better understanding and treatment of this process will likely improve outcomes as well.

References

1. Toner GC, Geller NL, Lin SY, Bosl GJ. Extragonadal and poor risk nonseminomatous germ cell tumors. Survival and prognostic features. *Cancer* 1991;67:2049–2057.
2. Hainsworth JD, Greco FA. Extragonadal germ cell tumors and unrecognized germ cell tumors. *Semin Oncol* 1992;19:119–127.
3. Moran CA, Suster S. Primary germ cell tumors of the mediastinum. *Cancer* 1997;80:681–690.
4. Moran CA, Suster S, Koss MN. Primary germ cell tumors of the mediastinum: III. Yolk sac tumor, embryonal carcinoma, choriocarcinoma, and combined nonteratomatous germ cell tumors of the mediastinum – a clinicopathologic and immunohistochemical study of 64 cases. *Cancer* 1997; 80:699–707.
5. Ganjoo KN, Rieger KM, Kesler KA, Sharma M, Heilman DK, Einhorn LH. Results of modern therapy for patients with mediastinal nonseminomatous germ cell tumors. *Cancer* 2000;88:1051–1056.

6. Walsh GL, Taylor GD, Nesbitt JC, Amato RJ. Intensive chemotherapy and radical resections for primary non-seminomatous mediastinal germ cell tumors. *Ann Thorac Surg* 2000;69:337–344.

7. Vuky J, Bains M, Bacik J, et al. Role of postchemotherapy adjunctive surgery in the management of patients with nonseminoma arising from the mediastinum. *J Clin Oncol* 2001;19:682–688.

8. Kesler KA, Rieger KM, Ganjoo KN, et al. Primary mediastinal nonseminomatous germ cell tumors: the influence of postchemotherapy pathology on long-term survival after surgery. *J Thorac Cardiovasc Surg* 1999;118:692–700.

9. International Germ Cell Consensus Classification: a prognostic factor-based staging system for metastatic germ cell cancers. International Germ Cell Cancer Collaborative Group. *J Clin Oncol* 1997;15:594–603.

10. Wright CD, Kesler KA, Nichols CR, et al. Primary mediastinal nonseminomatous germ-cell tumors – results of a multimodality approach. *J Thorac Cardiovasc Surg* 1990;99:210–217.

11. Bokemeyer C, Nichols CR, Droz JP, et al. Extragonadal germ cell tumors of the mediastinum and retroperitoneum: results from an international analysis. *J Clin Oncol* 2002;20:1864–1873.

12. Saxman SB, Nichols CR, Einhorn LH. Salvage chemotherapy in patients with extragonadal nonseminomatous germ cell tumors: the Indiana University experience. *J Clin Oncol* 1994;12:1390–1393.

13. Fizazi K, Culine S, Droz JP, et al. Primary mediastinal nonseminomatous germ cell tumors: results of modern therapy including cisplatin-based chemotherapy. *J Clin Oncol* 1998;16:725–732.

14. Bokemeyer C, Hartmann JT, Fossa SD, et al. Extragonadal germ cell tumors: relation to testicular neoplasia and management options. *APMIS* 2003;111:49–63.

15. Schneider BP, Kesler KA, Brooks JA, Yiannoutsos C, Einhorn LH. Outcome of patients with residual germ cell or non-germ cell malignancy after resection of primary mediastinal nonseminomatous germ cell cancer. *J Clin Oncol* 2004;22:1195–1200.

16. Gerl A, Clemm C, Lamerz R, Wilmanns W. Cisplatin-based chemotherapy of primary extragonadal germ cell tumors – a single institution experience. *Cancer* 1996;77:526–532.

17. Nichols CR, Saxman S, Williams SD, et al. Primary mediastinal nonseminomatous germ cell tumors: a modern single institution experience. *Cancer* 1990;65:1641–1646.

18. Bukowski RM, Wolf M, Kulander BG, Montie J, Crawford ED, Blumenstein B. alternating combination chemotherapy in patients with extragonadal germ-cell tumors – a Southwest Oncology Group Study. *Cancer* 1993;71:2631–2638.

19. Takeda S, Miyoshi S, Ohta M, Minami M, Masaoka A, Matsuda H. Primary germ cell tumors in the mediastinum – a 50-year experience at a single Japanese institution. *Cancer* 2003;97:367–376.

20. Hidalgo M, PazAres L, Rivera F, et al. Mediastinal non-seminomatous germ cell tumours (MNSGCT) treated with cisplatin-based combination chemotherapy. *Ann Oncol* 1997;8:555–559.

21. Bacha EA, Chapelier AR, Macchiarini P, Fadel E, Dartevelle PG. Surgery for invasive primary mediastinal tumors. *Ann Thorac Surg* 1998;66:234–239.

22. Lemarie E, Assouline PS, Diot P, et al. Primary malignant germ-cell tumors of the mediastinum – the results of a national retrospective inquiry. *Revue des Maladies Respiratoires* 1992;9:235–243.

23. Wright CD, Kesler KA, Nichols CR, et al. Primary mediastinal nonseminomatous germ cell tumors. *J Thorac Cardiovasc Surg* 1990;99:210–217.

59
Management of Malignant Pericardial Effusions

Nirmal K. Veeramachaneni and Richard J. Battafarano

The optimal treatment of patients with symptomatic pericardial effusion remains controversial. The goals of treatment are complete drainage of the effusion and acquisition of tissue and fluid for pathological analysis and microbiologic culture. Ideally, this should be performed using a method with minimal morbidity and a low risk for recurrence of the effusion. Therapeutic options include pericardiocentesis, percutaneous catheter drainage, open subxiphoid pericardial drainage (with or without the creation of a pericardioperitoneal window), and transthoracic drainage with creation of a pericardiopleural window. The choice of drainage procedure is significantly influenced by the physiological reserve of the patient and the need for a definitive diagnosis of the cause of the effusion.

The most likely cause of the pericardial effusion can often be determined by the patient's clinical history. Patients recovering from a myocardial infarction or recent cardiac procedure frequently develop transient effusions that respond to nonsteroidal anti-inflammatory agents and drainage of the effusion is not required. Pericardial effusions that develop in patients recently diagnosed with locally advanced or metastatic carcinoma are often a result of metastatic disease in the pericardium. In these cases, expedient drainage of the effusion by subxiphoid catheter drainage is often performed. However, a significant number of pericardial effusions occur in patients in whom the etiology is unclear. In these patients, the need for an accurate diagnosis will often influence the treatment strategy selected.

The majority of patients presenting with symptomatic pericardial effusion express dyspnea, cough, chest pain, fever, or edema.[1] The presence of clinical tamponade, characterized by tachycardia, hypotension, and jugular venous distension, is variable in different series. Although pericardial effusions are often identified on computed tomography (CT) scans of the chest, transthoracic and transesophageal echocardiography allows accurate assessment of the hemodynamic significance of the effusion. Right atrial or right ventricular compression during diastole, decreased left ventricle filling with inspiration leading to altered mitral valve mechanics, and persistent dilatation of the inferior vena cava with lack of respiratory variation suggest hemodynamic compromise and tamponade physiology.[2,3] Pericardial effusions may be the result of a variety of causes. The most common causes of pericardial effusions in developed nations are malignancy, postpericardiotomy, and autoimmune processes. In contrast, tuberculosis and uremia are more common causes worldwide.[1]

In determining the optimal therapy for a pericardial effusion, the surgeon must consider the value of obtaining an accurate diagnosis, the durability of the intervention, and the long-term prognosis of the patient. There have been no randomized studies evaluating the optimal diagnostic or therapeutic interventions to deal with this common problem. The available studies not only lack randomization of treatments, there have been no standardized treatments, and no consistent follow-up. However, available reports on the experiences of treating large numbers of patients with this problem provide useful information for determining the optimal diagnosis and treatment of pericardial effusions.

59.1. Patients with Malignant Pericardial Effusions Have Limited Survival

The optimal treatment of symptomatic malignant pericardial effusions is especially controversial due to the poor median survival (8–12 weeks) of patients reported in many series.[4-7] Case series and reports of single-institution experiences utilize an array of interventions including pericardiocentesis, pericardiocentesis with catheter drainage, balloon pericardiostomy, subxiphoid pericardial pericardiotomy, and video-assisted thoracoscopic approaches. The majority of the available literature focuses on two techniques: percutaneous catheter drainage and creation of a surgical subxiphoid pericardial pericardiotomy. The discussion will focus on these two approaches because they are readily available at many institutions and are the most widely utilized.

59.2. Diagnosis of Malignant Pericardial Effusion

Malignant pericardial effusions may be the result of direct tumor invasion into the pericardium, or by involvement of the mediastinal lymph nodes with subsequent spread into the epicardial lymphatic channels. Pericardial effusions in patients with a prior history of malignancy are often presumed to be malignant if other potential causes are excluded. Lung, breast, and hematological malignancies account for the majority of underlying cancers[4,7,8] and pericardial effusion cytology is positive in approximately half of the patients.[4,7]

Some authors have suggested that open drainage of a pericardial effusion may be the better procedure for diagnostic purposes, as both the effusion and the pericardial tissue may be biopsied and submitted for pathological evaluation. However, the available literature does not demonstrate a significant added benefit to pericardial biopsy evaluation in the diagnosis of the etiology of an effusion. In the setting of an effusion negative for malignancy on cytological evaluation, only 7% of patients in a large series had pericardial biopsies that were positive for malignancy.[7] Similarly, Cullinane demonstrated that no patient had a positive pericardial biopsy in the setting of negative fluid cytology.[5] In addition, 39% of patients with a presumed neoplastic effusion had biopsies of the pericardium and cytological evaluation of the fluid that were negative for malignancy.[7] In a smaller series of patients treated with catheter drainage for malignant effusion, Tsang reported positive cytology for malignancy in 53% of patients.[8]

It is important to obtain the treatment history of patients with malignancy associated pericardial effusion. Patients with breast or hematological malignancies who have received mediastinal radiation therapy are at risk for developing nonmalignant pericardial effusions. In our experience, these serous effusions typically develop within 6 months of completing radiation therapy and the fluid cytology is negative. These effusions respond well to drainage and infrequently recur.[9] In addition, the cause of pericardial effusions that develop in patients with a history of early-stage malignancies should be aggressively pursued. These effusions frequently develop from nonmalignant causes and are not a result of metastatic disease.

59.3. Significance of Positive Cytology

Although malignant cytology is not always identified in the clinical setting of a malignant pleural effusion, it is of considerable prognostic significance. Overall survival in patients with a malignancy-associated pericardial effusion is approximately 4 months. However, median survival is markedly shorter in patients with positive cytology. Whereas patients with underlying malignancy had median survival of 119 days and 31.6% survival at 1 year, proof of malignancy by pathological evaluation decreased median survival to 55 days and 1-year survival to 16.7%.[4,7,10] In the largest series of patients treated by catheter-based intervention, median survival was only 134 days in patients with a malignancy-associated effusion.[6]

In other series reporting survival of patients with malignant pericardial effusion according to malignancy type, patients with hematological malignancies had longer survival compared to all other patients with malignant disease.[11] Patients with lung cancer and a malignant pericardial effusion had the worst prognosis.[5]

59.4. Complications of Catheter-Based Drainage and Open Surgical Drainage

There are no randomized comparisons of different drainage procedures with respect to complication rate or risk of recurrence. In the last two decades, use and availability of ultrasound guidance has eliminated the need for non-image-guided pericardiocentesis. Uniformly, large series report a 3% to 5% complication rate utilizing catheter-based intervention. The most common complications include laceration of the heart, pneumothorax, and cardiac arrhythmia.[6,7] In the largest series, only 1% of patients suffered complications from catheter-based technique requiring operative intervention.[6] Similar results have been reported with Seldinger technique to introduce pericardial catheters.[4] An open surgical technique for a subxiphoid pericardiotomy has been reported to have an equally low complication rate. McDonald reported a single episode of arrhythmia in a series of 150 patients, and Allen reported a single case of postoperative bleeding in a series of 94 patients.[7,12] In the most recent analysis of 368 patients, Becit and colleagues reported three patients (0.8%) needing median sternotomy to control intraoperative bleeding caused by a subxiphoid approach.[1] In this study, the vast majority of patients underwent the procedure using a local anesthesia technique. The authors limited the use of general anesthesia to pediatric patients.

59.5. Recurrence of Effusion after Treatment

Simple pericardiocentesis is associated with the highest recurrence rate of 33%.[6,12] The efficacy of percutaneous catheter drainage is related to both the underlying cause of the pericardial effusion, and the duration of catheter placement. Use of prolonged drainage (defined as placement of the catheter until drainage decreases significantly) reduces the risk of recurrence to 14%.[6,8] Most authors recommend leaving a drain in place for a minimum of 4 to 5 days.[7,8,10] The presence of renal failure, large effusion, or malignant effusion increases the risk of recurrence in most series. While some authors have advocated the instillation of a sclerosing agent through the indwelling pericardial catheter,[4] the data suggesting a decreased risk of effusion recurrence are not compelling. Multiple investigators have found no relation between the use of sclerotherapy with either thiotepa or tetracycline and a decreased risk of recurrence.[6-8]

The efficacy of subxiphoid pericardial drainage has been demonstrated in a number of series. Dosios and colleagues report a low recurrence rate of 2% with open surgical drainage.[11] Retrospective review of our own experience in the management of patients with malignant pericardial effusion demonstrated that open surgical drainage (subxiphoid window with or without creation of a pericardial–peritoneal window) was associated with a 95% actuarial freedom from recurrence, whereas catheter drainage was associated with an 81% freedom from reintervention.[7]

59.6. Transthoracic Approaches to Pericardial Effusion Drainage

Some authors routinely perform transthoracic drainage of the pericardium with pericardial biopsy to diagnose and treat pericardial effusions[5,13] by either limited thoracotomy or video-assisted thorascopic techniques. Although this approach is clearly indicated for complex loculated effusions not amenable to the subxiphoid approach, it is not required for the management of most effusions. Computed tomography imaging is invaluable in planning the operative approach, and in determining which pleural cavity to enter. Unlike percutaneous drainage or open subxiphoid drainage, the transthoracic approach requires general anesthesia, and is facilitated by double-lumen intubation. Patients not able to tolerate general anesthesia and single-lung ventilation, or with tamponade physiology, are better treated with percutaneous catheter or open subxiphoid drainage under local anesthesia.

In summary, there are no randomized studies evaluating the optimal management of malignant pericardial effusions (Table 59.1). Given the paucity of such data, we may generalize that open surgical techniques and catheter interventions are equivalent in determining the etiology of a pericardial effusion (level of evidence 2+ to 2−; recommendation grade C), and that the complications of either technique are few using modern imaging techniques. Open drainage may have lower risk of recurrence and greatest freedom from re-intervention (level of evidence 2+ to 2−;

recommendation grade C), but the risk of recurrence is mitigated by the overall short life expectancy of patients with malignant pericardial effusion.

> Open surgical techniques and catheter interventions are equivalent in determining the etiology of a pericardial effusion (level of evidence 2+ to 2−; recommendation grade C).
>
> Open drainage may have lower risk of recurrence and greatest freedom from re-intervention (level of evidence 2+ to 2−; recommendation grade C), but the risk of recurrence is mitigated by the overall short life expectancy of patients with malignant pericardial effusion.

TABLE 59.1. Results of treatment for pericardial effusion.

Reference	Level of Evidence	Study design	Groups	Outcomes
Moores[10]	2−	Nonrandomized cases series	Subxiphoid window ($n = 155$)	Malignant cytology has poor prognosis; lung cancer–related effusion has the worst prognosis
Girardi[4]	2−	Nonrandomized cases series	Drainage catheter with sclerotherapy ($n = 37$); subxiphoid window ($n = 25$); other surgery ($n = 10$)	Malignant cytology has poor prognosis
Allen[12]	2−	Nonrandomized cases series	Percutaneous drainage ($n = 23$); subxiphoid window ($n = 94$)	Higher complication rate and recurrence rate with percutaneuous catheter drainage
Tsang[8]	2+	Nonrandomized cases series	Echo-guided pericardiocentesis only ($n = 118$); drainage catheter ($n = 139$); pericardiocentesis with planned surgery ($n = 18$)	Extended catheter placement reduces recurrence; sclerotherapy does not effect recurrence; positive cytology is associated with diminished survival
Tsang[6]	2+	Nonrandomized cases series	Echo-guided pericardiocentesis ($n = 1127$) and drainage catheter ($n = 640$)	Catheter placement has low complication rate and a 14% recurrence rate; malignant cytology has poor prognosis
Dosios[11]	2−	Nonrandomized cases series	Subxiphoid window ($n = 104$)	Patients with hematological malignancy–associated effusions have longest survival; recurrence rate of 2% with open technique
McDonald[7]	2−	Nonrandomized cases series	Percutaneous drainage ($n = 96$); subxiphoid drainage ($n = 150$)	Histopathology of pericardium did not augment cytological evaluation; positive cytology has poor prognosis; open surgery offers greatest freedom from recurrence; morbidity of either procedure is similar
Cullinane[5]	2−	Nonrandomized cases series	Thoracoscopic or subxiphoid window ($n = 63$)	Histopathology of pericardium did not augment cytological evaluation; positive cytology has poor prognosis; hematological malignancies have longest survival
Becit[1]	2+	Nonrandomized cases series	Subxiphoid window ($n = 368$)	Histopathology of pericardium is helpful in determining diagnosis; uremic pericarditis has highest risk of recurrence; malignancy determined by pathological evaluation is associated with highest mortality rate

59.7. Our Approach

The treatment algorithm for management of patients with pericardial effusions is depicted in Figure 59.1. For all hemodynamically unstable patients, immediate pericardiocentesis and catheter insertion is utilized to relieve tamponade physiology. Patients with pericardial effusion of unknown etiology or patients with a residual effusion undergo open pericardial drainage using the technique described below. This approach is most likely to determine the cause of the effusion and provides the lowest risk of recurrence.

In patients with a known history of malignancy and documented positive cytology, catheter drainage alone is often utilized given the overall short life expectancy. Open biopsy is reserved for patients with recurrent effusion or loculated effusion not amenable to catheter drainage. For patients with a history of locally advanced or metastatic cancer, the clinical status of the patient should be taken into account. If the clinical status is poor and life expectancy is limited, we favor catheter drainage of the effusion. In patients with good performance status, we favor open surgical subxiphoid pericardial window.

The technical aspects of performing a surgical subxiphoid window and placement of chest tube into the pericardium have been well described.[7,10] In an effort to decrease the risk of developing a recurrent pericardial effusion, we advocate the additional creation of a pericardioperitoneal window in patients without contraindications to this procedure (the presence of abdominal ascites or infectious etiology of effusion). After division

of the midline fascia overlying the xiphoid process and upper abdomen (6-cm incision), the pericardium is opened above the diaphragm and the fluid is drained and sent for culture and cytological analysis. The pericardial space is carefully inspected and palpated for the presence of malignant nodules. A 2-cm piece of pericardium is excised and sent for pathological analysis and culture. The peritoneum is opened just below the diaphragm and the epithelial surfaces of the pericardium and the peritoneum then are re-approximated creating a pericardioperitoneal window using interrupted suture over approximately 180° of the pericardial and peritoneal openings. A 28F right-angle chest tube is placed along the diaphragmatic surface of the pericardium, and is brought out through a separate stab wound in the fascia below the incision. The fascial incision is then closed using standard techniques.

59.8. Conclusion

Both minimally invasive techniques and surgical drainage of pericardial effusion are safe and effective means of treatment. Based upon the clinical facilities available, image-guided catheter drainage or subxiphoid window creation may be done expeditiously and safely. Given our understanding of the pathophysiology of pericardial effusion, the available data regarding long-term survival of patients, and the risk of recurrent effusion, we favor open surgical drainage for patients with persistent or recurrent effusions and no obvious etiology. We reserve catheter-based

Evaluation and treatment of malignant pericardial effusion

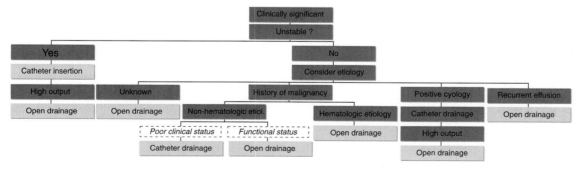

FIGURE 59.1. Algorithm for management of pericardial effusions.

drainage for hemodynamically unstable patients and in those with poor expectation for short-term survival.

References

1. Becit N, Unlu Y, Ceviz M, Kocogullari CU, Kocak H, Gurlertop Y. Subxiphoid pericardiostomy in the management of pericardial effusions: case series analysis of 368 patients. *Heart* 2005;91:785–790.

2. Tsang TS, Barnes ME, Hayes SN, et al. Clinical and echocardiographic characteristics of significant pericardial effusions following cardiothoracic surgery and outcomes of echo-guided pericardiocentesis for management: Mayo Clinic experience, 1979–1998. *Chest* 1999;116:322–331.

3. Beaulieu Y, Marik PE. Bedside ultrasonography in the ICU: part 2. *Chest* 2005;128:1766–1781.

4. Girardi LN, Ginsberg RJ, Burt ME. Pericardiocentesis and intrapericardial sclerosis: effective therapy for malignant pericardial effusions. *Ann Thorac Surg* 1997;64:1422–1427; discussion 1427–1428.

5. Cullinane CA, Paz IB, Smith D, Carter N, Grannis FW Jr. Prognostic factors in the surgical management of pericardial effusion in the patient with concurrent malignancy. *Chest* 2004;125:1328–1334.

6. Tsang TS, Enriquez-Sarano M, Freeman WK, et al. Consecutive 1127 therapeutic echocardiographically guided pericardiocenteses: clinical profile, practice patterns, and outcomes spanning 21 years. *Mayo Clin Proc* 2002;77:429–436.

7. McDonald JM, Meyers BF, Guthrie TJ, Battafarano RJ, Cooper JD, Patterson GA. Comparison of open subxiphoid pericardial drainage with percutaneous catheter drainage for symptomatic pericardial effusion. *Ann Thorac Surg* 2003;76:811–815; discussion 816.

8. Tsang TS, Seward JB, Barnes ME, et al. Outcomes of primary and secondary treatment of pericardial effusion in patients with malignancy. *Mayo Clin Proc* 2000;75:248–253.

9. Lee PJ, Mallik R. Cardiovascular effects of radiation therapy: practical approach to radiation therapy-induced heart disease. *Cardiol Rev* 2005;13:80–86.

10. Moores DW, Allen KB, Faber LP, et al. Subxiphoid pericardial drainage for pericardial tamponade. *J Thorac Cardiovasc Surg* 1995;109:546–551; discussion 551–552.

11. Dosios T, Theakos N, Angouras D, Asimacopoulos P. Risk factors affecting the survival of patients with pericardial effusion submitted to subxiphoid pericardiostomy. *Chest* 2003;124:242–246.

12. Allen KB, Faber LP, Warren WH, Shaar CJ. Pericardial effusion: subxiphoid pericardiostomy versus percutaneous catheter drainage. *Ann Thorac Surg* 1999;67:437–440.

13. Georghiou GP, Stamler A, Sharoni E, et al. Video-assisted thoracoscopic pericardial window for diagnosis and management of pericardial effusions. *Ann Thorac Surg* 2005;80:607–610.

60
Asymptomatic Pericardial Cyst: Observe or Resect?

Robert J. Korst

Pericardial cysts are congenital lesions of the mediastinum that are usually detected using chest imaging in the absence of symptoms. Historically referred to as spring-water cysts due to their clear fluid content,[1] the majority of published literature has suggested that surgical resection, traditionally via thoracotomy, be utilized only in symptomatic cases, with observation being sufficient for incidental, asymptomatic lesions.

Despite these recommendations for watchful waiting, life-threatening complications occurring in previously asymptomatic pericardial cysts have been reported. Given these reports, combined with the evolution of modern, minimally invasive techniques of resection, the question of surgical resection of asymptomatic pericardial cysts needs to be formally addressed.

60.1. Published Data

60.1.1. Grade of Existing Literature

The published literature regarding pericardial cysts and their treatment is limited to individual case reports or case series. No hypothesis-based experimental or interventional studies exist. Although some case series contain exclusively pericardial cysts,[1-4] most reports consist of patients who have undergone resection of mediastinal cysts, masses, or both, of which pericardial cysts represent a small fraction.[5-8] These tend to be surgical series, with data concerning the follow-up of unresected pericardial cysts sparse. Individual case reports usually describe complications of pericardial cysts,[9-24] or advances in operative techniques (e.g., thoracoscopy, robotics).[25,26] In published evidence-based guidelines, these studies represent level 3 data.[27]

60.1.2. Characterization, Prevalence, and Natural History of Pericardial Cysts

Pericardial cysts are mesothelium-lined cysts that are usually unilocular and filled with clear, transudative fluid.[1,3] Although not clearly delineated, these cysts are thought to arise from incomplete fusion of the mesenchymal lacunae during embryogenesis, a process which normally gives rise to the pericardial sac.[28] Pericardial cysts may be either intra- or extrapericardial.[29,30] The distinction between these two locations tends to be discernable using a variety of thoracic imaging modalities, including computed tomography (CT), magnetic resonance imaging, and echocardiography. Whereas intrapericardial lesions appear to be enveloped within the normal, globular contour of the pericardial sac (Figure 60.1A), extrapericardial cysts appear as pleural-based lesions which abut the pericardium, but are distinct from it (Figure 60.1B). The most common location of extrapericardial cysts are the cardiophrenic angles anteriorly, more frequently on the right.[3,4] However, they may also be found superiorly in the mediastinum as well.

The prevalence of pericardial cysts in the general population is essentially unknown. A figure frequently cited in the literature is one case in 100,000, however, this was an estimation based on a mass chest radiograph campaign in

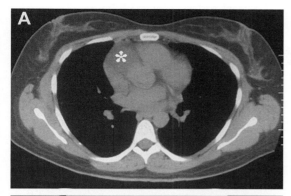

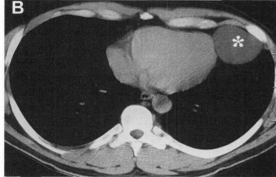

FIGURE 60.1. Differentiation between intra- and extrapericardial cysts on computed tomography. On both scans, the cyst is indicated by an asterisk. (A) A 3-cm asymptomatic, intrapericardial cyst. This cyst is in the most common location for an intrapericardial lesion, abutting the right atrium and ventricle. Note that the cyst is enveloped within the pericardial sac. Acute cyst enlargement in this position would result in severe compression of the right heart. (B) A 5-cm, extrapericardial cyst in the left hemithorax. The cyst clearly lies outside the pericardial sac in the left hemithorax. Even with acute cyst enlargement, symptoms may not become apparent until a massive size is attained.

Edinburgh in 1958,[1] and may not be accurate given obvious limitations in sensitivity and specificity. Data from large-scale, low-dose CT screening studies for lung cancer may provide a much more accurate estimate of the prevalence of pericardial cysts, but this information has yet to be published. Similar to their prevalence, little published data exist regarding the natural history of pericardial cysts. Although cyst enlargement,[31-33] as well as spontaneous resolution[34] and even asymptomatic rupture[35] have all been reported, there are no published case series describing long-term follow-up of unresected lesions.

60.1.3. Complications of Pericardial Cysts

Case series of pericardial cysts demonstrate that the majority of these lesions are asymptomatic, and are detected using chest imaging for an unrelated purpose. When symptoms do occur, however, they are typically mild and include chest discomfort, cough, and dyspnea.[1-8] Despite their generally innocuous clinical presentation, close examination of the English literature has revealed 17 case reports of severe, life-threatening complications of pericardial cysts (Table 60.1). Literature reports describing cases that appear not to be the result of congenital pericardial cysts, including postpericardiotomy tamponade, constrictive pericarditis, atrial fibrillation, and nonpericardial cystic lesions were not considered further and are not listed in the table. Although no cases of malignant degeneration have been reported, two complications resulted in mortality. The first involved acute hemorrhage into an extrapericardial cyst in an 84-year-old man, acutely compressing the heart into the left hemithorax,[12] while the second involved the sudden asystolic death of a 44-year-old man immediately following an exercise stress test. Postmortem examination revealed the absence of coronary disease, and the presence of a large (8.5cm), inflamed, intrapericardial cyst infiltrating into the wall of the heart in the region of the conduction system.[14]

Further examination of Table 60.1 reveals several interesting observations concerning life-threatening complications of pericardial cysts. First, these severe complications may occur at any age, including children, young and middle-aged adults, and the elderly. Second, the majority of complications occur in male patients. This may be a result of the natural gender distribution of pericardial cysts, but the ratio is generally higher than is reported in multiple surgical series of these lesions.[1-8] Third, although the clinical scenario is one of severe cardiac compression in the majority of cases, the inciting event seems to be the rapid expansion of the cyst or obvious intrapericardial rupture (causing tamponade) from either hemorrhage or inflammation. As stated previously, pericardial cysts normally contain clear, transudative fluid. In contrast, in nearly all cases listed in Table 60.1, the cysts

TABLE 60.1. Life-threatening complications of pericardial cysts.

Patient age (years)	Gender	Cyst size	Cyst type	Complication/etiology	Reference
8	M	7.5 cm	intra	Tamponade/hemorrhage	18
10	M	na	extra	Compression of right main bronchus	15
12	F	na	intra	Tamponade/hemorrhage	9
15	M	8 cm	intra	Tamponade/hemorrhage	16
17	F	15 cm	intra	Tamponade/hemorrhage	22
21	M	7 cm	intra	Erosion into heart/infected	17
29	M	5 cm	na	Hemodynamic compromise/pulmonary artery compression	24
36	M	7 cm	na	Cardiogenic shock/left atrial compression Sudden death/infected	24
44	M	8.5 cm	intra		14
47	F	5 cm	extra	SVC erosion/hemorrhage	20
52	M	8 cm	intra	Right heart failure/hemorrhage	10
57	F	10 cm	na	Hemodynamic compromise/hemorrhage	23
66	M	10 cm	intra	Hemodynamic compromise/cyst calcification	11
66	M	11 cm	na	Right heart failure/hemorrhage	13
68	M	8 cm	intra	Hemodynamic compromise/hemorrhage	19
82	M	12 cm	intra	Tamponade/hemorrhage	21
84	M	"large"	extra	Cardiac compression and death/hemorrhage	12

Abbreviations: intra, intrapericardial; extra, extrapericardial; na, information not apparent from the article; SVC, author, please provide definition.

contained either sanguinous fluid, frankly bloody material with clots, or exudative fluid with leukocytes and an inflammatory wall. Fourth, although pericardial cysts are detected in sizes ranging from 1 to 2 cm to well over 20 cm, complicated cysts tend to be generally large, with the majority being over 8 to 10 cm.

The final and perhaps most significant observation obtained from the cases listed in Table 60.1 is that the majority of complicated cysts are of the intrapericardial variety. Although not definitively stated in four reports, only two cases clearly involved extrapericardial cysts. The first was the previously described 84-year-old man who died from acute cardiac compression from massive hemorrhage into the cyst.[12] This cyst enlarged acutely to well over 20 cm in size, filling nearly the entire right hemithorax. The second was a 10-year-old boy with a completely collapsed right lung due to an extrapericardial cyst wrapping around the right main bronchus.[15] Because the vast majority of complicated cysts seem to be of the intapericardial variety, these lesions may be of more concern than extrapericardial cysts for the development of severe complications.

60.2. Treatment Guidelines for Asymptomatic Pericardial Cysts

Although most authors would agree that symptomatic pericardial cysts should be resected, no clear consensus exists for asymptomatic lesions. Opponents of the surgical approach to asymptomatic cysts argue that the vast majority are innocuous, and will never clinically affect the patient.[22,30] Advocates of resection, however, cite the occasional, life-threatening complications which can occur, as well as the relative ease of resection using modern, videothorascopic techniques.[8,36] What is clear is that given the poor grade of the published literature regarding pericardial cysts, it is difficult to provide concise, evidence-based guidelines regarding asymptomatic lesions.

Although the level of evidence of the published literature regarding pericardial cysts is poor, and data concerning the natural history of unresected lesions is virtually nonexistent, close examination of the details of the 17 reported cases of life-threatening complications associated with these lesions may allow the following statements to be made to assist with decision making:

> Asymptomatic extrapericardial cysts may be observed because life-threatening complications occurring with this type of cyst are extremely rare. Truly asymptomatic intrapericardial lesions warrant close observation; if cyst enlargement occurs, or imaging suggests bleeding into the cyst, resection should be undertaken, and may be best approached using an open procedure (level of evidence 3 to 4; recommendation grade D).

- Truly asymptomatic extrapericardial cysts may be observed because life-threatening complications occurring with this type of cyst are extremely rare. However, with regard to larger, extrapericardial cysts, it is important to determine if the lesion is indeed asymptomatic, as symptoms may be subtle and only occur only with exertion. Extrapericardial cysts are easily resected using videothorascopic techniques.
- Intrapericardial cysts are potentially more problematic. Because enlargement both with or without rupture of these cysts will affect hemodynamics more profoundly than extrapericardial cysts, truly asymptomatic intrapericardial lesions warrant close observation. If cyst enlargement occurs, or imaging suggests bleeding into the cyst (cyst contents become heterogeneous on imaging studies), resection should be undertaken. Given the close proximity of these intrapericardial lesions to the myocardium, sometimes incorporating muscle fibers into their walls, these lesions may be best approached using an open procedure.

In addition to the above statements regarding the management of asymptomatic intra- and extrapericardial cysts, the following caveats may also be considered, although they lack robust supporting data:

- Because the most frequent etiological factor in rare, life-threatening complications of pericardial cysts appears to be hemorrhage into the cyst, resulting in either compression of the heart or obvious cardiac tamponade, elective resection should be entertained for asymptomatic patients on chronic anti-coagulation. Although none of the patients in the existing case reports were chronically anti-coagulated,

the effects of acute bleeding, especially into an intrapericardial cyst, are profound.
- Elective resection should be entertained for patients in whom cyst enlargement is clearly demonstrated on imaging studies, especially if the cyst is intrapericardial. Enlargement of atypically located, extrapericardial cysts is also of concern because these lie in close proximity to the great vessels or bronchi. Cyst enlargement could imply either hemorrhage or conversion to an inflamed cyst, both of which have the potential to cause life-threatening complications.

60.3. Summary

Pericardial cysts are uncommon congenital anomalies of the pericardium that are primarily asymptomatic. Cysts may occur either inside or outside the pericardial sac, a characteristic which appears to impact their ability to present with rare, life-threatening complications. These complications are mainly due to rapid cyst expansion or rupture into the pericardial sac causing acute cardiac compression and/or tamponade. Most authors agree that symptomatic pericardial cysts should be resected, but proper treatment of asymptomatic lesions remains controversial. Although the quality of published evidence is poor, consisting of only case series and individual case reports, it is clear that hemorrhage into the cyst or conversion to an inflamed cyst are precipitating events leading to catastrophic complications, particularly for intrapericardial cysts. As a result, elective surgical resection should be considered for larger, asymptomatic, intrapericardial cysts, particularly for patients on chronic anti-coagulation, or if imaging studies suggest evidence of bleeding (cyst enlargement, heterogeneous cyst contents).

References

1. Le Roux BT. Pericardial coelomic cysts. *Thorax* 1959;14:27–35.
2. Mouroux J, Venissac N, Leo F, et al. Usual and unusual locations of intrathoracic mesothelial cysts. Is endoscopic resection always possible? *Eur J Cardiothorac Surg* 2003;24:684–688.
3. Lillie WI, McDonald JR, Claggett OT. Pericardial coelomic cysts and pericardial diverticula. A

concept of etiology and report of cases. *J Thorac Surg* 1950;20:494–504.

4. Kutlay H, Yavuzer I, Han S, et al. Atypically located pericardial cysts. *Ann Thorac Surg* 2001;72:2137–2139.

5. Ochsner JL, Ochsner SF. Congenital cysts of the mediastinum. 20-year experience with 42 cases. *Ann Surg* 1966;163:909–920.

6. Ovrum E, Birkeland S. Mediastinal tumors and cysts. A review of 91 cases. *Scand J Thorac Cardiovasc Surg* 1979;13:161–168.

7. Cohen AJ, Thompson L, Edwards FH, et al. Primary cysts and tumors of the mediastinum. *Ann Thorac Surg* 1991;51:378–386.

8. Takeda S, Miyoshi S, Minami M, et al. Clinical spectrum of mediastinal cysts. *Chest* 2003;124:125–132.

9. Shiraishi I, Yamagishi M, Kawakita A, et al. Acute cardiac tamponade caused by massive hemorrhage from pericardial cyst. *Circulation* 2000;101:e196–e197.

10. Komodromos T, Lieb D, Baraboutis. Unusual presentation of a pericardial cyst. *Heart Vessels* 2004;19:49–51.

11. Ng AF, Olak J. Pericardial cyst causing right ventricular outflow tract obstruction. *Ann Thorac Surg* 1997;63:1147–1148.

12. Nijveldt R, Beekl AM, Joost MHH, et al. Pericardial cysts. *Lancet* 2005;365:1960.

13. Borges AC, Gellert K, Dietel M, et al. Acute right-sided heart failure due to hemorrhage into a pericardial cyst. *Ann Thorac Surg* 1997;63:845–847.

14. Fredman CS, Parson SR, Aquino TI, et al. Sudden death after a stress test in a patient with a large pericardial cyst. *Am Heart J* 1994;127:946–950.

15. Davis WC, German JD, Johnson NJ. Pericardial diverticulum causing pulmonary obstruction. *Arch Surg* 1961;82:285–289.

16. Bandeira FC, de Sa VP, Moriguti JC, et al. Cardiac tamponade: an unusual complication of pericardial cyst. *J Am Soc Echocardiogr* 1996;9:108–112.

17. Chopra PS, Duke DJ, Pellet JR, et al. Pericardial cyst with partial erosion of the right ventricular wall. *Ann Thorac Surg* 1991;51:840–841.

18. Bava GL, Magliani L, Bertoli D, et al. Complicated pericardial cyst: atypical anatomy and clinical course. *Clin Cardiol* 1998;21:862–864.

19. Engle DE, Tresch DD, Boncheck LI, et al. Misdiagnosis of a pericardial cyst by echocardiography and computed tomographic scanning. *Arch Int Med* 1983;143:351–352.

20. Mastroroberto P, Chello M, Bevacqua E, et al. Pericardial cyst with partial erosion of the superior vena cava. An unusual case. *J Cardiovasc Surg* 1996;37:323–324.

21. Okubo K, Chino M, Fuse J, et al. Life-saving needle aspiration of a cardiac-compressing pericardial cyst. *Am J Cardiol* 2000;85:521.

22. Abad C, Rey A, Feijoo J, et al. Pericardial cyst. Surgical resection in two symptomatic cases. *J Cardiovasc Surg* 1996;37:199–202.

23. Koch PC, Kronzon I, Winer HE, et al. Displacement of the heart by a giant mediastinal cyst. *Am J Cardiol* 1977;40:445–448.

24. Antonini-Canterin F, Piazza R, Ascione L, et al. Value of transesophageal echocardiography in the diagnosis of compressive, atypically located pericardial cysts. *J Amer Soc Echocardiogr* 2002;15:192–194.

25. Satur CMR, Hsin MKY, Dussek JE. Giant pericardial cysts. *Ann Thorac Surg* 1996;61:208–210.

26. Bacchetta MD, Korst RJ, Altorki NK, et al. Resection of a symptomatic pericardial cyst using the computer-enhanced da Vinci surgical system. *Ann Thorac Surg* 2004;75:1953–1955.

27. Harbour R, Miller J. A new system for grading recommendations in evidence based guidelines. *BMJ* 2001;323:334–336.

28. Lambert AVS. Etiology of thin-walled thoracic cysts. *J Thorac Surg* 1940;10:1–7.

29. Mehta SM, Myers JL. Congenital heart surgery nomenclature and database project: diseases of the pericardium. *Ann Thorac Surg* 2000;69(suppl 4):S191–S196.

30. Losanoff JE, Richman BW, Curtis JJ, et al. Cystic lesions of the pericardium. Review of the literature and classification. *J Cardiovasc Surg* 2003;44:569–576.

31. Parienty RA, Fontaine Y, Dufour G. Transformation of a pericardial cyst observed on long-term follow-up. *J Comput Tomogr* 1984;8:125–128.

32. Stoller JK, Shaw C, Matthay RA. Enlarging, atypically located pericardial cyst. Recent experience and literature review. *Chest* 1986;89:402–406.

33. Patel J, Park C, Michaels J, et al. Pericardial cyst: case reports and a literature review. *Echocardiography* 2004;21:269–272.

34. Ambalavanan SK, Mehta JB, Taylor RA, et al. Spontaneous resolution of a large pericardial cyst. *Tenn Med* 1997;90:97–98.

35. King JF, Crosby I, Pugh D, et al. Rupture of pericardial cyst. *Chest* 1971;60:611–612.

36. Noyes BE, Weber T, Vogler C. Pericardial cysts in children: surgical or conservative approach. *J Pediatr Surg* 2003;38:1263–1265.

Part 8
Chest Wall

61
Optimal Approach to Thoracic Outlet Syndrome: Transaxillary, Supraclavicular, or Infraclavicular

Richard J. Sanders

Thoracic outlet syndrome (TOS) is not a single entity. By definition, TOS is compression of the neurovascular bundle in the thoracic outlet area eliciting symptoms in the upper extremity. The neurovascular bundle, comprising nerve, artery, and vein, gives rise to three types of TOS: neurogenic, arterial, and venous. When using the term TOS, most people are referring to the neurogenic form which comprises over 95% of all TOS patients; venous TOS makes up 3% and arterial TOS 1%. Because the optimal approach for each of the three types is different, it is important to define which type of TOS is being discussed.

The goal of treatment in arterial TOS (ATOS) is to repair or replace the subclavian artery and remove the abnormal cervical rib or first rib. This requires a supraclavicular approach, supplemented at times by an infraclavicular incision. In venous TOS (VTOS), the goal is to decompress the subclavian vein at the costoclavicular ligament which requires first rib resection, including the anterior part of the rib. This can be achieved via a transaxillary or infraclavicular approach, but not a supraclavicular one. In neurogenic TOS (NTOS) the goal is to decompress the brachial plexus. This can be done in several ways: transaxillary or infraclavicular first rib resection or by supraclavicular anterior and middle scalenectomy with or without first rib resection. The optimal approaches for each of the three types will be discussed individually.

61.1. Arterial Thoracic Outlet Syndrome

Subclavian artery pathology is necessary to produce ATOS. Arterial signs and symptoms can occur in the absence of ATOS. Some physicians use the term ATOS to describe symptoms of coldness and color changes in the hand; others use the term when the radial pulse is reduced in provocative positions such as Adson's[1] or 90° abduction external rotation (AER). These signs and symptoms do not establish a diagnosis of ATOS. Hand coldness and color changes are sympathetic nerve changes due to irritation of the sympathetic nerve fibers that accompany the lower trunk of the brachial plexus in the thoracic outlet area.[2] These are symptoms of NTOS that are usually relieved by surgical decompression of the plexus by scalenectomy or first rib resection.

Pulse reduction in provocative positions is a phenomenon that has been noted in 9% to 53% of normal (asymptomatic) controls[3-6] and is not indicative of arterial pathology. Pulse reduction is a very unreliable criterion for the diagnosis of NTOS; it is relying on an arterial sign to diagnose a neurological condition. Provocative maneuvers are helpful in diagnosing NTOS when these maneuvers produce nerve root irritation and symptoms of paresthesia, pain, and heaviness. The pulse change is not significant in making the diagnosis. It is important to distinguish arterial symptoms, which are often present with NTOS, from true ATOS as the treatment for each is different.

The term arterial TOS should be reserved for those patients who exhibit arterial insufficiency produced by pathological changes in the subclavian artery, namely stenosis or aneurysm formation, usually followed by thrombosis and embolization. As a rule, this only occurs in the presence of a cervical rib or anomalous first rib. These patients have a cold, discolored hand, an absent or reduced radial pulse at rest, pain and/or numbness in the fingers and hand, and often one or two ischemic fingers. The symptoms are constant and often associated with arm claudication. The diagnosis is established by suspicion, noting a rib abnormality on X ray, and confirmed by arteriography. Most patients with ATOS are asymptomatic until embolism occurs.

Treatment of ATOS is twofold: repair the artery and excise the abnormal rib. Even though a first rib and cervical rib can be removed through the axilla, the artery cannot be repaired from this approach. The supraclavicular route is the only approach for arterial repair, and it is also a very good approach through which to remove cervical and anomalous first ribs. Therefore, this route is preferred for treating ATOS.

Small subclavian artery aneurysms and small areas of stenosis can sometimes be excised and the two ends brought together with an end-to-end anastomosis. This is the easiest way to manage ATOS and it can be achieved through a single supraclavicular incision. However, many aneurysms extend below the clavicle or are too large to permit direct anastomosis. In these situations a graft is required, either vein or prosthetic, and an infraclavicular incision must be added to complete excision of the aneurysm and perform the distal anastomosis.

Claviculectomy is an alternative to the combined supra- and infraclavicular approach for managing ATOS. Because working around the clavicle is the challenge in exposure of the axillary and subclavian vessels, its removal can solve the problem. Removal of the medial two thirds of the clavicle provides excellent exposure of the subclavian and axillary arteries. It makes the operation much easier than working through two small incisions, one above and one below the clavicle. It has been advocated by a few surgeons who have pointed out that there is very little morbidity from removing the clavicle.[7,8] However, patients can develop instability of the shoulder when the clavicle has been excised, as was pointed out in a study of subclavian artery aneurysms where two of five patients undergoing claviculectomy had an unstable shoulder postoperatively.[9] In very large patients and in traumatic injury to subclavian or axillary arteries, claviculectomy may be necessary. The two options are either to excise and replace the medial two thirds with plates and screws or simply remove the clavicle without replacing it. The obvious advantage of replacing the clavicle is maintaining the integrity of the shoulder girdle; the disadvantage is the possibility of aseptic necrosis or infection requiring removal of the bone.

61.2. Venous Thoracic Outlet Syndrome

Venous TOS (VTOS) is subclavian vein obstruction with or without thrombosis. The pathology is compression of the subclavian vein at the point where the vein crosses over the first rib to join the innominate vein. At this point, the vein is surrounded medially by the costoclavicular ligament, superiorly by the subclavius tendon, posteriorly by the anterior scalene muscle, and inferiorly by the first rib. Adequate decompression of the vein requires that these four sides be divided and the subclavian vein freed of any remaining bands and ligaments. This can only be accomplished after the first rib has been excised, including the anterior end and the costal cartilage.

Once the vein has been freed, if there is intrinsic stenosis or residual thrombus, it may be desirable to open the vein, remove thrombus, correct stenosis, and close the vessel with a vein patch. If the surgical strategy is to consider opening the vein after rib resection, the infraclavicular incision is the preferred approach as it is easier to open and repair the vein through this route. If the surgical plan is to remove the rib and not open the vein, our preference is for the transaxillary route because by going through the axilla the arm can be elevated, which lifts the vein, artery, and lower trunk of the brachial plexus off the rib, making rib resection easier. Exposure is also a little better via the axilla when removing the costal cartilage and edge of the sternum.

As noted for ATOS, claviculectomy is another alternative for excellent exposure of the subclavian and axillary vessels. In very large patients or for very difficult reconstructions claviculectomy can provide the best visualization. Some surgeons have elected to use claviculectomy as their routine approach to all venous reconstructions.[10]

The supraclavicular approach for venous decompression has been used in the past. However, many now realize that this can decompress the brachial plexus, but not the subclavian vein. It is necessary to add an infraclavicular incision to excise the anterior end of the rib to adequately free the subclavian vein. Interestingly, a group that had been using the supraclavicular route noted in their latest communication that they were using the infraclavicular approach in their more recent cases.[11]

61.3. Neurogenic Thoracic Outlet Syndrome

Comprising over 95% of all TOS cases, NTOS can be treated surgically by either the supraclavicular, infraclavicular, or transaxillary routes. To date, there has been no data to strongly support the use of one route over another. The approach used depends in part on realization of the underlying etiology and pathology.

Neurogenic TOS is due most often to plexus compression by tight, scarred scalene muscles. The most common etiology is a hyperextension neck injury, frequently a whiplash. Occasionally a cervical rib or abnormal first rib is present, but even in these cases, symptoms are usually brought on by scalene muscle injury.[12] Thus, the goal of surgery is to either release or remove the scalene muscles. Transaxillary first rib resection is effective because it is one way to release the muscles. Results of transaxillary first rib resection from different authors are summarized in Table 61.1.

Transaxillary first rib resection has the advantage of performing anterior and middle scalenotomy through a route that stays out of the neck. While it is possible to also remove the lower 2cm of anterior scalene and divide its attachments to subclavian artery through this approach, the remaining muscle cannot be reached and can still adhere to the plexus.

Transaxillary rib resection is a difficult procedure to master, and even harder to teach.

TABLE 61.1. Transaxillary first rib.

Reference	Year	Operations	Excellent/good (%)	Fair (%)	Failed (%)	Length of follow-up (Months)	Level of evidence
McGough[16]	1979	113	80	13	7	6–60	4
Youmans[17]	1980	258	75	16	9	3–96	4
Roos[18]	1982	1315	92		8	Presumed 3–180	4
Batt[19]	1983	94	80		20	Not stated	4
Qvorfordt[20]	1984	97	79		21	4–48	3
Davies[21]	1988	115	89		11	6–180	4
Selke[22]	1988	460	79	14	7	6–240	4
Stanton[23]	1988	87	85	4	11	12–144	4
Lindgren[24]	1989	175	59		41	24	3
Lepantalo[25]	1989	112	52	25	23	1	3
Sanders[15]	1989	111	65	8	27	36–60 (life table)	3
Green[26]	1991	136	79		21	12–144	3
Martin[27]	1993	25	60		40	Not stated	3
Ellison[28]	1994	181	81	13	8	8–65	3
Cuypers[29]	1995	98	52		48	13–120	3
Mingoli[30]	1995	118	81	14	5	Average 99	4
Zatocil[31]	1997	112	45		55	Not stated	3
Leffert[32]	1999	282	69	16	15	6–253, average 55	3
Fulford[33]	1901	50	58	16	26	12–120, average 48	3
Yavuzer[34]	1904	127	83		17	Not stated	4
Alobelli[13]	1905	254	46		54	Average 25 (life table)	3
Toal (range)		4283	45%–92%	4%–25%	(6%–55%)	(0–41)	
Mean			77%	15%	21%		

Exposure is limited, even in experienced hands. Orientation can be misleading, not only for the surgeon who just occasionally ventures here, but also for the experienced surgeon. Many second ribs have been excised, mistaken for first ribs. Life-threatening complications of hemorrhage from subclavian artery or vein can occur. Once bleeding begins it is hard to dry up the field to find the bleeding spot; and once found, it is difficult to repair. There is often not enough room to position a needle holder until the first rib has been removed.

In addition to the bleeding complications, nerve injury is a significant risk. The T-1 and C-8 nerve roots lie against the neck of the first rib and are at risk when the posterior end of the rib is divided with heavy rib cutters. The difficulty is compounded by the location of the posterior rib in the deepest, narrowest corner of the wound. As bone shears are advanced they frequently block the surgeon's view of the nerves.

Other nerves at risk during transaxillary first rib resection are the phrenic and long thoracic. These nerves are usually not visualized during the operation, but are very close to the dissection.

A limitation of transaxillary first rib resection is that once the scalene muscles have been freed from the first rib, they still remain in the neck and are free to scar down to the subclavian artery and nerve roots of the plexus. This can cause recurrent symptoms, which occurs in a significant number of patients. In a recent study of 254 transaxillary rib resections where as much of the anterior scalene as possible was excised with the rib, 80 patients (31%) required reoperation by supraclavicular scalenectomy.[13]

Supraclavicular scalenectomy is another approach that has been gaining popularity since 1980. It has the advantage of allowing complete removal of the scalene muscles along with neurolysis of the five nerve roots with much better vision than through the axilla. It also provides good exposure of cervical ribs, bands, and ligaments. In addition, the first rib can be removed through this route with particularly good exposure of the neck of the rib, the area that is most difficult through the axilla. The results of scalenectomy with first rib resection via the supraclavicular approach are summarized in Table 61.2.

Proficiency with the supraclavicular approach to scalenectomy and first rib resection is a challenge to acquire. Exposure is facilitated with a self-retaining retractor system but still can be difficult. The phrenic is the most frequently injured nerve via this route, although it is almost always temporary. Nerve roots of the plexus are fairly easy to visualize and are rarely cut although they can be over stretched when retracted to excise the middle scalene muscle. At least two of the three forming branches of the long thoracic nerve frequently travel through the belly of the middle scalene muscle and are at risk during middle scalenectomy. Injury to subclavian artery or vein can also occur via this route, although these are easier to repair than via the transaxillary approach. Finally, the most difficult injury to prevent is a lymphatic leak in the left neck.

TABLE 61.2. Supraclavicular scalenectomy and first rib resection.

Reference	Year	Operations	Excellent/good (%)	Fair (%)	Failed (%)	Length of follow-up (months)	Level of evidence
Graham[35]	1973	78	91	5	4	4–84	4
Reilly[36]	1988	39	59	33	8	1–30	3
Sanders[15]	1989	278	64	8	28	36–60 (life table)	3
Baker[37]	1992	34	50	35	15	12	3
Cheng[14]	1995	125	69		31	24 (life table)	3
Thomas[38]	1995	210	75	15	10	6–26	3
Hempel[39]	1996	770	86	13	2	Not stated	4
Maxwell[40]	2001	126	72		28	"Long term"	3
Maxey[41]	2003	72	64	23	13	14–24	3
Total		1732					
Range			(50%–91%)	(5%–35%)	(2%–31%)		
Mean			72%	15%	13%		

Although the thoracic duct usually can be avoided, or if injured can be ligated, some patients have a plexus of small lymphatic channels along the internal jugular vein that can leak from multiple sites.

Scalenectomy must be differentiated from the older procedure, scalenotomy. Scalenotomy has a high failure rate, probably because the anterior scalene muscle has fibrous attachments to the subclavian artery and nerve roots of the plexus. As a result, simply dividing the muscle does not relieve its tension for very long. We have operated upon a few patients who had past histories of supraclavicular scalenotomies only to find the anterior scalene muscle had healed by reconstituting the muscle so that it looked and functioned normally. Scalenectomy is a different operation. If the entire muscle is excised, it can't reconstitute. However, scar tissue will replace the muscle and can form compressing envelopes of scar around the nerve roots, causing recurrent symptoms.

Realizing that the primary pathology is in the scalene muscles not the rib, the supraclavicular route has the advantage of permitting scalenectomy, without rib resection, and achieving the same success rate (Table 61.3). This approach permits easy excision of any ligaments, bands, or cervical ribs. At the time of scalenectomy, the relationship between first rib and lower trunk of the plexus can be observed. In those cases in which the trunk rests on the rib, the rib can be removed through the same supraclavicular incision.

The infraclavicular approach can also be used to perform first rib resection and scalenotomy. However, exposing the posterior rib and lifting the subclavian vein is more difficult than through the transaxillary route. The infraclavicular approach has no real advantage over the transaxillary one unless the subclavian vein is to be opened.

61.3.1. Evidence-Based Results

The results of the different approaches to NTOS are difficult to evaluate and compare. Although there have been several reports of each approach, there has been no standardization of success criteria. Because many patients operated upon for NTOS also have other diagnoses, such as cervical spine strain, cervical disc disease, or shoulder pathology, postoperative symptoms of pain may persist in the neck, shoulder, and arm even though paresthesia in the hand has been relieved. Some investigators will classify this as a good result because of relief of paresthesia, while others would call this fair or even failure because of the persistent pain. As a result, it is hard to compare the success rate of different studies.

Length of follow-up is very important in this evaluation because results are known to deteriorate over time, although 80% of failures will appear within the first 2 years. All approaches have success rates of over 90% for the first few months. Therefore, reports that include follow-ups of less than 1 year are not too meaningful. Accepting these limitations, one can still get an

TABLE 61.3. Scalenectomy without rib resection.

Reference	Year	Operations	Excellent/good (%)	Fair (%)	Failed (%)	Length of follow-up (months)	Level of evidence
Sanders[15]	1989	279	62	8	30	36–60 (life table)	3
Dellon[42]	1993	11	91		9	12–37	4
Razi[43]	1993	65	97		3	3–39	4
Gocke[144,*]	1994	107	63		37	24–132	3
Cheng[14]	1995	43	76		24	24 (life table)	3
Thomas[38]	1995	55	80	14	6	6–26	3
Jamieson[45]	1996	368	53	25	22	24 minimum	3
Axelrod[46]	2001	89	64		36	47 average	3
Total		1017	53%–97%	8%–25%	3%–37%		
Mean			70%	14%	23%		

* = scalenotomy.

idea of the success rate of supraclavicular and transaxillary approaches from the lists in Tables 61.1 through 61.3. Note that the studies that include some patients with follow-ups of under 12 months are the only ones with failure rates of under 10%. In those few studies with minimum follow-ups of 24 months, failure rates all exceed 20%. The results are about the same for all approaches. There is no statistically significant advantage of any one of the approaches. In two reports, different techniques are compared with the operations and criteria of evaluation being the same for all procedures. In one, there was no statistical difference between scalenectomy with or without rib resection[14] and in the other the results of all three approaches were virtually identical using life-table methods to 15 years[15] (Figure 61.1).

Grading each report on the basis of the evidence, which includes subjective criteria for success and length of follow-up, no study could be graded higher than a 3. Studies graded 4 were those that had a very small sample size, or success rates of over 89% or had follow-ups of only a few months. The three studies using life-table methods of follow-up [13–15] were graded 3.

Using evidence-based reports, the transaxillary and the supraclavicular approach have similar success rates. In selecting an approach, the training of the surgeon may be the deciding factor. Because this operation is one most surgeons seldom perform, familiarity with one approach is an advantage. The better approach may be the one the surgeon can perform with the least number of complications. However, it is worth noting a comparison of the two operations

by one group who performed 30 transaxillary first rib resections in a 15-year period between 1972 and 1987. There were 21 complications. Thirteen of these were pneumothoracies (9 requiring chest tubes), 3 were long thoracic nerve injuries (10%), and 3 were subclavian vein injuries with blood loss of 500 to 2400 mL (10%). Because of the high complication rate and difficulties of exposure, they began using the supraclavicular route. Among the 15 patients treated with anterior and middle scalenectomy (in one patient the first rib was also removed; in four others a cervical rib was also removed) there was only one complication, a urinary tract infection. Long-term results averaging 3 years revealed 83% improvement in the transaxillary group compared to 100% improvement in the supraclavicular group. They concluded that in addition to the poorer statistic, the transaxillary approach was more difficult to perform and much more difficult to teach.[47]

> The transaxillary and the supraclavicular approach have similar success rates (level of evidence 3; recommendation grade C). In selecting an approach, the training of the surgeon may be the deciding factor; familiarity with one approach is an advantage.

Our preference is for the supraclavicular approach. Over the past 35 years, we have tried both transaxillary and supraclavicular routes. We find the transaxillary approach technically more difficult. Moreover, even though the lower portion of the anterior scalene muscle can be

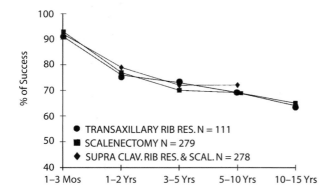

FIGURE 61.1. Results of three primary operations for TOS. *N*, number of operations. (Reproduced with permission from Sanders RJ, Haug CE. *Thoracic Outlet Syndrome: A Common Sequela of Neck Injuries*. Philadelphia: JB Lippincott Co; 1991:182.)

excised through this route, it is not possible to achieve a complete anterior or middle scalenectomy nor a complete neurolysis through the axilla. Our current operation for NTOS is supraclavicular anterior and middle scalenectomy with selective first rib resection through the same incision. The decision for rib resection is based on the relationship between first rib and lower trunk of the plexus. Using this approach, we have removed first ribs in only about 15% of the last 150 patients we have operated upon for NTOS during the past 2 years. We continue to note no difference in results between those with rib resections and those without rib resections. For VTOS we continue to use the transaxillary or the infraclavicular routes.

References

1. Adson AW, Coffey JR. Cervical rib: a method of anterior approach for relief of symptoms by division of the scalenus anticus. *Ann Surg* 1927;85: 839–857.
2. Telford ED, Stopford JSB. The vascular complications of cervical rib. *Br J Surg* 1930;18:557–564.
3. Rayan GM, Jensen C. Thoracic outlet syndrome: provocative examination maneuvers in a typical population. *J Shoulder Elbow Surg* 1995;4:113–117.
4. Gergoudis R, Barnes RW. Thoracic outlet arterial compression: prevalence in normal persons. *Angiology* 1980;31:538–541.
5. Colon E, Westdrop R. Vascular compression in the thoracic outlet: age dependent normative values in noninvasive testing. *J Cardiovasc Surg* 1988;29: 166–171.
6. Warrens A, Heaton JM. Thoracic outlet compression syndrome: the lack of reliability of its clinical assessment. *Ann R Coll Surg Engl* 1987;69:203–204.
7. Lord JW Jr, Urschel HC Jr. Total claviculectomy. *Surgical Rounds* 1988;11:17–27.
8. Maxey TS, Reece TB, Ellman PI, et al. Safety and Efficacy of the supraclavicular approach to thoracic outlet decompression. *Ann Thorac Surg* 2003;76:396–400.
9. Pairolero PC, Walls JT, Payne WS, Hollier LH, Fairbairn JF. Subclavian-axillary artery aneurysms. *Surgery* 1981;90:757–763.
10. Green RM, Waldman D, Ouriel K, Riggs P, Deweese JA. Claviculectomy for subclavian vein repair:

11. Schneider DB, Dimuzio PJ, Martin ND, et al. Combination treatment of venous thoracic outlet syndrome: open surgical decompression and intraoperative angioplasty. *J Vasc Surg* 2004;40:599–603.
12. Sanders RJ, Jackson CGR, Banchero N, Pearce WH. Scalene muscle abnormalities in traumatic thoracic outlet syndrome. *Am J Surg* 1990;159: 231–236.
13. Altobelli GG, Kudo T, Haas BT, Chandra FA, Moy JL, Ahn SS. Thoracic outlet syndrome: Pattern of clinical success after operative decompression. *J Vasc Surg* 2005;42(1)122–128.
14. Cheng SWK, Reilly LM, Nelken NA, et al. Neurogenic thoracic outlet decompression: rationale for sparing the first rib. *Cardiovasc Surg* 1995;3:617–623.
15. Sanders RJ, Pearce WH. The treatment of thoracic outlet syndrome: a comparison of different operations. *J Vasc Surg* 1989;10:626–634.
16. McGough EC, Pearce MB, Byrne JP. Management of thoracic outlet syndrome. *J Ther Cardiovasc Med* 1979;77:169–174.
17. Youmans CR Jr, Smiley RH. Thoracic outlet syndrome with negative Adson's and hyperabduction maneuvers. *Vasc Surg* 1980;14:318–329.
18. Roos DB. The place for scalenectomy and first rib resection in thoracic outlet syndrome. *Surgery* 1982;92:1077–1085.
19. Batt M, Griffet J, Scotti L, LeBas P. Le syndrome de la traversee cervico-brachiale. a proposde 112 cas: vers une attitude tactique plus nuancee. *J Chir Paris* 1983;120:687–691.
20. Qvarfordt PG, Ehrenfeld WK, Stoney RJ. Supraclavicular radical scalenectomy and transaillary first rib resection for the thoracic outlet syndrome: a combined approach. *Am J Surg* 1984;148:111–116.
21. Davies AL, Messerschmidt W. Thoracic outlet syndrome: a therapeutic approach based on 115 consecutive cases. *Del Med J* 1988;60:307–310.
22. Selke FW, Kelly TR. Thoracic outlet syndrome. *Am J Surg* 1988;156:54–57.
23. Stanton PE Jr, Vo NM, Haley T, Shannon J, Evans J. Thoracic outlet syndrome: a comprehensive evaluation. *Am Surg* 1988;54:129–133.
24. Lindgren SHS, Ribbe EB, Norgren LEH. Two year follow-up of patients operated on for thoracic outlet syndrome. Effects on sick-leave incidence. *Eur J Vasc Surg* 1989;3:411–415.
25. Lepantalo M, Lindgren K-A, Leino E, et al. Long term outcome after resection of the first rib for thoracic outlet syndrome. *Br J Surg* 1989;76:1255–1256.

26. Green RM, McNamara MS, Ouriel K. Long-term follow-up after thoracic outlet decompression: an analysis of factors determining outcome. *J Vasc Surg* 1991;14:739–746.

27. Martin GT. First rib resection for the thoracic outlet syndrome. *Br J Neurosurg* 1993;7:35–38.

28. Ellison DW, Wood VE. Trauma-related thoracic outlet syndrome. *J Hand Surg* 1994;19B:424–426.

29. Cuypers PWM, Bollen ECM, van Houtte HP. Transaxillary first rib resection for thoracic outlet syndrome. *Acta Chir Belg* 1995;95:119–122.

30. Mingoli A, Feldhaus RJ, Farina C, et al. Long-term outcome after transaxillary approach for thoracic outlet syndrome. *Surgery* 1995;118:840–844.

31. Zatocil Z, Gregor Z, Leypold J, et al. Resection of the first rib for the upper thoracic aperture syndrome–TOS. Long-term experience. *Rozhl Chir* 1997;76:242–245.

32. Leffert RD, Perlmutter GS. Thoracic outlet syndrome: results of 282 transaxillary first rib resections. *Clin Orthop* 1999;368:66–79.

33. Fulford PE, Baguneid MS, Ibrahim MR, Schady W, Walker MG. Outcome of transaxillary rib resection for thoracic outlet syndrome–a 10 year experience. *Cardiovasc Surg* 2001;9:620–624.

34. Yavuzer S, Atinkaya,C, Tokat O. Clinical predictors of surgical outcome in patients with thoracic outlet syndrome operated on via transaxillary approach. *Eur J Cardiothorac Surg* 2004;25:173–178.

35. Graham GG, Lincoln BM. Anterior resection of first rib for thoracic outlet syndrome. *Am J Surg* 1973;126:803–806.

36. Reilly LM, Stoney RJ. Supraclavicular approach for thoracic outlet syndrome. *J Vasc Surg* 1988;8:329–334.

37. Baker DM, Lamerton AJ. Surgical management of thoracic outlet compression syndrome. *Br J Surg* 1992;79:372.

38. Thomas GI. Diagnosis and treatment of thoracic outlet syndrome. *Perspect Vasc Surg* 1995;8:1–28.

39. Hempel GK, Shutze WP, Anderson JF, et al. 770 consecutive supraclavicular first rib resections for thoracic outlet syndrome. *Ann Vasc Surg* 1996;10:456–463.

40. Maxwell-Armstrong CA, Noorpuri BSE, Haque AS, Baker DM, Lamerton AJ. Long-term results of surgical decompression of thoracic outlet compression syndrome. *J R Coll Surg Edinb* 2001;46:35–38.

41. Maxey TS, Reece TB, Ellman PI, et al. Safety and Efficacy of the supraclavicular approach to thoracic outlet decompression. *Ann Thorac Surg* 2003;76:396–400.

42. Dellon AL. The results of supraclavicular brachial plexus neurolysis (without first rib resection) in management of post-traumatic "thoracic outlet syndrome". *J Reconstruct Microsurg* 1993;9:111–117.

43. Razi DM, Wassel HD. Traffic accident induced thoracic outlet syndrome: decompression without rib resection, correction of associated recurrent thoracic aneurysm. *Int Surg* 1993;78:25–27.

44. Gockel M, Vastamaki M, Alaranta H. Long-term results of primary scalenotomy in the treatment of thoracic outlet syndrome. *J Hand Surg* 1994;19B:229–233.

45. Jamieson WG, Chinnick B. Thoracic outlet syndrome: fact or fancy? A review of 409 consecutive patients who underwent operation. *Can J Surg* 1996;39:321–326.

46. Axelrod DA, Proctor MC, Geisser ME, Roth RS, Greenfield LJ. Outcomes after surgery for thoracic outlet syndrome. *J Vasc Surg* 2001;33:1220–1225.

47. Cikrit DF, Haefner R, Nichols WK, Silver D. Transaxillary or supraclavicular decompression for the thoracic outlet syndrome: a comparison of risks and benefits. *Am Surg* 1989;55:347–352.

62
Pectus Excavatum in Adults

Charles B. Huddleston

Pectus excavatum is a chest-wall deformity occurring in approximately 1 in 400 individuals and is identified four times more commonly in males than females. Based upon this figure, a region with 30,000 live births per year (approximately what would occur in an area with a population of 2,000,000) would expect to have 75 children born with pectus excavatum per year. The underlying etiology is unknown. More than 90% have some evidence of depression of the sternum at birth with progression of the severity of the deformity over the course of their growth and development.[1] Many patients will note that a family member also has this deformity, although no clear genetic predisposition to this as an isolated entity has been identified. Patients with connective tissue disorders, such as Marfan's syndrome, have a fairly high incidence of pectus excavatum or pectus carinatum.[2] Because these disorders are generally of genetic origin, there is likely a chromosomal correlation in this instance. It has also been noted in higher frequency in patients with abnormalities of the diaphragm, such as congenital diaphragmatic hernia.[3] In this case, the chest-wall deformity is likely related to mechanical forces exerted on the chest wall during development.

62.1. Assessment

Anatomically, pectus excavatum is characterized by depression of the sternum with posterior curvature of the attached ribs. It usually involves the inferior half of the sternum. There may be asymmetry of the deformity and when this is present the depression is more to the right than left side of the chest. The degree of the deformity is assessed radiographically. The most common assessment of the severity is the pectus index, a ratio of the transverse diameter of the chest divided by the distance from the posterior aspect of the sternum to the anterior aspect of the spine at its narrowest point. Normal is approximately 2.5.[4] Greater than 3.5 is considered abnormal and greater than 5.0 is severe. How that relates to symptoms or indications for operation varies from center to center. Certainly many patients with high pectus index will have few or no symptoms, whereas a patient with a pectus index of 3.5 may be quite symptomatic.

62.2. Indications for Repair

The controversial issues surrounding the care of patients with pectus excavatum relate to whether or not operation is warranted and what operation to perform. Most patients will seek care during childhood or teenage years. However, adults who were told that this was an insignificant deformity of cosmetic concern only during their childhood years may present for treatment as adults.

Patients generally present with symptoms of pain, exertional intolerance, or embarrassment over the appearance. Adults with this disorder often did not receive care for this because of the bias of the pediatrician or family physician serving as the primary caregiver, who may have held the notion that it poses no serious health problem and is of cosmetic importance only. Some believe that the child will grow out of it. For a variety of reasons, many children with pectus excavatum do not undergo repair and present as adults with this deformity.

62.3. Options for Management

There are a variety of operations available for these patients, although the two most commonly utilized procedures are the Ravitch procedure[5]

and the Nuss procedure.[6] The Ravitch procedure was introduced in the 1940s and has been modified by Welch[7] and others (Figure 62.1). This involves subperichondrial resection of the costal cartilages involved in the deformity, a so-called chondrectomy. The sternum is divided transversely at the point of posterior angulation of the sternum and a small wedge is removed anteriorly so that the inferior portion of the sternum can be

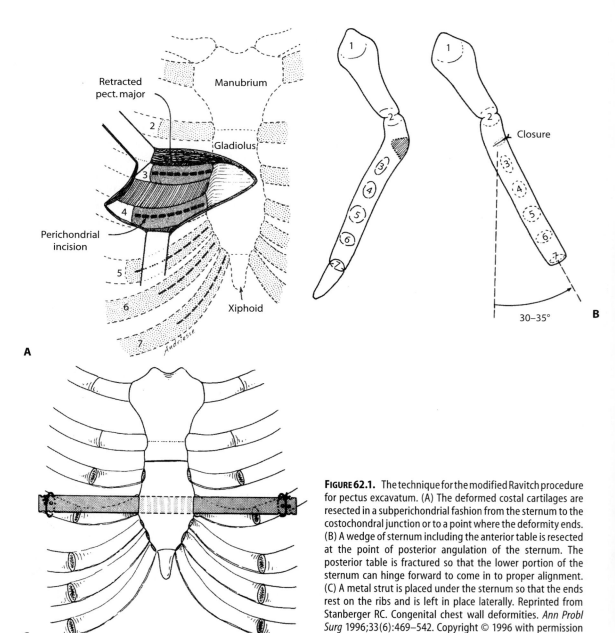

FIGURE 62.1. The technique for the modified Ravitch procedure for pectus excavatum. (A) The deformed costal cartilages are resected in a subperichondrial fashion from the sternum to the costochondral junction or to a point where the deformity ends. (B) A wedge of sternum including the anterior table is resected at the point of posterior angulation of the sternum. The posterior table is fractured so that the lower portion of the sternum can hinge forward to come in to proper alignment. (C) A metal strut is placed under the sternum so that the ends rest on the ribs and is left in place laterally. Reprinted from Stanberger RC. Congenital chest wall deformities. *Ann Probl Surg* 1996;33(6):469–542. Copyright © 1996 with permission from Elsevier.

hinged anteriorly. The sternum is stabilized with a metal strut placed behind the sternum, resting on the ribs present laterally. Generally, this strut is left in place for 3 to 6 months, during which time the resected ribs re-grow.

The Nuss procedure has been described as a minimally invasive repair (Figure 62.2) It is performed by passing a large clamp, from a small incision on one side, through the pleural space, under the sternum at the point where it is at its most posterior depression, through the pleural space on the other side and out through another skin incision on the opposite side. A preformed bar is grasped and pulled through the chest with the concavity facing posteriorly. Once positioned, the bar is rotated 180°, elevating the depressed sternum. The bar is fixed in place with metal stabilizers attached to the ribs laterally. One additional bar is occasionally necessary to completely correct the deformity. The bar is left in place for a minimum of 2 years to avoid the risk of recurrence.

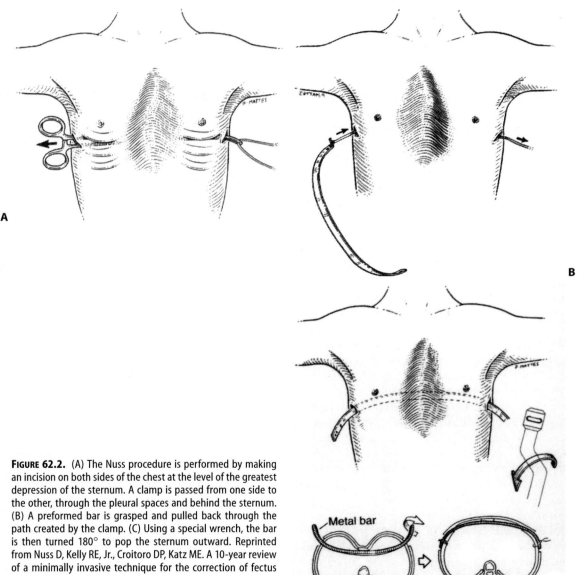

FIGURE 62.2. (A) The Nuss procedure is performed by making an incision on both sides of the chest at the level of the greatest depression of the sternum. A clamp is passed from one side to the other, through the pleural spaces and behind the sternum. (B) A preformed bar is grasped and pulled back through the path created by the clamp. (C) Using a special wrench, the bar is then turned 180° to pop the sternum outward. Reprinted from Nuss D, Kelly RE, Jr., Croitoro DP, Katz ME. A 10-year review of a minimally invasive technique for the correction of fectus excavation. *J Pediatr Surg* 1998;33(4):548. Copyright © 1998 with permission from Elsevier.

62.4. Results of Repair

There have never been any studies comparing operative repair to untreated patients with pectus excavatum. For the most part, prior studies use the patients as their own controls, comparing a variety of physiological parameters before and after repair, beginning with the first reported repair of pectus excavatum. Sauerbruch's patient, described in 1920, was 18 years old with dyspnea and palpitations associated with limited exercise; following repair he was working 12hs per day without tiring.[8] Anecdotes such as this have convinced many surgeons of the value of repairing pectus excavatum in patients complaining of exercise intolerance. Studies performed on series of patients in more recent decades evaluate more specific physiological parameters, including pulmonary function tests and various indicators of exercise tolerance. There is no question that some patients experiencing symptoms of exercise intolerance are improved following repair of pectus excavatum. Stamina is a complex issue with many potential contributing factors, but is certainly impacted by anything that might depress cardiac or pulmonary function. At first glance, one might assume that lung capacity is reduced with pectus excavatum and improved following relocation of the sternum to its normal position. In fact, pulmonary function tests generally show mildly restrictive lung volumes with total lung capacity and forced vital capacity (FVC) of approximately 80% predicted; forced expiratory volume in 1s (FEV_1)/FVC ratio is generally normal.[9–12] Evaluation of lung volumes at up to 3 years postrepair show that the lung volumes at best return to baseline,[12] with some studies showing a 10% decline from baseline values, presumably related to a reduction in chest-wall compliance[11,12] (Table 62.1) More sophisticated studies involving exercise evaluation of pulmonary function also failed to demonstrate objective improvement to correlate with the symptomatic improvement noted.

A study from the National Heart and Lung Institute was published in the *New England Journal of Medicine* in 1972 concerning cardiac function and exercise in patients with pectus excavatum.[13] These patients were older teenagers and young adults with what was described as a moderate pectus excavatum deformity. These

TABLE 62.1. Evaluation of lung volumes at up to 3 years postrepair.

	FVC^a	$FEV_1{}^a$	RV^a	Reference
Prerepair	81%		117%	Quigley[12]
Postrepair	80%		109%	
Prerepair	86%	85%	128%	Kaguraoka[11]
Postrepair	85%	85%	116%	
Prerepair	78%	79%	104%	Morshuis[9]
Postrepair	71%	73%	84%	

Abbreviations: FEV_1, forced expiratory volume in 1s; FVC, forced vital capacity; RV, residual volume.
^{a}Values expressed in percent predicted.

individuals were subjected to supine and upright exercise while instrumented, allowing for measurement of cardiac output, pulmonary artery oxygen saturation, heart rate, blood pressure, and arterial oxygen saturation. Measurements at baseline and during supine exercise were within normal limits and similar to a cohort of control individuals with normal chests. However, during upright exercise, the cardiac index fell significantly below that seen in the normal group. When these measurements were repeated 4 months following repair of the chest-wall deformity, the cardiac index during upright exercise had increased 38% compared to the preoperative measurements and was similar to that measured in the group of normal individuals. The heart rate was the same pre- and postrepair during exercise. It was therefore postulated that this increase was related to an improved stroke volume. It was further theorized that the sternal depression compressed the anterior wall of the right ventricle; when this was lifted away by the repair the right ventricle could respond normally to exercise.[13] Other studies have documented a marked decrease in symptoms after surgical correction of pectus excavatum in a regulated exercise protocol.[14] Further evidence supporting the notion of improved stroke volume following repair was forthcoming from a study on the echocardiographic features of pectus excavatum. In this study, it was noted that the right ventricular volume indices were depressed in patients with pectus excavatum and increased following repair.[15]

The subject of the relation of pectus excavatum to cardiopulmonary function remains controversial, however. In spite of conflicting data, the bottom line is that the vast majority of patients with symptoms of exercise limitations prior to repair feel subjectively improved after repair.[16] The role of conditioning and subjective response to surgery confound some of the studies showing a favorable response to repair and provide grist for those who doubt that there is any true physiological importance to this chest-wall deformity.

Although some studies have been reported comparing the Nuss and Ravitch procedures in children, such reports do not exist for adults. In general, the Nuss procedure takes less operative time, but is associated with greater need for postoperative narcotics, longer hospitalization, more complications, and more frequent re-operations.[17-19] The age range for patients in these studies is generally early-to-late teens. It is assumed that this information can be translated to the adult population. The original publication by Nuss and colleagues suggested that the ideal age for this procedure was before puberty, primarily because it was felt that a malleable chest wall was a necessary ingredient for success of the operation.[6] This assumption seemed to be confirmed by studies that demonstrated that the force necessary to elevate the sternum correlates directly with the age of the patient. Children under 11 years of age required approximately 15 pounds of pressure while adults over the age of 19 years required 41.2 pounds.[20] Subsequent reports have shown that the Nuss procedure can be successfully applied to adults.[21] Likewise, the modified Ravitch procedure has a long history of application in adults and is associated with results similar to those seen in children. However, the procedure is generally more difficult when performed in adults from a technical point of view.[22]

Having focused on the more objective issues with pectus excavatum, a rather subjective component with this deformity relates to its appearance and the impact that has on an individual. Many adults seek treatment primarily because they are embarrassed by the appearance of their chest with or without other symptoms. There is no question that patients are very satisfied with the postcorrection results and feel as though they are capable of leading a more enjoyable life. No study has attempted to quantify this in adults,

however. Another method of repair that produces a satisfactory cosmetic result involves placement of a Silastic mold into the subcutaneous space to alter the contour of the chest.[23] This obviously does nothing to the skeletal abnormalities and likewise would not be associated with any alteration in the physiological changes associated with pectus excavatum.

62.5. Recommendations

In summary, adults occasionally present with pectus excavatum seeking either treatment or advice regarding its consequences. This deformity can produce symptoms of intolerance to exertion that are often subjectively improved following repair. When the cosmetic appearance is the primary concern, operative repair is quite effective. The level of evidence supporting this is 2++ and the recommendation grade is B. Whether a surgeon chooses the Nuss or Ravitch procedure is based primarily on his or her experience and level of comfort with one procedure or another. It has been generally felt that the Nuss procedure is less likely to effectively treat this disorder because of the lack of malleability in the ribs seen in younger adults. The evidence level is 3 to 4 and the recommendation grade is C. The decision to repair this deformity rests primarily with the patient. He or she will have to balance the impact of symptoms, likelihood that they are related to the deformity, and the implications of a surgical procedure. These implications include the peri-operative risk, the length of hospitalization, time off work, and the rehabilitation involved. Pectus excavatum is not a life-threatening disorder.)

In adults with pectus excavatum in whom the cosmetic appearance is the primary concern, operative repair is quite effective (level of evidence 2++; recommendation grade B).

The Nuss procedure is less likely to effectively treat this disorder because of the lack of malleability in the ribs of older adults (level of evidence 3 to 4; recommendation grade C).

References

1. Shamberger RC, Welch KJ. Surgical repair of pectus excavatum. *J Pediatr Surg* 1988;23:615–622.
2. Arn PH, Haller JA, Pyeritz RF. Outcome of pectus excavatum in patients with Marfan syndrome and in the general population. *J Pediatr* 1989;115:954–958.
3. Brodkin HA. Congenital anterior chest wall deformities of diaphragmatic origin. *Dis Chest* 1953;24:259–277.
4. Haller JA, Kramer SS, Lietman SA. Use of CT scans in selection of patients for pectus excavatum surgery: a preliminary report. *J Pediatr Surg* 1987;22:904–906.
5. Ravitch MM. The operative treatment of pectus excavatum. *Ann Surg* 1949;129:429–444.
6. Nuss D, Kelly RE, Croitoru DP, Katz ME. A 10-year review of a minimally invasive technique for the correction of pectus excavatum. *J Pediatr Surg* 1998;33:545–552.
7. Welch KJ. Satisfactory surgical correction of pectus excavatum deformity in childhood: a limited opportunity. *J Thorac Surg* 1958;36:697–713.
8. Sauerbruch F. *Die Chirurgie der Brustorgane*. Berlin: Springer; 1920:440–444.
9. Morshuis W, Folgering H, Berentsz J, et al. Pulmonary function before surgery for pectus excavatum and at long-term follow-up. *Chest* 1994;105:1646–1652.
10. Synn SR, Driscoll DJ, Ostrom NK, et al. Exercise cardiorespiratory function in adolescents with pectus excavatum: observations before and after operation. *J Thorac Cardiovasc Surg* 1990;99:41–47.
11. Kaguraoka H, Ohnuki T, Itaoka T, et al. Degree of severity of pectus excavatum and pulmonary function in preoperative and postoperative periods. *J Thorac Cardiovasc Surg* 1992;104:1483–1488.
12. Quigley PM, Haller JA, Jelus KL, et al. Cardiorespiratory function before and after corrective surgery in pectus excavatum. *J Pediatr* 1996;128:638–643.
13. Beiser GD, Epstein SE, Stampfer M, et al. Impairment of cardiac function in patients with pectus excavatum, with improvement after operative correction. *N Engl J Med* 1972;287:267–272.
14. Peterson RJ, Young WG, Godwin JD, et al. Noninvasive assessment of exercise cardiac function before and after pectus excavatum repair. *J Thorac Cardiovasc Surg* 1985;90:251–260.
15. Kowalewski J, Brocki M, Dryjanski T, et al. Pectus excavatum: increase of right ventricular systolic, diastolic, and stroke volumes after surgical repair. *J Thorac Cardiovasc Surg* 1999;118:87–93.
16. Fonkalsrud EW, Beanes S. Surgical management of pectus carinatum: 30 years' experience. *World J Surg* 2001;25:898–903.
17. Molik KA, Engum SA, Rescorla FJ, et al. Pectus excavatum repair: experience with standard and minimal invasive techniques. *J Pediatr Surg* 2001;36:324–328.
18. Wu PC, Knauer EM, McGowan GE, Hight DW. Repair of pectus excavatum deformities in children: a new perspective of treatment using minimal access surgical technique. *Arch Surg* 2001;136:419–424.
19. Fonkalsrud EW, Beanes S, Hebra A, et al. Comparison of minimally invasive and modified Ravitch pectus excavatum repair. *J Pediatr Surg* 2002;37:413–417.
20. Fonkalsrud EW, Beanes S, Hebra A, et al. Force required to elevate the sternum of pectus excavatum patients. *J Am Coll Surg* 2002;195:575–577.
21. Park HJ, Lee SY, Lee CS, et al. The Nuss procedure for pectus excavatum: evolution of techniques and early results on 322 patients. *Ann Thorac Surg* 2004;77:289–295.
22. Fonkalsrud EW, DeUgarte D, Choi E. Repair of pectus excavatum and carinatum deformities in 116 adults. *Ann Surg* 2002;236:304–314.
23. Swart ACT, Alting MP, Specken TFJ, Morshuis WJ, Kung M. Pectus Excavation: cosmetic imporvement using preformed silicone implants. *European Journal of Plastic Surgery* 1996;19(6):284–288.

Index